AF783620

Clinical Echocardiography: Medical Diagnostic Techniques

Clinical Echocardiography: Medical Diagnostic Techniques

Edited by Aaron Jackson

hayle medical

New York

Hayle Medical,
750 Third Avenue, 9th Floor,
New York, NY 10017, USA

Visit us on the World Wide Web at:
www.haylemedical.com

© Hayle Medical, 2018

This book contains information obtained from authentic and highly regarded sources. Copyright for all individual chapters remain with the respective authors as indicated. All chapters are published with permission under the Creative Commons Attribution License or equivalent. A wide variety of references are listed. Permission and sources are indicated; for detailed attributions, please refer to the permissions page and list of contributors. Reasonable efforts have been made to publish reliable data and information, but the authors, editors and publisher cannot assume any responsibility for the validity of all materials or the consequences of their use.

ISBN: 978-1-63241-485-4

The publisher's policy is to use permanent paper from mills that operate a sustainable forestry policy. Furthermore, the publisher ensures that the text paper and cover boards used have met acceptable environmental accreditation standards.

Trademark Notice: Registered trademark of products or corporate names are used only for explanation and identification without intent to infringe.

Printed in China.

Cataloging-in-Publication Data

Clinical echocardiography : medical diagnostic techniques / edited by Aaron Jackson.
p. cm.
Includes bibliographical references and index.
ISBN 978-1-63241-485-4
1. Echocardiography. 2. Echocardiography--Digital techniques.
3. Heart--Diseases--Diagnosis. I. Jackson, Aaron.

RC683.5.U5 C55 2018
616.120 754 3--dc23

Table of Contents

Preface

The main aim of this book is to educate learners and enhance their research focus by presenting diverse topics covering this vast field. This is an advanced book which compiles significant studies by distinguished experts in the area of analysis. This book addresses successive solutions to the challenges arising in the area of application, along with it; the book provides scope for future developments.

Echocardiography is the procedure by which a sonogram of the heart is produced. This procedure allows cardiac physiologists to study in detail the structures of the heart as well as calculate blood flow and relaxation functions. The overall health of the heart can be studied by using this technique. Those who develop cardiovascular disorders and need to undergo surgeries greatly benefit from this technique. Transthoracic echocardiogram, transesophageal echocardiogram, stress echocardiogram, three-dimensional echocardiography, etc. are some common types of echocardiography. This book is a vital tool for all researching or studying echocardiography as it gives incredible insights into emerging trends and technologies. It is a collective contribution of a renowned group of international experts.

It was a great honour to edit this book, though there were challenges, as it involved a lot of communication and networking between me and the editorial team. However, the end result was this all-inclusive book covering diverse themes in the field.

Finally, it is important to acknowledge the efforts of the contributors for their excellent chapters, through which a wide variety of issues have been addressed. I would also like to thank my colleagues for their valuable feedback during the making of this book.

Editor

The Association between Atrium Electromechanical Interval and Pericardial Fat

Tze-Fan Chao[1,2], Yau-Huei Lai[3,4], Chun-Ho Yun[5], Chih-Hsuan Yen[3,4], Kang-Ling Wang[1,2], Yenn-Jiang Lin[1,2], Shih-Lin Chang[1,2], Li-Wei Lo[1,2], Yu-Feng Hu[1,2], Chung-Lieh Hung[3,4]*, Jen-Yuan Kuo[3,4], Hung-I Yeh[3,4], Shih-Ann Chen[1,2]*

1 Division of Cardiology, Department of Medicine, Taipei Veterans General Hospital, Taipei, Taiwan, **2** Institute of Clinical Medicine, and Cardiovascular Research Center, National Yang-Ming University, Taipei, Taiwan, **3** Division of Cardiology, Department of Internal Medicine, Mackay Memorial Hospital, Taipei, Taiwan, **4** Department of Medicine, Mackay Medical College, and Mackay Medicine Nursing and Management College, Taipei, Taiwan, **5** Division of Radiology, Department of Internal Medicine, Mackay Memorial Hospital, Taipei, Taiwan

Abstract

Objectives: Pericardial fat (PCF) may induce local inflammation and subsequent structural remodeling of the left atrium (LA). However, the adverse effects of PCF on LA are difficult to be evaluated and quantified. The atrial electromechanical interval determined by transthoracic echocardiogram was shown to be a convenient parameter which can reflect the process of LA remodeling. The goal of the present study was to investigate the association between the electromechanical interval and PCF.

Methods and Results: A total of 337 patients with mean age of 51.9±9.0 years were enrolled. The electromechanical interval (PA-PDI) defined as the time interval from the initiation of the P wave deflection to the peak of the mitral inflow A wave on the pulse wave Doppler imaging was measured for every patient. The amount of PCF was determined by multi-detector computed tomography. The PA-PDI interval was significantly correlated with the amount of PCF ($r = 0.641$, p value <0.001). Graded prolongation of PA-PDI interval was observed across 3 groups of patients divided according to the tertile values of PCF. The AUC for the PA-PDI interval in predicting an increased amount of PCF (third tertile) was 0.796. At a cutoff value of 130 ms identified by the ROC curve, the sensitivity and specificity of PA-PDI interval in identifying patients with a highest tertile of PCF were 63.4% and 85.3%, respectively.

Conclusions: The PA-PDI intervals were longer in patients with an increased amount of PCF. It may be a useful parameter to represent the degree of PCF-related atrial remodeling.

Editor: John Calvert, Emory University, United States of America

Funding: This work was supported by intramural grants (V96C1-049, V97C1-059, V98C1-037 and V99C1-120) from Taipei Veterans General Hospital, Taiwan and grants (NSC95-2314-B-010-017, NSC95-2314-B-010-025, NSC96-2314-B-010-006, NSC96-2628-B-010-036, NSC97-2314-B-010-037-MY3, NSC97-2314-B-010-038, NSC98-2314-B-010-031-MY3) from the National Science Council, Taiwan. The funders had no role in study design, data collection and analysis, decision to publish, or preparation of the manuscript.

Competing Interests: The authors have declared that no competing interests exist.

* E-mail: jotaro3791@gmail.com (CLH); epsachen@ms41.hinet.net (SAC)

Introduction

The pericardial fat (PCF), a unique fat deposit due to its proximity to cardiac structures, has been reported to serve as an abundant source of inflammatory mediators which directly damage the heart. [1] An increased amount of PCF has been linked with the presences of coronary calcification and coronary artery disease. [2,3] Besides, an increasing volume of literature has showed that PCF is significantly increased in patients with atrial fibrillation (AF). [4–6] The previous study suggested that PCF may induce local inflammation and subsequent structural remodeling of the left atrium (LA), which potentially contributes to AF genesis or perpetuation. [6] However, the adverse effects of PCF on LA are difficult to be evaluated and quantified clinically.

LA volume measured by transthoracic echocardiogram (TTE) was a non-invasive parameter which was commonly used to evaluate the structural change of LA. However, the measurements of LA volume are often limited by poor temporal and spatial resolution. Recently, a newly developed atrial electromechanical interval on transthoracic echocardiogram (TTE) was reported to be a useful parameter to estimate the total atrial conduction time. [7] Chao et al. further demonstrated that it can reflect the processes of both electrical (decreased voltage, prolonged total activation time) and structural remodeling (chamber enlargement) of LA. [8] In a previous study which enrolled 103 AF and 194 non-AF patients, atrial electromechanical interval, not LA size, is able to identify subjects with AF among those having a small LA. [9] Therefore, we hypothesized that the electromechanical interval may be longer in patients with an increased volume of PCF. It may serve as a convenient tool, which could be more sensitive than LA volume, in reflecting the extent of LA injury due to the adverse effects of PCF. The goal of the present study was to investigate the association between the atrial electromechanical interval and PCF.

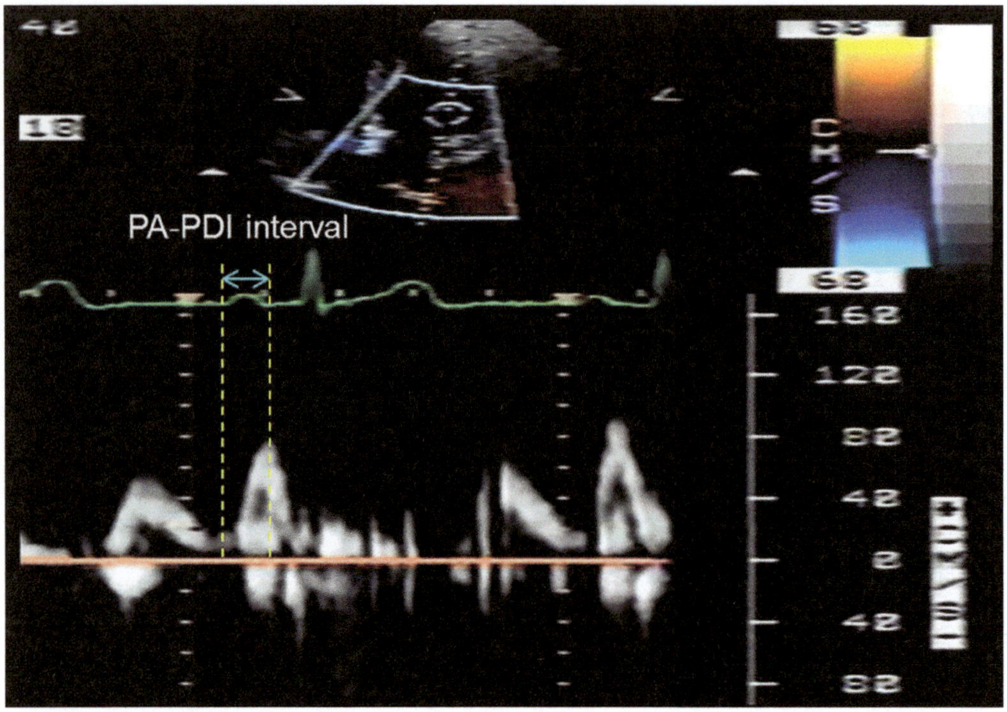

Figure 1. An example of the atrium electromechanical interval (PA-PDI interval) measurement. In the apical four chamber view, the pulse-wave Doppler sample was placed on the mitral inflow tract. The PA-PDI interval was defined as the time-interval from the initiation of the P wave from the electrocardiographic signal (lead II) provided by the echocardiographic machine to the peak of the mitral inflow A wave of the pulse wave Doppler imaging.

Methods

Study Population

In this retrospective study, a total of 337 subjects who received cardiovascular health examinations from 2006 to 2008 at the health examination center of Mackay Memorial Hospital in Taipei, Taiwan were included. In addition to blood tests, the health examination project included detailed cardiac examinations, including TTE and multi-detector computed tomography (MDCT). All subjects did not have overt cardiovascular diseases and received these examinations to evaluate their cardiac functions and detect any possibility of significant coronary diseases for screening purposes. All patients did not have the past history of AF, atrial flutter or atrial tachycardia. Subjects were excluded if they had left ventricular ejection fraction <50%, significant valvular heart disease (regurgitation or stenosis), more severe pulmonary hypertension (defined as systolic pulmonary arterial pressure higher than 60 mmHg), chronic lung diseases, existence of congenital heart diseases on echocardiography, known prior cardiac surgery history, and rheumatic heart disease. In addition, there was no previous implantation of pacemaker, overt renal insufficiency (creatinine >2.5 mg/dl), acute or symptomatic coronary events in our study subjects. Data of blood tests, TTE and MDCT were analyzed retrospectively in the present study.

Lab Data Acquisition

The blood samples were collected and examined for each patient in the fasting state. Lipid profiles and fasting glucose were obtained by a Hitachi 7170 automatic analyzer (Hitachi Corp. Hitachinaka, Ibaraki, Japan). High sensitivity - CRP (hs-CRP) levels were determined using a highly sensitive, latex particle-enhanced immunoassay (Elecsys 2010; Roche Diagnostics GmbH, Mannheim, Germany).

The Echocardiogram and Atrial Electromechanical Interval

TTE was performed using a multi-frequency transducer incorporated in a SONOS 5500 Echocardiograph (Hewlett Packard, Inc., Agilent Technologies, Andover, MA, USA) according to the standard techniques. [10] LA dimension was measured in parasternal long axis view at end systole. The LA volume was measured with a modified biplane area–length method with the echocardiographic tracings made in the apical two- and four-chamber views at end systole. [11] Left ventricular ejection fraction was assessed by Simpson's method. The atrium electromechanical interval (PA-PDI interval), defined as the time-interval from the initiation of the P wave from the electrocardiographic (ECG) signal (lead II) provided by the echocardiographic machine to the peak of the mitral inflow A wave of the pulse wave Doppler imaging in the apical four-chamber view (Figure 1), was measured in three consecutive cardiac cycles and averaged. The reproducibility of the measurement of the PA-PDI interval has been validated in our previous publication. [8].

MDCT Scanning Protocol and Measurements of Pericardial Fat

Scanning was performed using a 16-slice MDCT scanner (Sensation 16, Siemens Medical Solutions, Forchheim, Germany) with 16 mm × 0.75 mm collimation, rotation time 420 ms and tube voltage of 120 kV. In one breath-hold, images were acquired from above the level of tracheal bifurcation to below the base of heart using prospectively ECG triggering with the centre of the

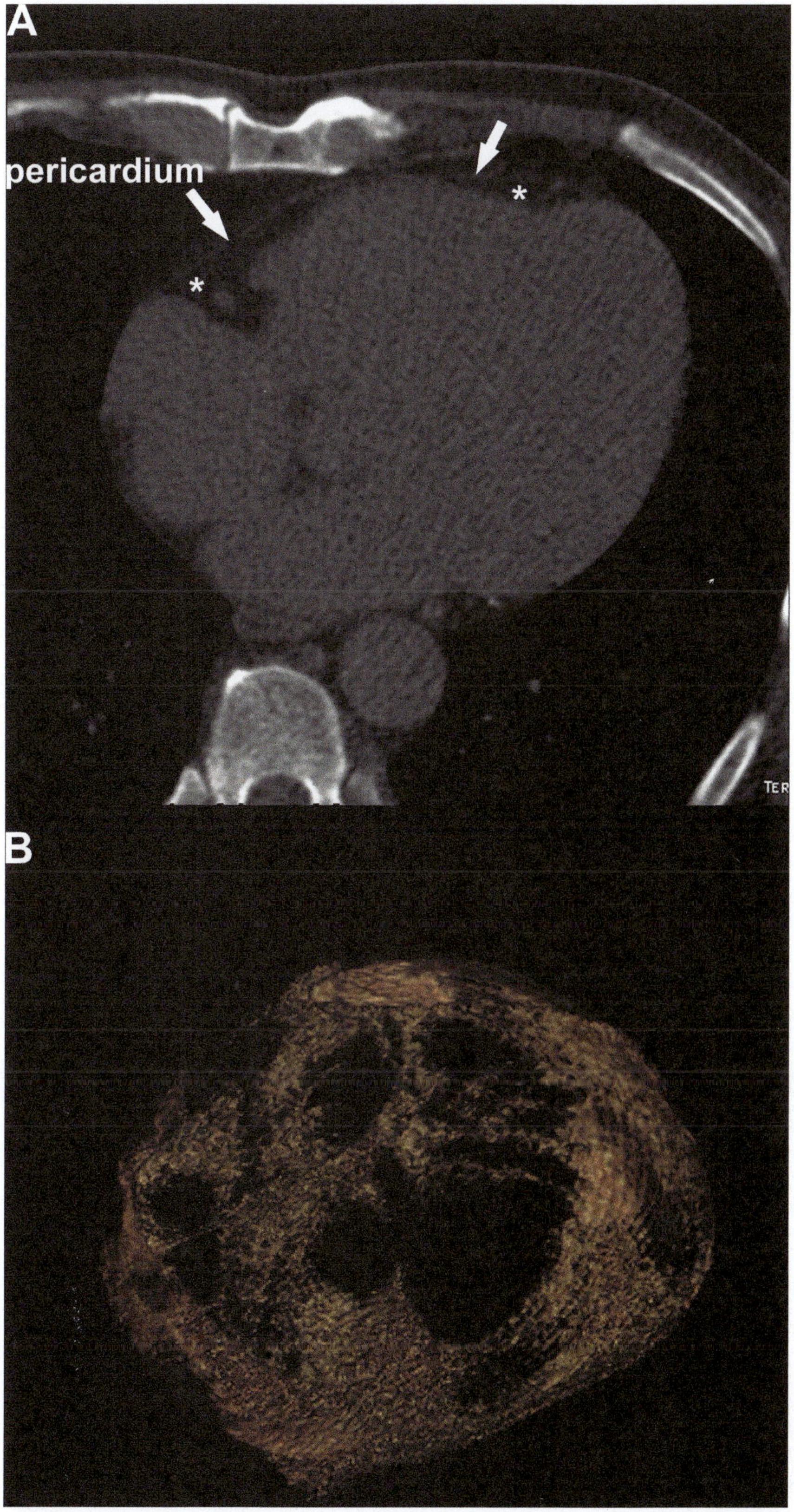

Figure 2. Measurement of pericardial adipose tissue. The PCF (*) was defined by the fat between the heart and the pericardium (arrow) as shown in axial view (A). Thick-slice (10 mm) 3D reconstruction axial view (B) demonstrated PCF. All pixels within a window of −195 to −45 HU and a window centre of −120 HU inside pericardial sac have been selected as PCF and reconstructed into the 3D image. PCF = pericardial fat.

Table 1. Clinical characteristics of the study population.

Variables	Study population, n = 337
Age, years	51.9±9.0
Male	68.5%
Body mass index, kg/m^2	24.6±3.0
Waist circumference, cm	84.4±9.0
Medical history	
Hypertension	27.6%
Diabetes mellitus	14.8%
Dyslipidemia	11.9%
Laboratory examinations	
WBCs count, cells/mm^3	4043±1813
Fasting glucose, mg/dL	100.1±20.0
Cholesterol, mg/dL	199.0±36.5
Triglyceride, mg/dL	142.0±83.4
hs-CRP, mg/dL	0.14±0.15
Transthoracic echocardiogram	
LV wall thickness, mm	9.6±1.2
LVIDD, mm	47.1±3.6
LVEF, %	68.7±3.3
Left atrial diameter, mm	31.3±4.3
Left atrial volume, mL	36.5±12.5
Peak E-wave velocity, cm/s	62.9±13.7
Peak A-wave velocity, cm/s	61.2±15.4
E/A ratio	1.02±0.33
PA-PDI interval, ms	125.3±14.0
Pericardial fat, mL	80.6±26.4

hsCRP = high sensitivity C-reactive protein; LV = left ventricle; LVEF = left ventricular ejection fraction; LVIDD = left ventricular internal dimension at end-diastole; WBCs = white blood cells; PA-PDI = the time interval from the initiation of the P wave deflection to the peak of the mitral inflow A wave on the pulse wave Doppler imaging.

acquisition at 70% of the R-R interval. From the raw data, the images were reconstructed with standard kernel in 3 mm thick axial, non-overlapping slices and 25 cm field of view.

PCF was quantified by MDCT using a dedicated workstation (Aquarius 3D Workstation, TeraRecon, San Mateo, CA, USA). The semi-automatic segmentation technique was developed for quantification of fat volumes. We traced pericardium in axial MDCT images manually from the level of left main coronary artery to diaphragm every four to six slices. The computer software then automatically interpolated and traced pericardium along the manually traced areas. All automatically traced slices were verified and modified if necessary for accuracy. The definition of fat tissue is pixels within a window of −195 to −45 HU and a window centre of −120 HU. PCF was defined as any adipose tissue located within the pericardial sac (Figure 2A and B).

Table 2. Linear regression models on the relationship between PA-PDI interval and pericardial fat.

Models	β±SE	P value
Model 1: adjusted for age and gender	0.672±0.082	<0.001
Model 2: adjusted for age, gender, body mass index and waist circumference	0.647±0.084	<0.001
Model 3: adjusted for all variables in model 2, and diabetes mellitus, hypertension and dyslipidemia	0.647±0.085	<0.001
Model 4: adjusted for all variables in model 3, and WBCs count, cholesterol, triglyceride, fasting glucose and hs-CRP	0.646±0.088	<0.001
Model 5: adjusted for all variables in model 4, and LV wall thickness, LVIDD, LVEF, left atrial diameter and E/A ratio	0.625±0.091	<0.001
Model 6: adjusted for all variables in model 4, and LV wall thickness, LVIDD, LVEF, left atrial volume and E/A ratio	0.585±0.089	<0.001

hs-CRP = high sensitivity C-reactive protein; LV = left ventricle; LVEF = left ventricular ejection fraction; LVIDD = left ventricular internal dimension at end-diastole; SE = standard error; WBCs = white blood cells.

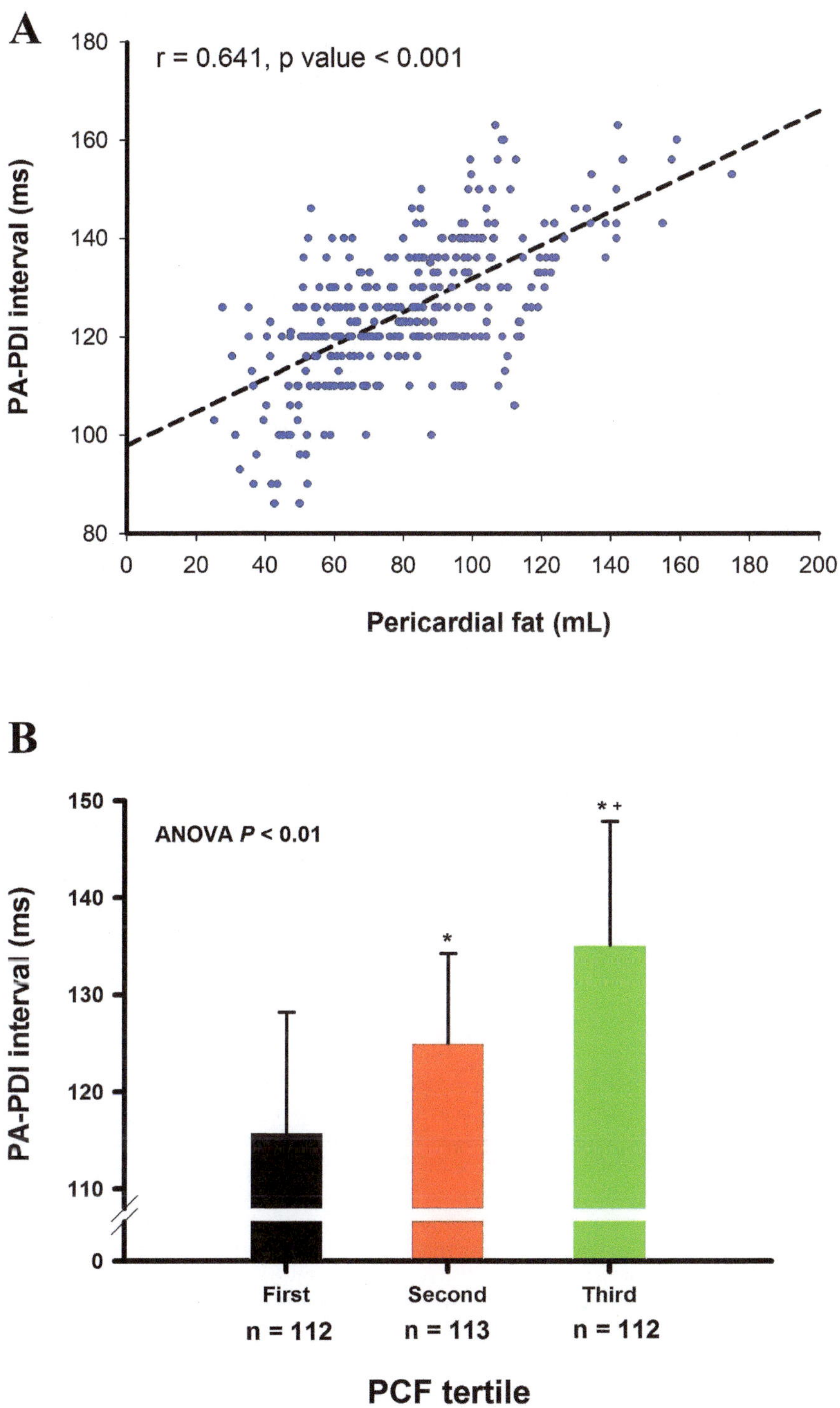

Figure 3. The association between PA-PDI interval and pericardial fat. The PA-PDI interval was significantly correlated with the amount of PCF (r = 0.641, p value <0.001) (A). When patients were divided into 3 groups according to the tertile values of PCF, the PA-PDI interval continuously lengthened from first (115.8±12.4 ms), second (125.0±9.3 ms) to third tertile (135.1±12.8 mm) (B). *P value <0.05, second or third tertile versus first tertile; +P value <0.05, third versus second tertile. PCF = pericardial fat.

The reproducibility of the measurement of the PCF has been validated in our previous publication. [12].

This study complies with the Declaration of Helsinki, and the study protocol was approved by the Institutional Review Board at Mackay Memorial Hospital, Taipei, Taiwan. Because the present study was a retrospective one, the Institutional Review Board agreed that the study can be performed without obtaining the informed consents of study subjects.

Statistical Analysis

The data are presented as mean values and standard deviations for normally distributed continuous variables, and proportions for

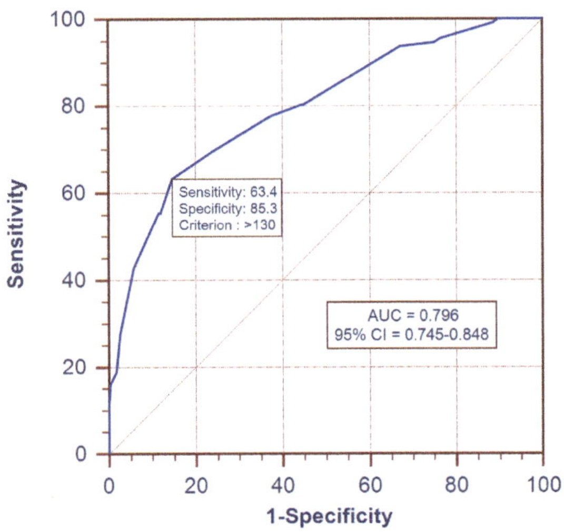

Figure 4. ROC curve for PA-PDI interval in predicting an increased amount of pericardial fat (third tertile). The AUC for the PA-PDI interval in predicting an increased amount of PCF (third tertile, ≥91.9 mL) was 0.796 (95% CI = 0.745–0.848, p value <0.001). At a cutoff value of 130 ms identified by the ROC curve, the sensitivity and specificity of PA-PDI interval in identifying patients with a highest tertile amount of PCF were 63.4% and 85.3%, respectively. AUC = area under the curve; CI = confidence interval; PCF = pericardial fat; ROC = receiver operating characteristic.

categorical variables. The differences between normally distributed continuous values are assessed using an unpaired 2-tailed t test or one-way analysis of variance (ANOVA) with Post Hoc Bonferroni test. The differences between nominal variables are compared using Chi-square test. The association of PA-PDI interval and PCF was analyzed with linear regression analysis. All statistical significances were set at $p<0.05$ and all statistical analyses were carried out by SPSS 17.0 (SPSS Inc. USA). The statistical powers of the analyses were higher than 80% based on the sample size and a two-sided alpha level of 0.05.

Results

Clinical Characteristics of the Study Population

The clinical characteristics of the study population were shown in Table 1. The mean PA-PDI interval was 125.3±14.0 ms with a range from 86 to 163 ms. The mean PCF was 80.6±26.4 mL with a range from 25.2 to 174.8 mL.

PA-PDI Interval and Pericardial Fat

The PA-PDI interval was significantly correlated with the amount of PCF (Figure 3A). When patients were divided into 3 groups according to the tertile values of PCF, the PA-PDI intervals continuously lengthened from first, second to third tertile (Figure 3B). The linear correlation between PA-PDI interval and PCF remained significant in different regression models adjusted for multiple variables, including age, gender, BMI, waist circumference, underlying diseases, biochemical data and echocardiographic parameters (Table 2). The results of these models demonstrated that the PA-PDI interval was significantly associated with PCF after taking obesity (model 2), comorbidities (model 3), systemic inflammation (model 4), left ventricular functions (model 5) and LA volume (model 6) into considerations.

The PA-PDI interval was useful in identifying patients with an increased amount of PCF (third tertile, ≥91.9 mL) with an odds ratio of 1.110 per 1 ms increment (95% confidence interval = 1.082–1.139, p value <0.001). The AUC for the PA-PDI interval in predicting an increased amount of PCF (third tertile) was 0.796 (95% CI = 0.745–0.848, p value <0.001)(Figure 4). At a cutoff value of 130 ms identified by the ROC curve, the sensitivity and specificity of PA-PDI interval in identifying patients with a highest tertile amount of PCF were 63.4% and 85.3%, respectively.

LA Volume and Pericardial Fat

We further compared the volume of LA in different groups of patients divided according to the tertile values of PCF. Similar to the PA-PDI interval, the LA volume was larger in third tertile compared to that of first or second tertile. However, the LA volume was not significantly different between first and second tertiles (Figure 5A). Linear regression analysis also showed significant correlation between LA volume and the amount of PCF (Figure 5B).

Discussion

Main Findings

In this study, we investigated the associations between the atrial electromechanical interval (PA-PDI interval) and PCF in 337 patients. The main findings were as follows: (1) The PA-PDI interval was positively correlated with the amount of PCF, and may be a useful parameter to quantify the degree of PCF-related LA remodeling. (2) The PA-PDI interval may serve as a more sensitive and convenient tool than LA volume to detect the PCF-related LA damages.

PCF, PA-PDI Interval and LA Remodeling

PCF represents a unique fat deposit because of its proximity to cardiac structures and its shared blood supply with the cardiac microcirculation. [13] It has been shown to have local inflammatory effects. [1,14] Tomasz et al. demonstrated that PCF exhibited significantly higher levels of several inflammatory cytokines (interleukin-1, interleukin-6, and TNF-alpha) than subcutaneous fat. [1] Besides, PCF has a threefold higher amount of the proinflammatory cytokine resistin, and fivefold lower amounts of the anti-inflammatory cytokine adiponectin when compared to gluteal adipose tissue. [14,15] In the study performed by Lin et al. which enrolled a total of 137 AF patients, systemic inflammation, represented by a higher level of hs-CRP, was associated with an abnormal and arrhythmogenic LA substrate. [16] Therefore, PCF serving as an abundant source of inflammatory mediators may increase the local inflammatory burden which directly damaged the LA. The hypothesis was supported by the observation that an increased amount of PCF was associated with a larger LA size, the presence of AF and a higher recurrence rate after AF ablation.[5,17–19].

However, the problem is how to quantify the adverse effects of PCF on LA easily and conveniently. The atrial electromechanical interval, PA-PDI interval, was reported to be able to reflect the degree of structural and electrical remodeling of LA, such as a LA enlargement, prolonged activation time and decreased voltage. [8] The prolongation of the interval was associated with new-onset AF and a higher recurrence rate after AF ablation. [8,20] In the present study, we demonstrated that the PA-PDI interval was longer in patients with an increased amount of PCF. It was significantly correlated with PCF volume even after adjusting for multiple factors. It may suggest that PA-PDI interval can be used to quantify the adverse effects of PCF on LA independently from obesity, systemic inflammation, left ventricular structures/functions

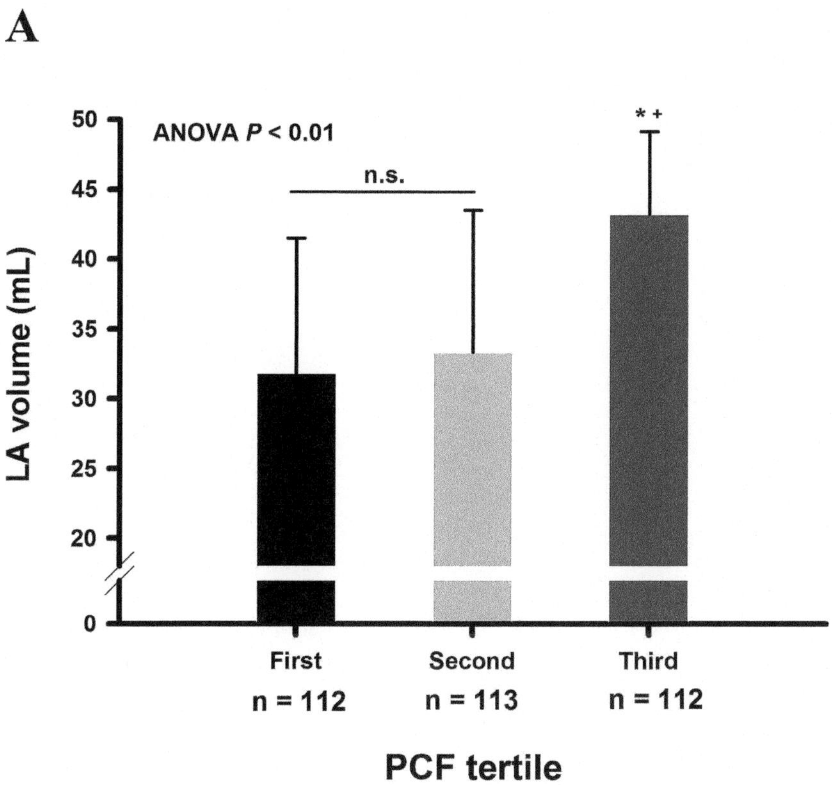

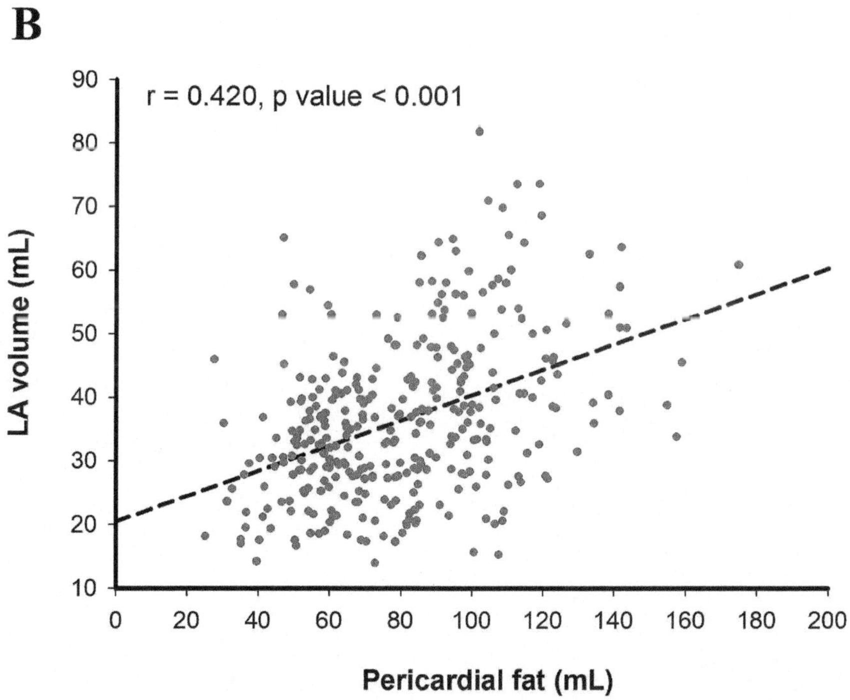

Figure 5. The association between LA volume and pericardial fat. Patients were divided into 3 groups according to the tertile values of PCF, and the LA volume was larger in third tertile compared to that of first or second tertile. However, the LA volume was not different between first and second tertiles (31.2±9.7 mL versus 33.3±10.2 mL, p value = 0.310) (A). LA volume was significantly correlated with the amount of PCF (r = 0.420, p value <0.001) (B). *P value <0.05, third tertile versus first tertile; $^{+}$P value <0.05, third versus second tertile; N.S. denotes non-significant p value. LA = left atrium; PCF = pericardial fat.

and LA size. At a cutoff value of 130 ms, the PA-PDI interval is helpful in identifying patients with a large amount of PCF (high tertile) with an odds ratio of 7.625 (95% confidence interval = 4.381–12.047). It may serve as a convenient parameter in evaluating the degree of PCF-related LA remodeling.

Comparisons of PA-PDI Interval and LA Volume in Evaluating PCF-related LA Remodeling

LA volume is a common parameter used in evaluating the process of LA remodeling. Compared with the LA volume calculation, the measurement of the PA-PDI interval was easier because manually traced two-dimensional echocardiographic LA areas are often limited by poor temporal and spatial resolution. The PA-PDI interval could be a alternative choice when precise measurement of the LA volume was difficult. In the present study, LA volume was not significantly different in patients with less amount of PCF (first and second tertiles), which may suggest that LA volume was not sensitive enough to detect the subtle changes of PCF-related LA remodeling. On the contrary, PA-PDI interval continuously lengthened when patients' PCF volume increased, and was still significantly different between patients with less amount of PCF (first and second tertiles). Besides, the PCF was correlated with PA-PDI interval ($r = 0.641$) more closely than with LA volume ($r = 0.420$). These findings suggested that PA-PDI interval, compared to LA volume, may be a better parameter to represent how severe the LA is affected by PCF. Since the subjects enrolled in the present study were those without AF and with a near normal LA size, the prolongation of PA-PDI interval in patients with an increased amount of PCF may imply that the LA has already been damaged in the pre-clinical stage without cardiac arrhythmias, and the PA-PDI interval may be sensitive enough to detect these subtle changes before the structural remodeling happened.

Limitations

There were several limitations of the present study. First, we analyzed the relationship between PA-PDI interval and the total amount, rather than regional distribution of PCF. Therefore, we were not able to investigate whether a specific site of PCF played a more important role in LA remodeling than other sites. Second, some precise echocardiographic parameters of LA, such as LA strain and strain rate, were not available in the present study. However, the purpose of our study was to provide a convenient and easy-measured clinical parameter with potentials in quantifying the degree of PCF-related atrial remodeling, rather than claiming that the PA-PDI interval was better than other echocardiographic tools. Third, the study subjects were patients who received cardiovascular health examinations at the medical center, and therefore a selection bias may exist. Lastly, since patients with atrial arrhythmias and overt cardiovascular diseases were not enrolled in the present study, whether the results presented here can be applied to patients with atrial arrhythmias or significant cardiac diseases remained uncertain.

Conclusion

The PA-PDI intervals were longer in patients with an increased amount of PCF. Compared to LA volume, the PA-PDI interval may be a more sensitive parameter to represent the degree of PCF-related atrial remodeling.

Author Contributions

Conceived and designed the experiments: CLH SAC. Analyzed the data: KLW YJL SLC LWL YFH. Contributed reagents/materials/analysis tools: YHL CH.Yun CH.Yen JYK HIY. Wrote the paper: TFC.

References

1. Mazurek T, Zhang L, Zalewski A, Mannion JD, Diehl JT, et al. (2003) Human epicardial adipose tissue is a source of inflammatory mediators. Circulation 108: 2460–2466.
2. Konishi M, Sugiyama S, Sugamura K, Nozaki T, Ohba K, et al. (2010) Association of pericardial fat accumulation rather than abdominal obesity with coronary atherosclerotic plaque formation in patients with suspected coronary artery disease. Atherosclerosis 209: 573–578.
3. Yerramasu A, Dey D, Venuraju S, Anand DV, Atwal S, et al. (2012) Increased volume of epicardial fat is an independent risk factor for accelerated progression of sub-clinical coronary atherosclerosis. Atherosclerosis 220: 223–230.
4. Thanassoulis G, Massaro JM, O'Donnell CJ, Hoffmann U, Levy D, et al. (2010) Pericardial fat is associated with prevalent atrial fibrillation: the Framingham Heart Study. Circ Arrhythm Electrophysiol 3: 345–350.
5. Al Chekakie MO, Welles CC, Metoyer R, Ibrahim A, Shapira AR, et al. (2010) Pericardial fat is independently associated with human atrial fibrillation. J Am Coll Cardiol 56: 784–788.
6. Shin SY, Yong HS, Lim HE, Na JO, Choi CU, et al. (2011) Total and interatrial epicardial adipose tissues are independently associated with left atrial remodeling in patients with atrial fibrillation. J Cardiovasc Electrophysiol 22: 647–655.
7. Merckx KL, De Vos CB, Palmans A, Habets J, Cheriex EC, et al. (2005) Atrial activation time determined by transthoracic Doppler tissue imaging can be used as an estimate of the total duration of atrial electrical activation. J Am Soc Echocardiogr 18: 940–944.
8. Chao TF, Sung SH, Wang KL, Lin YJ, Chang SL, et al. (2011) Associations between the atrial electromechanical interval, atrial remodelling and outcome of catheter ablation in paroxysmal atrial fibrillation. Heart 97: 225–230.
9. Chao TF, Sung SH, Wang KL, Tsao HM, Lin YJ, et al. (2011) Atrial electromechanical interval can identify patients with paroxysmal atrial fibrillation and is associated with CHADS2 score and peak velocity of left atrial appendage. J Cardiovasc Electrophysiol 22: 1325–1330.
10. Group TTACW, Douglas PS, Khandheria B, Stainback RF, Weissman NJ, et al. (2007) ACCF/ASE/ACEP/ASNC/SCAI/SCCT/SCMR 2007 appropriateness criteria for transthoracic and transesophageal echocardiography: a report of the American College of Cardiology Foundation Quality Strategic Directions Committee Appropriateness Criteria Working Group, American Society of Echocardiography, American College of Emergency Physicians, American Society of Nuclear Cardiology, Society for Cardiovascular Angiography and Interventions, Society of Cardiovascular Computed Tomography, and the Society for Cardiovascular Magnetic Resonance. Endorsed by the American College of Chest Physicians and the Society of Critical Care Medicine. J Am Soc Echocardiogr 20: 787–805.
11. Vandenberg BF, Weiss RM, Kinzey J, Acker M, Stark CA, et al. (1995) Comparison of left atrial volume by two-dimensional echocardiography and cine-computed tomography. Am J Cardiol 75: 754–757.
12. Yun CH, Lin TY, Wu YJ, Liu CC, Kuo JY, et al. (2012) Pericardial and thoracic peri-aortic adipose tissues contribute to systemic inflammation and calcified coronary atherosclerosis independent of body fat composition, anthropometric measures and traditional cardiovascular risks. Eur J Radiol 81: 749–756.
13. Sacks HS, Fain JN (2007) Human epicardial adipose tissue: a review. Am Heart J 153: 907–917.
14. Baker AR, Silva NF, Quinn DW, Harte AL, Pagano D, et al. (2006) Human epicardial adipose tissue expresses a pathogenic profile of adipocytokines in patients with cardiovascular disease. Cardiovasc Diabetol 5: 1.
15. Babcock MJ, Soliman EZ, Ding J, R AK, Goff DC Jr (2011) Pericardial fat and atrial conduction abnormalities in the Multiethnic Study of Atherosclerosis (MESA). Obesity (Silver Spring) 19: 179–184.
16. Lin YJ, Tsao HM, Chang SL, Lo LW, Tuan TC, et al. (2010) Prognostic implications of the high-sensitive C-reactive protein in the catheter ablation of atrial fibrillation. Am J Cardiol 105: 495–501.
17. Tsao HM, Hu WC, Wu MH, Tai CT, Lin YJ, et al. (2011) Quantitative analysis of quantity and distribution of epicardial adipose tissue surrounding the left atrium in patients with atrial fibrillation and effect of recurrence after ablation. Am J Cardiol 107: 1498–1503.
18. Wong CX, Abed HS, Molaee P, Nelson AJ, Brooks AG, et al. (2011) Pericardial fat is associated with atrial fibrillation severity and ablation outcome. J Am Coll Cardiol 57: 1745–1751.
19. Nagashima K, Okumura Y, Watanabe I, Nakai T, Ohkubo K, et al. (2011) Association between epicardial adipose tissue volumes on 3-dimensional reconstructed CT images and recurrence of atrial fibrillation after catheter ablation. Circ J 75: 2559–2565.
20. De Vos CB, Weijs B, Crijns HJ, Cheriex EC, Palmans A, et al. (2009) Atrial tissue Doppler imaging for prediction of new-onset atrial fibrillation. Heart 95: 835–840.

2

P Wave Area for Quantitative Electrocardiographic Assessment of Left Atrial Remodeling

Jonathan W. Weinsaft[1,2,3]*, Jonathan D. Kochav[1,4], Jiwon Kim[1,3], Sergey Gurevich[1], Samuel C. Volo[1], Anika Afroz[1], Maya Petashnick[1], Agnes Kim[1], Richard B. Devereux[1], Peter M. Okin[1]

1 Greenberg Cardiology Division/Department of Medicine, Weill Cornell Medical College, New York, New York, United States of America, **2** Department of Radiology, Weill Cornell Medical College, New York, New York, United States of America, **3** Memorial Sloan Kettering Cancer Center Department of Medicine, New York, New York, United States of America, **4** Duke University School of Medicine, Durham, North Carolina, United States of America

Abstract

Background: Left atrial (LA) dilation provides a substrate for mitral regurgitation (MR) and atrial arrhythmias. ECG can screen for LA dilation but standard approaches do not assess LA geometry as a continuum, as does non-invasive imaging. This study tested ECG-quantified P wave area as an index of LA geometry.

Methods and Results: 342 patients with CAD underwent ECG and CMR within 7 (0.1 ± 1.4) days. LA area on CMR correlated best with P wave area in ECG lead V1 ($r=0.42$, $p<0.001$), with lesser correlations for P wave amplitude and duration. P wave area increased stepwise in relation to CMR-evidenced MR severity ($p<0.001$), with similar results for MR on echocardiography (performed in 86% of patients). Pulmonary arterial (PA) pressure on echo was increased by 50% among patients in the highest (45 ± 14 mmHg) vs. the lowest (31 ± 9 mmHg) P wave area quartile of the population. In multivariate regression, CMR and echo-specific models demonstrated P wave area to be independently associated with LA size after controlling for MR, as well as echo-evidenced PA pressure. Clinical follow-up (mean 2.4 ± 1.9 years) demonstrated ECG and CMR to yield similar results for stratification of arrhythmic risk, with a 2.6-fold increase in risk for atrial fibrillation/flutter among patients in the top P wave area quartile of the population (CI 1.1–5.9, $p=0.02$), and a 3.2-fold increase among patients in the top LA area quartile (CI 1.4–7.0, $p=0.005$).

Conclusions: ECG-quantified P wave area provides an index of LA remodeling that parallels CMR-evidenced LA chamber geometry, and provides similar predictive value for stratification of atrial arrhythmic risk.

Editor: Giuseppe Schillaci, University of Perugia, Italy

Funding: This study was conducted with salary support as provided by the United States National Institutes of Health (grant number K23 HL102249-01). The funders had no role in study design, data collection and analysis, decision to publish, or preparation of the manuscript.

Competing Interests: The authors have declared that no competing interests exist.

* E-mail: jww2001@med.cornell.edu

Introduction

Left atrial (LA) chamber remodeling provides a physiologic substrate for mechanical and electrical alterations in cardiac performance. In population-based studies, LA size has been linked to clinical event risk, including heart failure and arrhythmias. [1–2] LA size has been shown to stratify prognosis for incident heart failure and mortality, with event risk independent of clinical indices. [3–4] Atrial fibrillation has also been closely linked to LA size,[5–7] consistent with the concept that LA remodeling alters electrical conduction and provides a physiologic substrate for arrhythmic events. Taken together, these findings provide a rationale for assessment of LA remodeling in at-risk patient populations.

Electrocardiography (ECG) is widely utilized as an initial screening test for patients with known or suspected heart disease. Unlike non-invasive imaging modalities (which directly measure LA geometry), ECG assesses LA physiology in relation to altered atrial electrical conductivity known to occur with chamber remodeling. P wave morphology is an established marker of atrial remodeling that has been used as an index of LA size for over a century. [8] However, conventional P wave criteria employ binary cutoffs for presence or absence of LA dilation,[9–11] rather than quantitative approaches that measure LA size as a continuum. Recent advances in ECG technology have facilitated quantification of constitutive components of the ECG waveform. Data from our group and others have shown quantitative analysis of the QRS complex to yield incremental utility over standard ECG approaches for assessment of LV remodeling and myocardial infarction. [12–13] P wave size and morphology can also be quantified in a similar manner, providing a quantitative index of LA remodeling that can be readily measured using standard data from the routine surface ECG.

This study tested the utility of P wave quantification as an index of LA remodeling among a broad cohort of subjects with ischemic heart disease. There were three aims: (1) to determine ECG based manifestations of LA chamber dilation as measured on cardiac magnetic resonance (CMR) imaging; (2) to identify alterations in P wave area that occur in relation to increasing magnitude of mitral regurgitation (MR) and pulmonary arterial hypertension; and (3) to test the predictive value of P wave area for stratification of longitudinal clinical endpoints related to LA remodeling – atrial fibrillation (AF) and atrial flutter (AFl).

Methods

Ethics Statement

The study protocol was approved by the Weill Cornell Institutional Review Board. For all subjects undergoing CMR and ECG exclusively for research purposes, written informed consent for study participation was obtained prior to data acquisition. For subjects meeting eligibility criteria but undergoing CMR and ECG for exclusively clinical purposes, data was retrospectively anonymized, with written informed consent for use of anonymized data waived.

Population

The study population comprised subjects with coronary artery disease (CAD) undergoing ECG and CMR within a 1 week interval at Weill Cornell Medical College. CMR was performed in both post-MI and heart failure (LVEF≤40%) subjects undergoing CMR for assessment of LV function and remodeling. In all subjects, CAD was defined as ≥70% stenosis of a major epicardial vessel (or ≥50% stenosis of the left main) based on invasive angiography. Patients with incomplete cine-CMR exams (i.e., with respect to LA imaging) were excluded from study participation.

ECG and CMR were performed at Weill Cornell Medical College (New York, NY) from 2005 to 2013. Transthoracic echocardiography (echo), if acquired within 1 week of ECG, was used as a supplemental test to measure MR severity and pulmonary arterial pressures, for which results were obtained via query of institutional databases. Baseline demographic indices were obtained using a standardized patient questionnaire, with results supplemented by review of electronic medical records (EMR). Clinical follow-up (concerning incident AF or AFl) was obtained from EMR record review, which was performed by a dedicated study investigator blinded to results of both ECG and imaging. Adequate follow-up was defined based on documented clinical evaluation occurring at least 60 days after ECG.

Data Acquisition

Electrocardiography. ECGs were acquired using a standard 12-lead surface electrode recording system (MAC 5000/5500, General Electric, Waukesha, WI). Recordings were performed at a sampling rate of 500 Hz. Data was stored digitally using a dedicated (GE Muse) archival system.

Cardiac magnetic resonance. CMR was performed by dedicated technologists using 1.5 Tesla scanners (General Electric, Waukesha, WI). Imaging consisted of two components: (1) cine-CMR for geometry/function, and (2) DE-CMR for myocardial infarction. Cine-CMR was performed using a steady-state free precession sequence (typical parameters: repetition time (TR) 3.5 msec, echo time (TE) 1.6 msec, flip angle 60°, in-plane spatial resolution 1.9 mm×1.4 mm). Following cine-CMR, gadolinium was intravenously administered (0.1–0.2 mmol/kg) to patients without renal contraindications. Delayed enhancement (DE-) CMR was performed 10–30 minutes thereafter using an inversion recovery pulse sequence (typical TI 250–350 msec).

Cine- and DE-CMR images were obtained in matching short and long-axis planes. Short-axis images were acquired throughout the LV from the mitral valve annulus through the apex. Long-axis images were acquired in standard two-, three- and four-chamber orientations.

Echocardiography. Transthoracic 2D echocardiograms were performed by experienced sonographers using commercially available equipment (e.g., General Electric Vivid-7, Philips ie33). Imaging was performed in parasternal, subcostal, as well as apical 2-, 3-, 4-, and 5- chamber orientations. Color Doppler was used to assess MR severity based on jet area, depth, vena contracta, and directionality. Pulsed wave Doppler included assessment of MR duration as well as pulmonary vein flow profiles.

Data Analysis

P wave assessment. ECGs were quantitatively analyzed using automated processing software (Magellan, GE Healthcare, Wauwatosa, WI, USA). Multiple aspects of P wave morphology in lead V1 were measured, including duration, amplitude, total geometric area subtended within the waveform (inclusive of both positive and negative deflections) and the area of the terminal negative component of the P wave (**Figure 1**).

Cardiac structure and function. CMR and echo indices of cardiac structure and function were measured to determine relationships between P wave characteristics and cardiac chamber remodeling. For cine-CMR, LA area was planimetered in 4-chamber orientation at ventricular end-systole (atrial end-diastole); left ventricular ejection fraction (LVEF), myocardial mass, and chamber volumes were measured via planimetry of contiguous short-axis images at ventricular end-diastole and end-systole. Corresponding echo measurements of LA and LV size were based on linear chamber dimensions in parasternal long axis views in accordance with consensus guidelines [14].

Mitral regurgitation. MR severity was graded on cine-CMR and echo in accordance with established conventions:

On cine-CMR, MR was graded based on maximal size of the regurgitant jet in relation to the left atrium (<1/3, 1/3–2/3, >2/3), with regurgitant severity scored using a 4 point scale (0 = none/trace, 1 = mild, 2 = moderate, 3 = severe) [15–16].

Echo was used as an additional test for MR, which was graded using a semi-quantitative 5-point scale. In accordance with established standards, [17] MR was primarily graded based on the farthest distance reached from the mitral orifice by the regurgitant jet (mild [1+]; ≤1.5 cm | moderate [2+]; 1.5–3.0 cm | moderately-severe [3+]; 3.0–4.5 cm | severe [4+]; ≥4.5 cm). MR severity was further confirmed based on jet area and vena contracta ([1+]; color jet <20% LA area, vena contracta <0.3 | [2+]; color jet 20–40%, vena contracta 0.3–0.69 | [3–4+]; color jet >40%, vena contracta ≥0.7) as well as jet density, mitral (E/A) and pulmonary vein flow pattern. [18] Pulmonary artery systolic pressure was calculated based on tricuspid valve regurgitant velocity and inferior vena cava caliber.

All imaging exams (both CMR and echo) were interpreted by experienced (ACC/AHA level III) investigators blinded to the results of ECG analysis.

Statistical Methods

Continuous variables (expressed as mean±standard deviation) were compared using paired Student's t-test for two-group comparisons. For multiple group comparisons, analysis of variance (ANOVA) was employed, as well as post-hoc (Tukey's) testing for comparison of differences between individual strata. Categorical variables were compared using Chi-square or, when fewer than 5 expected outcomes per cell, Fisher's exact test. ECG and imaging parameters were compared using bivariate correlation coefficients, with correlations further evaluated using Koenker's test for heteroscedasticity. Multivariate logistic regression was used to test clinical and imaging indices in relation to ECG parameters. Follow-up event rates were compared between groups using

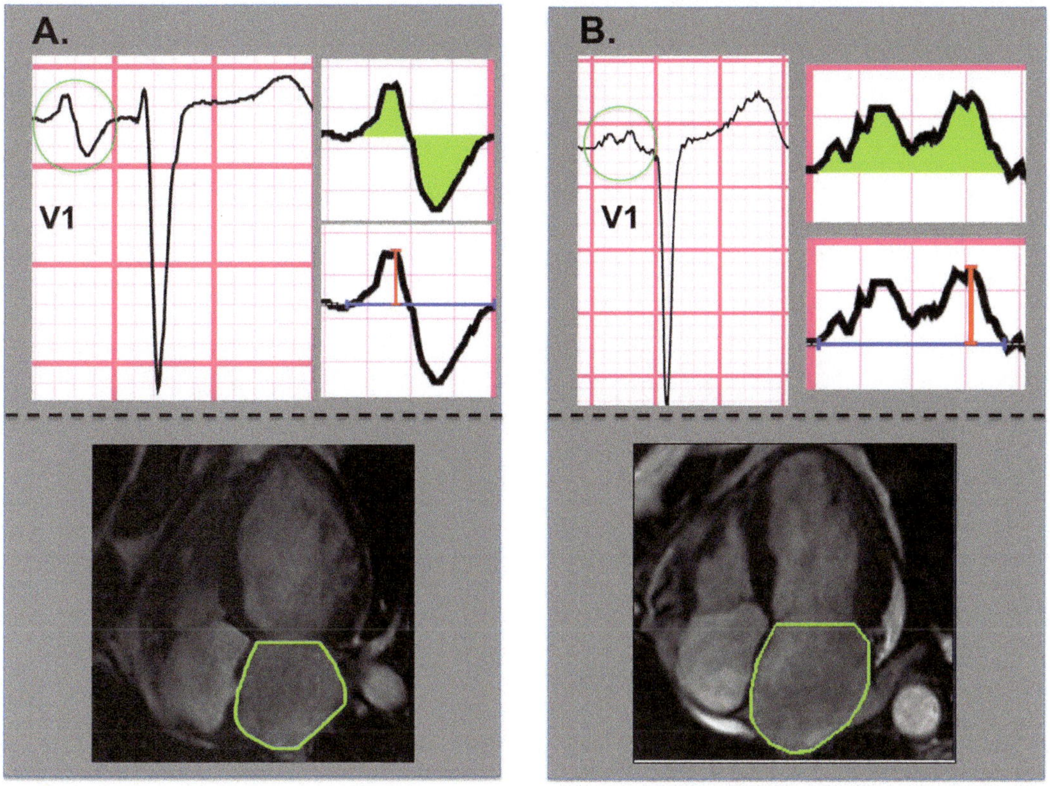

Figure 1. P wave and Left Atrial Area Quantification. Representative examples of LA quantification methods: For ECG (top), total P wave area was quantified based on geometric area (green shading) between the electrical waveform and the isoelectric line. Corresponding indices of amplitude (red line) and duration (blue line) were measured within the total P wave complex, as well as its positive and negative components. For CMR (bottom), LA area was measured by planimetry of chamber borders (green line) at ventricular end-systole. Note heterogeneity in P wave morphology among patients with LA enlargement: Whereas both patient examples demonstrate LA dilation by CMR, a bimodal P wave with large negative terminal component is present in **1A**, whereas a bifid but upright P wave is present in **1B**.

Kaplan-Meier survival curves and Cox regression analysis. Two-sided $p<0.05$ was considered indicative of statistical significance. Statistical calculations were performed using IBM SPSS Statistics Version 20 (IBM Corporation, Armonk, NY).

Results

Population Characteristics

The study population comprised 342 subjects with ischemic heart disease who underwent CMR and ECG within a 1-week interval (mean 0.1 ± 1.4 days); 94% had CMR and ECG performed within 1 day.

Table 1 details clinical and imaging characteristics of the population, stratified in relation to presence or absence of CMR-evidenced LA dilation (categorized based on an established CMR cutoff [15 cm^2/m^2]. [19] As shown, subjects with LA dilation were older, less likely to be male, and more likely to be hypertensive ($p< 0.01$), but were otherwise clinically similar to those without LA dilation. Body size indices, whether measured by height or weight alone or by aggregate body surface area, were smaller among subjects with LA dilation (all $p<0.001$). Regarding imaging parameters, LA size on CMR was, on average, 55% larger among subjects with (17 ± 2 cm^2/m^2), as compared to those without (11 ± 2 cm^2/m^2) LA dilation. [19] LA dilation was associated with global changes in LV structure and function, as evidenced by greater impairment of LVEF and more advanced chamber dilation (all $p<0.001$).

Electrocardiographic Markers of Left Atrial Dilation

Table 2 presents multiple indices of ECG-quantified P wave morphology in lead V1 stratified in relation to LA dilation on CMR. Mean P wave amplitude, duration, net area and terminal negative component area were all significantly greater in patients with LA dilation. Total P wave area, as quantified in lead V1, was 59% greater among patients with, as compared to those without, CMR-evidenced LA dilation, paralleling magnitude of difference in actual CMR-evidenced chamber size between groups. P wave area increased in association with prevalence of abnormal P wave morphology as classified using an established binary criterion (algebraic product of negative terminal amplitude and duration ≥ 40 mm•msec in lead V1). [20–22] However, whereas abnormal P wave morphology was associated with LA dilation in univariate analysis (OR 2.05 [CI 1.14–3.71], $p = 0.02$), forced entry of both P wave area and P wave morphology into a multivariate model demonstrated only P wave area to be positively associated with LA dilation.

Figure 2 provides scatterplots for P wave indices in relation to LA size. As shown, P wave area yielded the highest correlation with LA size ($r = 0.42$, $p<0.001$), although heteroscedasticity was present for this correlation ($p<0.001$), as well as for other ECG variables. Moreover, despite larger body size indices (which might be expected to attenuate measures of P wave dimensions)[23–24] among patients without LA dilation, P wave area yielded similar magnitude of correlation with both unadjusted ($r = 0.41$, $p<0.001$) and body surface area indexed ($r = 0.42$, $p<0.001$) left atrial area,

Table 1. Clinical and Imaging Characteristics in Relation to the Presence or Absence of Left Atrial Dilation.

Parameter	Overall (n = 342)	Left Atrial Dilation + (n = 66)	Left Atrial Dilation − (n = 276)	P
CLINICAL				
Age (years)	60±12	67±11	58±12	**<0.001**
Male gender	79% (271)	65% (43)	83% (228)	**0.002**
Anthropomorphic Indices				
Height (cm)	172±10	167±10	173±10	**<0.001**
Weight (kg)	83±20	72±15	85±20	**<0.001**
BSA (cm2)	2.0±0.2	1.8±0.2	2.0±0.2	**<0.001**
Coronary Artery Disease Risk Factors				
Hypertension	58% (199)	77% (51)	54% (148)	**<0.001**
Hypercholesterolemia	54% (186)	56% (37)	54% (149)	0.76
Diabetes Mellitus	33% (114)	36% (24)	33% (90)	0.56
Tobacco Use	44% (152)	55% (36)	42% (116)	0.07
Family History	18% (63)	9% (6)	21% (57)	**0.03**
IMAGING				
Cardiac Magnetic Resonance				
Left Ventricle				
Ejection fraction (%)	41±16	30±12	43±16	**<0.001**
Infarct Size (% LV myocardium)	17±12	17±12	16±11	0.98
End-diastolic volume (ml)	188±68	231±77	178±62	**<0.001**
ml/m^2	97±34	127±37	89±29	**<0.001**
End-systolic volume (ml)	118±70	166±74	107±63	**<0.001**
ml/m^2	61±36	91±37	54±31	**<0.001**
Stroke volume (ml)	70±20	66±18	71±20	**0.048**
Myocardial mass (gm)	162±56	184±54	157±55	**<0.001**
gm/m^2	83±27	101±27	79±25	**<0.001**
Left Atrium				
Diameter (cm)	3.9±0.6	4.5±0.6	3.8±0.6	**<0.001**
Area (cm^2)	24±6	31±5	22±4	**<0.001**
cm^2/m^2	12±3	17±2	11±2	**<0.001**

Left atrial dilation defined using established CMR normative cutoff (>15 cm^2/m^2) [19].
Numbers in boldface indicate p values <0.05.

with similarly minimal impact of body size adjustment for all other P wave indices. P wave area in lead V1 remained significantly associated with LA area ($p<0.001$) on CMR in both forced and stepwise linear regression analyses that controlled for P wave area in all other surface ECG leads.

Physiologic Indices in Relation to P Wave Area

Mitral regurgitation. P wave area in V1 was tested in relation to MR severity on cine-CMR in all patients. Echo,

Table 2. Lead V1 P wave Measurements in Relation to the Presence or Absence of Left Atrial Dilation.

A. Amplitude

Variable	Left Atrial Dilation +	Left Atrial Dilation −	Δmean (95% CI)	P
Amplitude (μV)	47.3±42.6	34.4±27.4	12.9 (2.0, 23.9)	**0.02**
Duration (ms)	114.8±16.0	107.7±17.1	7.2 (2.6, 11.8)	**0.002**
Area (mVm·sec)	4.3±2.5	2.7±1.3	1.5 (0.9, 2.2)	**<0.001**
Negative Component Area (mV·msec)	3.2±2.6	2.0±1.3	1.2 (0.5, 1.8)	**0.001**

Left atrial dilation defined using established CMR normative cutoff (>15 cm^2/m^2) [19].

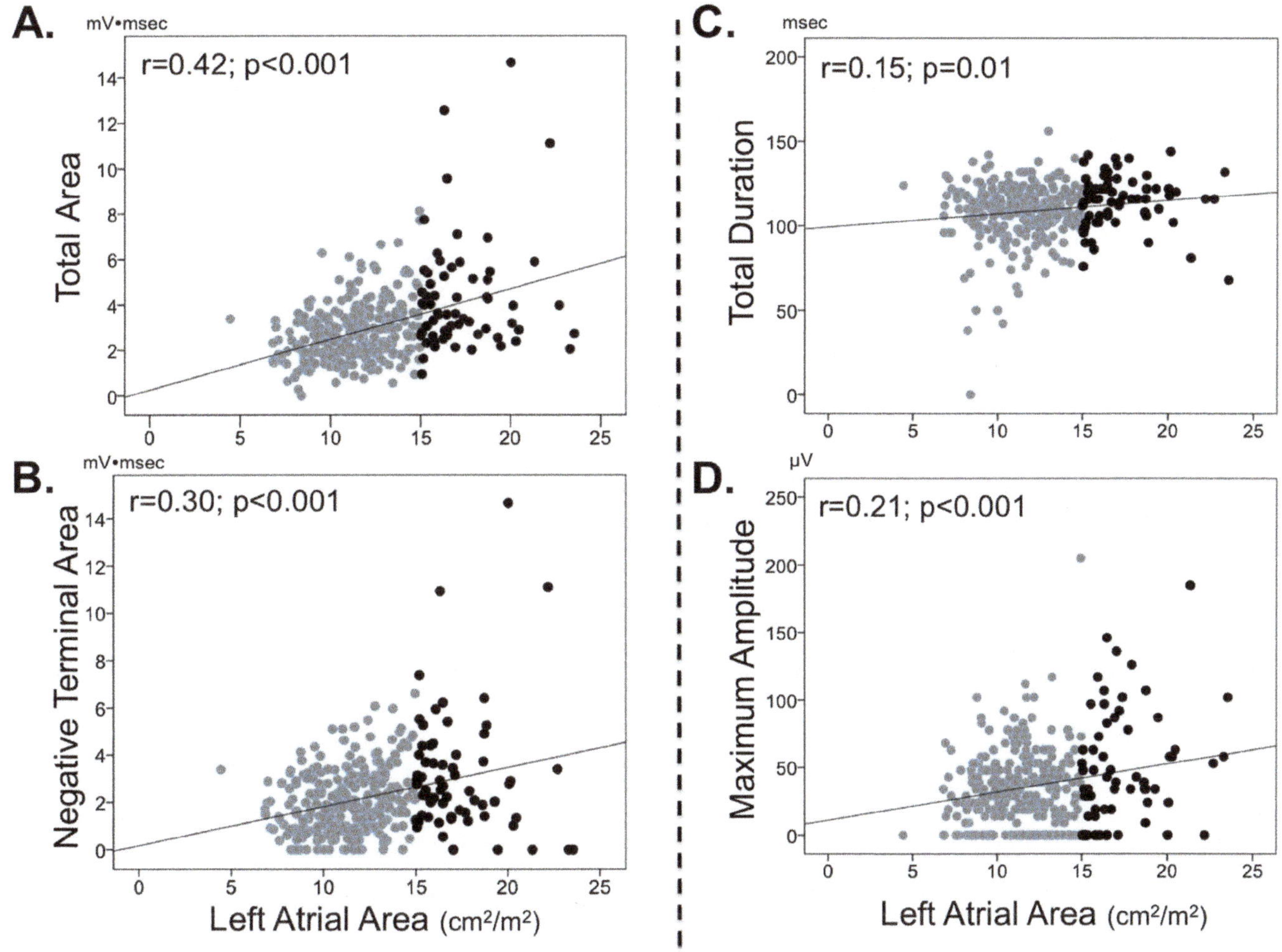

Figure 2. Left Atrial Size. Scatter plots relating CMR-quantified LA size to P wave morphology as measured in ECG lead V1. Data presented for total P wave area (**1A**), negative terminal area (**1B**), duration (**1C**), and maximum amplitude (**1D**). Patient data stratified based on normal (grey) and dilated (black) left atrial size on cine-CMR using an established diagnostic cutoff (>15 cm^2/m^2) [19].

performed within 7 days of ECG in 86% of the study population (n = 293), was used as an independent test for MR.

Figure 3A stratifies P wave area in relation to graded MR severity. Results demonstrate stepwise P wave area increases in relation to increasing MR on cine-CMR ($p<0.001$ for trend). Tukey's post-hoc testing revealed that all cine-CMR MR categories differed significantly with respect to P wave area ($p<0.05$), with exception of comparison between patients with moderate vs. those with severe MR ($p = 0.98$). Among the aggregate population, P wave area was nearly 1.5-fold higher among patients with MR graded as moderate or severe (3.7±1.9), as compared to those with mild or absent MR (2.6±1.5, $p<0.001$).

Figure 3B stratifies P wave area in relation to MR severity on echo. Echo similarly demonstrated P wave area to increase in relation to graded severity of MR ($p<0.001$ for trend). Tukey's post-hoc testing demonstrated significant differences in P wave area between patients with no MR as compared to each echo MR grade (all $p\leq0.01$), although comparisons between MR affected patients based on echo-assigned grade did not achieve significance (p = NS).

Pulmonary arterial pressure. Figure 4 examines mean PA systolic pressure, as measured by echo, among population-based quartiles stratified based on P wave area. As shown, PA pressure increased in association with P wave area ($p<0.001$ for trend), including a near 50% increase in mean PA systolic pressure among the highest (45±14 mmHg) as compared to the lowest (31±9 mmHg) P wave area quartile. Consistent with this, Tukey's post-hoc testing demonstrated significant differences between patients in the top P wave area quartile vs. all other groups (all $p<0.01$).

Markers of Increased P Wave Area

Logistic regression was used to assess the contribution of clinical and imaging variables to increased P wave area. Regarding clinical variables, patients in the highest quartile of P wave area (≥ 3.5 mV·msec) were more likely to be hypertensive (29% vs. 17%, $p = 0.008$) as compared to the remainder of the population, but were otherwise clinically similar with regard to age, gender, and prevalence of diabetes mellitus (all p = NS). Accordingly, hypertensive status, together with LA size as well as physiologic indices (MR, PA pressure) associated with P wave area in univariate analysis were tested in CMR and echo-specific multivariate logistic regression models.

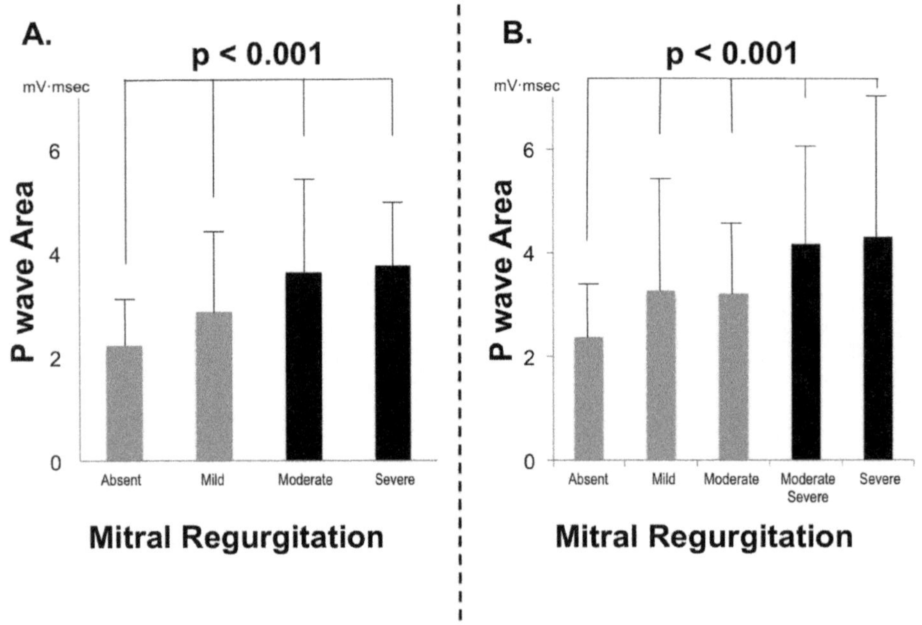

Figure 3. Mitral Regurgitation Severity. P wave area in lead V1 (mean ± standard deviation) in relation to MR severity on cine-CMR (**3A**) and echo (**3B**). Note that P wave area increased stepwise in relation to MR severity as measured by both modalities, with greatest magnitude of increase at a threshold of moderate-severe MR (black bars).

Tables 3–4 present multivariate models incorporating imaging variables from CMR (**3**) and echo (**4**). As shown, being in the upper quartile of P wave area was independently associated with LA size measured by either modality even after controlling for MR severity and hypertensive status. Applied clinically, results demonstrate that each 5 cm^2/m^2 increase in LA area by CMR resulted in a two-fold increased in likelihood of increased (i.e. top quartile) P wave area by ECG (odds ratio [OR] 1.21 per cm^2/m^2, $p<0.001$), with findings similar for echo-quantified left atrial diameter (OR 3.03 per cm/m^2, $p=0.03$). Regarding functional indices, echo results demonstrated PA systolic pressure to be independently associated with increased P wave area (OR 1.49 per 10 mmHg, $p=0.01$) even after controlling for LA diameter and graded severity of MR.

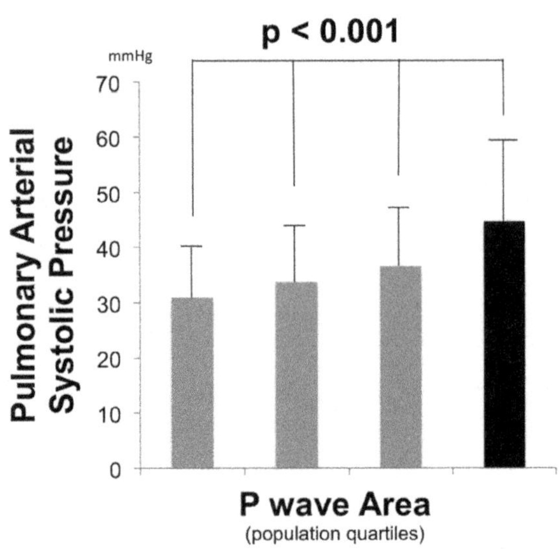

Figure 4. Pulmonary Arterial Pressure. Pulmonary arterial systolic pressure (mean ± standard deviation) among population subgroups stratified based on lead V1 P wave area quartiles (≤1.92 | 1.93–2.70 | 2.71–3.65 | >3.65 mV·msec). Black bar = top P wave area quartile.

Clinical Endpoints

Clinical follow-up was available in 64% (n = 218) of the study population. Study participants with follow-up were similar to those without follow-up with respect to age, gender, P wave area on ECG, and LA size on cine-CMR (all p = NS).

During a mean interval of 2.4±1.9 years following ECG, 11.5% (n = 25) of patients experienced atrial fibrillation (AF) or flutter (AFl). Incidence of the composite endpoint of AF/AFl increased in relation to P wave area as well as LA size, and was 4-fold higher among patients in the highest, as compared to the lowest, P wave area quartile (17.0% vs. 3.9%, $p=0.03$), with similar magnitude of difference when patient groups were compared based on quartiles of LA area (23.2% vs. 6.9%, $p=0.01$). As shown in **Figure 5**, both indices stratified arrhythmic risk ($p<0.05$). In Cox regression analysis, patients within the top quartile of P wave area manifested a 2.6-fold increase in risk for incident atrial fibrillation/flutter as compared to the remainder of the population (95% CI 1.1 to 5.9, $p=0.02$), whereas patients in the top quartile of LA area index manifested a 3.2-fold (95% CI 1.4 to 7.0, $p=0.005$) increase in risk. Similarly, when examined as continuous variables in univariate Cox regression models, both a one standard deviation increase in P wave area (1.54 mV·msec) as well as body surface area indexed LA area (3.19 cm^2/m2) conferred similar risk for incident AF/AFl during longitudinal follow-up: [P wave area hazard ratio 1.57 (95% CI 1.2–2.1), $p=0.003$/LA area hazard ratio 1.64 (CI 1.2–2.3), $p=0.005$].

Table 3. Multivariate Models for Prediction of Increased P wave Area in Lead V1* in Overall CMR Population.

Model chi-square = 48.08, p<0.001

Variable	Odds Ratio	95% Confidence Interval	P
Left Atrial Area (per cm^2/m^2)	1.21	1.10–1.34	**<0.001**
Mitral Regurgitation (CMR graded severity [0–III])	1.46	1.06–2.01	**0.02**
Hypertension	1.39	0.78–2.48	0.27

Discussion

This study, the first to test quantitative ECG assessment of LA remodeling in relation to both physiologic indices and clinical arrhythmic risk, offers several key findings: First, P wave area – as measured on routine surface ECG in lead V1– parallels LA size on CMR. Second, LA loading conditions influence P wave area, as evidenced by stepwise increases in relation to increasing graded MR severity. Association between P wave area and MR severity on CMR was independent of LA chamber size, supporting the concept that P wave area provides a composite marker of atrial stretch, rather than a simple index of chamber size alone. Finally, P wave area stratified longitudinal risk for atrial arrhythmias: risk of incident AF/AFl was nearly 3-fold higher among patients in the top quartile of P wave area as compared to the remainder of the population (hazard ratio [HR] 2.6, CI 95% 1.1 to 5.9, p = 0.02), paralleling a similar magnitude of risk among patients in the top quartile of LA area (HR 3.2, CI 1.4 to 7.0, p = 0.005).

Our findings build upon prior research concerning the link between ECG-evidenced P wave morphology and LA size. Established ECG criteria (such as P wave duration >0.11 sec, V1 negative terminal component >40 msec·mm, and prominent notching) have individually been shown to yield wide ranges of sensitivity (12 to 96%) and specificity (64 to 100%) for echo-evidenced LA dilation, possibly reflecting differences in study population, individual ECG criteria, and echo cutoffs for chamber enlargement. [9–11] CMR, which provides excellent endocardial definition and more reproducible chamber quantification than echo, [25] has also been used as a comparator for ECG. Consistent with prior echo studies, Tsao et al. reported that different ECG criteria yielded marked variability for assessment of CMR-evidenced LA enlargement (sensitivity 8 to 94%, specificity 21 to 90%). [26] However, despite differences in imaging modality, such prior studies share a common approach in that P wave data has been generally used to categorize LA dilation in a binary fashion, rather than to assess LA size as a continuous parameter. As evidenced in our study (**Figure 1**), P wave morphology can vary among patients with LA dilation, thereby compromising utility of established morphological criteria for LA enlargement, such as those predicated on P wave axis or terminal deflection component. Our results demonstrate that P wave area, a composite index of amplitude and duration, provides a continuous index of LA remodeling, reflecting physiologic changes in LA geometry.

It is important to recognize that whereas P wave area yielded higher correlation (r = 0.45) with LA size than did other P wave indices (r = 0.15–0.3), heteroscedasticity was present for all ECG indices. Limited correlation between P wave indices and LA area is consistent with our finding (**Tables 3–4**) that P wave area reflects a composite manifestation of both LA size and pressure volume/loading conditions, rather than a singular index of LA size alone. We note that our observed associations between P wave area and MR severity on CMR as well as estimated PA pressures on echo are consistent with prior physiologic studies that have examined the impact of both loading conditions and tissue properties on LA conductivity. Among patients with heart failure, LA dilation has been found to be accompanied by low voltage amplitudes on invasive electro-anatomic mapping, and prolonged P wave duration on surface ECG. [27] Similar findings have also been reported in conditions associated with LA remodeling, including mitral stenosis and atrial septal defect. [28–29] Changes in atrial conductivity have been shown to reflect alterations in tissue substrate. In a canine model of pacing-induced heart failure, regions of slow atrial conductivity had histology-evidenced interstitial fibrosis. [30] Atrial tissue characterization using delayed enhancement CMR has been used to demonstrate that areas of low voltage on electro-anatomic mapping correspond to regions of atrial fibrosis. [31] Of note, reverse LA remodeling has been shown to be capable of improving LA electrical properties. For example, among patients with mitral stenosis, commissurotomy has been shown to reduce both LA pressures and volumes, resulting in decreased P wave duration on ECG. [32] Taken together, these data demonstrate that that LA tissue substrate, geometry, and loading conditions all bear potential influence on

Table 4. Multivariate Models for Prediction of Increased P wave Area in Lead V1* in Echocardiography Sub-group.

Model chi-square = 33.85, p<0.001

Variable	Odds Ratio	95% Confidence Interval	P
Left Arial Diameter (per cm/m^2)	3.03	1.13–8.12	**0.03**
Pulmonary Arterial Systolic Pressure (per 10 mmHg)	1.49	1.14–1.86	**0.01**
Mitral Regurgitation (echo graded severity [0–IV])	1.38	0.84–2.27	0.20
Hypertension	1.04	0.45–2.42	0.93

(*top P wave area quartile ≥3.5 mV·msec).

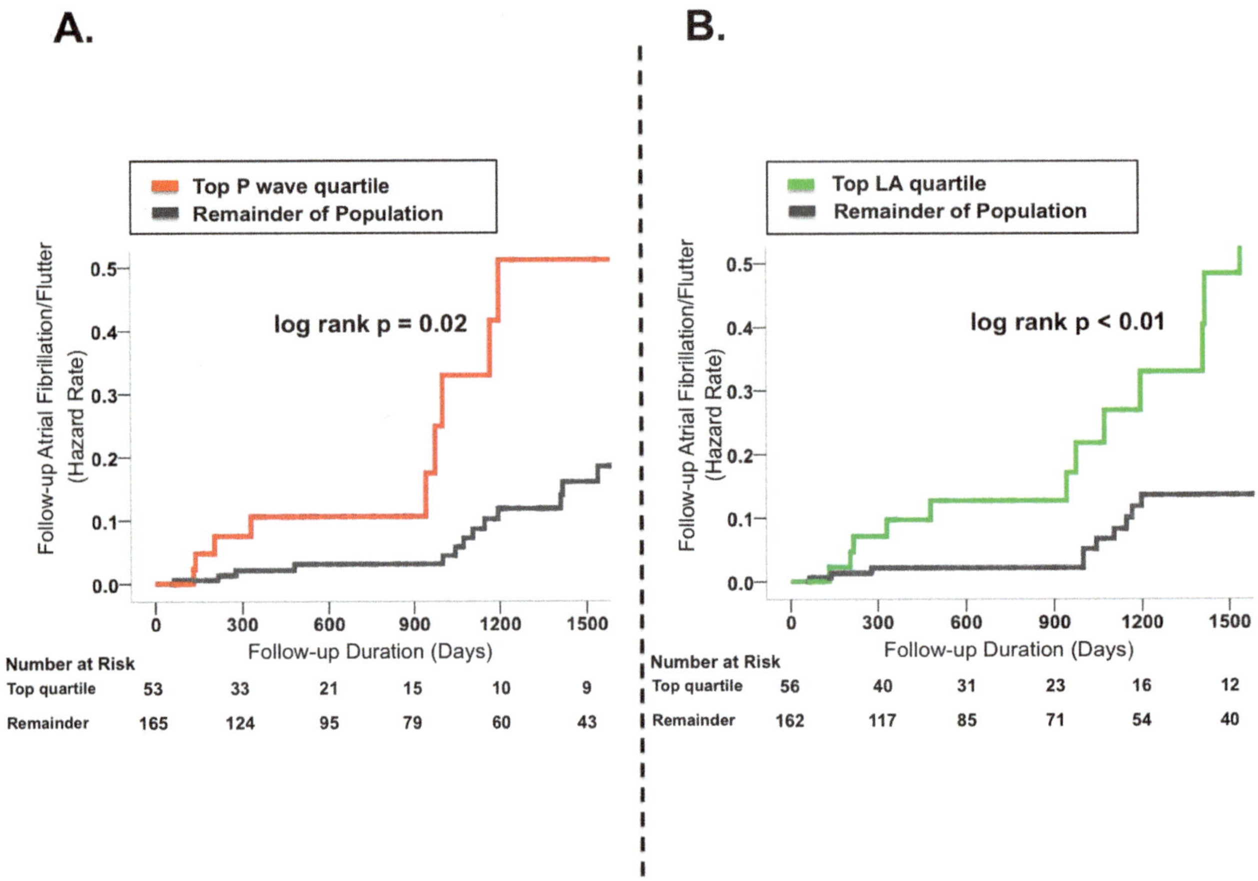

Figure 5. Atrial Fibrillation/Flutter Risk as Stratified by LA Remodeling Indices. Kaplan-Meier plots relating baseline P wave area (5A) and body surface area indexed LA area (5B) to follow-up risk for AF/AFl. Note that both ECG and CMR indices demonstrated increased risk for AF/AFl among patients in the highest quartile of LA remodeling.

ECG waveform indices, supporting the notion that P wave morphology offers a composite index for LA arrhythmic substrate.

Regarding clinical implications, our findings are consistent with prior literature linking P wave morphology to arrhythmic risk. Among 1550 subjects in the Framingham Heart Study, those in the top 5 percent of P wave duration had a 2.5-fold increase in relative risk for AF compared to the remainder of the population. [33] In the ARIC study, increased P wave duration (HR 3.9) and area (HR 2.8) were each associated with AF even after controlling for age, gender, and clinical risk factors for CAD. [34] Of importance, neither study examined the predictive value of P wave indices in relation to imaging parameters of LA dilation, which is itself a well-established predictor for AF. [5–7] Our results demonstrate the predictive value of P wave area to be near equivalent to that of CMR-quantified LA area for prediction of AF/AFl (HR 2.6 to 3.2). Applied clinically, these findings suggest that P wave data acquired from standard ECG, which is both inexpensive and widely available, can offer equivalent risk stratification for AF to that of sophisticated imaging via CMR.

Several limitations should be noted. First, whereas both ECG and CMR were performed within a narrow interval (mean Δ 0.1 ± 1.4 days), LA size itself can change dynamically due to transient alterations in loading conditions. Thus, differences between modalities may in part reflect interim changes in LA geometry. Second, whereas P wave area was tested in relation to a clinical endpoint of AF/AFl, event rates were captured based on clinical documentation, raising the possibility that clinically silent episodes were not captured via longitudinal follow-up. On the other hand, this potential source of ascertainment bias would not be expected to vary in relation to LA geometry as assessed by either ECG or imaging, and would therefore not impact our observed association between P wave area, LA geometry, and arrhythmic risk. Third, the number of clinical endpoints in this study were relatively low (n = 25), prohibiting definite conclusions regarding stratification of longitudinal risk for AF/AFl. Larger scale, population-based studies inclusive of subjects without ischemic heart disease or LV systolic dysfunction are necessary for more definitive assessment of P wave area for assessment of LA remodeling and stratification of atrial arrhythmic risk.

In conclusion, the current study demonstrates that ECG-quantified P wave area provides an index of LA remodeling that parallels CMR-evidenced LA chamber geometry and provides similar predictive value to imaging for stratification of longitudinal risk for AF/AFl among subjects with ischemic heart disease. Future studies are warranted to test this in other cohorts at risk for LA remodeling, such as subjects with non-ischemic cardiomyopathy, and to ascertain whether serial changes in P wave area may provide additional insights into changing LA chamber geometry, pressure and arrhythmic risk over time.

Author Contributions

Conceived and designed the experiments: JWW PMO JDK RBD. Performed the experiments: JWW JDK JK SG PMO SCV AK. Analyzed the data: JWW JDK JK AA MP SG PMO SCV AK. Wrote the paper: JWW JDK JK SCV RBD AA PMO.

References

1. Tsang TS, Barnes ME, Gersh BJ, Bailey KR, Seward JB (2002) Left atrial volume as a morphophysiologic expression of left ventricular diastolic dysfunction and relation to cardiovascular risk burden. Am J Cardiol 90: 1284–1289.
2. Gerdts E, Oikarinen L, Palmieri V, Otterstad JE, Wachtell K, et al. (2002) Correlates of left atrial size in hypertensive patients with left ventricular hypertrophy: the Losartan Intervention For Endpoint Reduction in Hypertension (LIFE) Study. Hypertension 39: 739–743.
3. Gardin JM, McClelland R, Kitzman D, Lima JA, Bommer W, et al. (2001) M-mode echocardiographic predictors of six- to seven-year incidence of coronary heart disease, stroke, congestive heart failure, and mortality in an elderly cohort (the Cardiovascular Health Study). Am J Cardiol 87: 1051–1057.
4. Benjamin EJ, D'Agostino RB, Belanger AJ, Wolf PA, Levy D (1995) Left atrial size and the risk of stroke and death. The Framingham Heart Study. Circulation 92: 835–841.
5. Vaziri SM, Larson MG, Benjamin EJ, Levy D (1994) Echocardiographic predictors of nonrheumatic atrial fibrillation. The Framingham Heart Study. Circulation 89: 724–730.
6. Berruezo A, Tamborero D, Mont L, Benito B, Tolosana JM, et al. (2007) Pre-procedural predictors of atrial fibrillation recurrence after circumferential pulmonary vein ablation. Eur Heart J 28: 836–841.
7. Olshansky B, Heller EN, Mitchell LB, Chandler M, Slater W, et al. (2005) Are transthoracic echocardiographic parameters associated with atrial fibrillation recurrence or stroke? Results from the Atrial Fibrillation Follow-Up Investigation of Rhythm Management (AFFIRM) study. J Am Coll Cardiol 45: 2026–2033.
8. Lewis T (1911) The Electrocardiographic Method and its Relationship to Clinical Medicine. Proc R Soc Med 4: 81–100.
9. Munuswamy K, Alpert MA, Martin RH, Whiting RB, Mechlin NJ (1984) Sensitivity and specificity of commonly used electrocardiographic criteria for left atrial enlargement determined by M-mode echocardiography. Am J Cardiol 53: 829–832.
10. Miller DH, Eisenberg RR, Kligfield PD, Devereux RB, Casale PN, et al. (1983) Electrocardiographic recognition of left atrial enlargement. J Electrocardiol 16: 15–22.
11. Waggoner AD, Adyanthaya AV, Quinones MA, Alexander JK (1976) Left atrial enlargement. Echocardiographic assessment of electrocardiographic criteria. Circulation 54: 553–557.
12. Kochav JD, Okin PM, Wilson S, Afroz A, Renilla A, et al. (2013) Usefulness of Q-wave area for threshold-based stratification of global left ventricular myocardial infarct size. Am J Cardiol 112: 174–180.
13. Okin PM, Roman MJ, Devereux RB, Pickering TG, Borer JS, et al. (1998) Time-voltage QRS area of the 12-lead electrocardiogram: detection of left ventricular hypertrophy. Hypertension 31: 937–942.
14. Lang RM, Bierig M, Devereux RM, Flachskampf FA, Foster E, et al. (2005) Recommendations for Chamber Quantification: A Report from the American Society of Echocardiography's Guidelines and Standards Committee and the Chamber Quantification Writing Group, Developed in Conjunction with the European Association of Echocardiography, a Branch of the European Society of Cardiology. J Am Soc Echocardiogr 18: 1440–1463.
15. Heitner J, Bhumireddy GP, Crowley AL, Weinsaft J, Haq SA, et al. (2012) Clinical application of cine-MRI in the visual assessment of mitral regurgitation compared to echocardiography and cardiac catheterization. PLoS One 7: e40491.
16. Lauren A, Simprini AA, Klem I, Jensen CJ, Kim RJ, et al. (2013) Routine cine-CMR for assessment of prosthesis-associated mitral regurgitation - a multicenter, multivendor study. Journal of Cardiovascular Magnetic Resonance 2013.
17. Jones EC, Devereux RB, Roman MJ, Liu JE, Fishman D, et al. (2001) Prevalence and correlates of mitral regurgitation in a population-based sample (the Strong Heart Study). Am J Cardiol 87: 298–304.
18. Zoghbi WA, Enriquez-Sarano M, Foster E, Grayburn PA, Kraft CD, et al. (2003) Recommendations for evaluation of the severity of native valvular regurgitation with two-dimensional and Doppler echocardiography. J Am Soc Echocardiogr 16: 777–802.
19. Maceira AM, Cosin-Sales J, Roughton M, Prasad SK, Pennell DJ (2010) Reference left atrial dimensions and volumes by steady state free precession cardiovascular magnetic resonance. J Cardiovasc Magn Reson 12: 65.
20. Morris JJ Jr, Estes EH Jr, Whalen RE, Thompson HK Jr, McIntosh HD (1964) P-Wave Analysis in Valvular Heart Disease. Circulation 29: 242–252.
21. Chirife R, Feitosa GS, Frankl WS (1975) Electrocardiographic detection of left atrial enlargement. Correlation of P wave with left atrial dimension by echocardiography. Br Heart J 37: 1281–1285.
22. Termini BA, Lee YC (1975) Echocardiographic and electrocardiographic criteria for diagnosing left atrial enlargement. South Med J 68: 161–165.
23. Nasir JM, Rubal BJ, Jones SO, Shah AD (2012) The effects of body mass index on surface electrocardiograms in young adults. J Electrocardiol 45: 646–651.
24. Maunganidze F, Woodiwiss AJ, Libhaber CD, Maseko MJ, Majane OH, et al. (2013) Obesity markedly attenuates the validity and performance of all electrocardiographic criteria for left ventricular hypertrophy detection in a group of black African ancestry. J Hypertens 31: 377–383.
25. Grothues F, Smith GC, Moon JC, Bellenger NG, Collins P, et al. (2002) Comparison of interstudy reproducibility of cardiovascular magnetic resonance with two-dimensional echocardiography in normal subjects and in patients with heart failure or left ventricular hypertrophy. Am J Cardiol 90: 29–34.
26. Tsao CW, Josephson ME, Hauser TH, O'Halloran TD, Agarwal A, et al. (2008) Accuracy of electrocardiographic criteria for atrial enlargement: validation with cardiovascular magnetic resonance. J Cardiovasc Magn Reson 10: 7.
27. Sanders P, Morton JB, Davidson NC, Spence SJ, Vohra JK, et al. (2003) Electrical remodeling of the atria in congestive heart failure: electrophysiological and electroanatomic mapping in humans. Circulation 108: 1461–1468.
28. John B, Stiles MK, Kuklik P, Chandy ST, Young GD, et al. (2008) Electrical remodelling of the left and right atria due to rheumatic mitral stenosis. Eur Heart J 29: 2234–2243.
29. Roberts-Thomson KC, John B, Worthley SG, Brooks AG, Stiles MK, et al. (2009) Left atrial remodeling in patients with atrial septal defects. Heart Rhythm 6: 1000–1006.
30. Li D, Fareh S, Leung TK, Nattel S (1999) Promotion of atrial fibrillation by heart failure in dogs: atrial remodeling of a different sort. Circulation 100: 87–95.
31. Oakes RS, Badger TJ, Kholmovski EG, Akoum N, Burgon NS, et al. (2009) Detection and quantification of left atrial structural remodeling with delayed-enhancement magnetic resonance imaging in patients with atrial fibrillation. Circulation 119: 1758–1767.
32. John B, Stiles MK, Kuklik P, Brooks AG, Chandy ST, et al. (2010) Reverse remodeling of the atria after treatment of chronic stretch in humans: implications for the atrial fibrillation substrate. J Am Coll Cardiol 55: 1217–1226.
33. Magnani JW, Johnson VM, Sullivan LM, Gorodeski EZ, Schnabel RB, et al. (2011) P wave duration and risk of longitudinal atrial fibrillation in persons >/= 60 years old (from the Framingham Heart Study). Am J Cardiol 107: 917–921 e911.
34. Soliman EZ, Prineas RJ, Case LD, Zhang ZM, Goff DC Jr (2009) Ethnic distribution of ECG predictors of atrial fibrillation and its impact on understanding the ethnic distribution of ischemic stroke in the Atherosclerosis Risk in Communities (ARIC) study. Stroke 40: 1204–1211.

3

Cardiac Impairment Evaluated by Transesophageal Echocardiography and Invasive Measurements in Rats Undergoing Sinoaortic Denervation

Raquel A. Sirvente[1,2]*, Maria C. Irigoyen[2], Leandro E. Souza[2], Cristiano Mostarda[2], Raquel N. La Fuente[2], Georgia O. Candido[2], Pamella R. M. Souza[2], Alessandra Medeiros[3], Charles Mady[1], Vera M. C. Salemi[1]

1 Cardiomyopathy Unit of the Heart Institute (InCor) do Hospital das Clínicas da Faculdade de Medicina da Universidade de São Paulo, São Paulo, Brazil, **2** Hypertension Unit of the Heart Institute (InCor) do Hospital das Clínicas da Faculdade de Medicina da Universidade de São Paulo, São Paulo, Brazil, **3** Federal University of São Paulo, Biosciences Department, Santos, São Paulo, Brazil

Abstract

Background: Sympathetic hyperactivity may be related to left ventricular (LV) dysfunction and baro- and chemoreflex impairment in hypertension. However, cardiac function, regarding the association of hypertension and baroreflex dysfunction, has not been previously evaluated by transesophageal echocardiography (TEE) using intracardiac echocardiographic catheter.

Methods and Results: We evaluated exercise tests, baroreflex sensitivity and cardiovascular autonomic control, cardiac function, and biventricular invasive pressures in rats 10 weeks after sinoaortic denervation (SAD). The rats (n = 32) were divided into 4 groups: 16 Wistar (W) with (n = 8) or without SAD (n = 8) and 16 spontaneously hypertensive rats (SHR) with (n = 8) or without SAD (SHRSAD) (n = 8). Blood pressure (BP) and heart rate (HR) did not change between the groups with or without SAD; however, compared to W, SHR groups had higher BP levels and BP variability was increased. Exercise testing showed that SHR had better functional capacity compared to SAD and SHRSAD. Echocardiography showed left ventricular (LV) concentric hypertrophy; segmental systolic and diastolic biventricular dysfunction; indirect signals of pulmonary arterial hypertension, mostly evident in SHRSAD. The end-diastolic right ventricular (RV) pressure increased in all groups compared to W, and the end-diastolic LV pressure increased in SHR and SHRSAD groups compared to W, and in SHRSAD compared to SAD.

Conclusions: Our results suggest that baroreflex dysfunction impairs cardiac function, and increases pulmonary artery pressure, supporting a role for baroreflex dysfunction in the pathogenesis of hypertensive cardiac disease. Moreover, TEE is a useful and feasible noninvasive technique that allows the assessment of cardiac function, particularly RV indices in this model of cardiac disease.

Editor: Luis Eduardo M. Quintas, Universidade Federal do Rio de Janeiro, Brazil

Funding: This work was supported by CNPq (Conselho Nacional de Desenvolvimento Científico e Tecnológico)(National Council for Scientific and Technological Development. The funders had no role in study design, data collection and analysis, decision to publish, or preparation of the manuscript.

Competing Interests: The authors have declared that no competing interests exist.

* E-mail: raquelsirvente@hotmail.com

Introduction

The arterial baroreflex (ABR) system is one of the most powerful and rapidly acting mechanisms for controlling blood pressure (BP) and heart rate (HR). Also, it has a prognostic value in many cardiovascular diseases. In arterial hypertension, sympathetic hyperactivity seems to be related to baro- and chemoreflex impairment and left ventricular (LV) dysfunction. One method of studying ABR dysfunction is the interruption of ABR by sinoaortic denervation (SAD) [1]. Previous studies have shown that traditional SAD may induce persistent high blood pressure variability (BPV) and mild LV hypertrophy, without an increase in mean BP [2–3]. Also, in this model, right ventricular (RV) hypertrophy secondary to pulmonary hypertension has been shown [4]. This could be caused by hypoxic pulmonary vasoconstriction, in response to hypoventilation-induced alveolar hypoxia, which possibly resulted from carotid body chemoreceptor denervation.

In the case of spontaneously hypertensive rats (SHR), which is a genetic model of hypertension, this disease has been accompanied by moderate BPV and severe LV hypertrophy. However, a relevant issue not previously shown in SHR that have undergone SAD is the noninvasive determination of detailed cardiac function, particularly RV function, the use of tissue Doppler indices, and the indirect estimation of pulmonary artery pressure.

Transesophageal echocardiography (TEE) can be performed in animals by using an intracardiac echocardiographic catheter (ICE) and may be useful for a comprehensive cardiac evaluation in small animal echocardiography [5–7]. Thus, the objective of our study was to evaluate the influence of denervation in SHR by noninvasive and invasive methods of cardiac function. In our study we found that baroreflex dysfunction could be related to the pathogenesis of hypertensive cardiac disease and TEE is feasable to demonstrate the cardiac compromising in small animals with hypertensive disease.

Methods

Experiments were performed in 2 month of age adult male Wistar (W) and spontaneously hypertensive rats (SHR) obtained from the Animal House of the University of São Paulo, São Paulo, Brazil. The rats (n = 32) were divided into 4 groups: 16 Wistar (W) with (n = 8) or without SAD (n = 8) and 16 SHR with (n = 8) or without SAD (SHRSAD) (n = 8). Ten weeks after SAD, cardiac function was evaluated by exercise testing (ET) at day 1, TEE and transthoracic (TTE, day 2), femoral artery and vein catheters were inserted for direct measurements of BP, HR, and drug administration at day 3, hemodynamic and autonomic measurements were performed at day 4 and 5, invasive evaluation of biventricular pressures were obtained at day 6, animal sacrifice and the heart was removed at day 7. Rats were housed in standard cages and fed with standard laboratory chow and water ad libitum. The animals were housed in collective polycarbonate cages in a temperature-controlled room (22°C) with a 12-hour dark-light cycle (light 07:00–19:00 h). The experimental protocol was approved by the institutional Animal Care and Ethics Committee of the University of São Paulo Medical School, and this investigation was conducted in accordance with the previously described ethical principles in animal research adopted by the Brazilian College of Animal Experimentation (COBEA) and the principles of the Declaration of Helsinki.

1. Sinoaortic Denervation

SAD was performed with the rats anesthetized with Ketamine (Parke-Davis, Brazil; 50 mg/kg, ip) and Xylazine (Bayer, Brazil; 12 mg/kg, ip). A 3-cm midline incision was made, and the sternocleidomastoid muscles were reflected laterally, exposing the neurovascular sheath [1]. The common carotid arteries and the vagal trunk were isolated, and the aortic depressor fibers either traveling with the sympathetic nerve or as an isolated aortic nerve were cut. The communicating branch of the aortic fibers was also resected. The third contingent of aortic baroreceptor fibers traveling with the inferior laryngeal nerve was interrupted by resection of the superior laryngeal nerve after the carotid bifurcation had been exposed extensively for carotid stripping. To complete the procedure, the sinus nerve, all carotid branches, and the carotid body were resected [1]. After surgery, all rats were given a single dose of penicillin (10 000 U/kg, im). The W and SHR were not submitted to fictitious surgery.

2. Maximal Exercise Test

Maximal exercise test was performed on a treadmill (Imbrasport, Porto Alegre, Brazil) using a protocol as previously described [11–12]. All animals were adapted to the exercise test procedure with light exercise (e.g. 0.3 km/h; 10 min/day) for 1 week. Forty-eight hours later the animals were submitted to a maximal progressive exercise test on a motor treadmill. All maximal protocol tests started with 0.3 km/h and increased 0.3 km/h each 3 min until the animals were unable to run further, as described in previous studies [13].

3. Echocardiography

3.1. Transesophageal echocardiography. The animals were anesthetized with Ketamine (Parke-Davis, Brazil; 50 mg/kg, ip) and Xylazine (Bayer, Brazil; 12 mg/kg, ip), had their chest shaved, were intubated and placed on small-animal ventilator model 683 (Harvard Apparatus, Holliston, MA, USA). Heart rate was evaluated by simultaneous electrocardiographic monitoring. After lubrication, a monoplane ICE (AcuNav, Siemens, Mountain View, CA, USA) with 10 F and multiple frequency of 5.5–10 MHz was inserted into the esophagus, posterior to the left atrium. This catheter has a transducer at its tips and generates M-mode, 2-dimensional, spectral Doppler and color Doppler images [5–7]. It was then connected to a Sequoia 512 echocardiographic machine (Siemens, Mountain View, CA, USA). Apical 4-chamber, 2-chamber, and 3-chamber views, and RV chamber and outflow images were acquired [14]. The sequence of echocardiographic examination was 2-dimensional apical views, color Doppler and pulsed-wave Doppler of the following variables: mitral inflow [peak velocity of early (E) and late (A) waves, E/A ratio, deceleration time of E wave, atrial filling fraction (AFF) obtained by velocity time integral of A wave/velocity time integral of mitral inflow], isovolumic relaxation time (IVRT) measured from aortic valve closure to the onset of mitral inflow, and LV outflow velocity measured just below the aortic valve, from an apical 5-chamber view. Tissue Doppler imaging (TDI) of the LV septum and lateral mitral annulus: systolic velocity (S'), early velocity (E'), late velocity (A'), and E'/A' ratio [15]. Also, RV maximum and minimum volume obtained by 2-dimensional echocardiography and RV ejection fraction (EF) was then calculated. Tricuspid inflow and TDI of the lateral tricuspid annulus were obtained, as described above for LV indices. Figure 1 shows RV diastolic dysfunction in SHR with tricuspid inflow E<A (B) and TDI tricuspid annulus E'< A' (C). Acceleration time (AcT) and duration of the RV outflow Doppler velocity profile (TT) and its ratio were obtained. Global cardiac function was evaluated by using the myocardial performance index (MPI), which is the ratio of total time spent in isovolumic activity (isovolumic contraction time and isovolumic relaxation time) to the ejection time (ET) [16]. These Doppler time intervals were measured from the mitral inflow and LV outflow time intervals. Interval "a", from the cessation to the onset of mitral inflow, is equal to the sum of the isovolumic contraction time, the ET and the isovolumic relaxation time. Ejection time "b" is derived from the duration of the LV outflow Doppler velocity profile. The MPI was calculated with the formula (a − b)/b. Also, MPI was obtained by TDI at the septum and lateral mitral annulus, and lateral tricuspid annulus. The advantage of these measurements over the conventional MPI is that TDI permits the evaluation of time intervals at the same cycle. All measurements were based on the average of 3 consecutive cardiac cycles. All study images were stored digitally and on VHS tapes.

3.2. Transthoracic echocardiography. Transthoracic echocardiography was performed in all the animals after TEE, with a Sequoia 512 machine (Siemens, Mountain View, CA) equipped with a 10–13 MHz multifrequency linear transducer, as previously described [17–18]. Images were obtained with the transducer placed on each animal's shaved chest. To obtain a more distinctive image display, a transmission gel was used between the transducer and the animal's chest (General Imaging Gel, ATL, Reedsville, PA). Wall thickness and LV dimensions were obtained from a short-axis view at the level of the papillary muscles by M-mode echocardiography [19]. LV mass was calculated by using the following formula, previously validated in rats [20]:

$$\mathbf{LV\ mass = 0.8 \times \{1{,}04[(LVd + PWd + IVSd)^3 - LVd^3]\} + 0.6,}$$

where LVd is LV end-diastolic diameter, PWd is end-diastolic

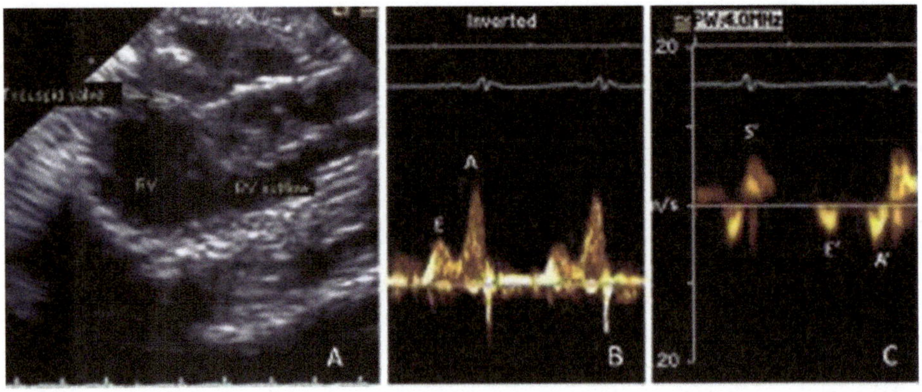

Figure 1. Transesophageal echocardiography of spontaneously hypertensive rats showing right ventricle (RV) (A), tricuspid inflow (B) and tissue Doppler imaging of the tricuspid annulus (C).

posterior wall thickness, and IVSd is end-diastolic interventricular septum thickness. In addition, the relative wall thickness (RWT), which is expressed by:

RWT = 2 ×PWd/LVd, was calculated.

LV fractional shortening (FS), was calculated as:

$$\mathbf{FS} = (LVd - LVs)/LVd \times 100,$$

where LVs is LV end-systolic diameter.

Acceleration time (AcT) and TT of the RV outflow and its ratio were obtained at parasternal short-axis view at the level of aorta/ left atrium.

4. Hemodynamic and Autonomic Measurements

Ten weeks after SAD, animals were anesthetized with Ketamine (Parke-Davis, Brazil; 50 mg/kg, ip) and Xylazine (Bayer, Brazil; 12 mg/kg, ip); femoral artery and vein catheters (PE-lO) filled with 0.06 mL saline solution were inserted for direct measurements of BP, HR, and drug administration. The rats were conscious and allowed to move freely in the cage during the experiments. Twenty-four hours after catheterization, the arterial catheter was connected to a transducer (Blood Pressure XDCR, Kent© Scientific, Litchfield, CT), and BP signals were recorded in conscious, freely moving rats, over a 30-minute period by a microcomputer equipped with an analog-to-digital converter board (Windaq, 2000 Hz sampling frequency, Dataq Instruments, Inc, Akron, OH). The recorded data were analyzed on a beat-to-beat basis to quantify changes in mean BP and HR. Both HR variability (HRV) and BPV were analyzed in time (SD PI = standard deviation of pulse interval, SD SBP = systolic blood pressure, PIV = pulse interval variance, SBPV = SBP variability) and frequency domains (spectral analysis) [8].

For baroreflex assessment, increasing doses of phenylephrine (0.25 to 32 ug/kg) and sodium nitroprusside (0.05 to 1.6 ug/kg) were given as sequential bolus injections (0.1 mL) to induce either an increase or decrease in BP, ranging from 5 to 40 mm Hg, and subsequent bradycardic or tachycardic responses to these BP changes [9]. The corresponding peak reflex change in HR was recorded for each dose of drug, and baroreflex sensitivity was calculated by a mean index relating changes in HR to changes in mean BP [8–10]. Both HR variability (HRV) and BPV were analyzed in time and frequency domains [8]. All 30-minute time series of pulse intervals and systolic BP were cubic spline interpolated (250 Hz) and decimated to be equally spaced in time. Following linear trend removal, power spectral density was obtained by fast Fourier transformation using Welch's method[8] over 16 384 points with a Hanning window (512) and 50% overlapping. Spectral power for very low frequency (VLF; 0–0.20 Hz), low frequency (LF; 0.20–0.75 Hz), and high frequency (HF; 0.75–3.0 Hz) bands were calculated by power spectrum density integration within each frequency bandwidth using a customized routine (MATLAB 6.0; Mathworks, Natick, MA, USA) [8].

5. Invasive Evaluation of Biventricular Pressures

Left ventricular and RV functions were measured invasively in anesthetized rats (pentobarbital sodium, 40 mg/kg). A polyethylene P50 catheter was inserted in the jugular vein to the RV, and signs of end-systolic (ESP) and end-diastolic pressures (EDP) of the RV were recorded for 5 minutes on a microcomputer equipped with a data acquisition system, at a sampling frequency of 2000 Hz per channel (Codas, DATAQ Instruments, Akron, OH, USA) [21–22]. Also, one catheter of PE-50 was inserted into the right carotid artery and advanced into the LV, and EDP of the LV, +dP/dt, -dP/dt and time constant of relaxation (Tau) were obtained.

6. Statistical Analysis

All data are expressed as mean ± SD. Comparisons of normally distributed continuous variables were performed with 2-way analysis of variance (ANOVA) then followed by Student-Newman-Keuls and Kruskal-Wallis tests for multiple comparisons. The Pearson or Spearman correlation coefficient was used to analyze the relation between noninvasive and invasive indices. Normality was determined by the Shapiro-Wilks test. $P<0.05$ was considered statistically significant. Statistical analysis was performed with SPSS v 17 (SPSS Inc. Chicago, IL, USA).

Results

1. Baroreflex Sensitivity and Cardiovascular Autonomic Control

Blood pressure and HR did not change between the groups with and without SAD, although SHR had higher BP levels compared with W. BP variability was increased in SHR groups compared to W. After SAD, BP variability increased in all groups compared to W (W: 15 $mmHg^2$; *SAD: 49 $mmHg^2$; *SHR: 60 $mmHg^2$; *SHRSAD: 137 $mmHg^2$, *$p<0.05$ vs. W, Table 1. As expected, hypertension induces impairment of bradycardic and tachycardic responses elicited by the increased and decreased BP by using vasoactive drugs. On the other hand, SAD reduced HR baroreflex-mediated responses in both normotensive and hypertensive animals, indicating the efficacy of denervation procedure. In addition, there was no baroreflex sensitivity difference between denervated animals (SAD and SHRSAD).

2. Maximal Exercise Test

Exercise test showed that the maximal velocity in the SHR group (1.4±0.3 Km/h) was increased compared to that in SAD (0.9±0.2 km/h). Similarly, SHRSAD (1.0±0.3 km/h) compared to SHR had decreased maximal velocity (1.4±0.3 km/h, $p<0.05$).

The W group had values intermediate between the other groups, did not have low values as the SAD and SHRSAD, nor high values as SHR, but did not differ between groups (1.16±0.11 km/h).

3. Echocardiography

3.1 Transesophageal data. RV maximal volume increased in SHR compared to W and SAD, and RV minimal volume increased in SHR and SHRSAD compared to W (Table 2). Right ventricular EF decreased in SHRSAD compared to W (Table 2).

LV diastolic function showed that SHR and SHRSAD increased IVRT compared to W. Also, SAD presented increased AFF compared to W (Table 2). RV diastolic function increased AFF in SAD and SHR compared to W (Table 2).

Tissue Doppler imaging showed that S' of the septum was reduced in SHRSAD compared to SAD and SHR. At the lateral mitral annulus, SHRSAD presented decreased S' compared to W. At the tricuspid annulus, SHRSAD showed diminished S' compared to W and SAD (Table 3). Also, the E'septum was reduced in SHRSAD compared to SHR. SAD augmented A' compared to W, whereas in SHR and SHRSAD it was reduced compared to SAD (Table 3).

Myocardial performance index increased in SHR compared to SAD. Also, MPI TDI of the lateral region of the mitral annulus increased in SHRSAD compared to SHR (Table 4).

All groups had a reduction of AcT compared to W and SHR, reflecting a possible increase in pulmonary artery pressure in all groups (Table 4).

3.2. Transthoracic data. The amount of data gathered from M-mode echocardiography suggests concentric hypertrophy in SHR and SHRSAD compared to the other groups (Table 5). Left atrium/weight increased in SHRSAD compared to SAD (Table 5).

Different from TEE, TTE showed that all groups had both reduced TAc and AcT/TT compared to W (Table 4).

4. Invasive Measurements and Relation of Noninvasive and Invasive Data

Biventricular EDP was increased in all groups compared to W (Table 4). Also, end-systolic pressure was increased in SHRSAD compared to the W group. -dP/dt RV and +dP/dt RV was decreased in all groups compared to W. Tau RV was increased in SHRSAD compared to all groups, except in SAD. -dP/dt LV and +dP/dt LV were decreased in SHRSAD and SAD compared to all groups. Tau LV was increased in SHRSAD compared to all groups, except SHR (Table 4).

There was a negative correlation between AcT of RV outflow velocity and RV EDP ($r=0.75$; $p=0.005$), a positive correlation between RV maximal volume and LV mass/weight ($r=0.5$;

Table 1. Blood pressure, heart rate, baroreflex sensitivity and cardiovascular autonomic modulation of normotensive and hypertensive groups.

Variables	Group			
	W	SAD	SHR	SHRSAD
HR (bpm)	334±10	327±8	347±6	358±9
PI (ms)	180±5	183±4	173±3	167±4
SD PI (ms)	9±0.6	7±0.4[a]	8±0.8	7±0.9[a]
SBP (mmHg)	126±4	119±3	190±4[a,b]	193±9[a,b]
SD SBP(mmHg)	4±3	7±0.8[a]	7±0.6[a]	11±1[a]
PIV (ms^2)	91±11	52±7	70±13	60±12
LF (ms^2)	2.0±0.9	3±0.9	12±3[a,b]	9±0.8[a,b]
HF (ms^2)	10±1	9±0.7	30±6[a,b]	25±6[a,b]
LF band (%)	17±1	23±6	27±4[a]	28±2[a]
HF band (%)	82±1	76±6	72±4[a]	72±2[a]
LF/HF	0.22±0.02	0.35±0.1	0.41±0.08	0.34±0.05
SBPV ($mmHg^2$)	16±2	50±11	60±10	137±28[a,b,c]
LF SBP($mmHg^2$)	3±0.6	6±2	14±2[a,b]	20±5[a,b]
BRI (bpm/mmHg)	2±0.09	0.7±0.04[a,c]	1±0.06[a]	0.6±0.03[a,c]
TRI (bpm/mmHg)	3.8±0.2	0.49±0.08[a,c]	1.29±0.15[a]	0.54±0.06[a,c]

Values are mean ± SD.
W = Wistar; SAD = sinoaortic denervation; SHR = spontaneously hypertensive rats; SHRSAD = spontaneously hypertensive rats with sinoaortic denervation.
HR = heart rate; PI = pulse interval; SD PI = standard deviation of pulse interval; SBP = systolic blood pressure; SD SBP = standard deviation of systolic blood pressure; PIV = pulse interval variance; LF (ms^2) = low-frequency band of heart rate variability; HF (ms^2) = high-frequency band of heart rate variability; LF band (%) = low-frequency band of heart rate variability; HF band (%) = high-frequency band of heart rate variability; SBPV = SBP variability; LF SBP ($mmHg^2$) = low frequency band of SBPV; BRI = bradycardic response index; TRI = tachycardic response index;
[a]$p<0.05$ vs. W, [b]$p<0.05$ vs. SAD, and [c]$p<0.05$ vs. SHR.

Table 2. Volumes and ejection fraction of the right ventricle, and biventricular diastolic function data obtained by transesophageal echocardiography.

Variables	W	SAD	SHR	SHRSAD
RV maximal volume (mL/kg)	1.50±0.14	1.51±0.18	1.76±0.22[a,b]	1.62±0.15
RV minimal volume (mL/kg)	0.75±0.32	0.85±0.16	1.04±0.15[a]	1.07±0.12[a]
LV diastolic	**function**			
E/A	1.99±0.50	1.38±0.44	2.29±0.88[b]	1.81±0.31
DT (ms)	40±4	47±8	43±7	47±8
IVRT (ms)	25±1	27°±2	37±5[a,b]	31±6[a,c]
AFF	0.25±0.04	0.37±0.10[a]	0.25±0.05[b]	0.31±0.04
RV diastolic	**function**			
E/A	1.67±0.35	1.00±0.42	1.06±0.68	1.44±0.76
DT (ms)	47±11	57±17	59±12	63±21
AFF	0.27±0.05	0.48±0.10[a]	0.44±0.11[a]	0.39±0.14

Values are mean ± SD.
W = Wistar; SAD = sinoaortic denervation; SHR = spontaneously hypertensive rats; SHRSAD = spontaneously hypertensive rats with sinoaortic denervation.
FE VD = right ventricular ejection fraction; E/A = ratio of peak velocity of E and A waves of mitral or tricuspid inflow; DT = deceleration time of E wave; IVRT = isovolumic relaxation time of LV; AFF = atrial filling fraction.
[a]$p<0.05$ vs. W, [b]$p<0.05$ vs. SAD and [c]$p<0.05$ vs. SHR.

p = 0.0016), and a positive correlation between AcT of RV outflow by TTE and TEE ($r = 0.53$; $p = 0.001$).

5. Relation between Invasive and Echocardiographic Indices

We performed the relation between invasive and echocardiographic indices (Table 6).

Discussion

In the present study, we found that 10 weeks after SAD, baroreflex sensitivity impairment significantly changed the morphological, functional, and hemodynamic cardiac variables in W and SHR. Also, denervated animals did not have altered BP and HR, but did have increased BP variability and decreased functional capacity. Also, baroreflex dysfunction participated in RV impairment, first demonstrated noninvasively here, by transesophageal echocardiography.

Table 3. Tissue Doppler imaging data of mitral and tricuspid annulus data obtained by transesophageal echocardiography.

Variables	W	SAD	SHR	SHRSAD
Mitral annulus - septum				
S′ (m/s)	0.048±0.015	0.064±0.019	0.054±0.013	0.038±0.008[b,c]
E′ (m/s)	0.039±0.010	0.045±0.013	0.049±0.008	0.038±0.007[c]
A′ (m/s)	0.026±0.005	0.043±0.015[a]	0.029±0.007[b]	0.025±0.008[b]
E′/A′	1.50±0.44	1.129±0.34	1.726±0.37	1.679±0.77
Mitral annulus – lateral region				
S′ (m/s)	0.055±0.015	0.046±0.011	0.041±0.011	0.036±0.014[a]
E′ (m/s)	0.035±0.01	0.039±0.015	0.034±0.011	0.035±0.009
A′ (m/s)	0.028±0.008	0.036±0.021	0.028±0.008	0.026±0.011
E′/A′	1.23±0.20	1.24±0.52	1.35±0.68	1.49±0.58
Tricuspid annulus – lateral region				
S′ (m/s)	0.060±0.018	0.058±0.014	0.047±0.011	0.035±0.009[a,b]
E′ (m/s)	0.042±0.010	0.044±0.012	0.038±0.006	0.036±0.008
A′ (m/s)	0.033±0.008	0.044±0.012	0.037±0.013	0.026±0.007[b]
E′/A′	1.28±0.26	1.08±0.45	1.15±0.48	1.48±0.56

Values are mean ± SD.
W = Wistar; SAD = sinoaortic denervation; SHR = spontaneously hypertensive rats; SHRSAD = spontaneously hypertensive rats with sinoaortic denervation.
S′ = peak velocity of systolic velocity obtained by tissue Doppler imaging; E′ = peak velocity of early diastolic velocity obtained by tissue Doppler imaging; A′ = peak velocity of late diastolic velocity obtained by tissue Doppler imaging.
[a]$p<0.05$ vs. W, [b]$p<0.05$ vs. SAD, and [c]$p<0.05$ vs. SHR.

Table 4. Myocardial performance index, right ventricular outflow by transesophageal, transthoracic echocardiography and invasive data.

Variables	W	SAD	SHR	SHRSAD
Pulsed-wave Doppler				
LV MPI	0.47±0.18	0.39±0.14	0.60±0.15[b]	0.54±0.16
RV MPI	0.35±0.08	0.34±0.15	0.35±0.17	0.47±0.12
Pulsed-wave tissue Doppler				
Septum MPI	1.08±0.48	0.98±0.38	0.78±0.19	0.96±0.51
Lateral LV MPI	1.39±0.23	1.02±0.36	0.85±0.32	1.30±0.56[c]
Lateral RV MPI	1,17±0.33	0.94±0.25	0.85±0.24	1.05±0.28
Right Ventricular outflow data TEE				
AcT (ms)	40±2.16	33±1.35[a]	32±1.03[a]	28±1.48[a,b]
AcT/TT	0.47±0.04	0.40±0.02	0.35±0.03[a]	0.32±0.02[a,b]
Right Ventricular outflow data TTE				
AcT (ms)	41±3	32±3[a]	32±3[a]	26±4[a,b,c]
AcT/TT	0.37±0.03	0.30±0.04[a]	0.29±0.05[a]	0.25±0.04[a,b,c]
Invasive data				
ESP RV (mmHg)	31.9±3.4	42.7±7.8	38.9±16.7	45.4±10.7[a]
EDP RV (mmHg)	3.03±0.39	4.7±0.52[a]	6.61±1.16[a,b]	7.8±0.87[a,b]
EDP LV (mmHg)	5.83±0.19	8.98±1.2[a]	12.51±4.73[a]	14.57±2.52[a,b]
−dp/dt RV (mmHg/s)	−1120.7±37.8	−783.5±4.9[a]	−780.7±32.3[a]	−691.8±24.5[a]
+dp/dt RV (mmHg/s)	1553.9±71.8	100.4±30.7[a]	1259.8±18.3[a,b]	1228.1±29[a,b]
Tau RV	16.28±0.42	23.14±0.79[a]	19.37±0.49[a,b]	25.37±0.62[a,c]
−dp/dt LV (mmHg/s)	−7424.2±206.2	−4824.1±206.2[a]	−7037.5±181.8[b]	−5530.7±192[a,c]
+dp/dt LV (mmHg/s)	9169.3±138.6	6021.2±138.6[a]	9273.7±122.2[b]	8510.8±129.6[a,b,c]
Tau LV	15.28±0.94	20±0.94[a]	22±0.83[a]	24.25±0.88[a]

Values are mean ± SD.
W = Wistar; SAD = sinoaortic denervation; SHR = spontaneously hypertensive rats; SHRSAD = spontaneously hypertensive rats with sinoaortic denervation.
MPI = myocardial performance index; LV = left ventricle; RV = right ventricle; AcT = aceleration time of right ventricular outflow; TT = time from the beginning to the end of right ventricular outflow; EDPRV = end-diastolic pressure of right ventricle; EDPLV = end-diastolic pressure of left ventricle; ESPRV = end-systolic pressure of the right ventricle.
[a]$p<0.05$ vs. W, [b]$p<0.05$ vs. SAD, and [c]$p<0.05$ vs. SHR.

Krieger first described SAD in rats in 1964, and this technique has been useful to assess the baroreflex role in both physiological and pathological situations [1–23;24]. In the first description, this model was considered to be neurogenic hypertension, but it is currently regarded as a BP variability model, because as shows hypertension in the acute phase (24 h), followed by tachycardia, but with a return to normal hemodynamic values in the chronic phase [25]. Likewise, the renal sympathetic hyperactivity detected in the acute phase returns to normal in the chronic phase. Nevertheless, increased BP variability occurs in chronic SAD [6]. These findings confirm the usefulness of SAD as a model of BP variability and baroreflex dysfunction. In our study, the denervated groups did not have altered basal BP and HR, and maintained the augmented BP variability. Additionally, W groups did not have a difference in sympathetic modulation, assessed by LF of HR in SAD and controls. On the other hand, SHR had an increase in this component and kept it augmented after SAD compared to the control group. Both groups had decreased PI variability and increased SBP variability. The latter was increased in SAD groups, and was additionally augmented in SHRSAD. Baroreflex sensitivity was decreased in SHR groups, and additionally reduced in SAD, with/without hypertension. Our findings highlight the level of autonomic dysfunction seen in these animals that probably contributed to the low performance during maximal exercise testing of SHRSAD compared to SHR. In addition to the limitation of the autonomic system to promote the necessary regulations during exercise test, possibly contributed to reducing the efficacy of the cardiovascular system [26]. It is important to emphasize that the peripheral control of sympathetic activity could be influenced not only by baroreceptor impairment, but also by concomitant aortic and carotid chemoreceptor impairment, characteristic of conventional SAD [24]. The evidence of autonomic dysfunction (increased sympathetic tonus, decreased baroreflex sensitivity, and augmented BP variability) may also explain the structural alterations in SHR and SAD groups. The increase in BP variability by interruption of aortic and carotid afferents, relieving the sympathetic from tonic inhibition, has been associated with target organ lesions, more than the constantly elevated BP itself has [24].

In our study, SHR with/without SAD had increased LV mass, relative wall thickness, indicating concentric LV hypertrophy [27]. In addition, there was a decrease in S' of the septum and lateral wall mitral annulus in SHRSAD compared to SHR and SAD groups, reflecting LV systolic segmental dysfunction, even in animals with LV preserved global systolic function. This is the first

Table 5. Cardiac morphology obtained by M-mode transthoracic echocardiography.

Variables	W	SAD	SHR	SHRSAD
Body weight (g)	351±13	401±44	304±21[a,b]	283±13[a,b]
Left ventricle				
LVd/weight (mm/kg)	1.84±0.30	1.71±0.17	1.71±0.19	1.79±0.44
LVs/weight (mm/kg)	0.80±0.39	0.85±0.14	0.73±0.22	0.74±0.42
IVSd/weight (mm/kg)	0.41±0.03	0.39±0.03	0.65±0.10[a,b]	0.61±0.08[a,b]
PWd/weight (mm/kg)	0.43±0.03	0.42±0.04	0.65±0.10	0.60±0.22
FS (%)	58±14	50±6.7	58±11	59±15
CI (mL/min/kg)	1.43±0.55	0.81±0.48	1.63±1.15	1.01±0.40
LVMass/weight (g/kg)	3.06±0.29	2.95±0.29	3.71±0.48[a,b]	3.54±0.43[a,b]
RWT	0.48±0.09	0.49±0.03	0.77±0.14[a,b]	0.76±0.27[a,b]
Left atrium				
Ao (mm)	0.35±0.05	0.37±0.03	0.34±0.04	0.33±0.04
LA (mm)	0.37±0.07	0.40±0.03	0.35±0.04	0.35±0.02
LA/weight (mm/kg)	1.06±0.20	1.03±0.15	1.16±0.15	1.23±0.10[b]
Ao/LA	0.96±0.13	0.93±0.06	0.96±0.09	0.94±0.11

Va1ues are mean ± SD.
W = Wistar; SAD = sinoaortic denervation; GSHR = spontaneously hypertensive rats; GSHRDSA = spontaneously hypertensive rats with denervation; LVd = left ventricular end-diastolic dimension; LVd = left ventricular end-systolic dimension; IVSd = interventricular septum thickness in diastole; PWd = posterior wall thickness in diastole; FS = fractional shortening; CI = cardiac index; LVMass = left ventricular mass; RWT = relative wall thickness; Ao = aortic dimension; LA = left atrium thickness in diastole.
[a]$p<0.05$ vs. W and [b]$p<0.05$ vs. SAD.

study to evaluate regional systolic and diastolic biventricular function by TEE in small denervated animals.

LV diastolic function showed that only IVRT was different between groups, which was greater in SHR with/without denervation compared to W, reflecting LV diastolic dysfunction in hypertension. This parameter was reduced in SHRSAD compared to SHR. This finding could indicate advanced diastolic dysfunction, as LA size was increased in SHRSAD, but not in SAD. A previous study from our group showed that diastolic function was worse in denervated normotensive animals, independent of BP variability [28].

Left ventricular global myocardial function by pulsed-wave MPI was increased in SHR compared to W, as expected. However, the same index analyzed by LV TDI was increased in SHRSAD compared to SHR, suggesting that baroreflex dysfunction could induce an additional impairment in this index. The importance of our findings is that the MPI has prognostic value in many cardiopathies, including pulmonary artery hypertension [29], which could allow the future use of this index for baroreflex dysfunction and its functional repercussion of the heart. Another advantage of this method is the high reproducibility and the fact that it is not based on geometric assumptions of ventricular morphology [30]. In our study, TDI MPI may have produced a more consistent finding, because, with this method, both systolic and diastolic functions are evaluated in the same cardiac cycle.

Different from our previous study, we did not find LV morphological alterations in SAD in the present study. This finding could be related to the denervation process, which is not always homogeneous in all animals, as some afferent fibers have a different path to the central nervous system, via the vagal nerve, for instance.

Considering the high BPV variability in hypertension, in SAD and the association of both, RV hypertrophy has been described [16], although not ever found. Van Vliet [4] reported RV hypertrophy, but this was associated with a reduction in body weight, which could falsely increase RV mass. In addition, in normotensive rats after SAD, Miao *et al* found an increase in RV mass of 22% and a decrease in 6% in body weight (unpublished data).

RV assessed by TEE showed increased maximum and minimum volumes in hypertensive animals, denervated or not, suggesting that hypertension associated or not with LV dysfunction may be related to RV dysfunction. Although previous guidelines have suggested that the RV area, and not volume, be measured, here we studied the volumes that could also reflect RV alterations, as they were obtained by 2-dimensional echocardiography [12]. In addition, there was a positive correlation between LV mass and RV volume, supporting the previous hypothesis. Moreover, RV function was reduced in SHRSAD, indicating greater compromise in this group.

End-diastolic RV pressure was greater in experimental groups compared to W, indicated that SAD with/without hypertension was related to right ventricular diastolic dysfunction.

Possibly, the decrease in acceleration time of RV outflow in SAD, SHR, and SHRSAD indicates increased pulmonary artery pressure and its consequent RV hypertrophy, especially because the denervation included the resection of the afferent chemoreceptors. Moreover, we agree with Van Vliet [4] hypotheses, indicating that in SAD the RV hypertrophy develops secondary to afferent chemoreceptor denervation, leading to consequences in pulmonary circulation and RV hypertrophy. In accordance with this, AcT obtained by TTE and TEE, associated with a decrease in RV ejection fraction and S' of tricuspid annulus, reinforces the indication of a possible increased pulmonary pressure in SHRSAD. Also, we found a good correlation of AcT between TEE and TTE ($r = 0.53$, $p = 0.001$). Our results showed that invasive parameters of systolic and diastolic RV and LV function

Table 6. Correlations between invasive and noninvasive data in all animals.

Comparison	Correlation coefficient (r)	P value
Right Ventricular Indices		
Comparison	**Correlation coefficient (r)**	**P value**
−dP/dt vs AFF	0.5985	P = 0.0016
−dP/dt vs E/E′	−0.5594	P = 0.0016
−dP/dt vs AcT/TT TTE	−0.6953	P<0.0001
−dP/dt vs AcT TTE	−0.8462	P<0.0001
−dP/dtvs AcT TEE	−0.6449	P = 0.0002
−dP/dt vs TT	−0.6724	P<0.0001
+dP/dt vs AFF	−0.5010	P = 0.0107
+dP/dt vs AcT TTE	0.5421	P = 0.0035
EDP vs E/E′	−0.5703	P = 0.0012
EDP vs TT	−0.5275	P = 0.0033
EDP vs AcT/TT	−0.7341	P<0.0001
EDP vs AcT TEE	−0.6080	P = 0.0005
EDP vs AFF	0.4258	P = 0.0338
EDP vs AcT TTE	−0.8302	P<0.0001
Tau vs AcT/TT	−0.7263	P<0.0001
Tau vs E/E′	−0.5732	P = 0.0014
Tau vs TT	−0.4164	P = 0.0275
Tau vs AcT TTE	−0.8117	P<0.0001
Tau vs AcT TEE	−0.4768	P = 0.0103
Left Ventricular Indices		
Comparison	**Correlation coefficient (r)**	**P value**
−dP/dt vs MPI	−0.3627	P = 0.0489
+dP/dt vs MPI	0.4892	P = 0.0061
+dP/dt vs LV weight	0.4318	P = 0.0396
+dP/dt vs LVMass/weight	0.4913	P = 0.0050
EDP vs CI	−0.4716	P = 0.0150
EDPvs EF	−0.6141	P = 0.0007
EDP vs LVMass	0.5459	P = 0.0018
EDP vs LV	0.5160	P = 0.0117
Tau vs EF	−0.6148	P = 0.0006

Values are mean ± SD.
AFF = atrial filling fraction; LV = left ventricle; AcT TTE = aceleration time of right ventricular outflow (transthoracic echocardiography); AcT TEE = aceleration time of right ventricular outflow (transesophageal echocardiography); TT = time from the beginning to the end of right ventricular outflow; CI = cardiac index; LVMass = left ventricular mass; MPI = myocardial performance index; EF = ejection fraction; E/E′ = ratio of peak velocity of E wave of mitral inflow and peak velocity of early diastolic velocity obtained by tissue Doppler imaging; EDP = end-diastolic pressure.

are more compromised in SHRSAD, thus, validating the noninvasive data (Table 4).

Conclusions

We found that baroreflex dysfunction impairs biventricular and LA functions, and increases pulmonary artery pressure, particularly in hypertensive rats, supporting a role for baroreflex dysfunction in the pathogenesis of hypertensive cardiac disease. Also, TEE is a useful and feasible noninvasive technique allowing the assessment of cardiac function, particularly RV indices in this model of cardiac disease. Our data was supported by concomitant invasive measurements.

Limitations of the Study

It was necessary to perform orotracheal intubation to perform TEE, because respiratory depression occurred by the manipulation of the TEE transducer in the esophagus. In humans, the assessment of RV volumetric quantification and the EF measurements have many limitations, because the complex RV shape limits performance of the required assessments [30]. This is even more challenging in small animals. In our study, the use of TEE allowed the acquisition of some RV conventional echocardiographic views, but we could not obtain all views frequently obtained in comprehensive evaluation of the right heart. Using TEE, we could detect change in global RV volumes in hypertensive groups (with/without SAD), but the position of the septum did not change. In addition, using TTE to analyze tricuspid inflow and TDI of the lateral tricuspid annulus in small animals is also challenging. But in our study, the use of TEE allowed this assessment.

Author Contributions

Conceived and designed the experiments: RAS MCI VMCS. Performed the experiments: RAS LES RNF GOC PRMS AM VMCS. Analyzed the data: RAS MCI CM VMCS. Contributed reagents/materials/analysis tools: MCI CM VMCS. Wrote the paper: RAS MCI CM VMCS.

References

1. Krieger EM, Marseillan RF (1963) Aortic depressor fibers in the rat: an electrophysiological study. Am J Physiol 05: 771–774.
2. Irigoyen MC, Moreira ED, Ida F, Pires M, Cestari IA, et al. (1995) Changes of renal sympathetic activity in acute and chronic conscious sinoaortic denervated rats. Hypertension 6: 1111–1116.
3. Miao CY, Yuan WJ, Su DF (2003) Comparative study of sinoaortic denervated rats and spontaneously hypertensive rats. Am J Hypertens 16: 585–591.
4. Van Vliet BN, Chafe LL, Montani JP (1999) Contribution of baroreceptors and chemoreceptors to ventricular hypertrophy produced by sino-aortic denervation in rats. J Physiol 516: 885–895.
5. Bruce CJ, Packer DL, O'Leary PW, Seward JB (1999) Feasibility study: transesophageal echocardiography with a 10F (3.2-mm), multifrequency (5.5- to 10-MHz) ultrasound catheter in a small rabbit model. J Am Soc Echocardiogr 12: 596–600.
6. Gao Z, Li J, Kehoe V, Davidson WR Jr, Sinoway L, et al. (2005) An initial application of transesophageal Doppler echocardiography in experimental small animal models. J Am Soc Echocardiogr 18: 626–631.
7. Li P, Dairywala IT, Liu Z, Stewart SR, Mathew B, et al. (2002) Anatomic and hemodynamic imaging using a new vector phased-array intracardiac catheter. J Am Soc Echocardiogr 15: 349–355.
8. Soares PP, da Nóbrega AC, Ushizima MR, Irigoyen MC (2004) Cholinergic stimulation with pyridostigmine increases heart rate variability and baroreflex sensitivity in rats. Auton Neurosci 113: 24–31.
9. Mostarda C, Rogow A, Silva IC, De La Fuente RN, Jorge L, et al. (2009) Benefits of exercise training in diabetic rats persist after three weeks of detraining. Auton Neurosci 145: 11–16.
10. Farah VM, Moreira ED, Pires MD, Irigoyen MC, Krieger EM (1999) Comparison of three methods for the determination of baroreflex sensitivity in conscious rats. Braz J Med Biol Res 2: 361–369.
11. Brum PC, Da Silva GJ, Moreira ED, Ida F, Negrão CE, et al. (2000) Exercise training increases baroreceptor gain sensitivity in normal and hypertensive rats. Hypertension 36: 1018–1022.
12. Silva GJ, Brum PC, Negrão CE, Krieger EM (1997) Acute and chronic effects of exercise on baroreflexes in spontaneously hypertensive rats. Hypertension 30: 714–719.
13. De Angelis K, Wichi RB, Jesus WR, Moreira ED, Morris M, et al. (2004) Exercise training changes autonomic cardiovascular balance in mice. J Appl Physiol 96: 2174–8.
14. Shanewise JS, Cheung AT, Aronson S, Stewart WJ, Weiss RL, et al. (1999) ASE/SCA guidelines for performing a comprehensive intraoperative multiplane transesophageal echocardiography examination: recommendations of the American Society of Echocardiography Council for Intraoperative Echocardiography and the Society of Cardiovascular Anesthesiologists Task Force for Certification in Perioperative Transesophageal Echocardiography. J Am Soc Echocardiogr 12: 884–900.
15. Nagueh SF, Appleton CP, Gillebert TC, Marino PN, Oh JK, et al. (2009) Recommendations for the evaluation of left ventricular diastolic function by echocardiography. J Am SocEchocardiogr 22: 107–133.
16. Tei C, Ling LH, Hodge DO, Bailey KR, Oh JK, et al. (1995) New index of combined systolic and diastolic myocardial performance: a simple and reproducible measure of cardiac function–a study in normals and dilated cardiomyopathy. J Cardiol 26: 357–366.
17. Ramires FJ, Salemi VM, Ianni BM, Fernandes F, Martins DG, et al. (2006) Aldosterone antagonism in an inflammatory state: evidence for myocardial protection. J Renin Angiotensin Aldosterone Syst 7: 162–1627.
18. Salemi VM, Bilate AM, Ramires FJ, Picard MH, Gregio DM, et al. (2005) Reference values from M-mode and Doppler echocardiography for normal Syrian hamsters. Eur J Echocardiogr 6: 41–46.
19. Lang RM, Bierig M, Devereux RB, Flachskampf FA, Foster E, et al. (2005) Chamber Quantification Writing Group; American Society of Echocardiography's Guidelines and Standards Committee; European Association of Echocardiography. Recommendations for chamber quantification: a report from the American Society of Echocardiography's Guidelines and Standards Committee and the Chamber Quantification Writing Group, developed in conjunction with the European Association of Echocardiography, a branch of the European Society of Cardiology. J Am Soc Echocardiogr 18: 1440–1463.
20. Devereux RB, Alonso DR, Lutas EM, Gottlieb GJ, Campo E, et al. (1986) Echocardiographic assessment of left ventricular hypertrophy: comparison to necropsy findings. Am J Cardiol 57: 450–458.
21. Jorge L, Rodrigues B, Rosa KT, Malfitano C, Loureiro TC, et al. (2011) Cardiac and peripheral adjustments induced by early exercise training intervention were associated with autonomic improvement in infarcted rats: role in functional capacity and mortality. Eur Heart J 32: 904–912.
22. Wichi R, Malfitano C, Rosa K, De Souza SB, Salemi V, et al. (2007) Noninvasive and invasive evaluation of cardiac dysfunction in experimental diabetes in rodents. Cardiovasc Diabetol 26: 6–14.
23. Ceroni A, Chaar LJ, Bombein RL, Michelini LC (2009) Chronic absence of baroreceptor inputs prevents training-induced cardiovascular adjustments in normotensive and spontaneously hypertensive rats. Exp Physiol 94: 630–640.
24. Miao CY, Xie HH, Zhan LS, Su DF (2006) Blood pressure variability is more important than blood pressure level in determination of end-organ damage in rats. J Hypertens 24: 1125–1135.
25. Norman RA Jr, Coleman TG, Dent AC (1981) Continuous monitoring of arterial pressure indicates sinoaortic denervated rats are not hypertensive. Hypertension 3: 119–125.
26. Moraes-Silva IC, De La Fuente RN, Mostarda C, Rosa K, Flues K, et al. (2010) Baroreflex deficit blunts exercise training-induced cardiovascular and autonomic adaptations in hypertensive rats. Clin Exp Pharmacol Physiol 37: e114–e120.
27. Carabello BA (2002) Concentric versus eccentric remodeling, J Card Fail 8: S258–S263.
28. Mostarda C, Moraes-Silva IC, Moreira ED, Medeiros A, Piratello AC, et al. (2011) Baroreflex sensitivity impairment is associated with cardiac diastolic dysfunction in rats. J Card Fail 17: 519–525.
29. Sebbag I, Rudski LG, Therrien J, Hirsch A, Langleben D (2001) Effect of chronic infusion of epoprostenol on echocardiographic right ventricular myocardial performance index and its relation to clinical outcome in patients with primary pulmonary hypertension. Am J Cardiol 88: 1060–1063.
30. Rudski LG, Lai WW, Afilalo J, Hua L, Handschumacher MD, et al. (2010) Guidelines for the echocardiographic assessment of the right heart in adults: a report from the American Society of Echocardiography endorsed by the European Association of Echocardiography, a registered branch of the European Society of Cardiology, and the Canadian Society of Echocardiography. J Am Soc Echocardiogr 23: 685–713.

4

CT-Angiography–Based Evaluation of the Aortic Annulus for Prosthesis Sizing in Transcatheter Aortic Valve Implantation (TAVI)–Predictive Value and Optimal Thresholds for Major Anatomic Parameters

Florian Schwarz[1]*, Philipp Lange[2], Dominik Zinsser[1], Martin Greif[2], Peter Boekstegers[3], Christoph Schmitz[4], Maximilian F. Reiser[1,5], Christian Kupatt[2,5], Hans C. Becker[1,5]

1 Institute for Clinical Radiology, Hospital of the Ludwig Maximilian University of Munich, Munich, Germany, **2** Medical Clinic I - Cardiology, Hospital of the Ludwig Maximilian University of Munich, Munich, Germany, **3** HELIOS Klinikum Siegburg, HELIOS Kliniken GmbH, Siegburg, Germany, **4** Department of Cardiac Surgery, Hospital of the Ludwig Maximilian University of Munich, Munich, Germany, **5** DZHK (German Centre for Cardiovascular Research), Partner Site Munich Heart Alliance, Munich, Germany

Abstract

Background/Objectives: To evaluate the predictive value of CT-derived measurements of the aortic annulus for prosthesis sizing in transcatheter aortic valve implantation (TAVI) and to calculate optimal cutoff values for the selection of various prosthesis sizes.

Methods: The local IRB waived approval for this single-center retrospective analysis. Of 441 consecutive TAVI-patients, 90 were excluded (death within 30 days: 13; more than mild aortic regurgitation: 10; other reasons: 67). In the remaining 351 patients, the CoreValve (Medtronic) and the Edwards Sapien XT valve (Edwards Lifesciences) were implanted in 235 and 116 patients. Optimal prosthesis size was determined during TAVI by inflation of a balloon catheter at the aortic annulus. All patients had undergone CT-angiography of the heart or body trunk prior to TAVI. Using these datasets, the diameter of the long and short axis as well as the circumference and the area of the aortic annulus were measured. Multi-Class Receiver-Operator-Curve analyses were used to determine the predictive value of all variables and to define optimal cutoff-values.

Results: Differences between patients who underwent implantation of the small, medium or large prosthesis were significant for all except the large vs. medium CoreValve (all p's<0.05). Furthermore, mean diameter, annulus area and circumference had equally high predictive value for prosthesis size for both manufacturers (multi-class AUC's: 0.80, 0.88, 0.91, 0.88, 0.88, 0.89). Using the calculated optimal cutoff-values, prosthesis size is predicted correctly in 85% of cases.

Conclusion: CT-based aortic root measurements permit excellent prediction of the prosthesis size considered optimal during TAVI.

Editor: Claudio Moretti, S. G. Battista Hospital, Italy

Funding: This work was supported by the DZHK (German Centre for Cardiovascular Research) and by the BMBF (German Ministry of Education and Research). The funders had no role in study design, data collection and analysis, decision to publish, or preparation of the manuscript.

Competing Interests: The authors have read the journal's policy and have the following conflicts: Professor Becker has received speaker honoraria from Siemens Healthcare. Professor Boekstegers is an employee of HELIOS Kliniken GmbH, yet his contribution to this study was made when he was an employee of the university hospital of the Ludwig-Maximilians-University of Munich.

* Email: Florian.Schwarz@med.uni-muenchen.de

Introduction

Aortic valve stenosis is the most common acquired valve disorder and symptomatic forms have dismal outcomes when treated medically [1,2]. For decades, surgical valve replacement has been the only curative treatment – however, due to comorbidities at the time of presentation up to one third of patients cannot undergo open heart surgery [3–5]. Transcatheter Aortic Valve Implantation (TAVI)/Transcatheter Aortic Valve Replacement (TAVR) is a novel, less invasive technique and is comparably safe even in patients with contraindications to surgery [6,7]. Results of the randomized controlled PARTNER-B-cohort comparing TAVI to best medical therapy have shown substantial survival benefits after 12 and 24 months [8,9]. In patients with a high surgical risk (PARTNER-A-cohort), TAVI was non-inferior to surgery after 12 months [10].

Unlike in surgical replacement, prosthesis sizing for TAVI significantly relies on imaging [11]. Imaging-derived measurements of the aortic root play the key role in patient and device selection. Transesophageal echocardiography and Multidetector

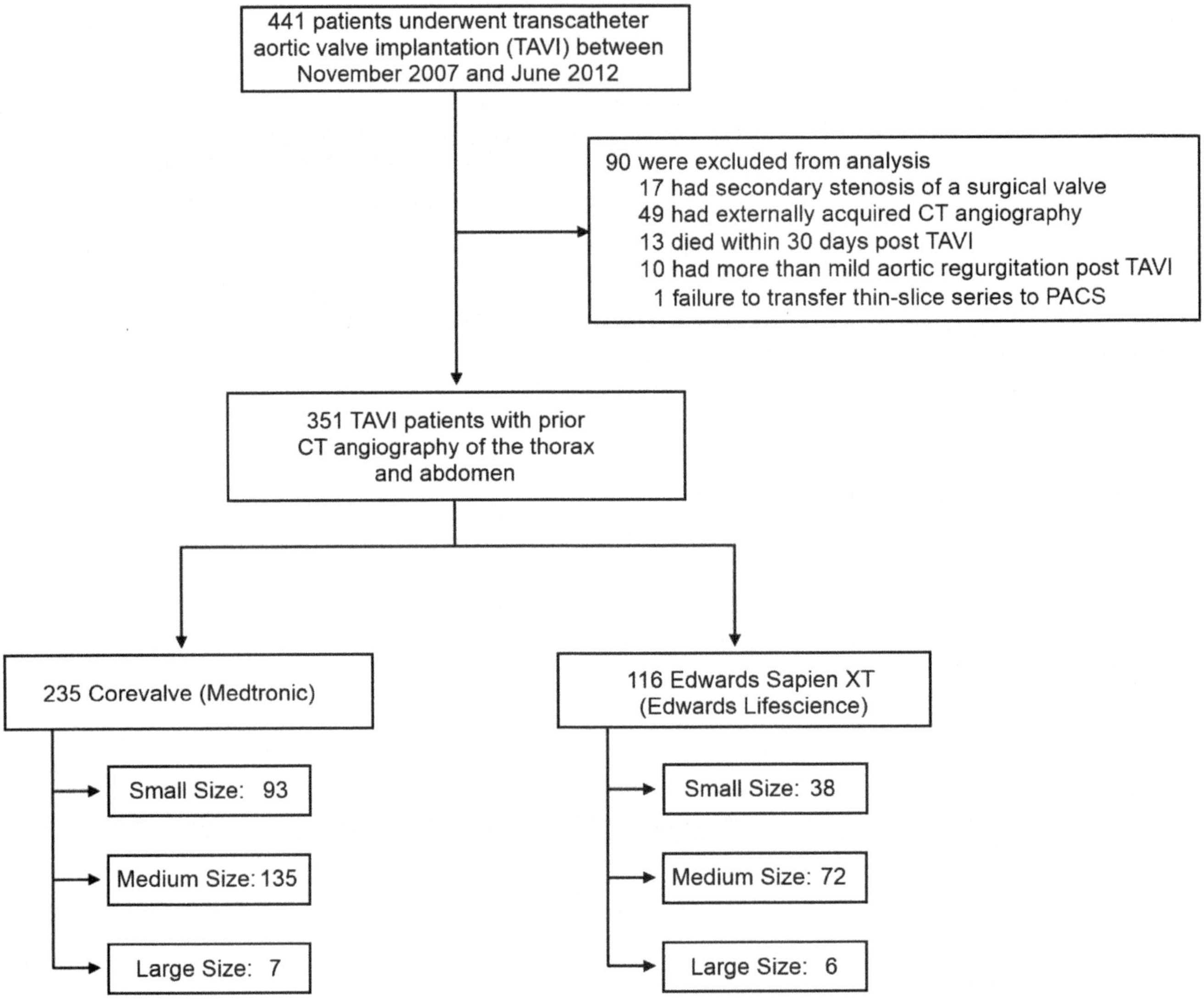

Figure 1. Inclusion chart for our analysis of 351 patients who underwent a successful TAVI procedure.

CT-angiography (CTA) have been applied extensively in this regard [12–14]. Several studies have consistently demonstrated that the aortic annulus has an elliptic shape described by a long and short axis with a wide range of reported eccentricities [15,16]. As a consequence, it is difficult to measure the true dimensions of the aortic annulus on the basis of a single plane obtained by 2D-echocardiography [17,18].

There is initial evidence favoring CTA over echocardiography for prosthesis selection. Recently, Jilaihawi et al had demonstrated for the SAPIEN XT valve (Edwards Lifesciences) that annular-sizing on the basis of CT resulted in lower rates of paravalvular regurgitation than sizing on the basis of 2D TEE [17]. Similar results had previously been reported by Hayashida et al for patients having undergone implantation of the Corevalve (Medtronic) or Sapien XT valve (Edwards Lifesciences) [19].

Several questions remain as to how select the optimal prosthesis size on the basis of CT-derived annulus parameters and most authors use a fixed algorithm suggesting certain annulus diameter ranges for distinct prosthesis sizes. Recently, Binder et al reported that the application of a CT-based annulus area sizing algorithm prior to TAVI resulted in the reduction of paravalvular regurgitation compared with simply providing quantitative results for anatomical parameters [20].

In this study, we analyzed all patients (n = 351) who had undergone dedicated CT-angiography prior to TAVI at our institution. We report descriptive statistics for the key anatomic parameters of the aortic root, determine interobserver reproducibility for CT-derived measurements and analyze various anatomic variables for their predictive value for the selection of optimal device size. Suggestions are provided for optimal cutoff values for CT-based measurements.

Methods

1. Patient Population

This analysis included patients with severe aortic valve stenosis who underwent a TAVI procedure at our institution between November 2007 and June 2012. Patients needed to have undergone CTA for the evaluation of aortic root anatomy within three months before TAVI. As all CT scans were performed as part of routine clinical workup and were analyzed anonymously,

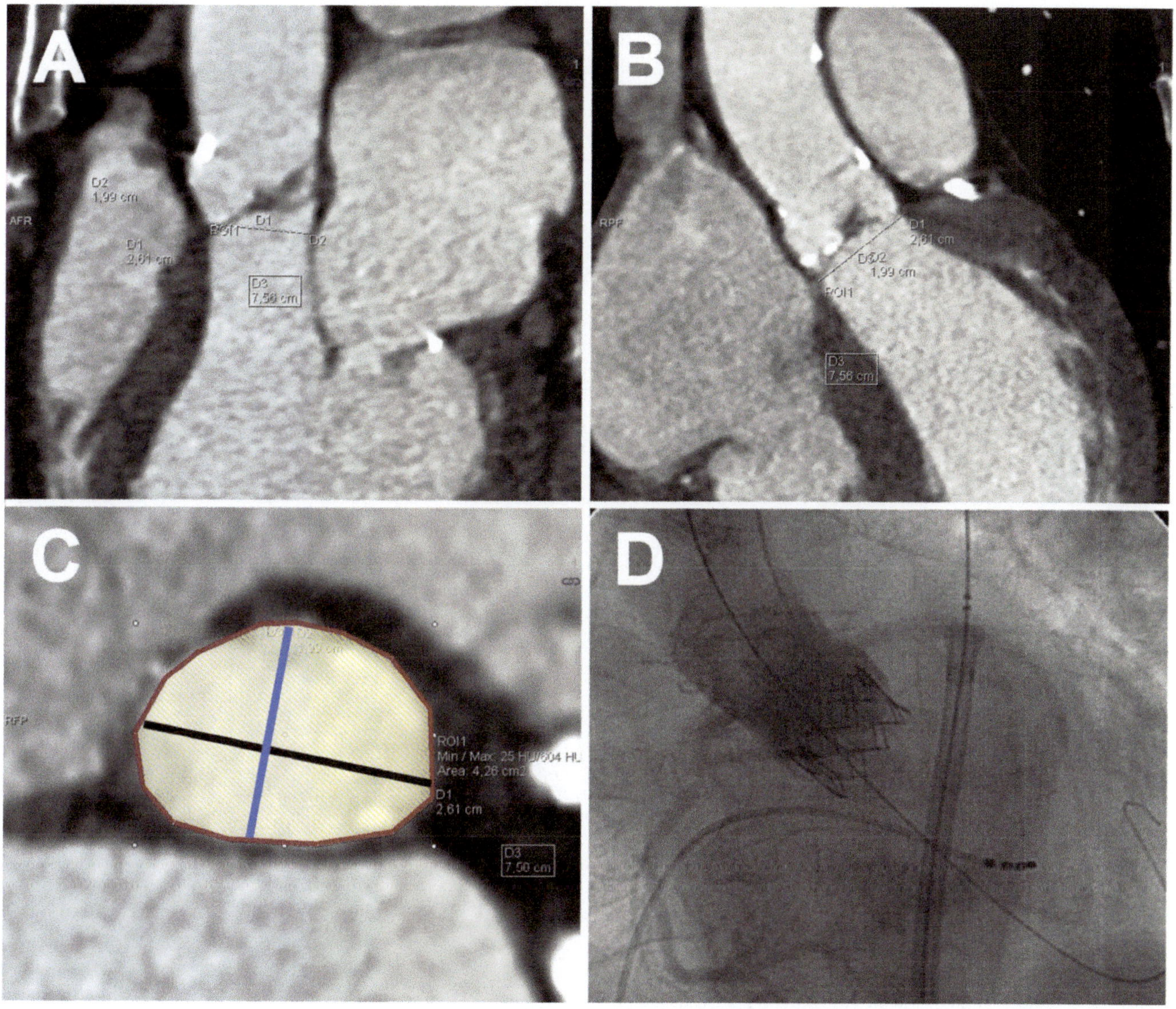

Figure 2. Examples of anatomic measurements at the aortic annulus performed for this study: isotropic small field-of-view CTA dataset of a 78 year old female patient with severe aortic stenosis, A) sagittal reformation and B) coronal reformation showing the orientation of the aortic annulus plane, C) double-oblique reformation of the aortic valve annulus, demonstrating the diameter of the long axis (black line), the diameter of the short axis (blue line), the annulus circumference (red polygonal), and annulus area (yellow shading). D) angiographic image after implantation of a 26 mm model of the Edward Sapien XT valve prosthesis demonstrates no paravalvular leakage.

the institutional review board of the Faculty of Medicine of the Ludwig Maximilian University of Munich waived the necessity to obtain consent beyond routine clinical requirements. All patients gave written consent to an anonymous analysis of the acquired data.

According to institutional policies patients with impaired renal function (glomerular filtration rate <30 ml/min), abnormal TSH-levels or a history of allergic reaction to iodine-containing contrast agents were excluded. After explicit education about the risks of iodinated contrast agents and exposure to x-rays, written informed consent was obtained (Figure 1).

2. CT Data Acquisition and Image Reconstruction

CT scans were performed either on a first-generation dual-source MDCT scanner (n = 49, Somatom Definition, Siemens Healthcare, Forchheim, Germany) or on a second-generation dual-source MDCT scanner (n = 302, Somatom Definition Flash, Siemens Healthcare) 3–90 days before TAVI. The ECG-signal was registered continuously throughout the scan. Images of the heart were acquired during diastole. Slice collimation was 2×64×0.6 mm (first generation) or 2×128×0.6 mm (second generation). Tube potential was 100 or 120 kV (depending on patient weight) and effective tube current-time product was 350–400 mAs/rotation. See Appendix S1 for detailed scan parameters.

In all patients, 90 ml of iomeprol 816.5 g/l (Imeron 400, Bracco Imaging, Milan, Italy) were administered via an ante-cubital vein at a flow-rate of 4 ml/s, followed by 100 ml of normal saline at the same flow rate. Contrast enhancement was controlled by bolus tracking within the ascending aorta.

Table 1. Patient parameters, N(%), mean ± SD or median [interquartile range] and summary of implanted valve sizes.

	All Patients	CoreValve Subgroup	Edward Sapien Subgroup	p
n	351 (100%)	235 (67%)	116 (33%)	
Female Patients	211 (58%)	132 (54%)	74 (62%)	0.18
Age at scan (yrs)	80.9±10.8	81.6±6.5	76.3±21.5	0.06
Height (cm)	165.7±8.9	165.5±13.9	163.2±18.2	0.125
Weight (kg)	72.9±14.7	72.6±15.0	72.1±17.0	0.83
BMI (kg/m²)	26.5±4.8	26.3±4.5	26.8±5.4	0.62
Aortic Valve Area (cm²)	0.70±0.15	0.69±0.16	0.72±0.13	0.21
Pressure gradient (mmHg)	66.9±22.4	67.3±23.8	66.0±19.6	0.65
Ejection fraction (%)	58.0±15.3	57.8±16.0	58.3±13.6	0.80
Logistic EuroSCORE	18.9 [13.4; 25.7]	19.6 [14.5; 26.7]	16.5 [11.0; 23.4]	<0.01
Valve Sizes:				
Small Size	131 (37%)	93 (40%)	38 (33%)	0.25
Medium Size	207 (59%)	135 (57%)	72 (62%)	0.44
Large Size	13 (4%)	7 (3%)	6 (5%)	0.52

Once intraluminal attenuation exceeded 150 HU, the table was repositioned for the desired scan range. Delay was 6 seconds (Somatom Definition) or 12 seconds (Somatom Definition Flash). Thereafter, the start of the scan was triggered by ECG automatically.

A medium-smooth convolution kernel was used to generate standard coronary CTA reconstructions (small field of view, slice thickness 0.75 mm, reconstruction increment 0.5 mm covering the entire heart). All series were pseudonymized and transferred to an external workstation.

3. CT Data Analysis

Two experienced readers analyzed all series independently using commercially available software (Syngo Via VA20, Siemens Healthcare, Germany). Readers determined subjective image quality and contrast enhancement on 4-point Likert scales (4: best image quality/contrast enhancement, 1: poor image quality/contrast enhancement). Furthermore, both readers measured the size of the aortic annulus according to techniques suggested by various authors [12,21–23]. Using multiplanar reformations, readers independently established the double-oblique plane defined by the three 'hinge' points (i.e. the most apical points of the valvular cusps, see Figure 2). On this plane, both readers manually determined the lengths of the long axis (LA), short axis (SA), circumference (C) and area (A) of the elliptical shape of the the aortic valve annulus (Figure 2). Three virtual diameters (d_{mean}, d_C *and* d_A) were derived from these parameters according to the following formulae:

$$d_{mean} = \frac{LA+SA}{2};\ d_C = \frac{C}{\pi};\ d_A = 2 \times \sqrt{\frac{A}{\pi}}$$

4. Clinical and procedural data

In all patients, TAVI was performed at the department of cardiology of this institution as part of routine clinical care. Patients were admitted at least 1 day prior to TAVI and transferred to a high-level intensive care unit for at least 24 hours afterwards. All patients underwent a routine transthoracic echocardiography exam within 7 days prior to TAVI.

Selection of valve type (CoreValve by Medtronic, Minneapolis, USA vs. Edward Sapien XT by Edwards Lifesciences, Irvine, CA, USA) and size was performed by the heart team members before and during TAVI. According to the standard operating procedures of this institution, an initial estimation of annulus size was performed based on all available imaging information. During the procedure, a balloon catheter with the estimated size was inflated at the annulus position and snug fit was evaluated by fluoroscopy and balloon pressures [24–26]. Depending on the appearance of the balloon and the recorded pressures, valve size was either confirmed or changed. In the latter case, a different balloon catheter was used and the changed size tested. Once optimal size had been established, the respective valve was implanted using the techniques recommended by manufacturers. Thereafter, conventional angiography was performed to test for aortic regurgitation, which was rated on a three point Likert scale (1: no, minimal or first degree regurgitation, 2: second degree regurgitation, 3: severe regurgitation).

5. Statistical Analysis

The D'Agostino-Pearson test was used to test for normal distribution of continuous variables. Continuous variables are reported as mean ± standard deviation when normally distributed, otherwise as median (interquartile range).

For categorical variables, Cohen's kappa was used to address observer agreement and was reported with 95% confidence interval. For continuous variables, the intraclass correlation coefficient (ICC) was used [27].

Differences in proportions were assessed using the Chi-squared test. To test for differences in means of interval variables, the Student's t-test (for independent or paired samples) was applied if variables followed normal distribution. For comparison of means of three or more variables, a one-way analysis of variance (ANOVA) was performed. If significant differences were found, variables were compared using the Tukey-HSD post-hoc test with

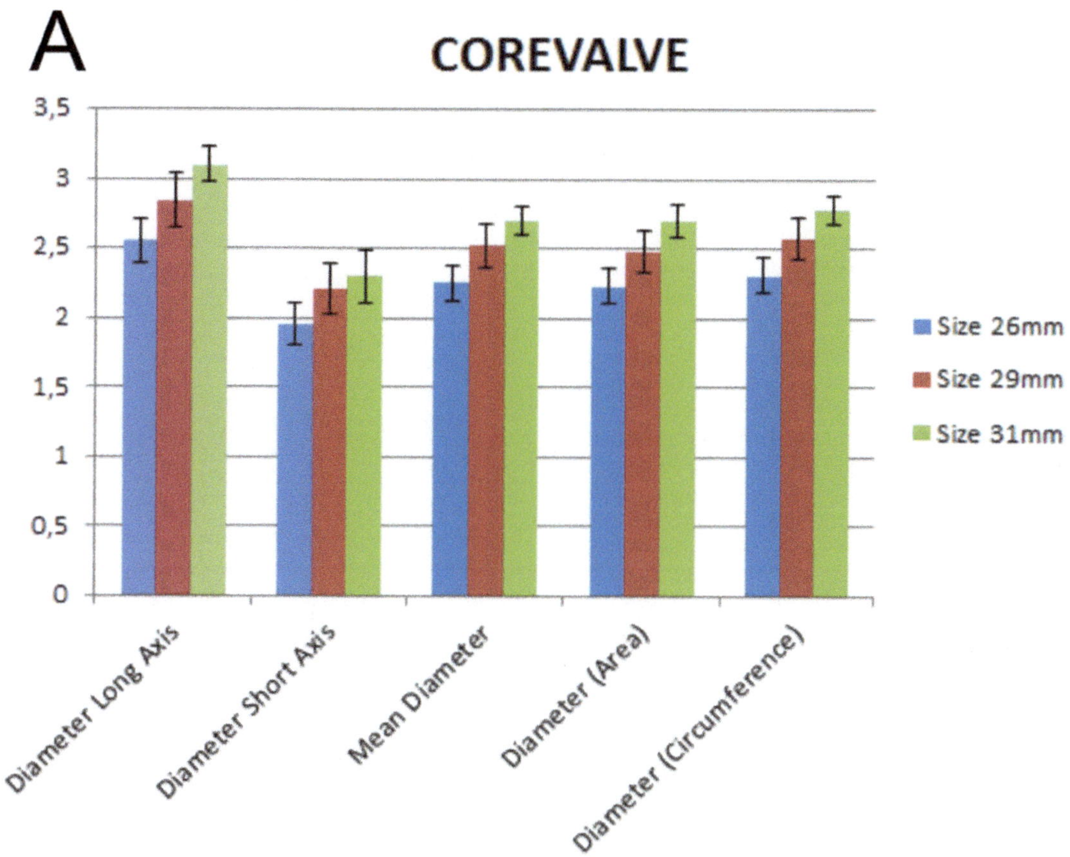
A
COREVALVE
3,5
3
2,5
2
1,5
1
0,5
0
Diameter Long Axis
Diameter Short Axis
Mean Diameter
Diameter (Area)
Diameter (Circumference)
Size 26mm
Size 29mm
Size 31mm

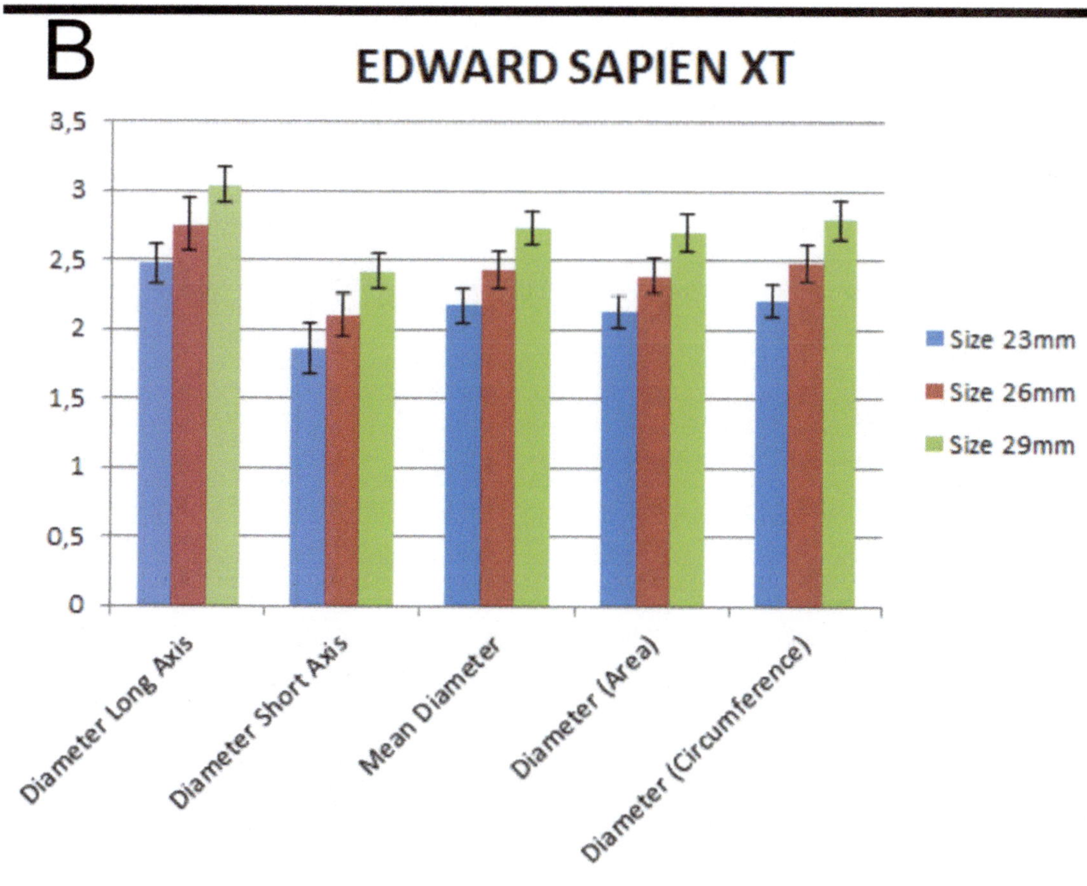
B
EDWARD SAPIEN XT
3,5
3
2,5
2
1,5
1
0,5
0
Diameter Long Axis
Diameter Short Axis
Mean Diameter
Diameter (Area)
Diameter (Circumference)
Size 23mm
Size 26mm
Size 29mm

Figure 3. Summary chart displaying major anatomic parameters (length of long and short axis; circumference-derived and area-derived virtual diameter) in patients in whom the small, medium or large size model was considered optimal for A) the CoreValve valve and the B) Edward Sapien XT valve. Except for the large vs. medium CoreValve size, all differences were statistically significant ($p<0.05$).

application of Bonferroni corrections to avoid errors due to multiple testing.

To compare means in variables not following normal distribution, a t-test was used if normal distribution was approximated after logarithmic transformation. In all other cases, non-parametric tests were used: the Mann-Whitney-test for independent variables and the Wilcoxon signed-rank test for paired variables.

To identify cut-off points that allow optimal prediction of implanted valve size on the basis of the particular anatomic parameter, and to estimate the associated generalization performance, we applied a 10-fold nested cross-validation approach. Details regarding this approach are included in Appendix S1.

P-values of 0.05 or less were considered statistically significant unless otherwise stated. Data were analyzed using MedCalc (Version 9.3.0.0, MedCalc Software, Mariakerke, Belgium), SPSS (21.0, IBM, Armonk, USA) and R [28].

Results

1. Patient Population

Between November 2007 and June 2012, 441 consecutive patients with high-grade aortic stenosis (mean AVA: 0.70 cm^2, SD: 0.15 cm^2) underwent a TAVI procedure at our institution. Of these, 17 patients were excluded as they presented with secondary stenosis of a surgical aortic valve prosthesis. Another 49 patients presented with externally acquired CT angiography datasets and were also excluded from this analysis. Of the remaining patients, 13 had died within 30 days after procedure and were not included into further analysis. 10 patients were excluded as they showed more than mild aortic regurgitation after valve implantation. Finally, one patient was excluded due to an error during archiving the small FOV (cardiac) series to PACS (Figure 1).

Of the remaining 351 patients, 235 had undergone implantation of a CoreValve prosthesis while in the remaining 116 patients the Edwards Sapien XT valve had been implanted. While differences in demographic parameters and preinterventional echocardiographic parameters between patients who underwent CoreValve vs. Edward Sapien XT valve implantation were not statistically significant, there was a difference in logarithmic Euro-Scores (19.6 [14.5; 26.7] vs. 16.5 [11.0; 23.4], $p<0.01$, see Table 1 for a summary of patient parameters) demonstrating a moderately less favorable risk profile in the CoreValve subgroup. In the entire cohort, no adverse events due to iv contrast administration during CT angiography were reported.

2. Subjective image quality and contrast enhancement of CTA datasets

There was substantial interobserver agreement for both subjective overall image quality (kappa = 0.76 [0.69–0.82]) and contrast enhancement (kappa = 0.72 [0.67–0.77]). Therefore, values from reader one were used for further analysis. Mean subjective image quality was 3.66 (SD: 0.58) and mean contrast enhancement was 3.88 (SD: 0.43).

3. CT-based anatomical measures of the aortic root

Interobserver agreement was excellent for all parameters with ICC-values consistently above 0.80. Bland-Altman-Analysis revealed no relevant systematic differences (Table 2 and Appendix S2). Therefore, arithmetic means between both observers were calculated for all variables.

Table 3 provides descriptive statistics on aortic valve measurements. Across all patients, length of the long axis and short axis were 2.70 [2.52; 2.90] and 2.05 [1.95; 2.25], respectively, and were slightly larger in the CoreValve subgroup than in the Edward Sapien subgroup (see Table 3). Median circumferences and median areas were 7.65 [7.28; 8.15] cm and 4.34 [3.90; 4.95] cm^2. There was a small but significant difference in average annulus diameters derived from circumference (2.44 [2.32; 2.60] cm) vs. those derived from annulus area (2.35 [2.23; 2.51] cm, $p<0.01$).

4. Annulus dimensions for different valve sizes

Of the 235 patients who underwent implantation of a CoreValve prosthesis, the 26 mm, 29 mm and 31 mm models were chosen in 93 (40%, 93/235), 135 (57%, 135/235) and 7 (3%, 7/235) cases. In 116 patients who received the Edward Sapien XT valve, the 23 mm, 26 mm and 29 mm were implanted in 38 (33%, 38/116), 72 (62%, 72/116) and 6 (5%, 6/118) cases.

Figure 3 provides details on long axis diameter, short axis diameter, circumference-derived and area-derived average annulus diameter measured for different sizes of CoreValve (Figure 3A) and Edward Sapien XT (Figure 3B). For all analyzed variables, one-way ANOVA showed significant differences between patients who underwent implantation of the small, middle or large valve (for the CoreValve: 26 mm, 29 mm, 31 mm; for the Edward Sapien XT: 23 mm, 26 mm, 29 mm, both p's<0.01). In Tukey-HSD post-hoc tests, differences between all size subgroups were statistically significant except for patients who underwent implantation of the CoreValve 31 mm vs. 29 mm ($p>0.05$), which was most likely due to the relatively small number of patients in the 31 mm CoreValve subgroup (n = 7).

Table 2. Interobserver Agreement for anatomical measurements of the aortic root reported as Intraclass Correlation Coefficient (ICC) and parameters of Bland-Altman-Analysis.

	Diameter long axis	Diameter short axis	$Diameter_{Mean}$	Annulus Circum-ference	Annulus Area
ICC [95% CI]	0.87 [0.84; 0.89]	0.86 [0.83; 0.88]	0.90 [0.88; 0.92]	0.92 [0.90; 0.93]	0.93 [0.92; 0.94]
Mean difference	0.00 cm	0.00 cm	0.00 cm	0.06 cm	0.03 cm^2
SD of differences	0.14 cm	0.12 cm	0.20 cm	0.54 cm	0.6 cm^2

Table 3. Primary anatomic parameters of the aortic annulus, N(%), mean ± SD or median [interquartile range] as well as "virtual diameters" derived from the mean of long axis and short axis, from annulus circumference and annulus area.

	All Patients	CoreValve Subgroup	Edward Sapien Subgroup	p
Diameter Long Axis [cm]	2.70 [2.52; 2.90]	2.75 [2.54; 2.90]	2.65 [2.50; 2.85]	0.049
Diameter Short Axis [cm]	2.05 [1.95; 2.25]	2.10 [1.95; 2.28]	2.05 [1.90; 2.20]	<0.01
Circumference [cm]	7.65 [7.28; 8.15]	7.73 [7.30; 8.25]	7.55 [7.05; 8.00]	<0.01
Area [cm^2]	4.34 [3.90; 4.95]	4.44 [3.98; 5.05]	4.19 [3.70; 4.75]	<0.01
Diameter$_{Mean}$ [cm]	2.40 [2.25; 2.55]	2.42 [2.27; 2.58]	2.35 [2.22; 2.52]	<0.01
Circumference- derived virtual diameter [cm]	2.44 [2.32; 2.60]	2.46 [2.32; 2.63]	2.40 [2.24; 2.55]	<0.01
Area-derived virtual diameter [cm]	2.35 [2.23; 2.51]	2.38 [2.25; 2.54]	2.31 [2.17; 2.46]	<0.01

5. Predictive value of different variables for device size selection and optimal cutoff values

Using multi-class ROC-analysis, the predictive value of all anatomic parameters for the size of prosthesis considered optimal was evaluated. For both valve types, all five analyzed parameters showed high predictive value for optimal prosthesis size (AUC: 0.75–0.91, Table 4). In particular, for the Medtronic CoreValve the short axis had a somewhat lower predictive value (multi-class AUC: 0.75) while there were no differences in predictive value between diameters of long axis, mean diameter, annulus area or annulus circumference (multi-class AUC's: 0.81, 0.80, 0.88, 0.9, $p>0.05$, Appendix S3). For the Edwards Sapien XT valve, differences in predictive value between the different parameters also did not reach statistical significance (multi-class AUC's: 0.83, 0.80, 0.88, 0.88, 0.89, $p>0.05$, Appendix S4). Application of the proposed cutoff-values in our sample of 351 patients results in the correct classification of 81.5% (286/351), 85.5% (300/351) and 82.9% (291/351) of cases if annulus circumference, annulus area or mean diameter are used.

Discussion

Transcatheter aortic valve implantation (TAVI) has been developed as a treatment strategy for patients with severe aortic stenosis who are at high risk or not eligible for heart surgery [29]. Several studies have demonstrated that MDCT is an ideal imaging modality prior to TAVI, providing isotropic datasets of the aortic root that can be reformatted in any spatial orientation [30–32]. There is some evidence favoring CT-derived annulus sizing over transthoracic echocardiography, particularly in regard to the incidence of postinterventional aortic regurgitation [17,19].

Several methods have been proposed to reduce the shape of the aortic annulus to a single measure for prosthesis sizing: calculation of the arithmetic mean between long and short axis [21], measurement of the length of the annulus circumference [12] or quantification of the annulus area [22,23]. To date, no consensus has been established on what the best technique is.

Binder et al have recently demonstrated for the Sapien XT valve that the recommendation of a particular prosthesis size on the basis of CT data results in more favorable outcomes than simply providing the annulus parameters [20]. In this regard

Table 4. Multi-Class AUC's as measures for the predictive value of the respective anatomic parameters for the valve size considered optimal by the implantation team.

	PARAMETER	OPTIMAL CUTOFF SMALL vs. MEDIUM	OPTIMAL CUTOFF MEDIUM vs. LARGE	MULTI-CLASS AUC
MEDTRONIC COREVALVE	Diameter Long Axis	2.70 cm	3.04 cm	0.8133
	Diameter Short Axis	2.05 cm	2.29 cm	0.7478
	Diameter$_{Mean}$	2.35 cm	2.70 cm	0.7974
	Annulus Area	4.30 cm^2	5.72 cm^2	0.8812
	Annulus Circumference	7.65 cm	8.60 cm	0.9146
EDWARDS SAPIEN XT	Diameter Long Axis	2.55 cm	3.05 cm	0.8347
	Diameter Short axis	1.95 cm	2.30 cm	0.7995
	Diameter$_{Mean}$	2.25 cm	2.55 cm	0.8793
	Annulus Area	3.85 cm^2	5.35 cm^2	0.8823
	Annulus Circumference	7.15 cm	8.20 cm	0.8884

Optimal cutoff values for the selection of the small, medium or large prosthesis size, defined as cutoff values that result in highest predictive accuracy.

however, uncertainty remains as to what the optimal size of prosthesis is for a given set of aortic annulus parameters.

In this analysis of over 350 patients who had undergone CT angiography prior to TAVI, we performed extensive anatomic measurements of the aortic root. Our results confirm previous analyses of Halpern et al [14], Gurvitch et al [12] and Delgado et al [33], since all relevant anatomic parameters can be measured in virtually all patients with excellent agreement between two experienced observers. Similar to the study by Gurvitch, observer agreement was highest for aortic annulus circumference and area (ICC's = 0.92, 0.93), even though in our study differences to observer agreement for long and short axis measurements were not significant.

In all patients included in this analysis, optimal prosthesis size was determined with the help of a sizing balloon catheter inflated during the implantation procedure [24–26]. Furthermore, all patients in whom this method might not have resulted in the selection of the correct prosthesis size – i.e. patients with more than mild regurgitation after TAVI (n = 10) and patients who died within 30 days after implantation (n = 13) – were deliberately excluded. No patient had to be excluded due to open heart surgery within 30 days. According to best professional judgment, prosthesis sizing was adequate in the remaining 351 patients. Thus, our data permit the unique opportunity to analyze the relation between different anatomic variables of the aortic root and the device size ultimately considered optimal. Even more importantly, the discriminatory power of different anatomic variables to predict prosthesis size as well as optimal cutoff values can be calculated.

Our results demonstrate that for all analyzed anatomic variables there are differences between patients who underwent implantation of the small, medium or large valve. Our results are both in line with but also extend those of Jilaihawi et al [17] and Delgado et al [34], demonstrating that on the basis of high-resolution MDCT datasets of the aortic root, the optimal valve size can be predicted. While in principle all evaluated anatomic parameters can be used for prosthesis sizing, the most favorable combination of high observer agreement and predictive value are observed for mean diameter, annulus area and annulus circumference (with multi-class AUC's of 0.88 and 0.91). Optimal thresholds for the selection of the small, medium or large size are given in Table 4. The use of these cutoff values in our cohort results in the correction prediction of valve size in 85% (300/351) of cases. In the remaining 15% (51/351), the application of a sizing balloon would result in a change of device size. Importantly, our 2-threshold-model does not take into account that a considerable number of patients will be suitable candidates for two valve sizes. Inclusion of the extent of aortic valve calcifications might further increase the predictive accuracy of our model.

Our single-center retrospective study has several limitations: first, the heart team members involved in valve implantation were not blinded towards the routine radiological reports derived from the CT dataset. While this would have been favorable from a scientific perspective, we feel that the information obtained from high-resolution CT angiography datasets prior to TAVI is of so essential a nature that withholding it would be clearly unethical. Furthermore, cardiologists integrated all available information regarding valve size, including transthoracic and transesophageal echocardiography and aortic angiography usually conducted before the TAVI procedure. In every single case, the presumed optimal valve size was simulated with a balloon catheter and changed if the size of the inflated balloon and the aortic annulus did not display the estimated ratio during aortography.

Second, we did not compare our measurements with a reference imaging modality such as 3D-echocardiography or MR angiography. However, our reference standard is the size of the implanted valve in those patients in whom – according to best professional judgment – prosthesis size turned out to be reasonably selected. For the purpose of this analysis we consider this outcome-oriented reference standard superior.

Third, we used only diastolic CT acquisitions to measure aortic annulus dimensions. However, it still is a matter of debate if systolic reconstructions are necessary for a reliable sizing of the aortic valve annulus: while some authors propose systolic reconstructions to avoid undersizing [35,36], others report no difference [37] or no substantial difference [38] between systolic and diastolic diameters. However, since we correlate our diastolic measures of annulus parameters with the prosthesis size considered optimal during implantation, a potential difference between systolic and diastolic dimensions is not a major concern; our results should rather be construed as a contribution to a prosthesis sizing algorithm from diastolic annulus parameters.

Fourth, we do not perform an analysis of the patients in whom valve implantation was not successful. However, the main intention of our manuscript is to perform a rigorous analysis of the dependencies between anatomical parameters of the aortic annulus and the implanted valve size for patients in whom the procedure was performed successfully. In that sense, we do not attempt to prove that an inadequate selection of prosthesis size increases the risk of a negative procedural outcome.

Finally, while our analysis suggests an ideal strategy to predict the appropriate valve size, we cannot answer the question how this strategy would perform in a prospective study context. However, the rate of excluded patients is comparatively small: only 23 patients had to be excluded due to either death within 30 days after the TAVI procedure (n = 13) or due to the development of more than mild aortic regurgitation (n = 10). Therefore, we are confident that our approach would permit a correct estimation of correct valve size in the vast majority of cases.

In conclusion, our analysis of 351 patients who successfully underwent TAVI shows that the valve size ultimately considered optimal can be predicted on the basis of CT-derived anatomic parameters of the aortic root. Mean diameter, annulus circumference and annulus area appear to have equally high reproducibility and predictive accuracy for both the Medtronic CoreValve and the Edwards Sapien XT prostheses. It remains to be shown that this approach holds up its predictive potential in a prospective study context.

Supporting Information

Appendix S1 Supplemental methods section including details on CT data acquisition, image reconstruction and statistical methods.

Appendix S2 Supplemental scatter plots and linear regression lines for the analysis of interobserver agreement.

Appendix S3 Extended results regarding the ANOVA analysis and post-hoc tests of differences in anatomic parameters of patients who underwent implantation of the large, middle or small version of either valve.

Appendix S4 Extended results regarding the analysis of differences in predictive values of the various anatomic

parameters for the valve size considered optimal by the TAVI team.

Author Contributions

Conceived and designed the experiments: FS PL DZ MG PB CS MFR CK HCB. Performed the experiments: FS PL DZ MG. Analyzed the data: FS PL DZ MG CK HCB. Contributed reagents/materials/analysis tools: MFR HCB. Wrote the paper: FS PL DZ MG PB CS MFR CK HCB.

References

1. Iung B, Baron G, Butchart EG, Delahaye F, Gohlke-Barwolf C, et al. (2003) A prospective survey of patients with valvular heart disease in Europe: The Euro Heart Survey on Valvular Heart Disease. Eur Hear J 24: 1231–1243. doi:S0195668X0300201X [pii].
2. Carabello BA, Paulus WJ (2009) Aortic stenosis. Lancet 373: 956–966. doi:S0140-6736(09)60211-7 [pii] 10.1016/S0140-6736(09)60211-7 [doi].
3. Bouma BJ, Van den Brink RBA, Van der Meulen JHP, Verheul HA, Cheriex EC, et al. (1999) To operate or not on elderly patients with aortic stenosis: the decision and its consequences. Heart 82: 143.
4. Iung B, Cachier A, Baron G, Messika-Zeitoun D, Delahaye F, et al. (2005) Decision-making in elderly patients with severe aortic stenosis: why are so many denied surgery? Eur Heart J 26: 2714.
5. Bach DS, Siao D, Girard SE, Duvernoy C, McCallister BD, et al. (2009) Evaluation of patients with severe symptomatic aortic stenosis who do not undergo aortic valve replacement. Circ Cardiovasc Qual Outcomes 2: 533.
6. Krishnaswamy A, Tuzcu EM, Kapadia SR (2010) Three-dimensional computed tomography in the cardiac catheterization laboratory. Catheter Cardiovasc Interv. doi:10.1002/ccd.22740.
7. Wood DA, Tops LF, Mayo JR, Pasupati S, Schalij MJ, et al. (2009) Role of multislice computed tomography in transcatheter aortic valve replacement. Am J Cardiol 103: 1295–1301. doi:S0002-9149(09)00110-6 [pii] 10.1016/j.amjcard.2009.01.034 [doi].
8. Leon M, Smith C, Mack M (2010) Transcatheter aortic-valve implantation for aortic stenosis in patients who cannot undergo surgery. N Engl J Med 363: 1597–1607. Available: http://www.nejm.org/doi/full/10.1056/nejmoa1008232. Accessed 2014 Jan 21.
9. Makkar RR, Fontana GP, Jilaihawi H, Kapadia S, Pichard AD, et al. (2012) Transcatheter aortic-valve replacement for inoperable severe aortic stenosis. N Engl J Med 366: 1696–1704. Available: http://www.ncbi.nlm.nih.gov/pubmed/23356420.
10. Smith CR, Leon MB, Mack MJ, Miller DC (2011) Transcatheter versus Surgical Aortic-Valve Replacement in High-Risk Patients. N Engl J Med 364: 2187–2198.
11. Achenbach S, Delgado V, Hausleiter J, Schoenhagen P, Min JK, et al. (2012) SCCT Expert Consensus Document on Computed Tomography Imaging Prior to Transcatheter Aortic Valve Implantation (TAVI)/Transcatheter Aortic Valve Replacement (TAVR). J Cardiovasc Comput Tomogr.
12. Gurvitch R, Webb JG, Yuan R, Johnson M, Hague C, et al. (2011) Aortic Annulus Diameter Determination by Multidetector Computed TomographyReproducibility, Applicability, and Implications for Transcatheter Aortic Valve Implantation. JACC Cardiovasc Interv 4: 1235–1245.
13. Wuest W, Anders K, Schuhbaeck A, May MS, Gauss S, et al. (2012) Dual source multidetector CT-angiography before transcatheter aortic valve implantation (TAVI) using a high-pitch spiral acquisition mode. Eur Radiol 22: 51–58.
14. Halpern EJ, Gupta S, Halpern DJ, Wiener DH, Owen AN (2012) Characterization and Normal Measurements of the Left Ventricular Outflow Tract by ECG-gated Cardiac CT: Implications for Disorders of the Outflow Tract and Aortic Valve. Acad Radiol.
15. Altiok E, Koos R, Schröder J, Brehmer K, Hamada S, et al. (2011) Comparison of two-dimensional and three-dimensional imaging techniques for measurement of aortic annulus diameters before transcatheter aortic valve implantation. Heart 97: 1578–1584.
16. Ng ACT, Delgado V, van der Kley F, Shanks M, van de Veire NRL, et al. (2010) Comparison of Aortic Root Dimensions and Geometries Before and After Transcatheter Aortic Valve Implantation by 2-and 3-Dimensional Transesophageal Echocardiography and Multislice Computed Tomography CLINICAL PERSPECTIVE. Circ Cardiovasc Imaging 3: 94–102.
17. Jilaihawi H, Kashif M, Fontana G, Furugen A, Shiota T, et al. (2012) Cross-sectional computed tomographic assessment improves accuracy of aortic annular sizing for transcatheter aortic valve replacement and reduces the incidence of paravalvular aortic regurgitation. J Am Coll Cardiol 59: 1275–1286.
18. Blanke P, Reinöhl J, Schlensak C, Siepe M, Pache G, et al. (2012) Prosthesis Oversizing in Balloon-Expandable Transcatheter Aortic Valve Implantation Is Associated With Contained Rupture of the Aortic Root. Circ Cardiovasc Interv 5: 540–548.
19. Hayashida K, Bouvier E, Lefevre T, Hovasse T, Morice M-C, et al. (2012) Impact of CT-guided valve sizing on post-procedural aortic regurgitation in transcatheter aortic valve implantation. J Am Coll Cardiol 59: E2142–E2142.
20. Binder RK, Webb JG, Willson AB, Urena M, Hansson NC, et al. (2013) The Impact of Integration of a Multidetector Computed Tomography Annulus Area Sizing Algorithm on Outcomes of Transcatheter Aortic Valve Replacement: A Prospective, Multicenter, Controlled Trial. J Am Coll Cardiol.
21. Leipsic J, Gurvitch R, LaBounty TM, Min JK, Wood D, et al. (2011) Multidetector Computed Tomography in Transcatheter Aortic Valve Implantation. JACC Cardiovasc Imaging 4: 416.
22. Schultz CJ, Moelker A, Piazza N, Tzikas A, Otten A, et al. (2010) Three dimensional evaluation of the aortic annulus using multislice computer tomography: are manufacturer's guidelines for sizing for percutaneous aortic valve replacement helpful? Eur Heart J 31: 849–856.
23. Blanke P, Siepe M, Reinöhl J, Zehender M, Beyersdorf F, et al. (2010) Assessment of aortic annulus dimensions for Edwards SAPIEN Transapical Heart Valve implantation by computed tomography: calculating average diameter using a virtual ring method. Eur J Cardio-Thoracic Surg 38: 750–758.
24. Babaliaros VC, Liff D, Chen EP, Rogers JH, Brown RA, et al. (2008) Can balloon aortic valvuloplasty help determine appropriate transcatheter aortic valve size? JACC Cardiovasc Interv 1: 580–586.
25. Babaliaros VC, Junagadhwalla Z, Lerakis S, Thourani V, Liff D, et al. (2010) Use of balloon aortic valvuloplasty to size the aortic annulus before implantation of a balloon-expandable transcatheter heart valve. JACC Cardiovasc Interv 3: 114–118.
26. Cerillo A, Mariani M, Berti S, Glauber M (2012) Sizing the aortic annulus. Ann Cardiothorac Surg 1: 245–256.
27. Bartko JJ (1966) The intraclass correlation coefficient as a measure of reliability. Psychol Rep 19: 3–11.
28. R Development Core Team (2010) R: A languae and environment for statistical computing. Available: http://www.r-project.org.
29. Cheung A, Soon JL (2011) Transcatheter aortic valve replacement: where will we be in 5 years? Curr Opin Cardiol 26: 106.
30. Schultz C, Moelker A, Tzikas A, Piazza N, De Feyter P, et al. (2010) The use of MSCT for the evaluation of the aortic root before transcutaneous aortic valve implantation: the Rotterdam approach. EuroIntervention 6: 505–511.
31. Del Valle-Fernandez R, Jelnin V, Panagopoulos G, Dudiy Y, Schneider L, et al. (2010) A method for standardized computed tomography angiography-based measurement of aortic valvar structures. Eur Hear J. doi:10.1093/eurheartj/ehq093.
32. Delgado V, Ng ACT, Shanks M, van der Kley F, Schuijf JD, et al. (2010) Transcatheter aortic valve implantation: role of multimodality cardiac imaging. Expert Rev Cardiovasc Ther 8: 113–123.
33. Delgado V, Ng ACT, Schuijf JD, van der Kley F, Shanks M, et al. (2011) Automated assessment of the aortic root dimensions with multidetector row computed tomography. Ann Thorac Surg 91: 716–723.
34. Delgado V, Ng ACT, Van De Veire NR, Van Der Kley F, Schuijf JD, et al. (2010) Transcatheter aortic valve implantation: role of multi-detector row computed tomography to evaluate prosthesis positioning and deployment in relation to valve function. Eur Heart J 31: 1114–1123.
35. Lehmkuhl L, Foldyna B, Von Aspern K, Lucke C, Grothoff M, et al. (2013) Inter-individual variance and cardiac cycle dependency of aortic root dimensions and shape as assessed by ECG-gated multi-slice computed tomography in patients with severe aortic stenosis prior to transcatheter aortic valve implantation: is it crucial for. Int J Cardiovasc Imaging 29: 693–703. doi:10.1007/s10554-012-0123-4.
36. Blanke P, Russe M, Leipsic J, Reinohl J, Ebersberger U, et al. (2012) Conformational pulsatile changes of the aortic annulus: impact on prosthesis sizing by computed tomography for transcatheter aortic valve replacement. JACC Cardiovasc Interv 5: 984–994. doi:10.1016/j.jcin.2012.05.014.
37. Bolen MA, Popovic ZB, Dahiya A, Kapadia SR, Tuzcu EM, et al. (2012) Prospective ECG-triggered, axial 4-D imaging of the aortic root, valvular, and left ventricular structures: a lower radiation dose option for preprocedural TAVR imaging. J Cardiovasc Comput Tomogr 6: 393–398. doi:10.1016/j.jcct.2012.10.006.
38. Bertaso AG, Wong DTL, Liew GYH, Cunnington MS, Richardson JD, et al. (2012) Aortic annulus dimension assessment by computed tomography for transcatheter aortic valve implantation: differences between systole and diastole. Int J Cardiovasc Imaging 28: 2091–2098.

Determinants and Improvement of Electrocardiographic Diagnosis of Left Ventricular Hypertrophy in a Black African Population

Ahmadou M. Jingi[1], Jean Jacques N. Noubiap[2]*, Philippe Kamdem[3], Samuel Kingue[1,4]

1 Department of Internal Medicine and Specialties, Faculty of Medicine and Biomedical Sciences, University of Yaoundé I, Yaoundé, Cameroon, 2 Internal Medicine Unit, Edéa Regional Hospital, Edéa, Cameroon, 3 Centre Médical de la Trinité, Bafoussam, Cameroon, 4 Department of Internal Medicine, Yaoundé General Hospital, Yaoundé, Cameroon

Abstract

Background: Left ventricular hypertrophy (LVH) is a major cardiovascular risk factor. The electrocardiogram (ECG) has been shown to be a poor tool in detecting LVH due to cardiac and extracardiac factors. We studied the determinants and possibility of improving the test performance of the ECG in a group of Black Africans.

Methods: We studied echocardiograms and electrocardiograms of 182 Cameroonian patients among whom 113 (62.1%) were having an echocardiographic LVH. Echocardiographic LVH was defined as Left Ventricular Mass Indexed to height $^{2.7}$(LVMI)>48 g/m$^{2.7}$ in men, and >44 g/m $^{2.7}$ in women or Body Surface Area ≥116 g/m^2 in men, and ≥96 g/m^2 in women. Test performances were calculated for 6 classic ECG criteria Sokolow-Lyon, Cornell, Cornell product, Gubner-Ungerleiger, amplitudes of R in aVL, V_5 and V_6.

Results: The most sensitive criteria were Cornell (37.2%) and Sokolow-Lyon index (26.5%). The most specific criteria were Gubner (98.6%), RaVL (97.1%), RV_5/V_6 (95.7%) and Cornell product (94.2%). The performance of the ECG in diagnosing LVH significantly increased with the severity of LVH for Cornell index ($r=0.420$, $p<0.0001$) and Sokolow index ($r=0.212$, $p=0.002$). It decreased with body habitus ($r=-0.248$, $p=0.001$) for Sokolow-Lyon index. Cornell index was less affected (age $p=0.766$; body habitus: $p=0.209$). After sex-specific adjustment for BMI, Cornell BMI sensitivity increased from 37.2% to 69% ($r=0.472$, $p<0.0001$), and Sokolow-Lyon BMI sensitivity increased from 26.5% to 58.4% ($r=0.270$, $p<0.001$).

Conclusion: The test performance of the ECG in diagnosing LVH is low in this Black African population, due to extracardiac factors such as age, sex, body habitus, and cardiac factors such as LVH severity and geometry. However, this performance is improved after adjustment for extracardiac factors.

Editor: Larisa G. Tereshchenko, Johns Hopkins University SOM, United States of America

Funding: The authors have no support or funding to report.

Competing Interests: The authors have declared that no competing interests exist.

* E-mail: noubiapjj@yahoo.fr

Introduction

Increased left ventricular mass (LVM) is an adaptation of the heart to increased hemodynamic burden, and alters cardiac functioning. It is often associated with hypertension and has been shown to be an independent cardiovascular risk factor [1]. Methods of diagnosing left ventricular hypertrophy (LVH) with increasing performance include a comprehensive clinical assessment, chest X-ray, electrocardiography (ECG), Cardiac ultrasound, CT scan, Nuclear Magnetic Resonance imaging (NMR). The ECG is the most cost-effective and is recommended for routine use in assessing LVH [2,3]. The test performance of the ECG has been shown to be influenced by race, gender, age and body habitus [4,5]. Adjustment of ECG LVH criteria for body mass index (BMI) and age has been shown to improve the classification accuracy in Caucasians [6]. Such studies are scarce in Sub-Saharan Africa and mostly looked at the test performance of the ECG [7,8]. Our objective was to study the test performance and determinants of some classic easy to use ECG criteria and the possibility of improvement.

Methods

Ethical Considerations

The study was granted ethical approval by the Institutional Review Board of the Health Science Foundation, Cameroon, and was performed in accordance with the guidelines of the Helsinki Declaration. Written informed consent was obtained from all the participants.

Study Design and Setting

The study was conducted between April and December 2011 in the "Centre Medical de la Trinité", one of the two cardiologic clinics in the West Region of Cameroon.

Study Population and Sampling

We included patients aged 18 years or more seen during the study period, consenting to participate, who underwent a Doppler echocardiography and an ECG on the same day. Eligible patients had to fulfil one of these criteria: **i)** normal LV size (Left Ventricular chamber size in end diastole (LVEDd) ≤59 mm and indexed LVEDd to BSA (indexed LVEDd) ≤31 mm/m^2 in men or ≤32 mm/m^2 in women) with normal LV or concentric LV remodeling or concentric LV hypertrophy; **ii)** minimally dilated LV (LVEDd ≤59 mm and indexed LVEDd >31 mm/m^2 in men or >32 mm/m^2 in women) with normal LV or concentric LV remodeling or concentric LV hypertrophy; **iii)** apparently dilated LV (LVEDd >59 mm and indexed LV ≤31 mm/m^2 in men or ≤ 32 mm/m^2 in women) with normal LV or concentric LV remodeling or concentric LV hypertrophy.

We excluded patients with: **i)** markedly dilated LV, LVEDd > 70 mm and indexed LVEDd >31 mm/m^2 in men or >32 mm/m^2 in women) as in LV aneurysm and dilated cardiomyopathy; **ii)** chronic obstructive pulmonary disease (COPD); **iii)** septal dyskinesia; **iv)** asymmetric septal hypertrophy (septum/posterior wall ratio >1.3); **v)** technically difficult echocardiography; **vi)** pericardial effusion; **vii)** chest deformity; **viii)** incomplete data (missing weight or height), discordant timing of tests (Echo/ECG).

A sample size of 90 patients was required, assuming the prevalence of 6.25% of LVH among patients with hypertension in Cameroon, a 5% margin of error and a 95% confidence level. The assumption of prevalence of 6.25% among was based on the prevalence of 25% of hypertension in Cameroon [9,10] and the prevalence of 25% of LVH among patients with hypertension [1].

Procedure

First, ECG was performed by a trained technician at rest in the supine position with a Mac 500 GE apparatus using standard procedure (speed and voltage regulation of 25 mm/s and 1 mV/10 mm respectively). Secondly, blinded to the ECG, the trans-thoracic echocardiography was performed with the patient in the left lateral decubitus position by an experienced cardiologist using commercially available echocardiography equipment (HP Sonos 2000 Color Doppler ver. A.2, HP Color) and a 4–7 Megahertz transducer.

Measurements

Subject identity (name, age, sex) were collected by a nurse. The blood pressure (BP) was measured with a mercury sphygmomanometer, the height measured with a stadiometer, and the weight with a clinical scale balance. The body surface area (BSA) was automatically calculated by the echocardiograph to nearest two decimals. The body mass index (BMI) calculated as Weight (kg)/height^2 (m^2) to nearest one decimal. Left ventricular measurements were done on long parasternal long axis 2-D guided M-mode using the ASE recommendations [11]. The LVM was calculated using the formula.

$$LVM = 0.8\left(1.04\left[(IVSd+LVPWd+LVEDd)^3-LVEDd^3\right]\right)+0.6g$$

LVM: Left Ventricular Mass
IVSd: Septal thickness in end diastole
LVPWd: Posterior wall thickness in end diastole
LVEDd: Left Ventricular chamber size in end diastole

LVH was defined based on ASE recommendations [11] as Indexed LVM (LVM per m^2 of BSA or LVM per m$^{2.7}$ of height) >115 g/m^2 (BSA) or >48 g/m$^{2.7}$ (height in case of obesity) in men and Indexed LVM >95 g/m^2 or >44 g/m$^{2.7}$ in women. The severity of Left Ventricular Mass (LVM) indexed to BSA was classified according to ASE recommendations as [11]:

- Mild (LVM: 116–132 g/m^2 in men and 96–109 g/m^2 in women)
- Moderate (LVM: 133–149 g/m^2 in men and 110–122 g/m^2 in women)
- Severe (LVM >149 g/m^2 in men and 122 g/m^2 in women).

The relative wall thickness (RWT) was calculated using the formula:

$$RWT=(IVSd+LVPWd)/LVEDd$$

The cut off 0.42 was used to define the LV geometry as:

- Normal: normal LVM and RWT ≤0.42
- Concentric remodeling: normal LVM and RWT >0.42
- Eccentric LVH: LVH and RWT ≤0.42
- Concentric LVH: LVH and RWT >0.42.

The ECG was then interpreted by the same cardiologist (PK). Voltage amplitude was measured to the nearest 0.05 mV and time to the nearest 0.02 s. The following voltage index criteria were evaluated.

- Sokolow-Lyon: SV1+ RV5 or RV6≥3.5 mV
- Cornell voltage index: RaVL+SV3≥2.8 mV in men and 2.0 mV in women
- Cornell product: (RaVL+SV3)×QRSd ≥0.244 mV.s
- Gubner index: RD1+ SD3≥2.5 mV.
- RaVL ≥1.1 mV
- RV5 or RV6≥2.7 mV.

Adjustment for body habitus was done by multiplying the voltage criteria and the BSA or BMI based on previous findings that body habitus has an inverse relationship with ECG voltage criteria.

Data Analysis

Data was coded, entered and analyzed using the Statistical Package for Social Science (SPSS) version 16.0 for Windows (SPSS, Chicago, Illinois, USA). We described continuous variables using means with standard deviations, and categorical variables using their frequencies and percentages. Pearson's correlation coefficient was used to associate LVMI (Left Ventricular Mass Index) and the several criteria that were analyzed. Sensitivity and specificity were calculated using 2×2 tables (Classifying ECG LVH as against Echo LVH as the standard). We calculated the specificity as true negatives divided by the sum of true negatives and false positives. Similarly, we calculated the sensitivity as true positives divided by the sum of true positives and false negatives. Regression lines were used to determine cut offs for the BSA or BMI adjusted criteria for two selected voltage criteria (Sokolow-Lyon and Cornell) when the LVM indexed to BSA ≥116 g/m2 for men, and ≥96 g/m2 for women). Mean values of demographic, electrocardiographic and echocardiographic variables were compared using 2-way ANOVA. The chi-square test or its equivalent was used to compare qualitative variables and a *p* value less than 0.05 was considered statistically significant.

Results

Clinical, ECG, and echocardiographic data were available and adequate for analysis in 182 patients aged 18 to 99 years with a mean age of 63 years (SD = 15.9). There was no significant age difference between sexes (males 61.7±15.8 years and females 64.1±16 years, p = 0.301). Most of the participants (81.9%) were aged ≥50 years. The most represented age groups were the 70 to 79 years (25.8%) and 60 to 69 years (24.2%) age groups (Figure 1). Fifty four point nine percent of patients (95% CI: 47.4–62) were females and 45.1% (95% CI: 37.7–52.6) were males. The prevalence of echocardiographic LVH was 62.1% (95% CI: 54.6–69.2) for LVM indexed to BSA (LVM ≥116 g/m2 for men, and ≥96 g/m2 for women). The prevalence of LVH when the LVM is indexed to height $^{2.7}$ (LVM >48 g/m $^{2.7}$ in men, and >44 g/m $^{2.7}$ in women) was 72.5% (95% CI: 65.4–78.9%). The concordance between indexing to BSA and height$^{2.7}$ was 87.4% (95% CI: 81.6–91.8). This was comparable between sexes and ages above or below 55 years. The LVH severity when the LVM is indexed to BSA is shown in figure 2.The proportions in the study population and mean values for the different LV geometry types are shown in table 1 and table 2 respectively.

Determinants of Test Performance

Table 3 shows the ECG voltage test performances with the severity of LVH. The sensitivity increased with the degree of LVH without a major decrease in the specificity. This was especially seen with the Cornell voltage criterion. Table 4 shows some other possible factors that could determine the test performance of the Sokolow-Lyon and Cornell voltage indices. The Sokolow-Lyon criterion is more sensitive in males though to a lesser extent than the Cornell criterion, which is more sensitive in females. Overall, Cornell voltage criterion performed better in both sexes. The test performance of the Sokolow-Lyon criterion significantly decreased with age (r = −0.159, p = 0.032), while the Cornell criterion showed a non-significant increase with age (r = 0.082, p = 0.766). The body habitus generally showed a significant negative effect on the Sokolow-Lyon criterion (r = −0.248, p = 0.001) while the Cornell criterion showed a non-significant positive effect (r = 0.094, p = 0.209). A positive effect was shown with the LV geometric pattern concordant with the pathologic evolution in both the Sokolow – Lyon and Cornell criteria.

Test Performances after Adjusting for Sex and Body Habitus

Table 5 shows the test performances of the un-adjusted and adjusted Sokolow-Lyon and Cornell indices with thresholds determined from regression equations at LV mass index ≥ 116 g/m^2 in males and ≥96 g/m^2 in females. The sensitivity doubled with both criteria with a decrease in the specificity by half and by a third with both the Sokolow-Lyon and Cornell criteria respectively. The test accuracy was better in the adjusted criteria.

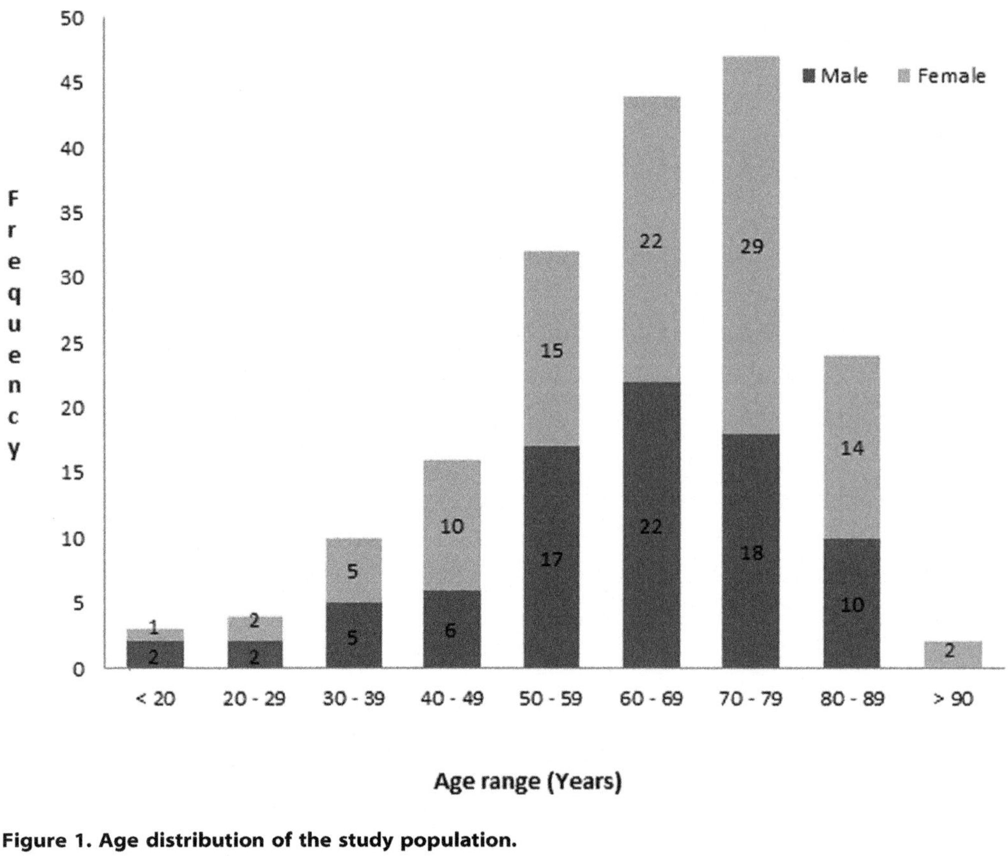

Figure 1. Age distribution of the study population.

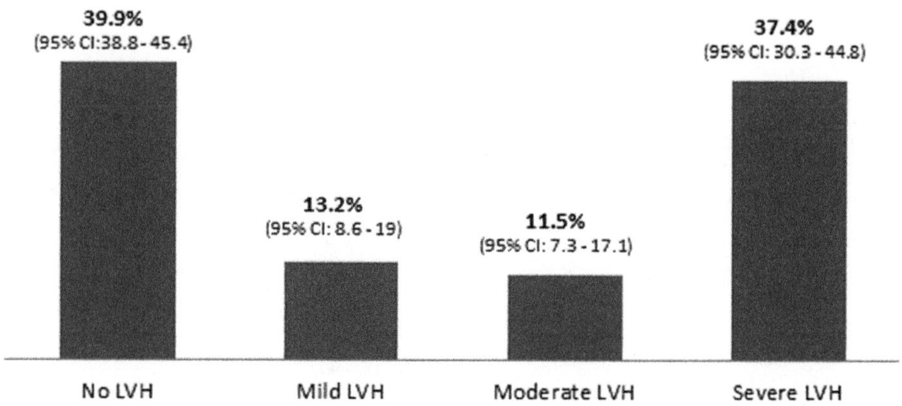

Figure 2. Left ventricular hypertrophy (LVH) severity when the left ventricular mass is indexed to the body surface area.

Table 1. Clinical, echocardiographic and electrocardiographic criteria (N = 182).

Characteristic	**Frequency (%)**
Body habitus (BMI)	
Underweight	7 (3.3)
Normal	66 (36.3)
Overweight	55 (30.2)
Obesity	54 (29.7)
Systolic blood pressure >140 mmHg	140 (76.9)
Diastolic blood pressure >90 mmHg	133 (73.1)
LV Chamber size	
Dilated	35 (19.2)
Normal	147 (80.8)
Pulmonary pressure >30 mmHg	61 (35.5)
LVH*	113 (62.1)
LVH**	132 (72.5)
LV Geometry	
Normal	13 (7.1)
Concentric remodeling	43 (23.6)
Concentric hypertrophy	96 (52.7)
Eccentric hypertrophy	30 (16.5)
Ejection fraction >50%	116 (63.7)
Heart rhythm	
Sinus	172 (94.5)
Atrial fibrillation	10 (5.5)
Sokolow LVH	44 (22.5)
Cornell LVH	51 (28)
Cornell product LVH	27 (14.8)
Gubner LVH	11 (6)
RaVL LVH	16 (8.8)
RV_5/RV_6 LVH	6 (3.3)

*(LVM Indexed to BSA ≥116 g/m^2 in men and ≥96 g/m^2 in women).
**(LVM Indexed to Height ≥49 $g/m^{2.7}$ in men and ≥45 $g/m^{2.7}$ in women).

Table 2. Clinical, electrocardiographic and echocardiographic characteristics comparing mean values relative to the left ventricular geometry type.

Characteristics	Normal N = 13	Concentric remodeling N = 43	Concentric hypertrophy N = 96	Eccentric hypertrophy N = 29	*p* value	Total	Range
Clinical							
Age (SD) years	49.9 (19.4)	60.1 (18.1)	66(13.7)	62.9(14.9)	0.003	62.98(15.9)	18–99
Systolic BP (SD)mmHg	147.9(24.6)	155.6(30.4)	169.5(33.1)	146.6(30.7)	<0.0001	160.45(33)	90–260
Diastolic BP(SD)mmHg	92.6(17.2)	94.3(15.9)	99(20.8)	89.2(19.5)	0.09	95.8(19.5)	50–177
BMI (SD) g/m^2	27.1(6.3)	26.8(5.7)	27.9(5.8)	25.7(5.6)	0.315	27.2(5.8)	16.3–43
BSA (SD) m^2	1.94(0.38)	1.89(0.26)	1.92(0.32)	1.84(0.32)	0.68	1.9(0.3)	1.27–2.89
Electrocardiogram							
Heart rate (SD): beats/min	75.5(11.4)	80.7(21)	76(19.1)	87.3(24)	0.057	78.9(20.3)	45–150
P wave duration (SD) s	0.1(0.01)	0.1(0.02)	0.1(0.02)	0.11(0.02)	0.283	0.10(0.02)	0.08–0.14
P-R (SD) s	0.17(0.03)	0.17(0.02)	0.17(0.03)	0.18(0.03)	0.428	0.17(0.03)	0.12–0.24
QRS							
Duration (s)	0.09 (0.02)	0.08(0.01)	0.08(0.01)	0.10(0.03)	<0.0001	0.08(0.02)	0.06–0.16
Axis	20.3(37.8)	31.5(42.6)	19.3(32)	10.4(36.1)	0.114	20.9	−46–120
QTc (s)	0.39(0.02)	0.39(0.03)	0.39(0.03)	0.38(0.04)	0.004	0.39 (0.03)	0.32–0.48
RaVL (mV)	0.54(0.26)	0.43(0.32)	0.65(0.42)	0.73(0.43)	0.004		
Sokolow (mV)	2.73(0.7)	2.55(0.79)	2.96(0.87)	3.02(0.97)	0.038	28.7(8.7)	6–55)
Cornell (mV)	1.36(0.58)	1.49(0.54)	1.95(0.72)	2.65(0.88)	<0.0001	19.2(8)	4–42
Cornell product (mV.s)	0.113(0.042)	0.115(0.045)	0.161(0.07)	0.261(0.129)	<0.0001	1.64(0.91)	0.32–6.72
Gubner - Ungerleiger(mV)	1.07(0.41)	0.96(0.56)	1.36(0.77)	1.51(0.79)	0.713	12.7(7.3)	0–42
Echocardiogram							
LA (cm)	3.6(0.8)	3.3(0.6)	4.1(0.9)	4.6(0.8)	<0.0001	3.97(0.88)	1.92–6.56
LVPWd (cm)	0.95(0.12)	1.09(0.13)	1.32(0.21)	1.15(0.15)	<0.0001	1.21(0.21)	0.79–2.2
IVSd (cm)	0.92(0.12)	1.17(0.12)	1.41(0.19)	1.15(0.15)	<0.0001	1.28(0.23)	0.74–2.11
DTDVg Index (cm/m^2)	2.59(0.3)	2.15(0.4)	2.49(0.5)	3.48(0.5)	<0.0001	2.58(0.63)	1.39–4.62)
EF (%)	63.6(12.3)	63.4(12.1)	57(13.3)	37.5(14.4)	<0.0001	55.76(15.6)	14–88
LVM Index (g/m^2)	80.72(16)	80.95(16.9)	136.26(38.2)	178.68(43.97)	<0.0001	126.22(48)	52.4–280.6
RVSP mmHg	34(10.7)	38.2(15.9)	43.9(17.6)	44.2(20.6)	0.485	42.3(17.5)	14–90

Table 3. Sensitivity and specificity at different thresholds for Left Ventricular Hypertrophy Mass Indexed to Body Surface Area (ASE).

Index	Mild LVH* (N = 24)		Moderate LVH** (N = 21)		Severe LVH*** (N = 68)		r	*p* value
	Sensitivity	Specificity	Sensitivity	Specificity	Sensitivity	Specificity		
Sokolow-Lyon	26.5%	84.1%	27.8%	82.6%	28.4%	80.9%	0.212	0.004
Cornell	37.2%	87%	42.2%	85.9%	49.3%	84.3%	0.420	<0.0001
Cornell product	20.4%	94.2%	23.3%	93.5%	31.3%	94.8%	0.419	<0.0001
Gubner-Ungerleiger	8.8%	98.6%	6.7%	93.5%	6%	93.9%	0.165	0.027
RaVL	11.5%	95.7%	4.9%	91.3%	10.4%	92.2%	0.179	0.016
RV_5/V_6	3.5%	97.1%	1.6%	97.8%	4.5%	97.4%	0.082	0.269
All combined	55.8%	73.9%	60%	70.7%	67.2%	68.7%	NA	NA

Mild LVH*: For at least LVM ≥116 g/m^2 for men and ≥96 g/m^2 for women.
Moderate LVH**: For at least LVM ≥133 g/m^2 for men and ≥110 g/m^2 for women.
Severe LVH***: For at least LVM ≥149 g/m^2 for men and ≥122 g/m^2 for women.

Discussion

These findings demonstrate that the test performance of the ECG in diagnosing LVH is low in this Black African population. This is affected by a number of extracardiac factors such as age, sex, body habitus, and cardiac factors such as LVH severity and geometry. Sex specific adjustment to body habitus improves the test sensitivity. Dzudie et al. reported a similar finding of performance in a similar population [7]. Dada et al. reported a high test performance in a neighboring community [8]. The poor performance of the ECG in detecting LVH has been shown in several studies [4,12,13,14].

ECG and Sex

Sex is a major determinant of body structure and function. The Sokolow-Lyon criterion performed better in males. This could be attributed to the fixed voltage criterion that does not take account of structural body difference. Levy et al. reported an overall better performance in males where most indices used are non-sex specific [4]. Cornell criterion had an overall better performance especially in females. Rodrigues et al. reported a similar finding [14].

ECG and Age

Sokolow-Lyon and Cornell indices test performance decreased with advancing age. This was particularly significant with the Sokolow-Lyon criterion. The Cornell criterion showed a very weak but non-significant positive trend with age. Left axis shift and precordial voltages have been shown to decrease with age in men and left axis shift in women [15]. This could explain the trend observed with both criteria. Sokolow-Lyon index depends only on precordial leads while Cornell index depends on a precordial and limb leads. Left axis shift might lead to a higher R voltage in the augmented unipolar left limb lead used in Cornell index, thus a positive but non-significant trend. Aging is associated with physical changes such as a reduction in height. The enlarged heart then deviates to the left with changes in the cardiac vector as explained by Levy et al. [15]. Voltage changes associated with age cancel out with the Cornell index, thus less affected by age. The overall lower sensitivity with age could be attributed to lower tissue conductance, a point for further investigations.

ECG and Body Habitus

Sokolow-Lyon index showed a significant negative trend with increasing body size while Cornell index showed a non-significant positive trend. Levy et al. reported an overall negative trend [4]. Compared with normal weight patients, overweight and obese patients had a higher sensitivity and specificity with the Cornell index. This shows that the Cornell index is more accurate in diagnosing LVH in overweight and obese patients than Sokolow-Lyon index. Okin et al. reported a similar finding [5,16]. This could be explained by the high prevalence of LVH with obesity and attenuating effects of obesity on precordial voltages [17]. The less affected augmented limb lead in Cornell index will pull the voltage towards higher values for LVH. Sokolow-Lyon criterion depends on the precordial leads that undergo significant attenuation in overweight and obese patients, thus a decrease in its sensitivity.

ECG and LV Geometry

The sensitivity progressively increased with the severity of LVH and with the pathologic evolution of the LV with both indices. This was higher with the Cornell index. Levy et al. and Schillaci et al. reported a similar finding of increased sensitivity with LVH [4,13].

Table 4. Factors influencing the specificity and sensitivity for two selected index criteria: Sokolow-Lyon and Cornell indices.

Index	Sokolow-Lyon				Cornell			
	Sensitivity	**Specificity**	**r**	***p* value**	**Sensitivity**	**Specificity**	**r**	***p* value**
Sex								
Male	27.6%	83.3%	NA	NA	23.1%	90%	NA	NA
Female	24.3%	88.5%	–		49.2%	84.6%	–	–
Age								
≤55 years	35%	82.6%	–0.160	0.032	47.2%	87.1%	0.082	0.766
>55 years	26%	88.9%	–	–	32.5%	86.8%	–	–
Body habitus								
Underweight	40%	–	–0.248	0.001	20%	–	0.094	0.209
Normal	31.8%	72.7%	–	–	27.3%	86.4%	–	–
Overweight	29%	91.7%	–	–	45.2%	83.3%	–	–
Obesity1	15.6%	90.9%	–	–	28.1%	90.9%	–	–
LV geometry								
Normal	–	84.6%	0.172	0.020	–	100%	0.472	<0.0001
Remodeling	–	87.4%	–	–	–	87.8%	–	–
Concentric LVH	25.9%	73%	–	–	30.9%	73.4%	–	–
Eccentric LVH	30%	–	–	–	56.7%	–	–	–

NA: not applicable.

Table 5. Test performance of unadjusted and adjusted indices when the Left Ventricular Mass is indexed to the Body Surface Area.

Index	Threshold (Male/Female)	Sensitivity	Specificity	PPV	NPV	Accuracy	Likelihood ratio	r	*p* value
Sokolow-Lyon									
Unadjusted (mV)	3.5	26.5%	84.1%	73.2%	41.1%	48.4%	1.66	0.162	0.029
Adjusted to BSA (mV.m^2)	5.17/5.1	55.8%	46.4%	63%	39%	52.2%	1.04	0.283	<0.001
Adjusted to BMI (mV.Kg/m^2)	72.82/71.49	58.4%	40.6%	61.7%	37.8%	51.7%	0.98	0.270	<0.001
Cornell									
Unadjusted (mV)	2.8/2.0	37.2%	87%	82.4%	45.8%	56%	2.86	0.424	<0.0001
Adjusted to BSA (mV.m^2)	3.11/3.02	68.1%	52.2%	70%	50%	62.1%	1.43	0.501	<0.0001
Adjusted to BMI (mV.Kg/m^2)	44.23/42.74	69%	49.3%	69%	50%	61.5%	1.36	0.472	<0.0001
Combined indices									
Unadjusted	NA	50.4%	76.8%	78.1%	48.6%	60.4%	2.08	NA	NA
Adjusted to BSA	NA	77%	38.1%	62.1%	38.1%	56.6%	1.24	NA	NA
Adjusted to BMI	NA	79.6%	23.1%	62.9%	39.5%	57.7%	1.04	NA	NA

PPV: positive predictive value; NPV: negative predictive value; NA: not applicable.

Unadjusted and Adjusted Criteria

Sex specific adjustment to body habitus markedly increased the sensitivity by 2 fold with both Sokolow-Lyon and Cornell indices, with a fall in the specificity by a third and by half with Cornell and Sokolow-Lyon criteria. The highest increase was noted with Cornell index or combined indices adjusted to body mass index. With a fall in specificity, the predictive values were comparable (Table 5). Okin et al. and Norman et al. reported similar effects [5,6]. We used thresholds estimated from regression equations, which are considered to be the mean in the measured parameters. Sensitivity and specificity move in opposite directions [18]. Specificity increases with the set threshold, with a concomitant decrease in the sensitivity. Concomitant high sensitivity and specificity are seen in measurements with less spread about the mean (very strong correlation). This is however difficult to achieve with biological measurements especially when reproducibility is not perfect. Biological parameters have a high variability and are less reproducible. This gives sensitivities and specificities wide apart. The cut-off point between normal and abnormal of a test may therefore be varied to increase sensitivity or specificity (with concomitant decrease in the other) according to what we are using the test for [19]. LVH has been shown to be an independent cardiovascular risk factor and as well treatable [1,16]. It is best not to miss the diagnosis thus, the need for a test with a high sensitivity as the sex specific adjusted criteria [19]. Rodrigues et al. proposed a lower sex specific threshold for the Cornell index with the aim of improving the sensitivity [14]. This will be particularly useful in high risk patients. Further analysis using the ROC curve will give a clearer view of the situation with optimal cut-offs.

One of the limitations of our study is that only a single observer made the diagnosis of LVH both in the echocardiography and ECG. Echocardiography measurements are observer-dependent and no agreement test was carried out. The study was a specialist clinic based with selection bias of patients with heart disease. There is the risk of generalizing our findings. The echocardiography was used for comparison instead of more accurate tools like the CT scan and MRI. These are however very expensive, highly technical and not widely available. The echocardiography is widely available and user friendly, and has been shown to have a strong correlation with autopsy findings [20]. Not all possible determinants of electrocardiographic diagnosis of LVH were studied such as the cardiovascular risk factors and ethnicity. Moreover, our study is limited by the small number of subjects aged less than 40 years, as there is a significant difference in voltage between this younger age group and the more elderly. Hence the relationship between age and ECG test performance should be considered with caution. Notwithstanding, our work has some implications. We have contributed in paving the way for the ECG to be more accurate, since it is widely available and more user friendly than the echocardiography, and more accurate than the clinical method and X-ray in diagnosing LVH. Similar studies need to be carried out in the general population. A combined adjustment for age, sex, and body habitus with optimal cut-offs derived from the ROC curve is necessary for a clearer view of the possibility of improving the ECG. Fewer ECG criteria were studied further. Our choices were motivated by their better performance and are easier to use in routine clinical practice.

Conclusion

These findings demonstrate that the test performance of the ECG in diagnosing LVH is low in this black African population. This is affected by a number of extracardiac factors such as age, sex, body habitus, and cardiac factors such as LVH severity and geometry. Cornell voltage criteria had a higher performance and less affected than the Sokolow-Lyon voltage criteria. Sex specific adjustment to body habitus improves the test sensitivity by two fold and a fall in the specificity.

Author Contributions

Conceived and designed the experiments: AMJ JJNN. Performed the experiments: AMJ PK. Analyzed the data: AMJ JJNN. Contributed reagents/materials/analysis tools: AMJ JJNN SK. Wrote the paper: AMJ JJNN. Revised the manuscript: JJNN AMJ SK.

References

1. Levy D, Garrison RJ, Savage DD, Kannel WB, Castelli WP (1990) Prognostic implication of echocardiographically determined left ventricular mass in the Framingham Heart Study. N Engl J Med 322: 1561–1566.
2. National High Blood Pressure Education Program (1998) The sixth report of the Joint National Committee on Prevention, Detection, Evaluation, and Treatment of High Blood Pressure. Arch Intern Med 157: 241–46.
3. Chobanian AV, Bakris GL, Black HR, Cushman WC, Green LA, et al. (2003) The Seventh Report of the Joint Committee on Prevention, Detection, Evaluation, and Treatment of High Blood Pressure: the JNC 7 report. JAMA 289 (19): 2560–72.
4. Levy D, Labib SB, Anderson KM, Christianson JC, Kannel WB, et al. (1990) Determinants of Sensitivity and Specificity of Electrocardiographic Criteria for Left Ventricular Hypertrophy. Circulation 81: 815–820.
5. Okin PM, Roman MJ, Devereux RB, Kligfield P (1996) ECG identification of left ventricular hypertrophy. Relationship of test performance to body habitus. J Electrocardiol 29 Suppl: 256–61.
6. Norman JE Jr, Levy D (1996) Adjustment of ECG left ventricular hypertrophy criteria for body mass index and age improves classification accuracy. The effects of hypertension and obesity. J Electrocardiol 29 suppl: 241–7.
7. Dzudie A, Muna W, Kingue S, Akono M, Ouankou M, et al. (2006) Electrocardiograms to assess left ventricular hypertrophy in black African hypertensives. Abstract 005. First PanAfrican congress on hypertension organized by International Forum for Hypertension Prevention and Control in Africa (IFHA).
8. Dada A, Adebiyi AA, Aje A, Oladapo OO, Falase AO (2005) Standard Electrocardiogrphic Criteria for Left Ventricular Hypertrophy in Nigerian Hypertensives. Ethn Dis 15(4): 578–84.
9. Mbanya JCN, Minkoulou EM, Salah JN, Balkau B (1998) The prevalence of hypertension in rural and urban Cameroon. Int J Epidem 27: 181–185.
10. Kingue S, Befidi-Mengue R, Angwafo F III, Abbenyi AS, Wansi E, et al. (2000) Prevalence of hypertension in Cameroon. Preliminary results of the Cameroon National Health Survey (Abstract). Proc 12th Natn Med Conf Cameroon, Yaounde.
11. Lang RM, Biering M, Devereux RB, Flachskampf FA, Foster E, et al. (2005) Recommendations for chamber quantification: a report from the American Society of Echocardiography's guidelines and standards committee and the Chamber quantification writing group, developed in conjunction the European Association of Echocardiography, a branch of the European Society of Cardiology. J Am Soc Echocardiogr18: 1440–63.
12. Verdecchia P, Dovellini EV, Gorini M, Gozzelino G, Milletich A, et al. (2000) Comparison of eletrocardiographic criteria for diagnosis of left venricular hypertrophy in hypertension: the MAVI study. Ital Heart J 1(3): 207–15.
13. Schillaci G, Verdecchia P, Borgioni C, Ciucci A, Guerrieri M, et al. (1994) Improved electrocardiogrphic diagnosis of left ventricular hypertrophy. Am J Cardiol 74 (7): 714–9.
14. Rodrigues SL, D'Angelo L, Pereira AC, Krieger JE, Mill JG (2008) Revision of the Sokolow-Lyon-Raappaport and Cornell voltage criteria for left ventricular hypertrophy. Arq Bras Cardiol 90(1): 46–53.
15. Levy D, Bailey JJ, Garrison RJ, Horton MR, Bak SM, et al. (1987) Electrocardiographic changes with advancing age. A cross-sectional study of the association of age with QRS axis, duration and voltage. J Electrocardiol 20 Suppl: 44–7.
16. Okin PM, Jern S, Devereux RB, Kieldsen SE, Dahlof B, et al. (2000) Effect of Obesity on Electrocardiographic Left Ventricular Hypertrophy in Hypertensive Patients: the Losartan Intervention For Endpoint (LIFE) reduction in hypertension study. Hypertension 35(1pt 1): 13–8.
17. De Simone G, Devereux RB, Roman MJ, Aliderman MH, Laragh JH (1994) Relation of obesity and gender to left ventricular hypertrophy in normotensive and hypertensive adults. Hypertension 23: 600–606.
18. Akobeng AK (2007) Understanding diagnostic tests 1: Sensitivity, Specificity, and Predictive values. Acta Paediatr 96(3): 338–41.
19. Akobeng AK (2007) Understanding diagnostic tests 3: Receiver Operating Characteristics curves. Acta Paediatr 96(5): 644–7.
20. Devereux RB, Alonso DR, Lutas EM, Gottlieb GJ, Campo E, et al. (1986) Echocardiographic assessment of left ventricular hypertrophy: comparison to necropsy findings. Am J Cardiol 57: 450–80.

6

Noninvasive Technique for the Diagnosis of Patent Ductus Arteriosus in Premature Infants by Analyzing Pulse Wave Phases on Photoplethysmography Signals Measured in the Right Hand and the Left Foot

Sabrina Goudjil[1,3]*, Fatiha Imestouren[1], Aurelie Armougon[1], Lucie Razafimanantsoa[2], Mahdi Mahmoudzadeh[3], Fabrice Wallois[3], André Leke[1], Guy Kongolo[1,3]

1 Neonatal Intensive Care Unit, Amiens University Hospital, Amiens, France, **2** Pediatric Cardiology, Amiens University Hospital, Amiens, France, **3** INSERM U1105, GRAMFC, Jules Verne University of Picardie, Amiens, France

Abstract

Objective: To evaluate the impact of patent ductus arteriosus (PDA) on the pulse phase difference (PPD) between the left foot (postductal region) and the right hand (preductal region).

Materials and Methods: PPD was determined from arterial photoplethysmography signals (pulse waves) measured by infrared sensors routinely used for pulse oximetry in 56 premature infants less than 32 weeks gestation. Only infants with significant PDA (sPDA) diagnosed by echocardiography were treated with ibuprofen (for 3 days). Patients were classified according to whether or not they responded (Success/Failure) to this treatment. The Control group was composed of infants in whom ductus had already closed spontaneously at the time of the first echocardiography. The 3 groups were compared in terms of PPD at the beginning (T1) and at the end (T2) of the study. For patients in the Failure (n = 17) and Success groups (n = 18), T1 corresponded to the first day of treatment and T2 to the day after completion of the course of ibuprofen. In the Control group (n = 21), T1 corresponded to 1 to 3 days of life (DOL), and T2 to 4–6 DOL.

Results: Compared to the Control group, PPD was higher in the Failure (at T1 and T2) and Success (at T1) groups characterized by sPDA. After ibuprofen therapy, PPD in the Success group decreased to about the level observed in the Control group. The area under the ROC curve of PPD for the diagnosis of sPDA was 0.98 (95% CI 0.96–1); for an optimal cut-off of PPD ≥1.65 deg/cm, the sensitivity was 94.2% and the specificity was 98.3%.

Conclusion: In this study, PPD was correlated with ductus arteriosus status evaluated by echocardiography, indicating involvement of the ductal shunt in the mechanism of redistribution in systemic vascular territories. PPD can be considered for the diagnosis of hemodynamically significant PDA.

Editor: Vincenzo Lionetti, Scuola Superiore Sant'Anna, Italy

Funding: The authors have no funding or support to report.

Competing Interests: The authors have declared that no competing interests exist.

* E-mail: goudsab2002@yahoo.fr

Introduction

Patent ductus arteriosus is common in premature infants born before 32 weeks and is associated with high morbidity (i.e., pulmonary hemorrhage, necrotizing enterocolitis, acute renal failure, intraventricular hemorrhage, etc.) and mortality, especially in neonates with a birthweight less than 1000 g [1], [2]. This condition is characterized by a ductal shunt that diverts part of the aortic blood flow towards the pulmonary circulation, resulting in pulmonary vascular overload and decreased blood flow to systemic organs. Recent data suggest that the decrease in systemic blood flow is more pronounced in postductal regions than in preductal regions [3]. Treatment with ibuprofen or indomethacin is prescribed only in infants with significant patent ductus arteriosus and surgical ligation is proposed in the case of failure or contraindication to medical treatment. The characteristics of arterial pulse wave propagation are dependent on the mechanical properties of the blood vessel (inner diameter and wall thickness) and blood viscosity, according to the Moens-Korteweg law [4]. The fact that local hemodynamic conditions have an influence on blood vessel mechanics suggests that, in the presence of significant patent ductus arteriosus, pulse wave propagation properties would probably be impacted to varying degrees on preductal and postductal vessels [5], [6].

Some authors consider that blood oxygen saturation is low in congenital heart diseases and suggest to perform screening in newborn by criteria of postductal arterial oxygen saturation <95%

or a difference > 3% between pre and postductal saturation [7], [8].

The present study, using photoplethysmography signals recorded by conventional pulse oximetry technology measured the arterial pulse wave phase [9] in the right hand (preductal vascular area) and left foot (postductal vascular area) and then calculated the difference between these two values, corresponding to the pulse phase difference (PPD).

The objective of this study was to evaluate the impact of PDA on the PPD and to analyze PPD as a marker of ductal shunt severity (as classified by echocardiographic criteria).

Materials and Methods

This pilot study was conducted during the first week of life in premature infants, at the time of diagnosis and evaluation of patent ductus arteriosus in the Amiens University Hospital neonatal intensive care unit between August 2010 and July 2013.

Ethics Statement

The study protocol was approved by the Amiens University Medical Center Institutional Review Board (CPP Nord Ouest II-France, IDRCB: 2008-A00704-51). Infants between 26 and 32 weeks of gestational age investigated by echocardiography for the diagnosis of ductus arteriosus were eligible to participate in the study after obtaining written informed consent from their parents. The Institutional Review Board approved this consent procedure.

Study protocol

The study started at the time of echocardiographic assessment of ductus arteriosus status (T1). Patients with significant PDA were treated with a 3-day course of ibuprofen. A second echocardiography was performed on the day after completion of ibuprofen therapy to confirm ductus closure (T2). Photoplethysmography signals were recorded at T1 and T2 in the right hand and left foot, corresponding to preductal and postductal regions, respectively. Patients treated by catecholamine infusion were not included in this study. Clinical characteristics of the patients are summarized in Table 1.

Doppler echocardiography

Echocardiography protocols and diagnostic criteria for PDA complied with those published by several authors in many specialized journals [10], [11]. Patent ductus arteriosus was diagnosed on echocardiography by visualization of a left-to-right ductal shunt between the aortic isthmus and the pulmonary artery [12], [13]. In our study, patent ductus arteriosus was considered to be significant when it was associated with at least one of the two main echocardiographic criteria of severity (ductal diameter > 2 mm and/or left atrial-to-aorta diameter ratio (LA/Ao) >1.4) with at least one other criterion of severity (ductal shunt flow velocity (V_{ductus}) <1.2 m/s, mean left pulmonary artery flow velocity (LPAV) >0.40 m/s and end-diastolic LPA flow velocity (EDLPAV) >0.20 m/s). In our study, echocardiographic assessments were performed by neonatologists and were systematically reviewed by a pediatric cardiologist, who was not informed of PPD finding, to validate the results.

Photoplethysmography signals acquisition and extraction from the bedside monitor

Photoplethysmography signals were acquired in the right hand (preductal territory) and left foot (postductal territory) (Figure 1) using pulse oximetry infrared sensors [9], [14].

Electrocardiogram and thoracic respiratory movements were also recorded at the same time and were then extracted from the bedside monitor (MP40, Philips) to a laptop for further processing (Figure 2). The photoplethysmography signal sampling frequency was 125 Hz.

Empirical Mode Decomposition (EMD) of photoplethysmography signals

The technique developed in this study is based on determination and comparison of instantaneous angular position - the phase - of the arterial wave pulse in the hand and foot. This operation is only possible with mono-component signals such as those obtained by applying empirical decomposition [15], [16]. EMD is an adaptive technique for non-linear and non-stationary signal analysis based on the signal characteristics. In our study, EMD decomposed the photoplethysmography signal into stationary components with a very narrow frequency band corresponding to Intrinsic Mode Functions (IMF):

Table 1. Clinical characteristics of the study population.

	Failure group (n = 17)	Success group (n = 18)	Control group (n = 21)	p
GA, median (IQR), wks	27 (26.7–29)	28.9 (27–30)	29.4 (28–31)	ns
PNA, median (IQR), d	2.2 (1.2–2.9)	2.4 (1.6–2.8)	1.9 (1.4–2.5)	ns
BW, median (IQR), g	1080 (870–1280)	1230 (900–1410)	1250 (1000–1440)	ns
CRIB II, median (IQR)	8.1 (7.8–9.7)	8.3 (4.5–9)	7.7 (4.2–10)	ns
Hb, median (IQR)	10.7 (9.9–13.1)	12.6 (10.9–16)	12.4 (11.8–15.5)	ns
FiO2, median (IQR), %	21 (21–29)	21 (21–26)	23 (23–27)	ns
Vaginal delivery, %	52.9	55.5	57.1	ns
Antenatal steroids, %	70.6	61.5	71.4	ns
Tracheal ventilation, %	64.7	55.5	52.4	ns
Midazolam, %	17.6	16.7	19.0	ns
Sufentanyl, %	35.3	33.3	33.3	ns

GA, gestational age; PNA, Postnatal age; BW, Birth weight; CRIB II, clinical risk index for babies score; Hb, Hemoglobin; FiO_2, Fractional inspired concentration of oxygen; IQR, interquartile interval

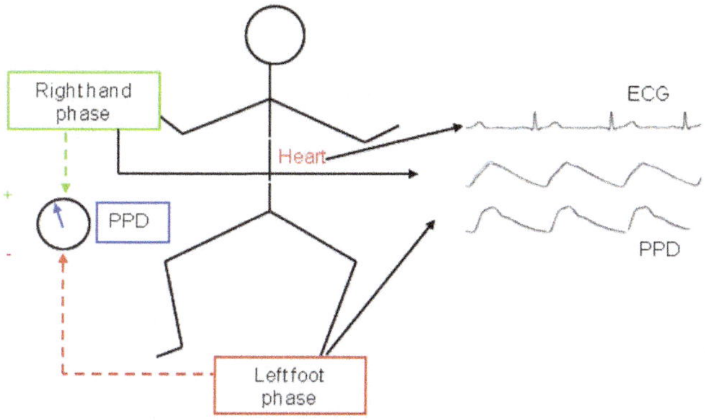

Figure 1. Photoplethysmography signals acquisition technique using infrared sensors. Acquired signals were used to compute pulse phases corresponding to preductal (right hand sensor) and postductal (foot sensor) regions and their difference, the PPD.

$$\mathbf{X(t)} = \sum_{n=1}^{N} \mathbf{c_n(t)} + \mathbf{r_N(t)} \qquad (1)$$

In this expression, X(t) corresponds to the original data; $c_n(t)$ are intrinsic mode functions (IMF) of specific time-scale obtained after sifting the original data; and $r_N(t)$ is the residue. In this study, extended EMD (EEMD) was applied to avoid mode mixing problems resulting from intermittent signals that can induce instability of EMD operations. In the EEMD version, many trials (n = 100) were repeated, each with a different sequence of white noise ($\sigma = 0.2$ times the amplitude of X(t)) added to the original signal X(t) before performing decomposition.

IMFc then represented the mean of a set of 100 trials. Technical and computational details on EMD and the improved EEMD version can be found in the papers by Huang *et al.* [17] and Lo *et al.*[16].

Figure 3 shows the results of decomposition of signals from the foot (A) and hand (B) after the EMD sifting operations. Each line corresponds to a distinct IMF related to physiologic phenomena with a specific time-scale.

In Figure 3, the intrinsic mode functions are organized in ascending order of time-scales from top to bottom. Depending on its complexity, a signal can be decomposed into a large number of IMF, each related to phenomena with a specific time-scale. In this study, the EMD features allowed identification of components (IMFc) whose energy was mostly concentrated around the time-scale corresponding to the patient's cardiac activity, which also allowed elimination of all global trends due to respiratory cycles, and artifacts from active body movements and other experimental errors.

Instantaneous phase of photoplethysmography signals

The IMFc was derived from decomposition of the signals recorded in the foot and hand. The IMFc was then submitted to Hilbert transformation [17] to obtain the amplitude and instantaneous phase of their analytic signals.

$$\mathbf{y(t)} = \frac{1}{\pi}\mathbf{P}\int_{-\infty}^{+\infty} \frac{\mathbf{c(t')}}{\mathbf{t-t'}}\mathbf{dt'} \qquad (2)$$

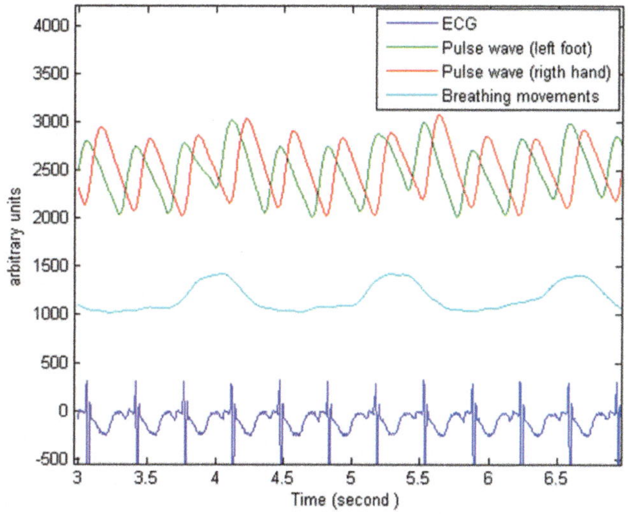

Figure 2. Raw photoplethysmography signals. These photoplethysmography traces show a delay between the recordings from the right hand and left foot in an infant with PDA.

where P indicates the Cauchy principal value, and y(t) the result of Hilbert transformation of the IMF signal c(t).

The analytic signal can be expressed as:

$$\mathbf{z(t)} = \mathbf{c(t)} + \mathbf{iy(t)} = \mathbf{A(t)e^{-\varphi(t)}} \qquad (3)$$

where A(t) is the instantaneous amplitude,

$$\mathbf{A(t)} = \sqrt{\mathbf{c^2(t)} + \mathbf{y^2(t)}} \qquad (4)$$

and φ(t), the instantaneous phase:

$$\varphi(\mathbf{t}) = \mathbf{a}\tan\left[\frac{\mathbf{y(t)}}{\mathbf{c(t)}}\right] \qquad (5)$$

Figure 4 shows the curves of instantaneous unwrapped phases of cardiac component (IMFc) in pulse signals from the hand (red) and foot (green). The graph on the left (Figure 4A) shows two very close phase curves corresponding to recordings from an infant in the Control group with closed ductus; the graph on the right (Figure 4B) shows a more marked difference between the two phase curves that were recorded in an infant of the Failure group with significant patent ductus arteriosus.

Determination of the pulse wave phase difference (PPD)

The pulse wave phase difference (PPD) was obtained by subtracting the phase of the signals recorded in the right hand from that recorded in the left foot (Figure 5).

PPD can also be analyzed on a simple statistical histogram (Figure 6) or on a Rose diagram angular graph.

In this study, PPD was determined 3 times for each investigation on randomly selected segments of photoplethysmography signals during quiet periods with regular electrocardiogram complexes and breathing movements. The three estimations were applied to compute the mean value of PPD for further analyses and were also used for determination of the coefficient of variation to confirm the reproducibility of the PPD technique [18].

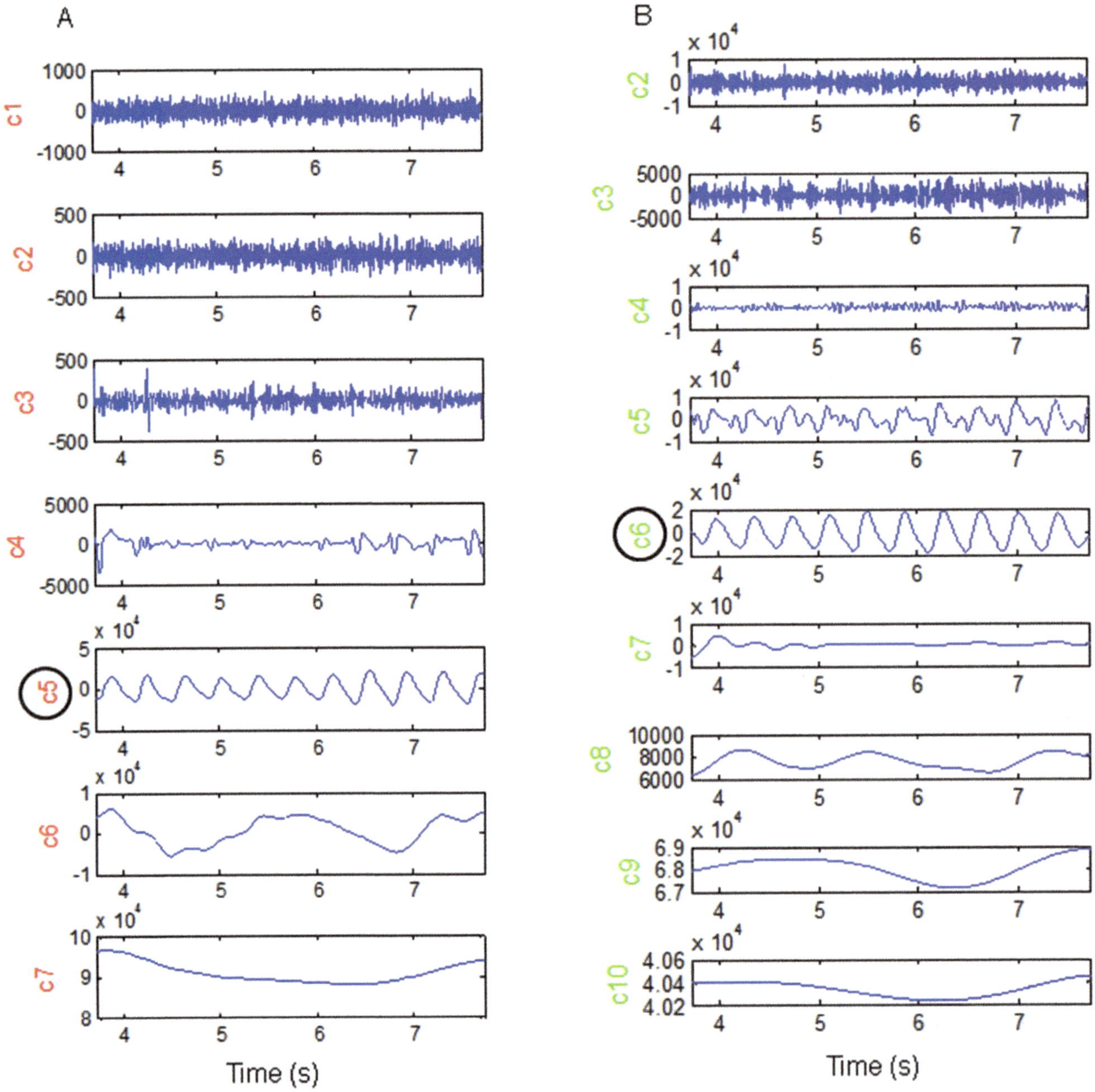

Figure 3. Intrinsic Mode Functions resulting from empirical decomposition of photoplethysmography signals. This figure shows the decomposition of signals recorded in the left foot (A) and right hand (B) in elementary functions (IMF) characterized by selective time-scale. This allowed the identification of components relating to cardiac activity (c5 in figure 3A and c6 in figure 3B). In these graphs, IMFs are organized in ascending order from top to bottom.

Patient classification

All patients with PDA were treated by intravenous ibuprofen according to the usual treatment protocols used in our neonatal unit (*Pedea*, 3 days of intravenous treatment: 10 mg/kg on the first day, 5 mg/kg on the 2nd and 3rd days). Echocardiography was repeated after ibuprofen therapy to confirm PDA closure.

Patients in whom ductus arteriosus was closed or constricted after ibuprofen therapy were classified in the Success group and those with persistent significant PDA despite medical treatment were classified in the Failure group.

A Control group was composed of infants with spontaneous closure of the ductus since the first echocardiographic assessment at 1–3 days and at the follow-up assessment performed at 4–6 days of life. Patients of Control group did not receive any treatment.

Statistical analysis

Quantitative variables were expressed as the median (IQR, 25th–75th percentile) and qualitative variables were expressed as number (percentage). Nonparametric Kruskal-Wallis ANOVA was performed to compare PPD between the three groups (Failure, Success and Control) and the Wilcoxon test was used

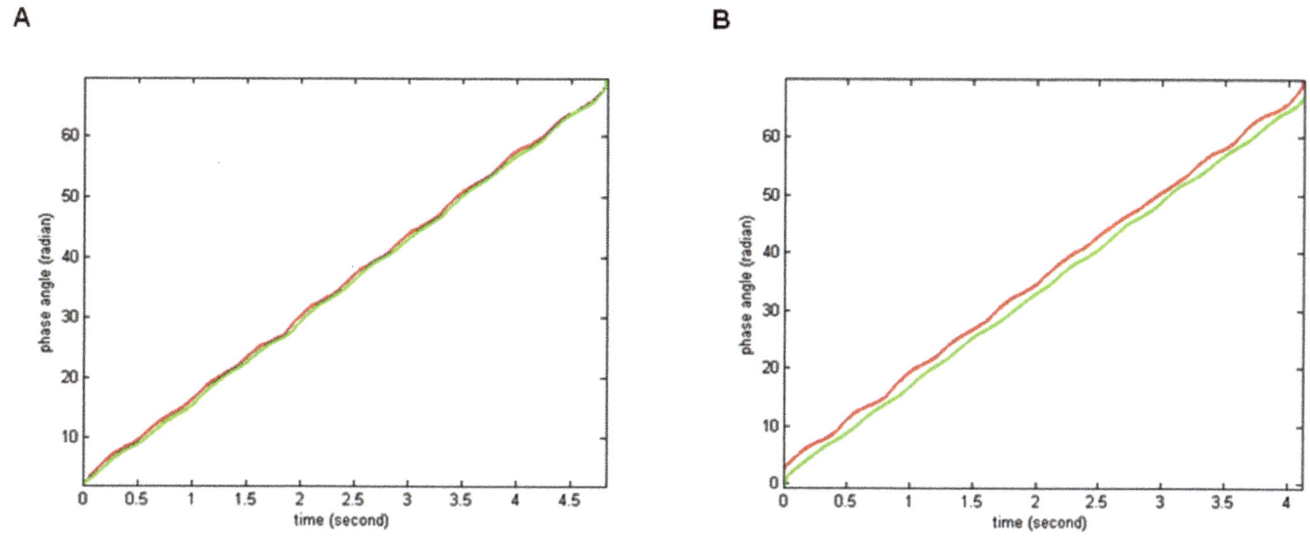

Figure 4. Unwrapped phase obtained by applying Hilbert transform to cardiac IMF. The phase curves obtained from an infant in the Control group (A) are very close, while those recorded in an infant from the Failure group are more distinct (B).

for comparison of paired observations between the first (T1) and second (T2) evaluation time-points. Statistical significance was defined as $p<0.05$.

Results

Clinical characteristics of the study population and management

A total of 56 premature infants were included in the study. Thirty five infants presented significant PDA diagnosed by echocardiography and were treated by ibuprofen. Following the 3-day intravenous ibuprofen therapy, constriction or closure of the ductus arteriosus was observed on echocardiography in 18 of these infants (6F/12M) (Success group). Seventeen patients (5F/12M) still had significant PDA after ibuprofen therapy (Failure group).

The clinical characteristics of the 21 infants (10F/11M) in the Control group, and those in Success and Failure groups are summarized in Table 1.

Echocardiographic characteristics of ductus arteriosus

Echocardiographic characteristics are summarized in Table 2. Ductus diameter was >2 mm in the Success and Failure groups at T1. At T2, ductus diameter in the Success group had decreased to very low values (about 0.5 mm).

As expected in the SUCCESS group at T2, ductal flow velocity became very high (2.6 m/s) and end-diastolic LPA velocity became lower than the values measured when the ductus was

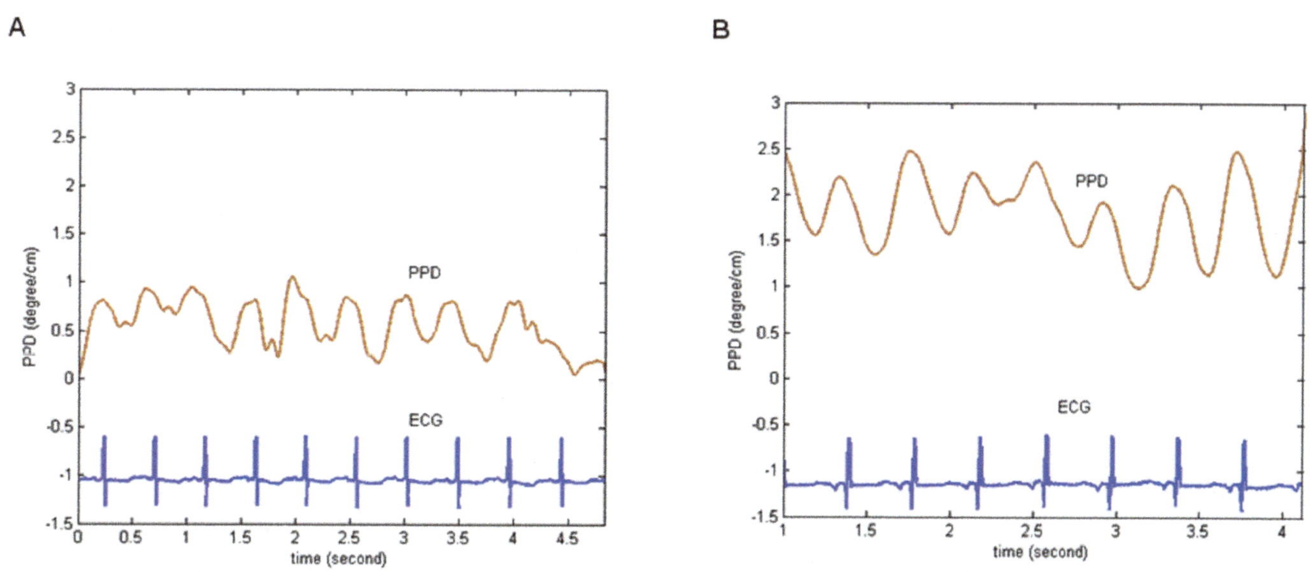

Figure 5. Time-course of PPD (deg/cm) normalized with respect to body height. (A) Infant with closed ductus; (B) Infant with patent ductus arteriosus. ECG, electrocardiogram; PPD, the pulse phase difference.

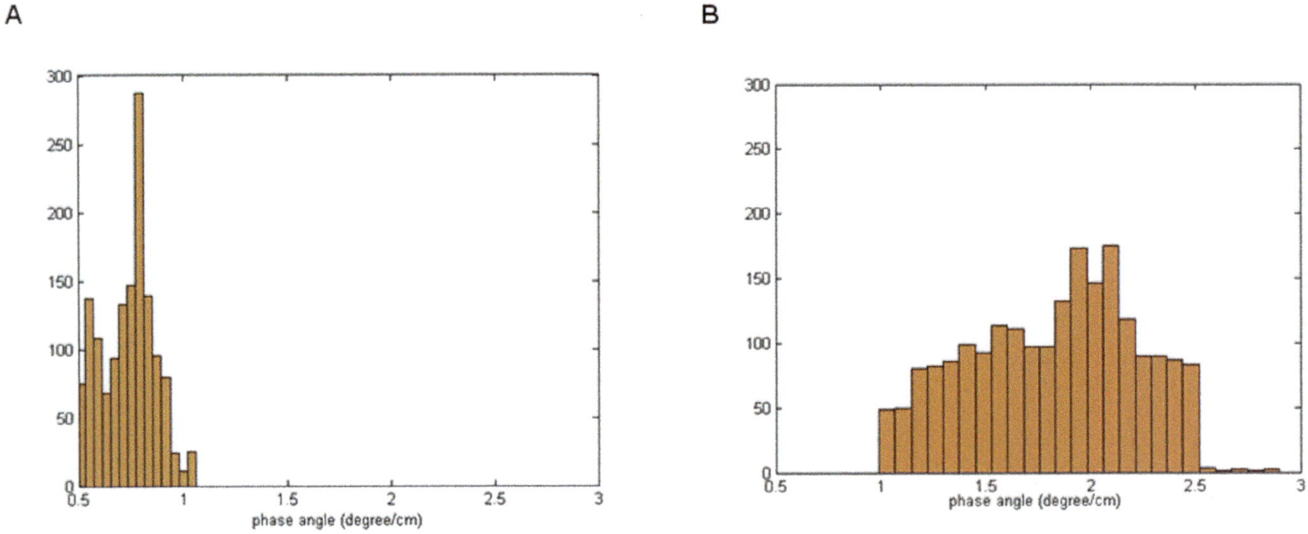

Figure 6. Histogram of distribution of PPD values (deg/cm). (A) Infant with closed ductus: the histogram of PPD is narrow and concentrated to segment less than 1 degree/cm; (B) Infant with patent ductus arteriosus: the histogram of PPD is broad, with values above 1 degree/cm.

fully patent (i.e, in the Failure group at T1 and T2, and in the Success group at T1).

Pulse wave phase difference (PPD) between the right hand and the left foot

In this study, the coefficient of variation of PPD was 11.6% for all measurements.

PPD results for each group are summarized in Figure 7.

The 3 groups were not homogeneous in terms of PPD at T1 (Kruskal-Wallis, $H(2, N=56)=35.6$; $p<0.001$. The PPD value in the Control group (T1: median, IQR: 0.74 (0.44–1.12)) was lower than those observed in the Failure group (T1: median, IQR: 2.46, 2.30–2.75; $p<0.001$) and in the Success group (T1: median, IQR: 2.48, 1.95–2.89; $p<0.001$). PPD was not significantly different between the Failure and Success groups.

The 3 groups also differed in terms of PPD at T2 (Kruskal-Wallis, $H(2, N=56)=35.3$; $p<0.001$). PPD decreased significantly between T1 and T2 in the Success group (T2: median, IQR: 1.03, 0.61–1.30; $p<0.001$, Wilcoxon) and became similar to the PPD values observed in the Control group (T2: median, IQR: 0.68, 0.59–1.16; $p=0.19$). PPD did not change between T1 and T2 in the Failure group (T2: median, IQR: 2.38, 2.24–2.76; $p=0.24$, Wilcoxon). The PPD value at T2 in the Failure group was higher than that measured in the Success ($p<0.001$) and Control groups ($p<0.001$). PPD did not change between T1 and T2 in the Control group ($p=0.77$).

Analysis of the PPD technique for the diagnosis of hemodynamically significant patent ductus arteriosus showed an optimal PPD cut-off of ≥1.65 deg/cm, with an area under the ROC curve of 0.98 (95% confidence interval, 0.96–1), a sensitivity of 94.2% and a specificity of 98.3% (Figure 8).

Discussion

The primary objective of this study was to analyze the pulse wave phase difference (PPD) between the preductal (right hand) and postductal (left foot) regions as function of the significant or closed-constricted status of the ductus arteriosus in preterm infants.

Table 2. Echocardiographic characteristics of the study population, median (IQR).

Group (n)	Failure (n = 17)		Success (n = 18)		Control (n = 21)	
	T1	T2	T1	T2	T1	T2
Ductal diameter (mm)	2.5 (2.3–2.5)	2.6 (1.8–2.9)	2.4 (2.2–2.6)	0.55 (0–0.9)**‡	-	-
V. ductus (m/s)	1.0 (0.8–1.9)	1.4 (1.0–2.4)	1.3 (1.1–2.3)	2.6 (2.1–2.9)*‡	-	-
LPAV (m/s)	0.67 (0.5–0.8)	0.77 (0.7–0.9)	0.55 (0.5–0.7)	0.3 (0.3–0.51)	0.3 (0.2–0.5)	0.38 (0.3–0.5)
EDLPAV (m/s)	0.3 (0.2–0.35)	0.22 (0.1–0.4)	0.25 (0.2–0.4)	0.1 (0.0–0.3)*	0.03 (0–0.04)	0.02 (0–0.05)
LA/Ao	1.42 (1.3–1.8)	1.36 (1.2–1.7)	1.4 (1.3–1.6)	1.2 (1.1–1.3)*	1.3 (1.1–1.4)	1.3 (1.2–1.4)

(‡): Data only for patients with constrictive ductus; **V. ductus**, Maximal ductal flow velocity; **LPAV**, Mean left pulmonary artery flow velocity; **EDLPAV**, End diastolic left pulmonary artery flow velocity; **LA/Ao**, Left atria-to-Aorta diameter ratio; **IQR**, Interquartile interval; **T1**, the day of diagnosis by echocardiography; **T2**, the day after the end of treatment with ibuprofen. For patients in the Control group, T1: 1–3 day of life and T2: 4–6 days of life; paired comparison T1 vs T2 in the same infants, (*): $p<0.05$, (**): $p<0.01$.

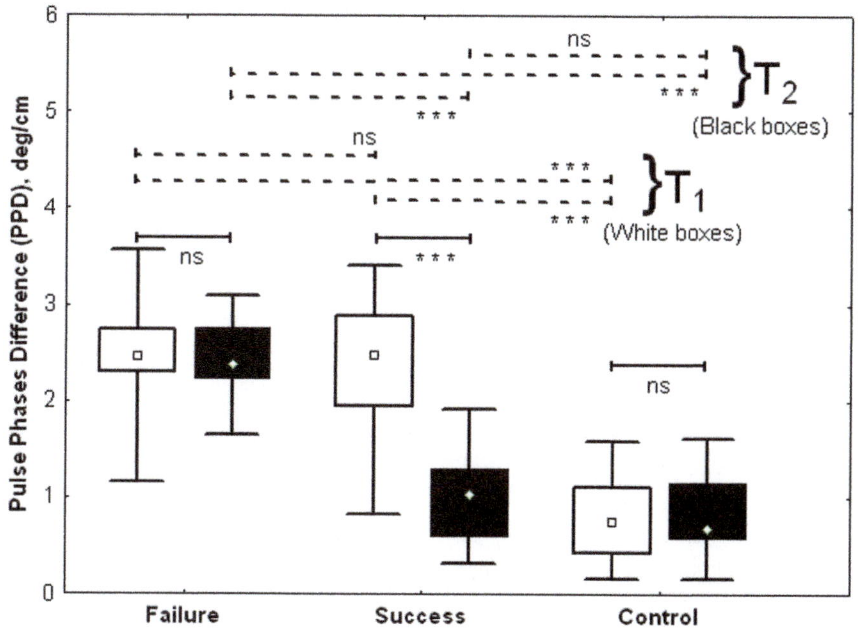

Figure 7. PPD during the study in function of classification in Failure, Success and Control groups (Median; Box: 25th -75th percentile; Whisker: Minimum-Maximum). The values of PPD (deg/cm) at the beginning of the study at T1 are represented with white boxes and at the end of the study (T2), with black boxes (***: $p<0.001$; ns: non significant).

PPD and ductus arteriosus status

The main findings from this study are that closed ductus is associated with low PPD values and significant patent ductus arteriosus is associated with high PPD values.

This is corroborated by the lower PPD values observed in patients of the Control and Success group at T2 after ibuprofen therapy. In these patients, the closed status of the ductus was confirmed by echocardiography. Moreover, in the Success group, ductus status changed from open to closed between the start and end of treatment while PPD decreased from high (about 2.4 deg/cm) to low values (about 1 deg/cm).

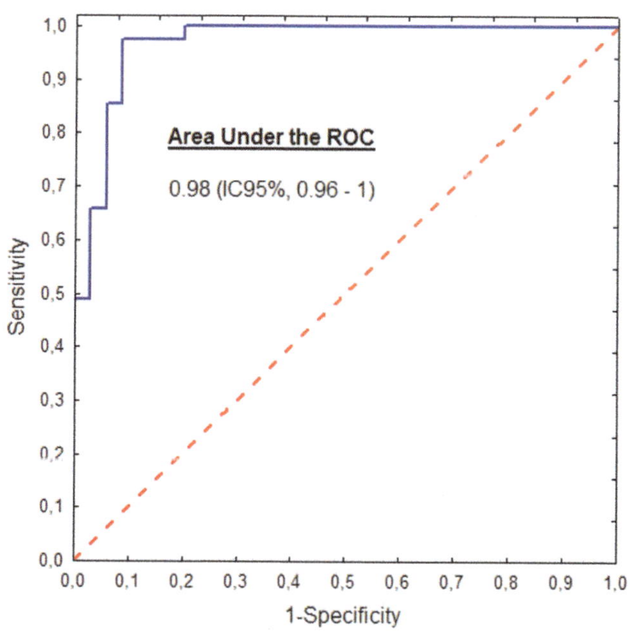

Figure 8. ROC curve of PPD for discrimination of infants with or without significant patent ductus arteriosus. For the optimal cut-off of PPD ≥1.65 deg/cm, the area under ROC curve was 0.98 (0.96–1) with a sensitivity of 94.2% and a specificity of 98.3%.

The highest PPD values were measured in patients with significant patent ductus arteriosus, corresponding to patients of the Success group at the start of the study (T1), and patients of the Failure group at both T1 and T2. As the study groups mainly differed in terms of closure of the ductus and not in terms of any other of the characteristics analyzed (Table 1), these results suggest an impact of ductus status on PPD. To our knowledge, such data have not been previously reported in the literature.

Other potential determinants of PPD

The pharmacologic effects of ibuprofen are less likely to be associated with the PPD differences observed between patients in the Control group and patients with PDA, as, at time-point T2, PPD was very high in Failure group but low in the Success group; however, patients in both groups received ibuprofen therapy.

In the Moens-Korteweg equation [19], wave velocity is dependent on blood viscosity, blood vessel diameter, wall thickness and wall elasticity: $\mathbf{C}=\sqrt{\mathbf{Eh}/\rho\mathbf{D}}$ (C = pulse velocity, D = vessel diameter, E = wall elasticity, h = wall thickness and ρ = blood viscosity).

Other factors such as mean blood flow in the vessel and mean blood pressure also influence pulse wave velocity, but via indirect mechanisms [20].

PDA is known to alter the distribution of blood flow to various organs, causing pulmonary vascular overload and decreased blood flow in the systemic circulation [1], [21]. Redistribution disorders are also observed in the various regions of the systemic circulation [22], [23]. The blood volume supplying the brain and upper limbs would be relatively preserved [5], as it is derived from large arteries arising from the aortic arch proximal to the ductus arteriosus [24]. Therefore, as vessel diameter is proportional to mean blood flow in a given territory [25], artery diameter would remain unchanged in preductal regions and would be significantly decreased only in postductal regions due to a more marked reduction of perfusion in postductal regions due to the ductal shunt [25].

Several other factors may also affect the elastic properties of vessels [26]: as catecholamine infusion can alter vascular tone [27], patients treated with catecholamines were therefore excluded from this study.

Blood viscosity influences arterial pulse propagation properties [20]. No significant change in hemoglobin was observed between the first (T1) and second examinations (T2) in any of the patients of this study, suggesting that blood viscosity remained unchanged. Moreover, no patient received blood transfusions during the study period. Some potential determinants of the PPD were recognized starting from speculation on the equation of Moens-Korteweg. However this model was validated on adults, it has been only few applications in neonates [28].

The pulse wave propagation time to a given territory also depends on the distance traveled from the heart. For this reason, in our study, PPD was normalized to the patient's body height prior to interpretation [29].

We believe that modulation of the autonomic nervous system (ANS) is also a determinant of pulse wave propagation properties due to its influence on vascular tone [30], [31].

In the Success group (responder patients), PPD decreased after closure of the ductus, but remained slightly higher (but not significantly) than the PPD value observed in the Control group (Figure 7). This aspect of PPD dynamics during treatment may suggest a memory process reflecting either a local phenomenon involving blood vessel wall mechanisms (histological, humoral.) or probably the influence of autonomic nervous system adaptations, which sometimes take many hours or days to completely resolve. Further appropriate studies are necessary to explore these hypotheses.

Technical specificities

In our study, we used a sampling frequency of 125 Hz for the acquisition of plethysmographic signal. The determination of the sampling frequency must meet the criterion of Shannon which states that its value must be at least twice the highest frequency of its spectrum [32], [33]. Studies have shown that the upper limit of the pulse plethysmographic signal spectrum remains below 25 Hz [34], [35]. In these conditions, the sampling frequency of 125 Hz performed in our study was adequate for the plethysmographic pulse signal.

Pulse wave phase characteristics are not usually analyzed for the purposes of PDA diagnosis and this analysis requires certain mathematical and engineering skills. This technique must therefore be automated before it can be used in routine clinical practice. The PPD method requires strict symmetry of the acquisition channels used to record the two photoplethysmography signals (hand and foot), since the main property of interest in this technique corresponds to the pulse wave phase difference. If this requirement is not met, it could lead to bias in PPD results. In the present study, this problem was avoided by using 2 symmetric modules in the MP40 monitor (Philips) originally designed to measure oxygen saturation by pulse oximetry from 2 different anatomic sites.

In our study the minimum value of PPD measured between the right hand and the left foot was 0.2 deg/cm; this was observed in the control group, in infants in whom the ductus arteriosus was closed. The manufacturer of MP40 monitor (Philips) ensures that recordings are symmetrical and synchronous when the two pulse oximetry modules (Philips M3001A and Philips M1020B # A01) used are original, as in our study [36].

The PPD technique developed in our study presents a number of advantages over conventional methods based on pulse transit time, as in the study by Oishi *et al.* [37]. In the present study, the EMD algorithm used to calculate PPD operates in the phase domain taking into account nonlinearities and nonstationarities usually contained in the photoplethysmography signals [38]. Based on permanent photoplethysmography waves, it was then possible to continuously estimate PPD in contrast with the conventional pulse transit time technique, which can provide only 1 estimation per cardiac cycle, dependent on R-peak detection on electrocardiogram (event-related approach) [39], [40].

Study limitations

PPD values are difficult to interpret due to the absence of reference values from large populations of healthy preterm infants. In this pilot study, the reproducibility of PPD was only estimated by the coefficient of variation (CV = 11.6%). In fact, when introducing a new measurement's system, reproducibility should be evaluated in terms of inter/intra operator and inter/intra session variability. This precaution was not respected in our study because it was difficult to impose repeated examinations (cardiac echography.) to these tiny premature infants hospitalized in the NICU, as they were in very critical clinical state.

In future studies, efforts should be undertaken to provide a more complete analysis of the variability associated with the PPD technique.

Photoplethysmography signals were recorded only from the right hand and left foot. The decision to place a pulse oximetry sensor at the right hand was justified by its location in the arterial preductal territory. For compliance with the study protocol and to minimize the uncontrollable sources of variations, the left foot was chosen as the postductal position in all infants. However, measurements of the postductal position could be the right foot.

In future studies, it would be interesting to verify the sensitivity of this technique when measurement sites are changed from right to left hand since the origin of the left subclavian artery from the aortic arch is also proximal to the ductus arteriosus [3], [24].

The echocardiography technique consists of detection of ultrasound energies reflected on measured structures enabling measurement of distances and flow velocities used to determine the severity of patient ductus arteriosus. In contrast, PPD is based on the temporal properties of pulse wave propagation and could therefore provide original information on PDA hemodynamics, independent of the parameters measured by echocardiography.

The post-hoc analysis of the statistical power

This pilot study provided the first quantitative data on the interest of PPD in the diagnosis of patent ductus arteriosus. Hence, it became possible to perform a post-hoc analysis of the statistical power for the PPD technique.

The design of our study was an anova model with within-effects (repeated measurements of PPD before and after ibuprofen treatment) and between-effects (the 3 groups: Failure, Success, Control) and within-between interactions.

When we considered that each of the 3 groups comprised only 17 patients (size of the smallest group), the statistical power was > 80% for the within, the between and the within-between effects.

Using equal size groups is recommended to avoid overestimating the statistical power when in actually, the anova study involves unequal groups [41]. Moreover, this is a requirement in the GPower3 program used in this study for calculation of the statistical power [42]. The results of this analysis (statistical power >80%) suggest that a total population of 56 infants should be adequate for this study.

Conclusion

PPD is a new noninvasive approach for the evaluation of PDA which proceeds in the analysis of photoplethysmography waves recorded in the right hand and the left foot using conventional pulse oximetry sensors. In this study, PPD measurements demonstrated good correlations with ductus status and were very reproducible: PPD was higher in patients with significant patent ductus arteriosus than in those with restricted or closed ductus. PPD can therefore be considered in addition to echocardiography which is the reference technique for diagnosis and evaluation of the ductus arteriosus. Automation of the PPD technique is required before considering its use in routine clinical practice.

Author Contributions

Conceived and designed the experiments: SG GK. Performed the experiments: SG GK FI AA. Analyzed the data: SG GK LR MM AL. Contributed reagents/materials/analysis tools: SG GK FW MM. Wrote the paper: SG GK MM.

References

1. Evans N, Kluckow M (1996) Early ductal shunting and intraventricular haemorrhage in ventilated preterm infants. Arch Dis Child Fetal Neonatal Ed 75: F183–186.
2. Beuchée A, Pladys P, Senhadji L, Bétrémieux P, Carré F (2003) Beat-to-beat blood pressure variability and patent ductus arteriosus in ventilated, premature infants. Pflugers Arch 446: 154–160.
3. Hiedl S, Schwepcke A, Weber F, Genzel-Boroviczeny O (2010) Microcirculation in preterm infants: profound effects of patent ductus arteriosus. J Pediatr 156: 191–196.
4. Wang JJ, Parker KH (2004) Wave propagation in a model of the arterial circulation. J Biomech 37: 457–470.
5. Hoodbhoy SA, Cutting HA, Seddon JA, Campbell ME (2009) Cerebral and splanchnic hemodynamics after duct ligation in very low birth weight infants. J Pediatr 154: 196–200.
6. De Felice C, Mazzieri S, Pellegrino M, Del Pasqua A, Toti P, et al. (2004) Skin reflectance changes in preterm infants with patent ductus arteriosus. Early Hum Dev 78: 45–51.
7. de-Wahl Granelli A, Wennergren M, Sandberg K, Mellander M, Bejlum C, et al. (2009) Impact of pulse oximetry screening on the detection of duct dependent congenital heart disease: a Swedish prospective screening study in 39,821 newborns. BMJ 338: a3037.
8. Zuppa AA, Riccardi R, Catenazzi P, D'Andrea V, Cavani M, et al. (2014) Clinical examination and pulse oximetry as screening for congenital heart disease in low-risk newborn. J Matern Fetal Neonatal Med 0: 1–5.
9. Millasseau SC, Guigui FG, Kelly RP, Prasad K, Cockcroft JR, et al. (2000) Noninvasive assessment of the digital volume pulse. Comparison with the peripheral pressure pulse. Hypertension 36: 952–956.
10. Evans N, Iyer P (1994) Assessment of ductus arteriosus shunt in preterm infants supported by mechanical ventilation: effect of interatrial shunting. J Pediatr 125: 778–785.
11. Skinner J (2000) Ductal shunting. In: Skinner J, Alverson D, Hunter S, editors. Echocardiography for the neonatologist. London: Churchill-Livingstone. pp. 151–167.
12. Evans N (2008) Functional Echocardiography in the Neonatal Intensive Care Unit. In: Kleinman C, Seri I, editors. Hemodynamics and Cardiology. Philadelphia: Saunders. pp. 83–109.
13. El Hajjar M, Vaksmann G, Rakza T, Kongolo G, Storme L (2005) Severity of the ductal shunt: a comparison of different markers. Arch Dis Child Fetal Neonatal Ed 90: F419–422.
14. Pologe JA (1987) Pulse oximetry: technical aspects of machine design. Int Anesthesiol Clin 25: 137–153.
15. Huang NE, Shen Z, Long S, Wu M, Shih H, et al. (1998) The empirical mode decomposition and the Hilbert spectrum for non-linear and non-stationary time series analysis. Proc R Soc Lond A 454: 903–995.
16. Lo MT, Hu K, Liu Y, Peng CK, Novak V (2008) Multimodal Pressure Flow Analysis: Application of Hilbert Huang Transform in Cerebral Blood Flow Regulation. EURASIP J Adv Signal Process 2008: 785243.
17. Huang NE, Shen Z, Long S (1999) A new view of non-linear water waves: the Hilbert spectrum. Annu Rev Fluid Mech 31: 417–457.
18. Armitage P (2002) Measure of variation. Description data. In: Armitage P, Berry G, Matthews J, editors. Statistical method in medical research. 4 ed. Massachusetts, USA: Blackwell Sciences. pp. 43–44.
19. Fung Y (1981) Mechanical properties of blood vessels. Wave propagation. In: Fung Y, editor. Biomechanics: Mechanical Properties of Living Tissues. New York: Springer-Verlag. pp. 282–283.
20. Caro C, Pedley T, Schroter R, Seed W (2012) Wave propagation in arteries. In: Caro C, Pedley T, Schroter R, Seed W, editors. The Mechanics of the Circulation. 2 ed. Cambridge: Cambridge University Press. pp. 268–278.
21. Teixeira L, McNamara P (2006) Enhanced intensive care for the neonatal ductus arteriosus. Acta Paediatr 95: 394–403.
22. Agata Y, Hiraishi S, Misawa H, Hirota H, Nowatari M, et al. (1994) Regional blood flow distribution and left ventricular output during early neonatal life: a quantitative ultrasonographic assessment. Pediatr Res 36: 805–810.
23. Shimada S, Kasai T, Konishi M, Fujiwara T (1994) Effects of patent ductus arteriosus on left ventricular output and organ blood flows in preterm infants with respiratory distress syndrome treated with surfactant. J Pediatr 125: 270–277.
24. Szpinda M (2007) Morphometric study of the ascending aorta in human fetuses. Ann Anat 189: 465–472.
25. Peters J, Mack GW, Lister G (2001) The importance of the peripheral circulation in critical illnesses. Intensive Care Med 27: 1446–1458.
26. Kelly RP, Millasseau SC, Ritter JM, Chowienczyk PJ (2001) Vasoactive drugs influence aortic augmentation index independently of pulse-wave velocity in healthy men. Hypertension 37: 1429–1433.
27. Freyschuss U, Hjemdahl P, Juhlin-Dannfelt A, Linde B (1986) Cardiovascular and metabolic responses to low dose adrenaline infusion: an invasive study in humans. Clin Sci (Lond) 70: 199–206.
28. Cheung YF, Wong KY, Lam BC, Tsoi NS (2004) Relation of arterial stiffness with gestational age and birth weight. Arch Dis Child 89: 217–221.
29. Yasmin, Brown MJ (1999) Similarities and differences between augmentation index and pulse wave velocity in the assessment of arterial stiffness. QJM 92: 595–600.
30. Allen J (2007) Photoplethysmography and its application in clinical physiological measurement. Physiol Meas 28: R1–39.
31. Ahn JH, Kong M (2011) The Relationship among Pulse Wave Velocity, Ankle-Brachial Pressure Index and Heart Rate Variability in Adult Males. Korean J Fam Med 32: 406–411.
32. Oppenheimer A, Schafer R (1989) Discrete-time signal processing; Oppenheimer A, editor. New York: Prentice Hall.
33. Stoica P, Moses R (2005) Power spectral density of random signals. In: Stoica P, Moses R, editors. Spectral analysis of signals. New Jersey: Prentice Hall. pp. 4–8.
34. Sherebrin MH, Sherebrin RZ (1990) Frequency analysis of the peripheral pulse wave detected in the finger with a photoplethysmograph. IEEE Trans Biomed Eng 37: 313–317.
35. Chowienczyk PJ, Kelly RP, MacCallum H, Millasseau SC, Andersson TL, et al. (1999) Photoplethysmographic assessment of pulse wave reflection: blunted response to endothelium-dependent beta2-adrenergic vasodilation in type II diabetes mellitus. J Am Coll Cardiol 34: 2007–2014.
36. Philips (2007) Manuel d'utilisation. Moniteur Patient IntelliVue MP20/30, MP40/50, MP 60/70/80/90. Allemagne: Philips.
37. Oishi M, Nishida H, Kabe K, Hoshi J (1993) Monitoring neonatal peripheral circulation by electrocardiogram-to-oximeter pulse velocity. Pediatr Res 33: 653–657.
38. Landsverk SA, Hoiseth LO, Kvandal P, Hisdal J, Skare O, et al. (2008) Poor agreement between respiratory variations in pulse oximetry photoplethysmographic waveform amplitude and pulse pressure in intensive care unit patients. Anesthesiology 109: 849–855.
39. Pagani J, Villa M, Calcagnini G, Alterio A, Ambrosio R, et al. (2003) Pulse transit time as a measure of inspiratory effort in children. Chest 124: 1487–1493.
40. Smith R, Argod J, Pépin J, Lévy P (1999) Pulse transit time: an appraisal of potential clinical applications. Thorax 54: 452–457.
41. Cohen J (1988) The analysis of variance. In: Cohen J, editor. Statistical power analysis for the behavioral sciences. 2 ed. New York: Psychology Press, Taylor & Francis Group. pp. 273–403.
42. Faul F, Erdfelder E, Lang AG, Buchner A (2007) G*Power 3: a flexible statistical power analysis program for the social, behavioral, and biomedical sciences. Behav Res Methods 39: 175–191.

7

Speckle-Tracking Echocardiography Elucidates the Effect of Pacing Site on Left Ventricular Synchronization in the Normal and Infarcted Rat Myocardium

Michal Mor[1◎], Wesam Mulla[1◎], Sigal Elyagon[1], Hovav Gabay[1,2], Shani Dror[1], Yoram Etzion[1,3¶*], Noah Liel-Cohen[4¶]

1 Cardiac Arrhythmia Research Laboratory, Department of Physiology and Cell Biology, Faculty of Health Sciences, Ben-Gurion University of the Negev, Beer-Sheva, Israel, **2** Department of Emergency Medicine, Recanati School for Community Health Professions, Faculty of Health Sciences and PREPARED Center for Emergency Response Research, Ben-Gurion University of the Negev, Beer-Sheva, Israel, **3** Division of Internal Medicine, Soroka University Medical Center, Beer-Sheva, Israel, **4** Cardiology Department, Soroka University Medical Center, Beer-Sheva, Israel

Abstract

Background: Right ventricular (RV) pacing generates regional disparities in electrical activation and mechanical function (ventricular dyssynchrony). In contrast, left ventricular (LV) or biventricular (BIV) pacing can improve cardiac efficiency in the setting of ventricular dyssynchrony, constituting the rationale for cardiac resynchronization therapy (CRT). Animal models of ventricular dyssynchrony and CRT currently relay on large mammals which are expensive and not readily available to most researchers. We developed a methodology for double-site epicardial pacing in conscious rats. Here, following post-operative recovery, we compared the effects of various pacing modes on LV dyssynchrony in normal rats and in rats with ischemic cardiomyopathy.

Methods: Two bipolar electrodes were implanted in rats as follows: Group A ($n=6$) right atrial (RA) and RV sites; Group B ($n=7$) RV and LV sites; Group C ($n=8$) as in group B in combination with left coronary artery ligation. Electrodes were exteriorized through the back. Following post-operative recovery, two-dimensional transthoracic echocardiography was performed during pacing through the different electrodes. Segmental systolic circumferential strain (Ecc) was used to evaluate LV dyssynchrony.

Results: In normal rats, RV pacing induced marked LV dyssynchrony compared to RA pacing or sinus rhythm, as measured by the standard deviation (SD) of segmental time to peak Ecc, SD of peak Ecc, and the average delay between opposing ventricular segments. LV pacing and, to a greater extend BIV pacing diminished the LV dyssynchrony compared to RV pacing. In rats with extensive MI, the effects of LV and BIV pacing were markedly attenuated, and the response of individual animals was variable.

Conclusions: Rodent cardiac pacing mimics important features seen in humans. This model may be developed as a simple new tool to study the pathophysiology of ventricular dyssynchrony and CRT.

Editor: Alena Talkachova, University of Minnesota, United States of America

Funding: This work was supported by a research grant from the Clalit Research Institute, Clalit health services, Israel (Yoram Etzion and Noah Liel-Cohen). The funders had no role in study design, data collection and analysis, decision to publish, or preparation of the manuscript.

Competing Interests: The authors have declared that no competing interests exist.

* E-mail: tzion@bgu.ac.il

◎ These authors contributed equally to this work.

¶ These authors also contributed equally to this work.

Introduction

Dyssynchronous contraction of the left ventricle (LV) can markedly worsen the outcome of heart failure (HF) independently of traditional risk factors [1,2]. This pathophysiology is often derived from or exacerbated by native conduction delay, such as left bundle branch block (LBBB) or artificial pacing of the right ventricle (RV) [3–5]. Based on QRS widening, it is estimated that at least 25–30% of patients with HF exhibit dyssynchronous LV contraction [6,7]. Clinical studies employing biventricular (BIV) pacing (cardiac resynchronization therapy; CRT) to treat HF patients with dyssynchronous contraction have revealed significant benefits in terms of contractile performance, improved quality of life, and long-term survival [8].

Although dyssynchronous heart failure (DHF) has been extensively studied in mechanical terms and although the clinical effectiveness of CRT is remarkable, there are multiple issues that remain ill-defined at present. It is, for example, estimated that around 30% of patients do not benefit from CRT, and the clinical criteria to identify CRT non-responders remain obscure and controversial. In addition, there is variability in individual patient vulnerability to DHF progression in response to conventional RV pacing, which is difficult to predict at present [4,9]. Only recently has the impact of dyssynchrony and BIV pacing on molecular signaling and the ionic properties of the myocardium been realized [9,10]. Animal studies have shown that DHF is associated with regional molecular changes (collectively termed 'molecular polarization'), including downregulation of Ca^{2+} handling proteins and connexin 43, activation of stress response kinases and increased expression of tumor necrosis factor in the lateral LV wall. Most of these changes can be reversed by CRT [11]. Additional studies identifying regional changes in ionic channels and multiple gene transcripts [12,13] have revealed a highly complicated picture in which multiple players are involved. Therefore, comprehensive understanding of the effects of various pacing modes at the molecular level will require extensive additional scientific efforts.

One of the problems hampering progress in this field of research is the lack of suitable animal models that can be utilized for routine experimentation. Current studies almost exclusively utilize large animals (mainly dogs) and are based on the implantation of human devices. Such an experimental setting is highly demanding. In addition, the large animal models can not be manipulated genetically, an issue that is becoming increasingly critical when it is necessary to reveal molecular mechanisms. While rat and mouse models are extensively used in research on HF [14], these animal models are largely missing in research on DHF and CRT, mainly due to technical difficulties in electrode implantation. Two independent studies using M-mode echocardiography have managed to demonstrate dyssynchrony between the septum and the LV lateral wall in the murine heart [13,15]. In addition, in the pioneering study of Bilchick et al. 2006 mice were implanted with a single pacing electrode on the RV free wall and were paced for seven days using an implanted miniature pacemaker. Using microarray analysis, this study demonstrated indications for molecular polarization as a result of prolonged RV pacing [13,15]. Thus, it appears that rodents may mimic important features that are seen in large mammals in regard to the mechanical effect of ventricular pacing. However, to the best of our knowledge, the mechanical effect of RV pacing as compared with LV and BIV pacing has not yet been defined in rodents.

In the present study, using an implanted device that was developed for pacing and recordings in conscious rodents [16], we acutely evaluated the effect of pacing site on LV synchronization in normal and infarcted rats following post operative recovery. We hypothesized that the mechanical effects of LV pacing and BIV pacing should be favorable compared to RV pacing. Elucidation of this issue seems critical in order to clarify whether rodent models may be further developed as simple experimental tools to study the molecular biology of DHF and CRT. Utilizing speckle-tracking 2-dimensional echocardiography, a method that has been repeatedly validated in rats for segmental strain analysis over the past decade [17–20], we confirmed the existence of mechanical dyssynchrony when RV pacing was applied. In addition, we elucidated the electrical and mechanical effects of LV pacing and BIV pacing. Overall, our results support the notion that the effects of pacing in rodents can recapitulate important features observed in large animal models and humans.

Methods

Ethics statement

All animal studies reported in this article were approved by the institutional ethics committee, Faculty of Health Sciences, Ben-Gurion University of the Negev, Israel. At the end of all experiments animals were killed using IV KCl injection under deep isoflurane anesthesia.

Implantable rat pacing device

The implantable device that was used to pace the heart at different locations was originally designed for long-term atrial pacing and recording in freely moving rats [16]. In this device, the electrical connections to the epicardial surface are achieved using miniature-bipolar hook electrodes, which have been described in detail previously [16]. The specific design of the miniature-bipolar hook electrode allows it to be positioned on a desired location on the epicardial surface of the atria or ventricles through a small lateral thoracotomy without the need of additional suturing [16]. The implantable device consists of an 8-pin 'female' connector that is attached by flexible insulated electrical wires to a set of two miniature bipolar hook electrodes (Figure 1a). Peripheral electrodes that are implanted on the back for pseudo ECG measurements also exist (Figure 1a,c). Before implantation, the 8-pin 'female' connector was covered with a latex sheath to prevent direct contact with the subcutaneous tissue during the operation. Electron beam radiation was applied for sterilization of the device before use.

Surgical procedures

Adult male Sprague-Dawley rats (250–300 g) were anesthetized (ketamine/xylazine 75/5 mg/kg, IP) and mechanically ventilated. The animals were placed supine on a warmed heating and under sterile conditions a skin incision in the left thorax was performed and a subcutaneous tunnel was extended posteriorly to the upper back of the animal. The 8-pin 'female' connector (covered with a latex sheath) was inserted through the subcutaneous tunnel. Thereafter, lateral thoracotomy was performed and the two miniature -bipolar hook electrodes were positioned as follows: Group A; on the right atrium (RA) and RV apex (RV). Group B; on the RV and on the posterobasal aspect of the left ventricle (LV). Group C; similar electrode implantation as in group B, as well as proximal left anterior descending coronary artery ligation to induce myocardial infarction (MI). In order to insert electrodes on the right side (for positioning on the RA and RV) a small subcutaneous tunnel was done in the chest wall through which the electrodes were moved to the right side of the thorax. The coronary artery was ligated by 6/0 surgical suture and MI was confirmed by the presence of regional cyanosis in the myocardial surface. Following chest closure, each animal was placed in a prone position and the back connector was exteriorized through the skin of the back (Figure 1B). Postoperative recovery and analgesia were done as described previously [16].

Cardiac pacing and echocardiograpy

Normal rats were evaluated 6–8 days following the surgical procedure. MI rats were evaluated 14 days following the surgical procedure. For the echocardiograpic analysis, each animal was sedated (isoflurane 1%) and placed on a heating pad. ECG recordings (Nihon Kodhen, RMC1100) were monitored online throughout the experiment and were also digitized and stored for offline analysis in each pacing mode (PCI-6024E, National Instruments, Austin, TX, USA). Electrical stimulation (2 ms square pulses) was applied through isolation units (Iso-Flex, AMPI, Israel) at a double diastolic threshold. The cycle length that was used to induce override pacing in the normal rats was set to 150 ms (400 bpm) which invariably induced override pacing in these animals. In the MI rats, baseline heart rate was sometimes slightly higher than 400 bpm. Therefore, the override pacing cycle length was set to 140 ms (428 bpm), which managed to override

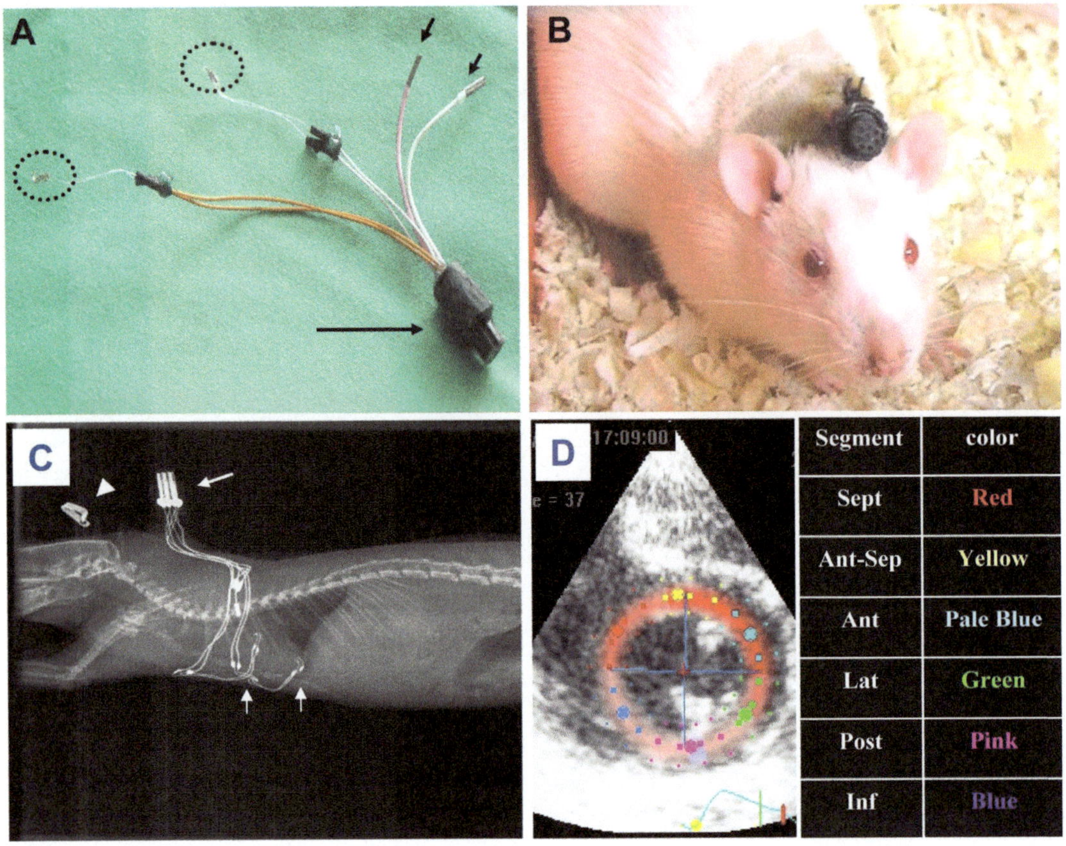

Figure 1. Experimental setup for LV strain analysis in paced rats. A: An implanted pacing device consisting of two miniature-bipolar hook electrodes (dotted circles). Long arrow; 8-pin back connector. Short arrows; peripheral electrodes for optional pseudo ECG measurements in conscious animals [16]. **B**: A rat with an exteriorized back connector following the implantation procedure. **C**: X-ray lateral view of an implanted rat. The two miniature-bipolar hook electrodes (vertical arrows at the bottom) were inserted on the RV and the LV as described in the text. The X-ray view is shown for illustration and was not utilized to access the position of the electrodes on the heart. D: Short axis mid-level echocardiographic view of an implanted rat and standard separation map of the LV into six segments for circumferential strain (Ecc) analysis.

the spontaneous heart rate of these animals. During BIV pacing, two independent isolation units were used for simultaneous but independent RV apical and LV pacing. A program developed by YE [16] was used to control data acquisition, electrical stimulation and off-line analysis. QT interval measurements were manually done off-line on the digital signals under high time and voltage magnification scales. These measurements were performed using dedicated cursors which marked the isoelectric line and stressed out the time of return of the ECG signal to this line. The measured QT intervals of five independent complexes were averaged in each condition to reduce sampling error. Two-dimensional transthoracic echocardiography was performed with a Vivid 7 echocardiography system (GE Healthcare, Milwaukee WI, USA) by short-axis mid-ventricular scans at the level of the papillary muscle tips. Images were obtained with a 10 S transducer (5.4~11.8 MHz) using an image depth of 2.5 cm and a frame rate of 225 frames/s as was repeatedly validated in the literature in rat studies [17-20]. The acquisition protocol was as follows: Following optimal positioning of the transducer on the chest wall, it was fixed in place by the operator, while 2D clips (20 s each) were sequentially recorded in sinus rhythm followed by override pacing at the different pacing sites. Of note, we took special care that the transducer will stay in the exact same position throughout the experiment to allow for accurate comparison between the different pacing modes in each animal. The procedure was always done by two experimentalist, one acquiring there echocardiography clips and the other controlling the pacing and confirming continuous electrical capture in each pacing mode. At the end of each experiment, the animal was sacrificed and correct positioning of the epicardial electrodes was confirmed by post mortem operation. Offline analysis of LV fractional area shortening (LV-FAS) was done by calculating the LV areas during maximal systole (LVAs) and during maximal diastole (LVAd) and then expressing LV-FAS as: (LVAd-LVAs)/LVAd×100.

Circumferential 2-dimensional strain analysis

Based on the existing literature in rodents, we restricted our current analysis to circumferential strain (Ecc) which is more reliable than radial strain in the small heart of rats [18,19]. Ecc was evaluated as described in the literature [17-19]. Briefly, analysis of mid-level short-axis images was done with dedicated software ("2D-strain", EchoPAC, GE healthcare, Vingmed, Norway). Endocardial border at end-systole and the region of interest from the endocardium to the epicardial edge were determined by the user (Figure 1d). Thereafter, an automatic speckle tracking analysis was performed for the short-axis images to track the motion of speckles contained within the region of interest on a frame-to-frame basis [21]. Ecc curves, expressed in percentage values as a function of time were exported to a customized program (MATLAB software, MathWorks) to calculate the time from onset of QRS to peak Ecc (time to peak Ecc) and the value of maximal Ecc (across the six mid-level segments (Figure 1d, Figure 2a). The values of maximal Ecc are shown as % of segmental length at onset QRS complex. At least five consecutive beats were analyzed under each pacing condition in each animal. Initial determination of the region of interest from the endocardium to the epicardial edge was performed under no pacing conditions and was kept as constant as possible during the different pacing conditions. Analysis of all rats in each group was done by a single observer (MM - normal rats, WM - MI rats). An independent observer who is highly experienced in echocardiographic methodologies including 2D strain analysis (NLC) confirmed the consistency of the analysis performed by the two observers.

Statistical analysis

Values are expressed as means ±SE. Due to the relatively small sample size in each group, analysis of the difference between pacing conditions was done using Kruskal-Wallis one way analysis of variance on ranks with Student-Neuman-Keuls post hoc test. All statistical tests were done using SigmaStat 3.1 (Systat Software, Inc, Point Richmond, CA). The criterion for significance was set at $P<0.05$.

Results

RV pacing versus RA pacing or sinus rhythm in normal rats

As a first step we aimed to compare the effect of RV pacing to both no pacing and RA pacing modes. This analysis was done in order to confirm that the override pacing itself does not induce rate-dependent LV dyssynchrony compared to the no pacing mode (sinus rhythm). For that purpose, group A (n = 6) was instrumented with a bipolar RA pacing electrode and a bipolar RV pacing electrode, and override pacing in these two locations (150 ms CL) was compared to the no pacing state. The obtained Ecc traces of the different LV segments typically demonstrated no major differences between RA pacing and sinus rhythm. In contrast, RV pacing invariably induced marked changes in the segmental strain pattern. The RV pacing typically produced an early systolic contraction in the inferior or posterior segments, which was associated, in some cases, with a clear stretching effect in opposing segments (Figure 2A). Summary of the segmental time to peak Ecc and the segmental peak Ecc patterns under the different pacing modes is presented figure 2B. Analysis of important global parameters derived from the segmental Ecc analysis under the different pacing modes is shown in Figure 3. The global time to peak Ecc was found to be slightly shorter during RA pacing compared to no pacing (85.6±4.1%, $p<0.05$) an was also shorter compared to RV pacing (Figure 3A). Global peak Ecc (Figure 3B) was not different between RA pacing and no pacing but was markedly attenuated during RV pacing (61.0±3.7% compared to no pacing, $p<0.01$ compared to both RA pacing and no pacing). While the Ecc analysis identified a marked effect of RV pacing on strain parameters, concurrent analysis of LV-FAS did not identify a significant effect of the different pacing modes on this parameter (Figure 3C, see discussion). Specific analysis of LV dyssynchrony variables indicated marked deleterious effects of RV pacing on all the calculated parameters, including standard deviation of time to peak Ecc (Figure 3D), standard deviation of peak Ecc (Figure 3E) and the average time difference between the peak Ecc of opposing segments (Delta TP opposing segments, Figure 3F). There was no statistical difference in these parameters between RA pacing and sinus rhythm.

Effects of different ventricular pacing modes in normal rats

In the next stage, we evaluated group B (n = 7) rats, which had bipolar pacing leads in the RV and LV. The effect of override pacing in these two locations alone or simultaneously (BIV pacing) was compared to the no pacing mode. In terms of electrical activity, the ECG recording indicated QRS prolongation during RV pacing as compared to LV and BIV pacing (Figure 4A). However, the unclear separation between the QRS and the T-wave in the rodent heart [22,23], did not allow quantitative analysis of QRS width during the various pacing modes. Nevertheless, an analysis of QT duration indicated marked QT prolongation during RV pacing (138.3±5.3%, $p<0.01$) as compared to the no pacing mode. This marked QT prolongation was reduced by LV pacing (124.9±2.9%) and even further reduced by BIV pacing (109.1±3.6%), as shown with detailed statistical analysis in Figure 4B. In addition, recordings of epicardial electrograms from the RV electrode when pacing the LV and vice versa, was performed in two animals from group B. These recordings supported a longer sequence of activation during RV pacing compared to LV pacing (Figure 4C).

We next evaluated the mechanical dyssynchrony during the various pacing modes. Summary of the segmental time to peak Ecc and the segmental peak Ecc under the different pacing modes in group B are presented figure 5. Analysis of important global parameters derived from the segmental Ecc analysis under the different pacing modes is shown in Figure 6. RV pacing significantly reduced both the global time to peak Ecc and the global peak Ecc as compared to no pacing. These parameters recovered significantly during LV and BIV pacing (Figure 6A, B). In addition, while a prominent increase in all the parameters of LV dyssynchrony was noted during RV pacing, LV pacing and particularly BIV pacing markedly improved all three parameters of LV dyssynchrony (Figure 6 D–E). Of note, the segmental pattern of the time to peak Ecc during RV pacing (Figure 5) was somewhat different from that observed in group A (Figure 2), possibly due to variability in the positioning of the RV electrode on the epicardial surface of the RV (see limitations section in our discussion). As in group A (Figure 3), we could not detect significant changes in LV-FAS during the different pacing modes (Figure 6C).

Effects of different ventricular pacing modes in rats with ischemic-induced heart failure

To elucidate the influence of ischemic HF on the electromechanical results of our model, group C (n = 8) was subjected to a combined procedure of electrode implantation and left coronary artery ligation. We analyzed the effect of pacing two weeks following surgery, at a time when prominent scar tissue and myocardial remodeling were present (Figure 7A, B). Out of the eight animals with confirmed MI, one had electrical capture only in the LV and was excluded from analysis. Two additional animals had electrical capture only in the RV and were therefore analyzed only in the no pacing and RV pacing modes. Final statistical analysis was done only on the five MI rats that exhibited electrical capture in both RV and LV sites. In electrophysiological terms, the MI rats demonstrated baseline prolongation of the QT interval compared to the normal rats (94.0±4.4 ms vs. 70.5±4.4 ms, $p<0.001$). However, the effect of pacing on the QT interval followed a similar trend to that in the normal rats. Indeed, RV pacing

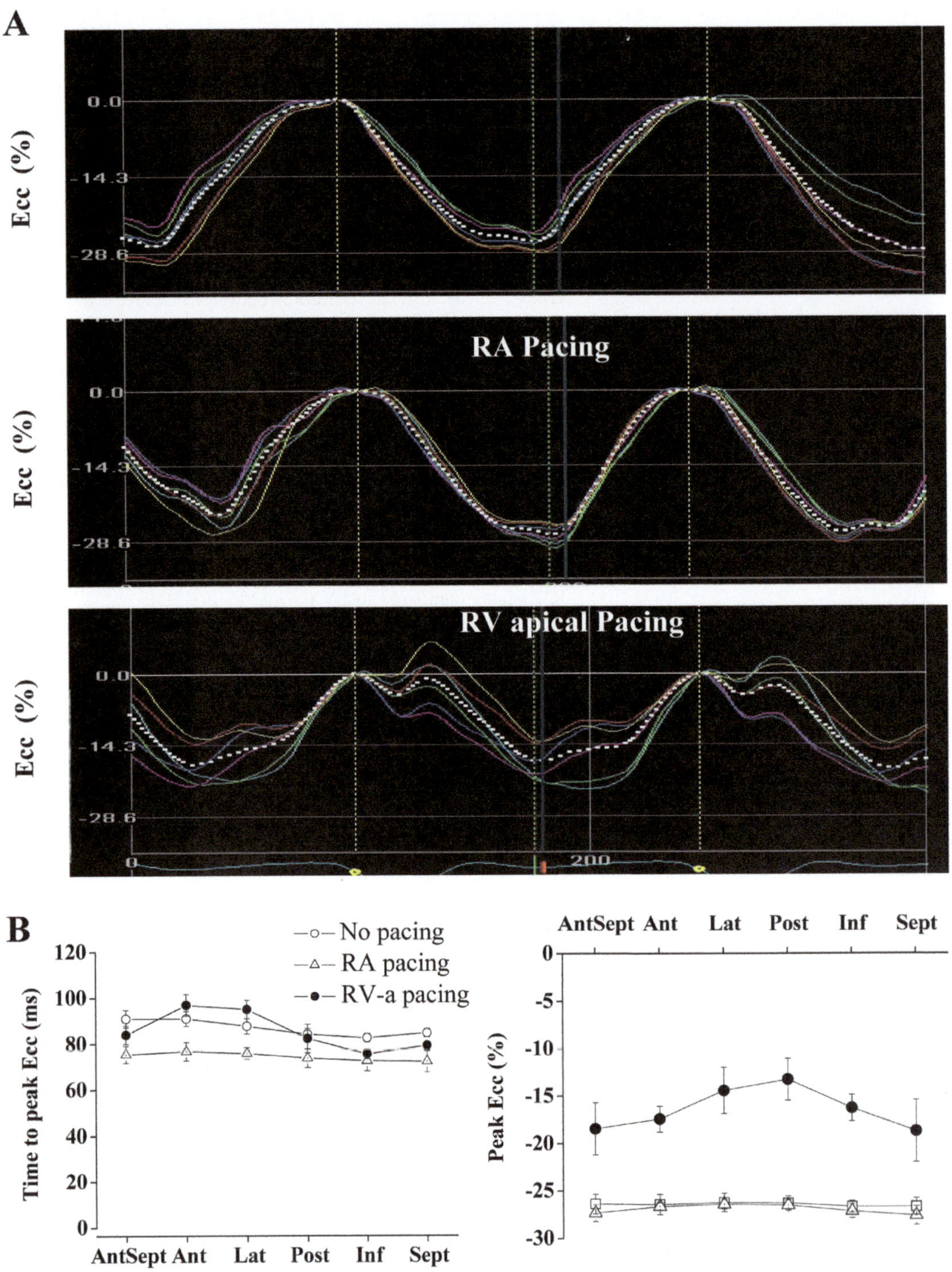

Figure 2. Segmental Ecc analysis during RA and RV pacing. A: Representative strain waveforms in an instrumented rat subjected to no pacing (upper), RA pacing (middle) and RV (lower). The colors of the different waveforms match those in the segmental map in Figure 1D. White dotted lines represent the global (average) strain of all six segments. **B**: Average segmental time to peak Ecc (left) and peak Ecc (right) in seven animals subjected no pacing, RA pacing, and RV pacing.

statistically increased the QT interval as compared with no pacing mode (118.6±3.7%, $p<0.05$), while the QT during LV and BIV pacing did not differ from sinus rhythm (113.9±4.7% and 106.2±3.9%, respectively, see details in Figure 7C).

Evaluation of segmental Ecc in group C revealed typical akinesia or dyskinesia in the anteroseptal, anterior and lateral segments at baseline (Figure 7D). No apparent effect of pacing on the magnitude and temporal pattern of the peak Ecc was observed in these rats (Figure 7E, Figure 8 A,B). In addition, while dyssynchrony parameters were much higher in the MI animals at baseline, there were no apparent effects of the different pacing modes on these parameters, excluding a non-significant tendency

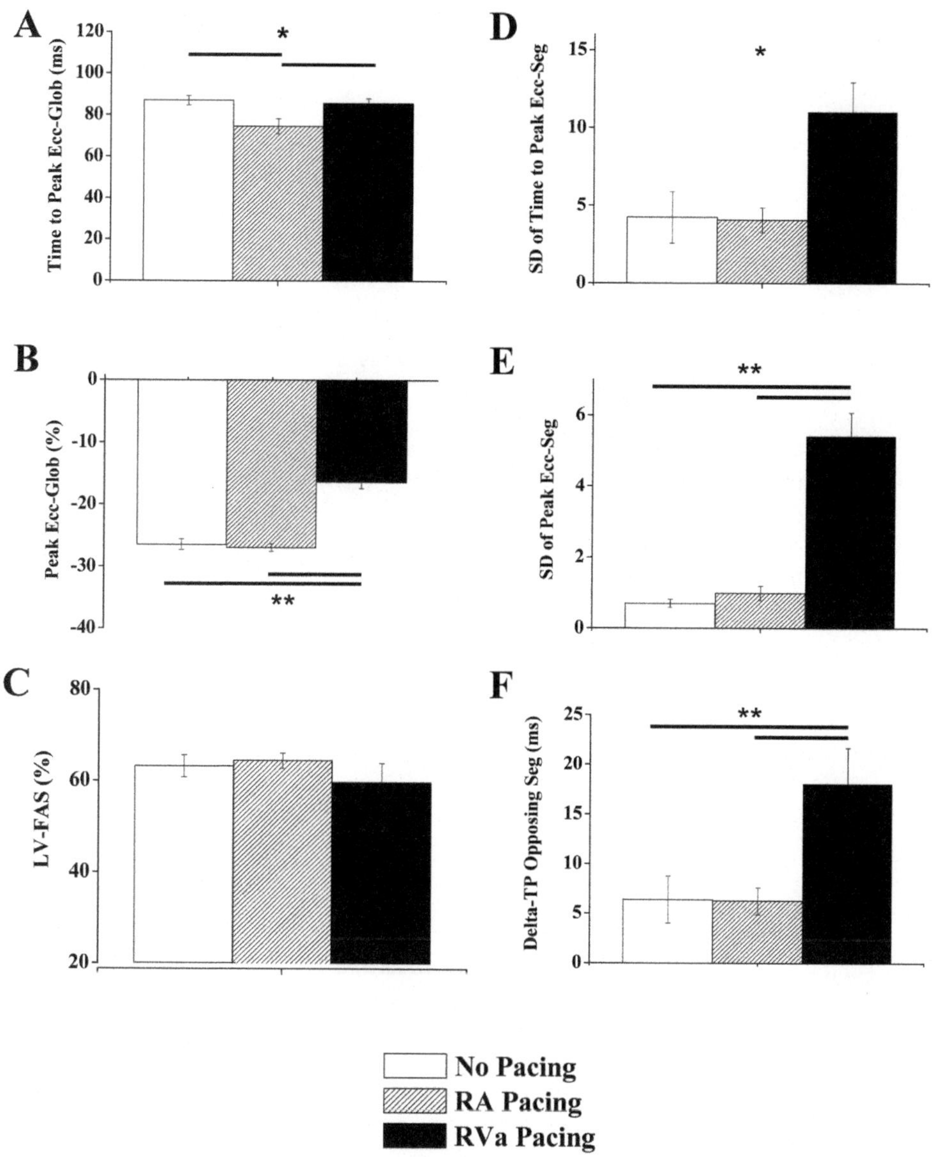

Figure 3. RV pacing induces marked LV dyssynchrony compared to RA pacing. Summary of echocardiographic parameters in group A subjected to no pacing, RA pacing, and RV pacing. **A**: Average time to peak Ecc of all six segments (global). **B**: Average peak Ecc of all six segments (global). **C**: LV fractional area shortening. **D**: Standard deviation of the time to peak Ecc of different segments. **E**: Standard deviation of the peak Ecc of different segments. **F**: Analysis of 'delta TP opposing segments', i.e., the average time difference between the peak Ecc of opposing segments. * $P < 0.05$, ** $P < 0.01$. Horizontal lines above\below the bar graphs indicate significant differences between pacing modes in the post-hoc analysis. Note that in **D** the Kruskal-Wallis test was significant. However, the post-hoc analysis could not reveal the source of difference between the groups.

to increase in the 'delta TP opposing segments' parameter during RV pacing (Figure 8 D–F). Looking more closely at the effect of pacing on the 'delta TP of opposing segments' in individual rats (Figure 9 A), we observed a consistent tendency for this parameter to increase during RV pacing in 6 out of the 7 evaluated animals. Compared with RV pacing the effects of LV pacing and BIV pacing on the delta TP of opposing segments were variable. While these pacing modes seemed to have a beneficial effect in some cases (e.g., animals 2 and 3), there was a worsening of this parameter in animal 5 when LV and BIV pacing were applied (Figure 9 A). An additional analysis specifically focusing on the two opposing segments that had maximal temporal dyssynchrony during RV pacing detected a rather similar pattern (Figure 9 B, C).

Discussion

The present study introduces a new model of ventricular pacing in an instrumented rat, which allowed us for the first time to systematically evaluate the effects of pacing site on LV synchronization in the rodent heart. We used speckle-tracking echocardiography analysis of Ecc, which has been reported to reliably and sensitively detect changes in LV dyssynchrony under various clinically relevant conditions in the rat heart [17–20]. The speckle-tracking echocardiographic methodology has previously been applied extensively in large animal models and in people and has been shown to be much more sensitive to changes in LV dyssynchrony than global echocardiographic measures, such as fractional shortening [24]. Therefore, in the present study, it is not

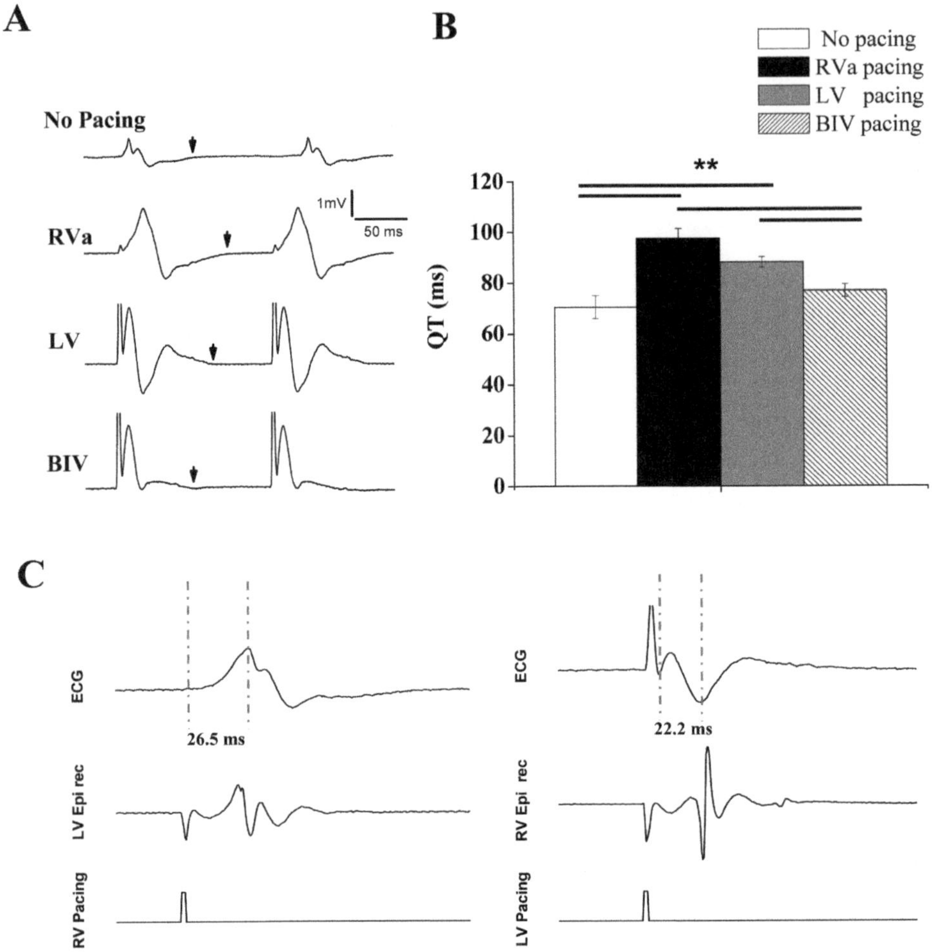

Figure 4. RV pacing induces electrical dyssynchrony compared to LV and BIV pacing. A: Representative ECG recordings from an instrumented rat during sinus rhythm (no pacing) and during RV, LV and BIV pacing. Arrows indicate the termination of the T wave in each trace. **B**: Summary of QT interval analysis in six instrumented rats. ** P<0.01. Horizontal lines above the bar graph indicate significant differences between pacing modes in the post-hoc analysis. **C**: Example of epicardial electrograms during RV pacing (left) and LV pacing (right). In each recording upper trace is a peripheral ECG signal (Lead I), middle trace is the epicardial electrogram and lower trace shows the time of cardiac pacing. Note that the epicardial activation in the RV electrode correlates with a late negative vector in the ECG signal. In contrast, the epicardial activation during RV pacing is correlated with a late positive vector in the ECG signal. Measurements of the time from end of stimulus artifact to the peaks of these late vectors in the ECG (dash vertical lines) indicate shorter activation time during LV pacing. Analysis of epicardial electrograms in an additional animal from group B demonstrated similar findings (not shown).

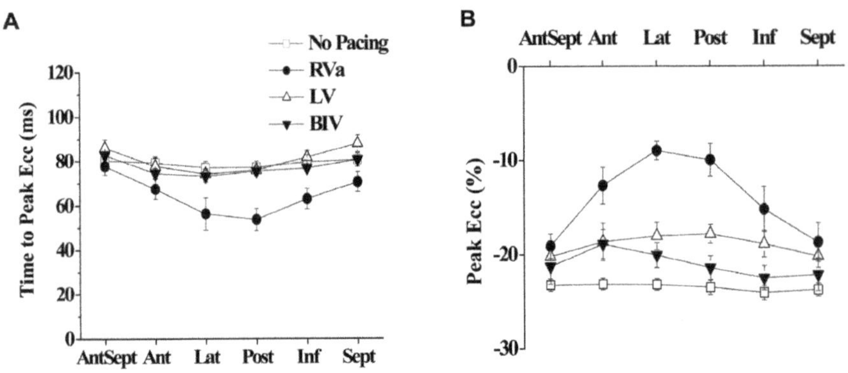

Figure 5. Segmental Ecc analysis during RV, LV and BIV pacing. Average segmental time to peak Ecc (**A**) and peak Ecc (**B**) in seven animals from group B subjected to no pacing, RV pacing, LV pacing and BIV pacing.

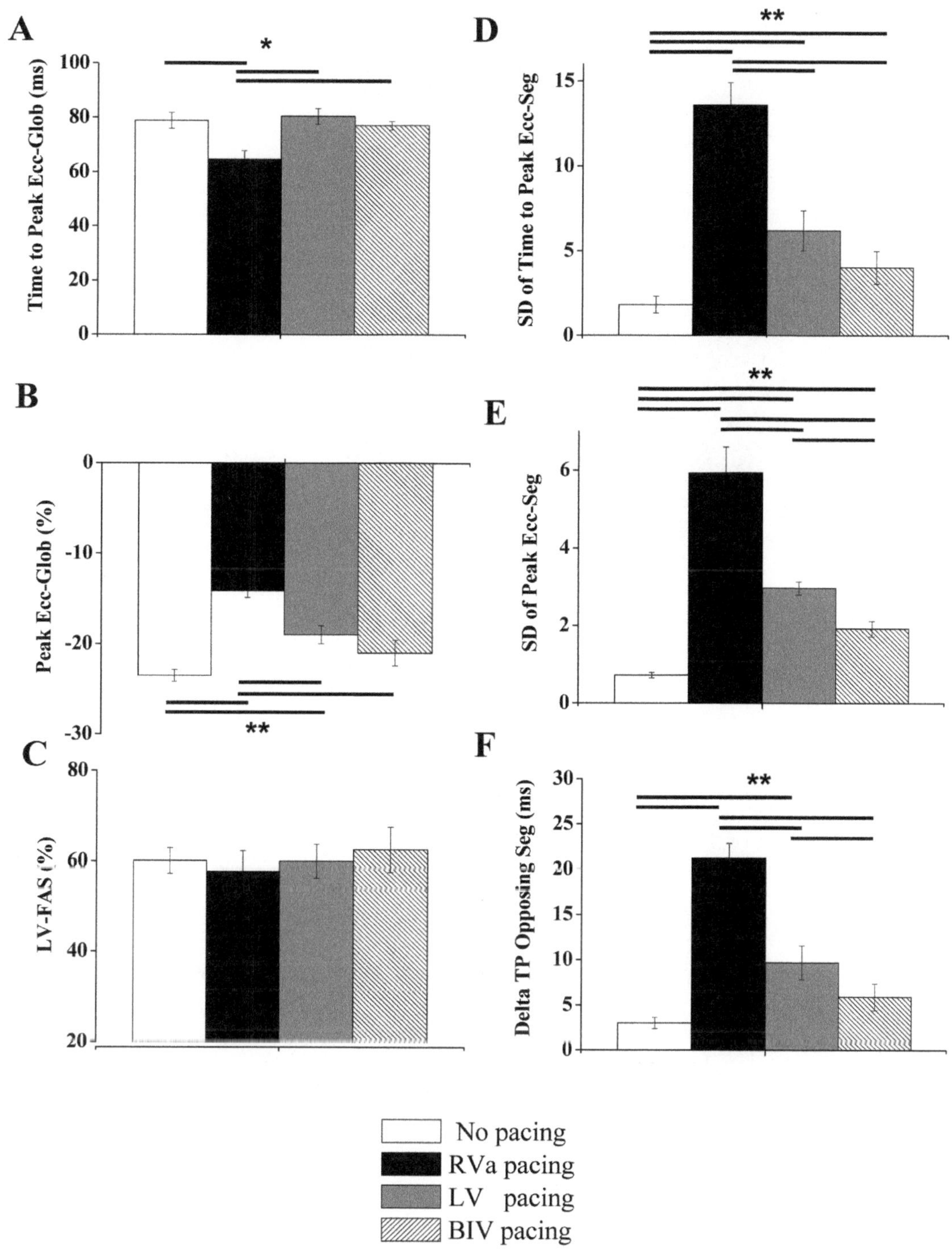

Figure 6. RV pacing induces mechanical dyssynchrony compared to LV and BIV pacing. Summary of echocardiographic parameters in six animals subjected to no pacing, RV, LV and BIV pacing. **A**: Average time to peak Ecc of all six segments (global). **B**: Average peak Ecc of all six segments (global) **C**: LV fractional area shortening **D**: Standard deviation of the time to peak Ecc of different segments. **E**: Standard deviation of the peak Ecc of different segments. **F**: Average time difference between the peak Ecc of opposing segments ('delta TP opposing segments', see Figure 3 for details). * $P<0.05$, ** $P<0.01$. Horizontal lines above\below the bar graphs indicate significant differences between pacing modes in the post-hoc analysis.

surprising that there were no significant effects of pacing on LV-FAS, while the effects of pacing site on segmental and global Ecc pattern were consistent and significant.

The main findings of our Ecc analysis indicate that while the rodent heart has some clear differences compared to the human heart in aspects such as action potential repolarization and calcium handling [22,23,25], its mechanical response to the effect of various pacing modes seems to have important similarities to the large mammalian heart. While previous studies in the mouse heart have already demonstrated negative effects of acute RV pacing on

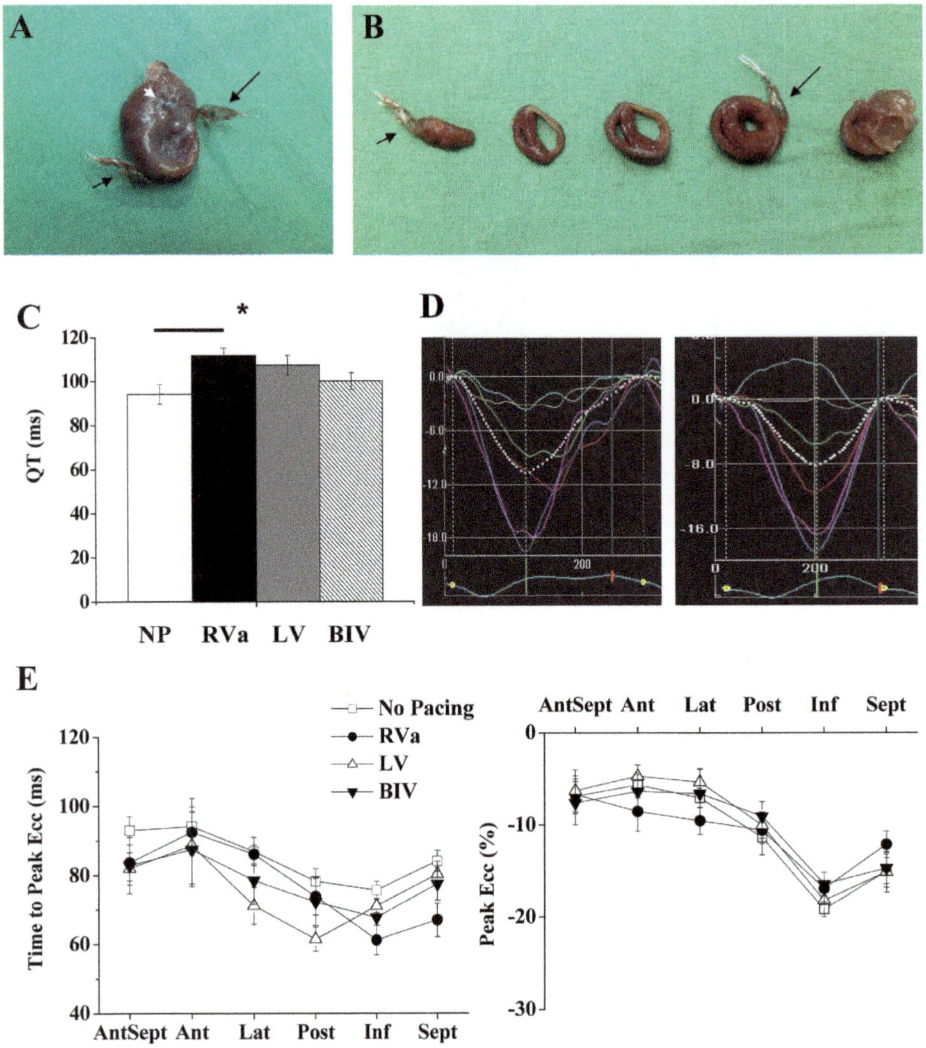

Figure 7. Combined model of pacing and ischemic heart failure. A: Anterior image of a heart subjected to electrodes implantation in combination with left coronary ligation. RV electrode and LV electrode are marked by short and long black arrows, respectively. White arrow; coronary artery ligation site. **B**: Transverse sections of the heart shown in A. Apical to basal sections are ordered from left to right. **C**: Summary of QT interval analysis in five instrumented rats with MI. * P<0.01. Horizontal line above the bar graph indicate significant difference in the post-hoc analysis. **D**: Representative strain waveforms of two instrumented rats with MI under control conditions. **E**: Average segmental time to peak Ecc (left) and peak Ecc (right) in five rats with ischemic heart failure subjected to no pacing, RV, LV and BIV pacing.

LV synchrony using M-mode echocardiography, [13,15] our study is the first to utilize speckled tracking analysis under various pacing modes in order to view the full segmental pattern during RA, RV, LV and BIV pacing. The results show clear beneficial effects of LV and to a greater extend BIV pacing on LV synchrony compared to RV pacing. In terms of electrical synchrony, we found it difficult to reliably measure the QRS duration during the different pacing modes due to the absence of apparent differentiation between the QRS complex and the T wave in the rat ECG. However, the effects of different pacing modes on the QT duration, which were consistent and significant (Figure 4 A,B), seem to reflect, at least partially, changes in QRS duration that are embedded in the QT interval. In addition, analysis of epicardial electrograms also supports longer activation time during RV pacing compared to LV pacing (Figure 4 C). Thus, LV and BIV pacing appear to induce beneficial effects on electrical synchrony compared with RV pacing in the rat heart. In terms of mechanical synchrony our results demonstrate that LV-only pacing has favorable outcome which is almost similar to the effect of BIV pacing. While many studies support the notion that LV-only pacing may have beneficial effects in HF patients [26], recent data in children with normal cardiac function and complete AV block demonstrated striking similarity to the results of our rat model in regard to LV-only pacing [27]. Moreover, LV-only pacing appears to be associated with good clinical outcome in this and other studies in the pediatric population [28,29]. It should be mentioned that the segmental findings of our study as well as the pediatric studies stated above appear to contrast the findings of [30], which demonstrated reduced Ecc near the LV pacing site compare to remote sites near the RV in the dog model of acute pacing. However, the segmental Ecc analysis in the above study was done by MRI using a much higher spatial resolution dividing the mid LV into 24 segments and 8 longitudinal segments. Thus the analysis focused on segments which are not in the same transverse plane and are much more refined to the actual vicinity of the pacing electrodes.

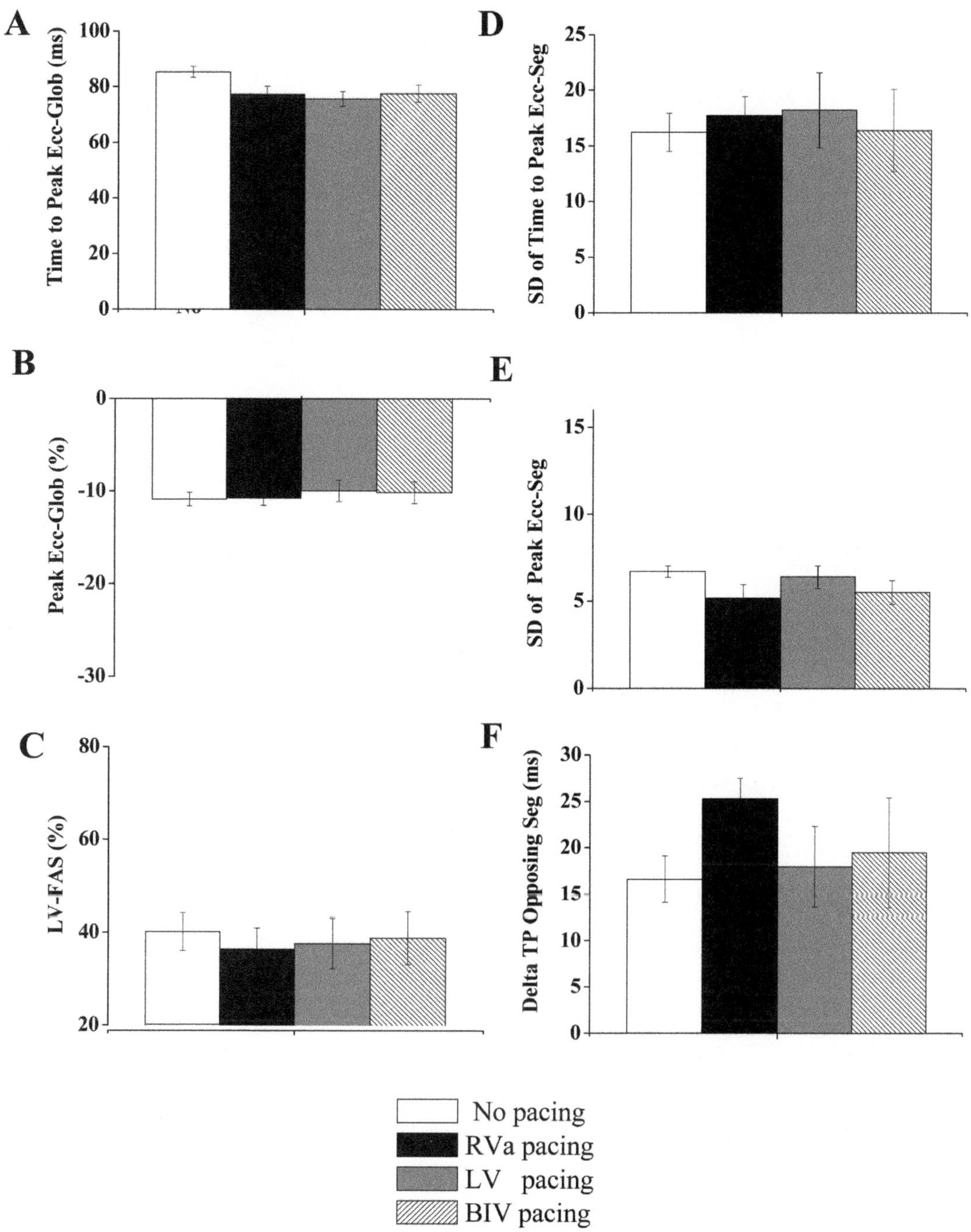

Figure 8. Attenuated effects of pacing in rats subjected to extensive MI. Summary of echocardiographic parameters in five rats with ischemic heart failure subjected to no pacing, RV pacing, LV pacing, and BIV pacing. **A**: Average time to peak Ecc of all six segments (global). **B**: Average peak Ecc of all six segments (global) **C**: LV fractional area shortening **D**: Standard deviation of the time to peak Ecc of different segments. **E**: Standard deviation of the peak Ecc of different segments. **F**. Average time difference between the peak Ecc of opposing segments ('delta TP opposing segments', see Figure 3 for details). Kruskal-Wallis test did not reveal a significant difference between the different pacing modes for any of the presented parameters.

The addition of MI-induced HF to the double site ventricular pacing model was performed as a proof of concept for the usefulness of our rat model in simulating a scenario that is clinically relevant. Our results indicate decreased beneficial effect of LV or BIV pacing in animals with extensive MI. These results are consistent with various clinical results indicating that the beneficial effect of CRT is highly dependent on the scar burden and is lost when the scar burden passes a certain limit [31,32]. A recent study in a dog model indicated, however, a clear beneficial effect of CRT in the setting of ~20% scar burden [33]. In this context, a limitation of our current analysis was the lack of a quantitative measurement of scar burden. However, based on the echocardiographic analysis of akinetic/dyskinetic segments, LV-FAS analysis (Figure 8C), and the macroscopic view of the MI in

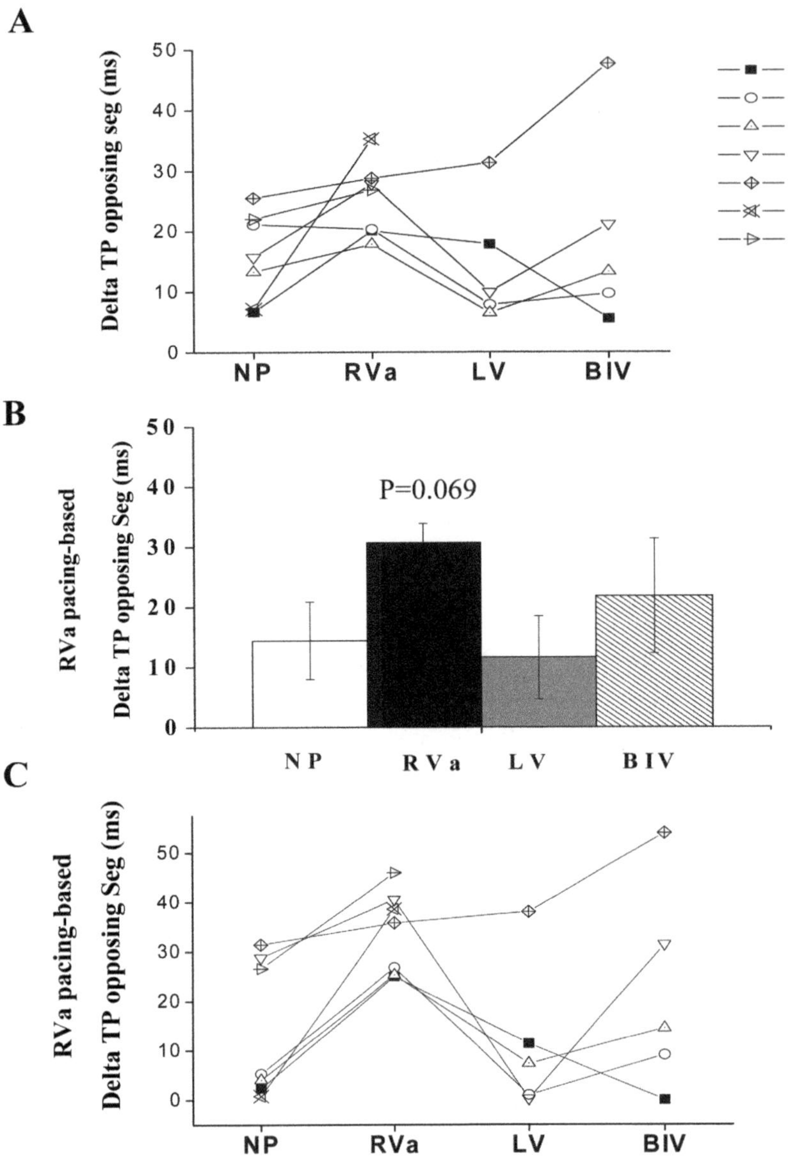

Figure 9. Individual variability in the effect of pacing in rats subjected to extensive MI. A: Average time difference between the peak Ecc of opposing segments in seven individual rats with MI (MI1 to MI7). Note the tendency of increased delta TP in all rats during RV pacing. **B**: Analysis of delta TP in each animal focused solely on the two opposing segments presenting maximal dyssynchrony during RV pacing. **C**: Delta TP focused on the two opposing segment presenting maximal dyssynchrony in seven individual rats with MI (as in Figure 9B).

the hearts (Figure 7A, B), it appears that the MIs of the present study were rather extensive in nature and were far beyond the 20% scar burden that was calculated in the dog model of Rademakers et al. [33]. Importantly, our initial analysis did not detect a marked deleterious effect of RV pacing in the MI animals when LV dyssynchrony parameters were compared to the no pacing mode (Figure 8). This phenomenon may be partially attributed to the nature the dyssynchrony parameters that were selected in our study, which may lose their sensitivity when high values are already present at the baseline. Nevertheless, it may also be possible that in the presence of an extensive MI, the effect of RV pacing on LV dyssynchrony is indeed small due to the high LV dyssynchrony that is already present at baseline. Looking specifically at the temporal synchrony of opposing segments, which appears to be specifically useful both clinically and experimentally [19,34], the picture that we obtained was somewhat different. Indeed, using this measure, we could identify a tendency of increased dyssynchrony during RV pacing in the majority of rats (Figure 9), a finding suggesting that this pacing still imposes a deleterious effect in the extensive MI setting but is harder to detect and analyze in this context. An examination of opposing segments also revealed marked variability in the response of individual rats with ischemic HF to the effect of LV and BIV pacing. While, in some animals, these modes of pacing seemed to be favorable compared to RV pacing, an opposite tendency was clearly noted in one out of the five fully analyzed rats. Clearly, more extensive work is required to further define the parameters that are responsible for the observed variability in the setting of MI. Quantitative analysis of scar burden and precise post mortem analysis of the location of LV pacing site in relation to the scar tissue, as well as invasive hemodynamic measurements during the different pacing modes, would all make a valuable contribution to further analysis in this complex setting.

The current rat model opens a window of opportunity for various studies regarding DHF and CRT using a rather simple and economically efficient model. The study might also pave the way to the application of double site pacing in genetically engineered mice models. New technical advances in the development of wireless pacing for mice, [35] imply that such studies may indeed become more feasible in the near future.

Limitations

There are several limitations to the present model. The absence of atrial sensing electrode and dependence on override pacing prevents atrioventricular synchrony. However, since the main comparisons of different ventricular pacing modes all rely on override pacing, this confounder should be equal in the different ventricular pacing modes. In addition, the pseudo LBBB pattern induced by RV pacing may not necessarily represent all the features of true LBBB. In this context, the epicardial location of our RV electrodes is also important to note, since this setting differs from the most common clinical RV pacing situation, where the RV lead is endocardial. Finally, the patterns of LV dyssynchrony observed in different animals are not completely identical, as can be appreciated by comparison of the segmental time to peak patterns in Figure 2 (group A) and Figure 5 (group B). The source of this variability between the groups was not clear to us. One of the things we suspect is that although the position of electrode implantation seems identical to the operator, the small size of the rat heart did not allow for detection of subtle differences in the position of the implantation, specifically in the anterior-posterior dimension. Such difference may affect the electrical activation sequence. Thus, if an electrode is positioned in a more anterior position close to the apex, the first LV segment that is activated is the inferior one as seen in the summary of animals in group A (Figure 2C). On the other hand, if the electrode is positioned in a more posterior location then the first LV segment that is activated is the posterior one as was dominantly observed in the animals of group B (Figure 5). This possibility implies that more attention to the exact location of the RV electrode should be used in future studies. Nevertheless, our current analysis also indicates that regardless of the exact segmental pattern of the time to peak strain, the variability of this parameter is remarkably larger during RV pacing compared to LV pacing and BIV pacing.

Conclusions

The present study shows the feasibility of an electrodes implantation procedure for double site epicardial pacing in rats, and the ability to combine this technique with conventional MI surgery. By the use of ECG recordings and speckle-tracking echocardiography we found that rodent pacing mimics important electromechanical features seen in large mammals and in people. Thus, this model may become a simple new tool to study the pathophysiology of ventricular dyssynchrony and CRT.

Supporting Information

Checklist S1 NC3Rs ARRIVE Guidelines Checklist.

Acknowledgments

The authors thank Prof. Amos Katz for important scientific insights. We also thank Yossi Tsadok and Dr. Noa Bachner-Hinenzon for technical assistance with the 2DS analysis.

Author Contributions

Conceived and designed the experiments: MM WM YE NLC. Performed the experiments: MM WM SE HG SD. Analyzed the data: MM WM SE SD. Contributed reagents/materials/analysis tools: MM WM HG. Wrote the paper: MM WM YE NLC.

References

1. Bader H, Garrigue S, Lafitte S, Reuter S, Jais P, et al. (2004) Intra-left ventricular electromechanical asynchrony. A new independent predictor of severe cardiac events in heart failure patients. J Am Coll Cardiol 43: 248–256.
2. Cho GY, Song JK, Park WJ, Han SW, Choi SH, et al. (2005) Mechanical dyssynchrony assessed by tissue Doppler imaging is a powerful predictor of mortality in congestive heart failure with normal QRS duration. J Am Coll Cardiol 46: 2237–2243.
3. Ludwig DR, Tanaka H, Friehling M, Gorcsan J, 3rd, Schwartzman D (2013) Further deterioration of LV ejection fraction and mechanical synchrony during RV apical pacing in patients with heart failure and LBBB. J Cardiovasc Transl Res 6: 425–429.
4. Rickard J, Cheng A, Spragg D, Cantillon D, Chung MK, et al. (2013) QRS narrowing is associated with reverse remodeling in patients with chronic right ventricular pacing upgraded to cardiac resynchronization therapy. Heart Rhythm 10: 55–60.
5. Tops LF, Schalij MJ, Bax JJ (2009) The Effects of Right Ventricular Apical Pacing on Ventricular Function and Dyssynchrony: Implications for Therapy. J Am Coll Cardiol 54: 764–776.
6. Bleeker GB, Bax JJ, Steendijk P, Schalij MJ, van der Wall EE (2006) Left ventricular dyssynchrony in patients with heart failure: pathophysiology, diagnosis and treatment. Nat Clin Pract Cardiovasc Med 3: 213–219.
7. Kashani A, Barold SS (2005) Significance of QRS complex duration in patients with heart failure. J Am Coll Cardiol 46: 2183–2192.
8. Leclercq C, Singh JP (2011) Cardiac resynchronization therapy: from treatment to prevention. Eur Heart J 32: 1580–1582.
9. Cho H, Barth AS, Tomaselli GF (2012) Basic science of cardiac resynchronization therapy: molecular and electrophysiological mechanisms. Circ Arrhythm Electrophysiol 5: 594–603.
10. Saba S, Mehdi H, Mathier MA, Islam MZ, Salama G, et al. (2010) Effect of Right Ventricular Versus Biventricular Pacing on Electrical Remodeling in the Normal Heart. Circ Arrhythm Electrophysiol 3: 79–87.
11. Chakir K, Daya SK, Tunin RS, Helm RH, Byrne MJ, et al. (2008) Reversal of global apoptosis and regional stress kinase activation by cardiac resynchronization. Circulation 117: 1369–1377. doi: 1310.1161/CIRCULATIONAHA.1107.706291. Epub 702008 Mar 706293.
12. Barth AS, Aiba T, Halperin V, DiSilvestre D, Chakir K, et al. (2009) Cardiac Resynchronization Therapy Corrects Dyssynchrony-Induced Regional Gene Expression Changes on a Genomic Level. Circ Cardiovasc Genet 2: 371–378.
13. Bilchick KC, Saha SK, Mikolajczyk E, Cope L, Ferguson WJ, et al. (2006) Differential regional gene expression from cardiac dyssynchrony induced by chronic right ventricular free wall pacing in the mouse. Physiol Genomics 26: 109–115.
14. Houser SR, Margulies KB, Murphy AM, Spinale FG, Francis GS, et al. (2012) Animal models of heart failure: a scientific statement from the American Heart Association. Circ Res 111: 131–150.
15. Kontogeorgis A, Kaba RA, Kang E, Feig JE, Gupta PP, et al. (2008) Short-term pacing in the mouse alters cardiac expression of connexin43. BMC Physiol 8:8: 10.1186/1472-6793-1188-1188.
16. Etzion Y, Mor M, Shalev A, Dror S, Etzion O, et al. (2008) New insights into the atrial electrophysiology of rodents using a novel modality: the miniature-bipolar hook electrode. Am J Physiol Heart Circ Physiol 295: H1460–1469. Epub 2008 Jul 1425.
17. Popovic ZB, Benejam C, Bian J, Mal N, Drinko J, et al. (2007) Speckle-tracking echocardiography correctly identifies segmental left ventricular dysfunction induced by scarring in a rat model of myocardial infarction. Am J Physiol Heart Circ Physiol 292: H2809–2816.
18. Bachner-Hinenzon N, Ertracht O, Leitman M, Vered Z, Shimoni S, et al. (2010) Layer-specific strain analysis by speckle tracking echocardiography reveals differences in left ventricular function between rats and humans. Am J Physiol Heart Circ Physiol 299: H664–672.
19. Bonios M, Chang CY, Pinheiro A, Dimaano VL, Higuchi T, et al. (2011) Cardiac resynchronization by cardiosphere-derived stem cell transplantation in an experimental model of myocardial infarction. J Am Soc Echocardiogr 24: 808–814.
20. Bachner-Hinenzon N, Ertracht O, Malka A, Leitman M, Vered Z, et al. (2012) Layer-specific strain analysis: investigation of regional deformations in a rat

model of acute versus chronic myocardial infarction. Am J Physiol Heart Circ Physiol 303: H549–558.
21. Rappaport D, Adam D, Lysyansky P, Riesner S (2006) Assessment of myocardial regional strain and strain rate by tissue tracking in B-mode echocardiograms. Ultrasound Med Biol 32: 1181–1192.
22. Salama G, London B (2007) Mouse models of long QT syndrome. J Physiol 578: 43–53.
23. Nerbonne JM (2004) Studying cardiac arrhythmias in the mouse–a reasonable model for probing mechanisms? Trends Cardiovasc Med 14: 83–93.
24. Dandel M, Hetzer R (2009) Echocardiographic strain and strain rate imaging–clinical applications. Int J Cardiol 132: 11–24.
25. Kaese S, Verheule S (2012) Cardiac electrophysiology in mice: a matter of size. Front Physiol 3: 345.
26. Strik M, van Deursen CJ, van Middendorp LB, van Hunnik A, Kuiper M, et al. (2013) Transseptal conduction as an important determinant for cardiac resynchronization therapy, as revealed by extensive electrical mapping in the dyssynchronous canine heart. Circ Arrhythm Electrophysiol 6: 682–689.
27. Tomaske M, Breithardt OA, Bauersfeld U (2009) Preserved cardiac synchrony and function with single-site left ventricular epicardial pacing during mid-term follow-up in paediatric patients. Europace 11: 1168–1176.
28. Tomaske M, Breithardt OA, Balmer C, Bauersfeld U (2009) Successful cardiac resynchronization with single-site left ventricular pacing in children. Int J Cardiol 136: 136–143.
29. Janousek J, van Geldorp IE, Krupickova S, Rosenthal E, Nugent K, et al. (2013) Permanent cardiac pacing in children: choosing the optimal pacing site: a multicenter study. Circulation 127: 613–623.
30. Prinzen FW, Hunter WC, Wyman BT, McVeigh ER (1999) Mapping of regional myocardial strain and work during ventricular pacing: experimental study using magnetic resonance imaging tagging. J Am Coll Cardiol 33: 1735–1742.
31. Adelstein EC, Tanaka H, Soman P, Miske G, Haberman SC, et al. (2011) Impact of scar burden by single-photon emission computed tomography myocardial perfusion imaging on patient outcomes following cardiac resynchronization therapy. Eur Heart J 32: 93–103.
32. Ypenburg C, Roes SD, Bleeker GB, Kaandorp TA, de Roos A, et al. (2007) Effect of total scar burden on contrast-enhanced magnetic resonance imaging on response to cardiac resynchronization therapy. Am J Cardiol 99: 657–660. Epub 2007 Jan 2004.
33. Rademakers LM, van Kerckhoven R, van Deursen CJ, Strik M, van Hunnik A, et al. (2010) Myocardial infarction does not preclude electrical and hemodynamic benefits of cardiac resynchronization therapy in dyssynchronous canine hearts. Circ Arrhythm Electrophysiol 3: 361–368.
34. Prinzen FW, Vernooy K, De Boeck BW, Delhaas T (2011) Mechano-energetics of the asynchronous and resynchronized heart. Heart Fail Rev 16: 215–224.
35. Laughner JI, Marrus SB, Zellmer ER, Weinheimer CJ, Macewan MR, et al. (2013) A fully implantable pacemaker for the mouse: from battery to wireless power. PLoS One 8: e76291.

8

Validation of a Novel Clinical Prediction Score for Severe Coronary Artery Diseases before Elective Coronary Angiography

Zhang-Wei Chen[1]ᶿ, Ying-Hua Chen[2]ᶿ, Ju-Ying Qian[1]*, Jian-Ying Ma[1], Jun-Bo Ge[1]*

1 Department of Cardiology, Zhongshan Hospital affiliated to Fudan University, Shanghai, China, 2 Department of Endocrinology Medicine, East Hospital affiliated to Tongji University, Shanghai, China

Abstract

Objectives: Coronary artery disease (CAD) severity is associated with patient prognosis. However, few efficient scoring systems have been developed to screen severe CAD in patients with stable angina and suspected CAD before coronary angiography. Here, we present a novel scoring system for CAD severity before elective coronary angiography.

Methods: Five hundred fifty-one patients with stable angina who were admitted for coronary angiography were enrolled in this study. Patients were divided into training (n = 347) and validation (n = 204) cohorts. Severe CAD was defined as having a Gensini score of 20 or more. All patients underwent echocardiography (ECG) to detect ejection fraction and aortic valve calcification (AVC). Multivariable analysis was applied to determine independent risk factors and develop the scoring system.

Results: In the training cohort, age, male sex, AVC, abnormal ECG, diabetes, hyperlipidemia, high-density lipoprotein cholesterol, and low-density lipoprotein cholesterol were identified as independent factors for severe CAD by multivariable analysis, and the Severe Prediction Scoring (SPS) system was developed. C-indices of receiver operating characteristic (ROC) curves for severe CAD were 0.744 and 0.710 in the training and validation groups, respectively. The SPS system also performed well during calibration, as demonstrated by Hosmer-Lemeshow analysis in the validation group. Compared with the Diamond-Forrester score, the SPS system performed better for severe CAD prediction before elective coronary angiography.

Conclusions: Severe CAD prediction was achieved by analyzing age, sex, AVC, ECG, diabetes status, and lipid levels. Angina patients who achieve high scores using this predicting system should undergo early coronary angiography.

Editor: Renate B. Schnabel, University Heart Center, Germany

Funding: This work was supported by the National Natural Science Foundation of China (Grant Nos: 81200146, 30901383 and 30671998), Zhongshan Hospital Youth Science Funding (Grant No: 2012ZSQN12), New Teacher Foundation of Ministry of Education (Grant No: 20120071120061), and Scientific Research for Young Teacher of Fudan University (Grant No: 20520133177). The funders had no role in study design, data collection and analysis, decision to publish, or preparation of the manuscript.

Competing Interests: The authors have declared that no competing interests exist.

* E-mail: Ge.junbo@hotmail.com (J-BG); Qian.juying@zs-hospital.sh.cn (J-YQ)

ᶿ These authors contributed equally to this work.

Introduction

Coronary artery disease (CAD) is a leading cause of morbidity and mortality worldwide, and the costs of invasive and noninvasive diagnostic methods, which are performed to identify the presence and severity of CAD, are increasing dramatically. The severity of CAD, which can be analyzed by Gensini score [1] or Syntax score [2], has been shown to be associated with short- and long-term cardiovascular risk [3]. Both of these scoring systems consider coronary anatomy, artery morphology, and severity of stenosis in lesions [4]. Therefore, in order to identify severe CAD (defined as ≥70% stenosis in the proximal left anterior descending artery, equal to a Gensini score ≥20 points) and help cardiologists make treatment decisions, several clinical risk models have been developed. These models, including the EuroHeart score, Clinical SYNTAX score, Mayo clinic risk score, etc., predict long-term cardiovascular risk by analyzing clinical risk factors and severity of CAD [2,5–7]. However, all of these models require the results of coronary angiography or coronary computed tomography angiography. Because many patients with atypical chest pains or even asymptomatic patients may be at risk of severe CAD, it is not feasible to suggest that every patient undergo coronary angiography in this setting. Several clinical scoring systems, such as Diamond-Forrester score [8], Framingham risk score (FRS), and systematic coronary risk evaluation (SCORE) have been established to assess CAD risk by analyzing classical risk factors, such as chest pain type, age, gender, blood pressure, smoking status, diabetes status, and cholesterol level [9–10]. However, the effectiveness of these models for prediction of severe CAD by clinical risk factors is not sufficient. While the Diamond-Forrester

Table 1. Demographic data of patients with and without severe coronary artery disease.

	Severe CAD (n = 202)	Non-severe CAD (n = 145)	*P*
Clinical factors:			
Male (%)	149 (73.8%)	89 (61.4%)	**0.014**
Age (year)	65.1±9.6	62.4±8.9	**<0.01**
Hypertension (%)	144 (71.3%)	97 (66.9%)	0.381
Hyperlipidemia (%)	80 (39.6%)	34 (23.4%)	**<0.01**
Diabetes (%)	76 (37.6%)	31 (21.4%)	**<0.01**
Smoking (%)	92 (45.5%)	60 (41.4%)	0.441
Laboratory test (admission):			
Serum Creatinine (μmol/L)	78.9±18.8	73.7±17.2	**<0.01**
Serum Uric acid (mmol/L)	352.2±88.1	342.1±86.2	0.287
Fibrinogen (g/L)	293.4±59.7	275.1±58.2	**<0.01**
Total cholesterol (mmol/L)	4.33±1.27	4.11±0.88	0.055
Triglyceride (mmol/L)	1.91±1.35	1.79±1.29	0.409
LDL-C (mmol/L)	2.45±1.11	2.16±0.69	**<0.01**
HDL-C (mmol/L)	1.08±0.25	1.19±0.29	**<0.01**
Lipoprotein-a (mmol/L)	208.4±186.7	175.4±170.5	0.089
Apo-A (mmol/L)	1.09±0.22	1.09±0.24	0.878
Apo-B (mmol/L)	0.86±0.23	0.76±0.22	**<0.01**
Electrocardiography			
Abnormal ECG (%)	117 (57.9%)	52 (35.9%)	**<0.01**
Echocardiography			
Ejection fraction (%)	62.4	64.5	0.465
AVC	85 (42.1%)	34 (30.6%)	**<0.01**
Coronary angiography:			
Gensini score	46.3±28.0	7.1±6.0	**<0.01**
Number of stenosed vessels	2.26±0.88	0.6±0.6	**<0.01**

AVC: aortic valve calcification; CAD: coronary artery disease; ECG: electrocardiography;
HDL-C: high density lipoprotein cholesterol; LDL: low density lipoprotein cholesterol;

score has been recommended to predict CAD before coronary angiography, its performance in severe CAD prediction is unknown. Therefore, it is necessary to develop a highly efficient and convenient screening model for severe CAD without requiring coronary angiography results.

The aim of this study was to develop a novel risk scoring system to guide early invasive coronary angiography in angina patients using analysis of clinical risk factors, electrocardiography (ECG), and echocardiography. Additionally, we attempted to demonstrate whether this risk scoring system was effective to predict severe CAD before coronary angiography, and we compared the performance of this system with that of the Diamond-Forrester score for prediction of CAD and severe CAD. Further analyses were also carried out to detect the association between scores from our novel system and Gensini scores.

Methods

1. Study Population and Grouping

From October 2011 to September 2012, a total of 551 angina patients referred to our hospital for elective coronary angiography were enrolled in this study. The inclusion criteria were as follows: (1) 18 to 85 years of age; (2) providing a complete clinical history; and (3) normal preprocedural troponin T (below the 10% coefficient of variation [CV] value, <0.03 ng/mL [11]) and creatine kinase (CK)-MB (<23 U/L). The exclusion criteria were as follows: (1) underwent coronary angiography or computerized tomography angiography previously; (2) diagnosed with acute coronary syndrome; (3) evidence of elevated cardiac troponin T (≥ 0.03 ng/mL) or CK-MB (≥23 U/L) before coronary intervention; (4) presence of heart failure, diagnosed by clinical presentation, echocardiography (ejection fraction [EF] <40%), and N-terminal-pro-brain natriuretic peptide (>300 pg/mL); (5) presence of cardiomyopathy, congenital heart disease, or heart valve disease; (6) underwent recent surgery or trauma; (7) presence of active chronic inflammation, renal failure, dysfunction of hematological and immunological systems, carcinoma, or a condition treated with immunosuppressive agents.

From this patient population, 347 patients (continuously enrolled by hospitalization time) were enrolled into the training cohort for risk factor identification and predicting system development, while the other 204 patients were enrolled for validation of the prediction system. First, the training cohort was subjected to univariate and multivariate analyses to identify independent risk factors for severe CAD (defined in section 2.6). Each prediction score was evaluated by determining the odds ratio (OR) of each risk factor in multivariate analysis, and the total prediction score for severe CAD was calculated by summating all

Table 2. Multivariate logistic regression analysis for severe CAD in patients with chest pain.

	r	95% confidence intervals	*P*
AVC	2.580	1.538–4.329	**<0.01**
Abnormal ECG	2.148	1.333–3.460	**<0.01**
diabetes	1.966	1.149–3.365	**0.014**
Male	1.880	1.095–3.226	**0.022**
Hyperlipidemia	1.794	1.054–3.053	**0.031**
LDL-C	1.516	1.136–2.024	**<0.01**
HDL-C	0.310	0.116–0.827	**0.019**

AVC: aortic valve calcification; CAD: coronary artery disease; ECG: electrocardiography; HDL-C: high density lipoprotein cholesterol; LDL: low density lipoprotein cholesterol;

prediction scores. In order to demonstrate the clinical practicality and efficacy of this new prediction score for severe CAD screening, receiver operating characteristic (ROC) curves and Hosmer-Lemeshow analysis were analyzed in the validation cohort to examine model performance in terms of discrimination and calibration.

2. Ethics Statement

We provided a written informed consent form to participants in our study and explained the entire study procedure to each patient. This study and consent procedure were approved by our local ethics committee (Ethics Committee of Zhongshan Hospital affiliated to Fudan University), and were carried out in accordance with the principles of the Declaration of Helsinki.

3. Medical History Records and Laboratory Measurements

The clinical characteristics of all patients, including gender, age, and previous histories of smoking, hypertension, diabetes, and hyperlipidemia, were recorded before coronary angiography. Fasting blood samples were collected before angiography to detect blood biochemistry, and complete blood cell counts was performed. All biochemical parameters, including total cholesterol, total triglycerides, low-density lipoprotein cholesterol (LDL-C), high-density lipoprotein cholesterol (HDL-C), apolipoprotein-A, apolipoprotein-B, uric acid, and creatinine concentrations, were analyzed.

Patients were defined as hypertensive (JNC VII Guidelines), if they had a systolic pressure greater than 140 mmHg or a diastolic pressure greater than 90 mmHg, or if they were being treated with an antihypertensive medication. Patients were considered to have type II diabetes mellitus (DM) if they were previously diagnosed or following the 2010 American Diabetes Association (ADA) diabetes diagnostic criteria. The definition of hyperlipidemia was taken from the NHLBI ATP III prevention guidelines.

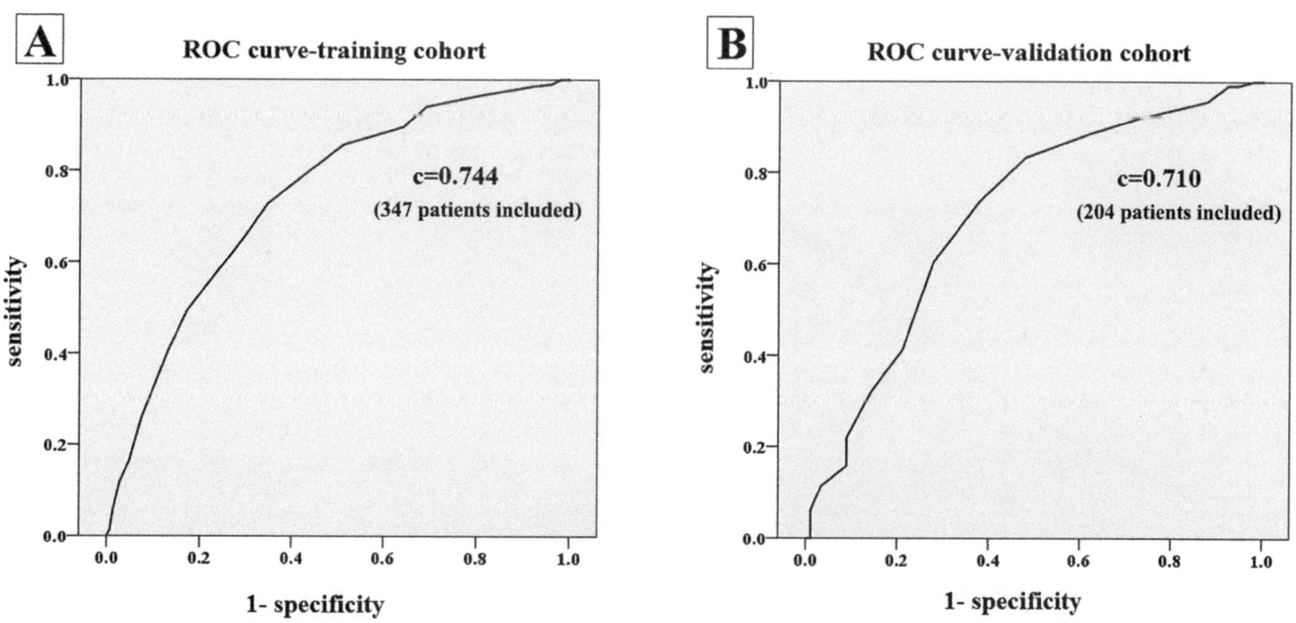

Figure 1. Receiver operating characteristic (ROC) curve in training (A) and validation (B) cohort. (347 and 204 patients were analyzed in training and validation cohorts respectively).

Table 3. Scoring system predicting for severe CAD in patients with chest pain.

Risk factor	Range	Single score
AVC	yes	3
Abnormal ECG	yes	3
Diabetes	yes	2
Male	yes	2
Hyperlipidemia	yes	2
LDL-C (mmol/L)	<1.8	0
	1.8–2.2	1
	≥2.2	2
HDL-C (mmol/L)	≥1.2	0
	1.0–1.2	1
	<1.0	2
Age (years)	<65	0
	≥65	2
Severe Predicting Score		18

AVC: aortic valve calcification; CAD: coronary artery disease; ECG: electrocardiography; HDL-C: high density lipoprotein cholesterol; LDL: low density lipoprotein cholesterol;

4. Electrocardiography and Echocardiography

Admission ECG was performed for each patient. Abnormal ECG was defined as having Q waves in multiple leads, ST-T-wave inversions, left/right bundle-branch blockage, or left ventricular hypertrophy [12]. Echocardiography was performed in all patients using a Philips IE33 instrument (Philips, Netherlands) with a 2–3.5 MHz transducer (X3-1), and left ventricular EF and aortic valve calcification (AVC) were detected. Two-dimensional assessment of the aortic valve was performed on the basis of the parasternal long-axis and short-axis views, where abnormalities of the aortic valve were coded as representing AVC, aortic stenosis, a bicuspid aortic valve, or aortic-valve regurgitation. AVC was defined as focal areas of increased echogenicity and thickening of the aortic valve leaflets without restriction of leaflet motion on transthoracic echocardiography [13–14]. Observers who made the diagnosis of AVC were blinded to the results of coronary angiography.

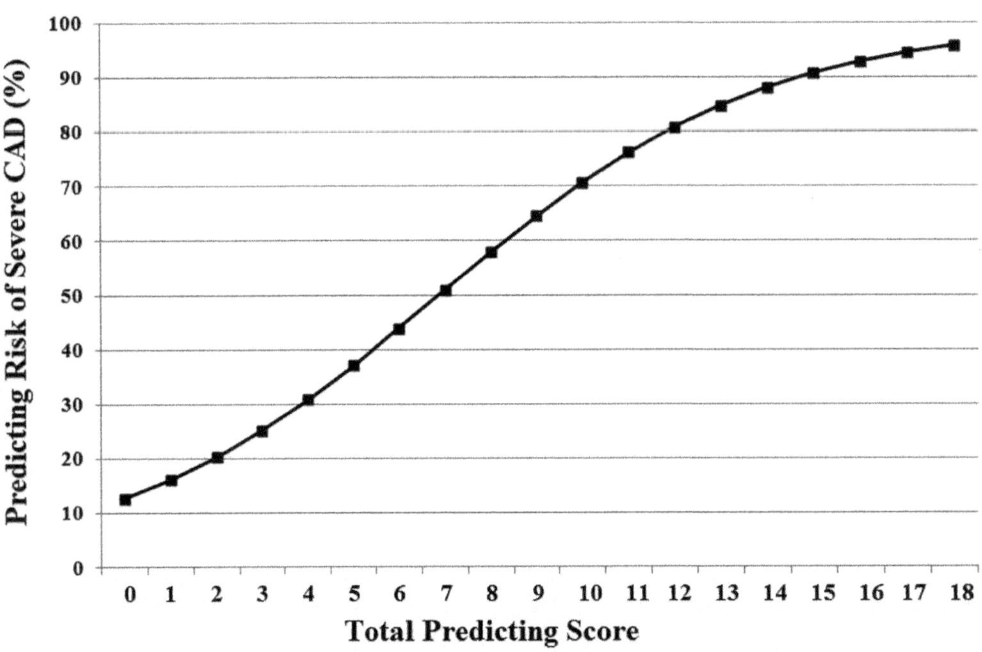

Figure 2. Predicting risk of severe coronary artery disease by this scoring model.

Table 4. Subgroup analysis for the scoring system in the whole cohort.

Risk factor	Subgroup	Severe CAD/Sample	C-index	H-L p-value
Gender	Male	236/379	**0.690***	0.308
	Female	80/172	**0.778***	0.477
Age (year)	≥65	165/259	0.706*	0.291
	<65	151/292	0.734*	0.459
Hypertension	Hypertension	235/390	0.719*	0.390
	Non-hypertension	81/161	0.749*	0.848
Diabetes	Diabetes	117/170	0.715*	0.770
	Non-diabetes	199/381	0.718*	0.288
Serum creatinine (μmol/L)	≥80	136/214	**0.639***	0.747
	<80	180/337	**0.774***	0.710

*means the p-value <0.05; CAD: coronary artery disease; H–L: Hosmer–Lemeshow;

5. Coronary Angiography and Severity CAD Identification

Elective coronary angiography was performed in all patients after admission. A patient was considered to have CAD when a stenosed lesion resulting in a 50% or greater reduction in lumen diameter existed in at least one of the coronary arteries. Furthermore, the total number of stenosed vessels was represented as the number of major stenoses in epicardial arteries with at least one stenosed lesion (≥50% reduction of lumen diameter), including the left anterior descending artery (LAD), left circumflex artery (LCX), right coronary artery (RCA), and left main artery (LM).

The severity of CAD was evaluated by Gensini score [1]. Gensini score grades narrowing of the lumen as follows: 1, 1%–25% occlusion; 2, 26%–50% occlusion; 4, 51%–75% occlusion; 8, 76%–90% occlusion; 16, 91%–99% occlusion; and 32, total occlusion. This score is multiplied by a factor accounting for the importance of the lesion position in the coronary arterial tree, such as 5 for LM, 2.5 for proximal LAD, and 1 for proximal RCA. The severity of the disease is expressed as the sum of the scores for individual lesions. Gensini score and number of stenosed vessels were recorded by observers who were blinded to the results of laboratory testing and study grouping.

Patients with Gensini scores of 20 or more were defined as having severe CAD, which was approximately equal to one stenosed lesion of 70% or more in the proximal left anterior descending artery.

6. Calculation of the Diamond-Forrester Score

First, we classified angina type as typical, atypical, or nonspecific [15]. Typical chest pain was defined as having (i) substernal chest pain or discomfort; (ii) pain provoked by exertion or emotional stress; and (iii) pain relieved by rest and/or nitroglycerine. Atypical chest pain was defined as having 2 of the above-mentioned criteria. If one or none of the criteria was present, the patient was classified as having nonspecific chest pain. The Diamond Forrester model was developed to calculate the probability of CAD and considers age (only patients 30 to 70 years old were considered for this model), sex, and type of chest pain [8].

7. Statistical Analysis

All statistical analyses were performed with SPSS software 19.0. Data were presented as the percentage or mean ± standard deviation (SD). The database was randomly divided into 2 parts. The first part was used to develop the scoring system (i.e., the training cohort). The second part was used to validate the scoring system (i.e., the validation cohort). In the training cohort, chi-squared tests were used to compare the frequencies of categorical variables, and Student's *t* or correction *t* tests were used to compare means for continuous variables. Multivariate analysis (logistic) was performed to identify independent risk factors for severe CAD patients (variables with a significance level of $P<0.05$ in a univariate test were used in multivariate analysis). According to each OR of independent variables, we set each prediction score and calculated the total prediction score. Then, a prediction risk curve of severe CAD was established. The area under the ROC curve was used to test the discriminatory capability of the total prediction score, and Youden's index was applied to establish the optimal cutoff. ROC and Hosmer-Lemeshow analyses were also applied in the validation cohort to demonstrate the goodness of fit for the novel prediction scoring system. Correlation analysis (Spearman test) was performed to evaluate correlations between this prediction score and the Gensini score. All *P*-values were 2-

Table 5. Prevalence and severity of CAD in different novel scoring groups.

	A: 0–3 points (n = 51)	B: 4–7 points (n = 185)	C: 8–11 points (n = 218)	D: >11 points (n = 97)	*P*
CAD (%)	30 (58.8%)	130 (70.3%)	190 (87.2%)	90 (92.8%)	**<0.01**
Severe CAD patients (%)	12 (23.5%)	73 (39.5%)	153 (70.2%)	78 (80.4%)	**<0.01**
Gensini score	14.1±19.3	20.3±22.3	33.6±28.1	43.9±33.6	**<0.01**
Stenosed vessels	0.9±0.9	1.2±1.0	1.8±1.1	2.2±1.0	**<0.01**

CAD: coronary artery disease;

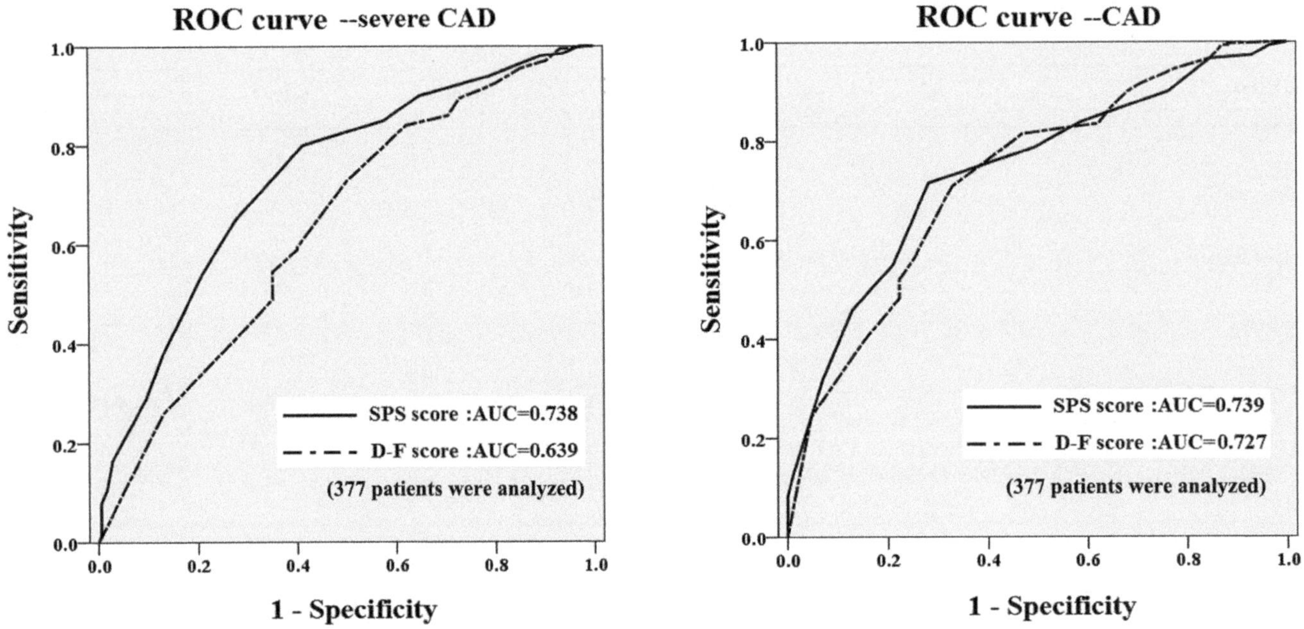

Figure 3. Compared receiver operating characteristic (ROC) curve between our SPS system and Diamond-Forrester score in severe CAD and CAD predicting. (377 patients were analyzed).

sided, and $P<0.05$ was considered to indicate statistical significance.

Results

1. Population Baseline Characteristics

A total of 551 patients with exertional chest tightness or chest pain were enrolled in this study for selective coronary angiography. There were 379 men (average age, 62.7±9.8 years) and 172 women (average age, 66.2±8.9 years). The prevalences of hypertension, diabetes, hyperlipidemia, and AVC were 70.8% (390 patients), 30.9% (170 patients), 30.7% (169 patients), and 34.3% (189 patients), respectively. A total of 440 (79.8%) patients were diagnosed as having CAD by coronary angiography.

In the training cohort (n = 347), there were 202 patients diagnosed with severe CAD by Gensini score (≥20), and the average Gensini score was significantly higher in the severe CAD group than in the mild/moderate CAD group (46.3±28.0 vs. 7.1±6.0, respectively, $P<0.01$). The baseline characteristics of patients with or without severe CAD are shown in Table 1. Compared to patients with nonsevere CAD, patients with severe CAD were older (65.1 vs. 62.4 years, $P<0.01$) and had higher prevalences of hyperlipidemia (39.6% vs. 23.4%, $P<0.01$), diabetes (37.6% vs. 21.4%, $P<0.01$), and AVC (42.1% vs. 30.6%, $P<0.01$).

2. Identification of Determinants of Severe CAD by Multivariate Logistic Regression

In the training cohort, multivariate logistic regression analysis was used to evaluate the association between severe CAD and risk factors. In this analysis, severe CAD was employed as a dependent variable, while age, male sex, AVC, abnormal ECG, diabetes, hyperlipidemia, HDL-C, LDL-C, and serum creatinine were set as independent variables (Table 2). After adjustment for other associated factors, we found that the risk of severe CAD was increased independently in patients who were male or had AVC, abnormal ECG, diabetes, hyperlipidemia, or abnormal LDL-C. Serum levels of HDL-C were associated with a 69% risk reduction

Table 6. Prevalence of CAD and risk score in different types of chest pain (377 patients met 30–70 years condition for Diamond–Forrester score).

	Typical angina n = 190	Atypical angina n = 132	Non-specific CP n = 55	P
CAD (%)	168 (88.4%)	95 (72.0%)	29 (52.7%)	**<0.01**
Age (years)	59.9±6.6	58.5±6.6	55.2±7.9	**<0.01**
Male (%)	33 (60.0%)	99 (75.0%)	141 (74.2%)	0.106
D-F score	91.0±4.6	56.9±11.1	17.9±6.4	**<0.01**
SPS score	8.1±3.2	7.1±3.4	5.9±3.0	**<0.01**

CAD: coronary artery disease; CP: chest pain; D-F score: Diamond–Forrester score;
SPS score: Severe Predicting Score.

for severe CAD (OR = 0.310, 95% confidence interval [CI] = 0.116–0.827, P=0.019).

3. New Prediction Scoring System and Risk Curves for Severe CAD

According to each OR of independent variables in multivariate logistic regression analysis, we set the prediction score of each risk factor (Table 3). The total prediction score was determined by summating the 7 individual prediction scores. Then, ROC curve analysis was applied to detect the efficacy of the new prediction score, and the area under the ROC curve (AUC) was analyzed. Using the 7 defined factors, the AUC was 0.734 (P<0.01). After adding age (>65 years), the AUC was increased to 0.744 (P<0.01), as shown in Figure 1-A. Therefore, age was added as a risk factor for predicting severe CAD.

In order to calculate the prediction risk score for severe CAD, we set severe CAD as a dependent variable and set the new total prediction score as an independent variable in multivariate analysis. Then, "Y = constant+βX" was obtained from logistic analysis, and each prediction risk score for severe CAD was calculated. Figure 2 demonstrates the prediction risk score curve for severe CAD according to each score. For example, an angina patient with a new score of 3 points had less than 25% risk of severe CAD, and this risk increased to 60% when the score was 9 points. The optimal cutoff for prediction of severe CAD was 8 points, with a sensitivity of 72.8% and a specificity of 65.5%.

4. Validation Test in the Validation Cohort

In order to demonstrate the clinical practicality and efficacy of this new prediction score for severe CAD screening, the scoring system and prediction risk curves were retested in the validation cohort. First, the total prediction score was calculated according to Table 3. Then, an ROC curve was established. The AUC of the ROC in the validation cohort was 0.710 (P<0.01, Figure 1B). Hosmer-Lemeshow analysis was also performed in the validation cohort to evaluate the goodness of fit for the prediction score. The Hosmer-Lemeshow P-value was 0.425 (>0.05), which indicated that the prediction risk curve was effective for severe CAD screening.

We also investigated the model performance in different subgroups, as shown in Table 4. The results demonstrated that this scoring system had similar performance in older, hypertensive, and diabetic patients. However, it performed less well in male (0.690 vs. 0.778 in female) patients and patients with kidney dysfunction (0.639 vs. 0.774 in patients with normal kidney function).

5. Extent of CAD and the New Scoring System

Patients were also classified into 4 groups by different Severe Prediction Scoring (SPS) results in the whole cohort: A, low-risk group, 0–3 points; B, intermediate-risk group, 4–7 points; C, high-risk group, 8–11 points; and D, very-high-risk group, more than 12 points. In higher scoring groups, the prevalences of CAD, severe CAD, and multivessel stenosis were increased significantly, as shown in Table 5. The association between SPS and Gensini scores was also analyzed in the whole cohort. We found that SPS scores were positively associated with Gensini scores for each patient (r=0.414, P<0.01).

6. Compare with Diamond-Forrester Scores for Predicting Performance.

As a classic scoring system for CAD prediction, the Diamond-Forrester score was calculated in patient ages 30–70 years (only 377 patients met this age condition for Diamond-Forrester score calculation). The average Diamond-Forrester score was 68.3±27.3 in these 377 patients. After dividing patients according to the type of chest pain, we found that patients with typical chest pain had significant associations between the prevalence of CAD and the SPS score, as shown in Table 6. As compare to the Diamond-Forrester score, our SPS system seemed to perform better for prediction of severe CAD (C-index, 0.738 vs. 0.639, respectively), while they had similar performance for prediction of nonsevere CAD (C-index, 0.739 vs. 0.727, respectively), shown in Figure 3.

Discussion

As we have discussed, several clinical scoring systems, including the Diamond-Forrester score [8], FRS [9], and SCORE [10], have been established to assess CAD risk by classical risk factors; however, the usefulness of these systems in predicting severe CAD before coronary angiography has not been established. In our study, we developed a novel risk scoring system for severe CAD screening by clinical risk factors, ECG, and echocardiography before coronary anatomic analysis. ROC and Hosmer-Lemeshow analysis in both the training and validation cohorts demonstrated that this model had good performance in terms of discrimination (C-indices of 0.744 and 0.710, respectively) and calibration (Hosmer–Lemeshow P-values of 0.824 and 0.425, respectively). Therefore, our results suggested that this system could help cardiologists identify severe CAD in a great number of angina patients before coronary angiography, thereby indicating whether early invasive coronary angiography should be performed. Especially in the setting where catheter lab resources are scant and waiting time for the examination is long, this score system could screen sever CAD patients by higher score conveniently. As low and intermediate score cohort, other non-invasive examinations and further follow-up could be considered.

Distinguished from conventional scoring systems for CAD risk prediction or prognosis in patients with CAD [3,5,9], our scoring system employed AVC, an echocardiography characteristic, for evaluation of CAD severity. As a characteristic of aging, AVC is also considered a frequent cause of aortic stenosis [16]. However, recent data have challenged this concept, showing that AVC is an active and highly regulated process, with histological similarities to atherosclerosis [14,17–18]. In our previous cross-sectional study [19,20], we found that AVC was still associated with CAD and CAD severity even after adjustment for aging itself. However, few other studies have considered using AVC for evaluation of CAD or CAD severity. As demonstrated by the multivariate analysis in this study, AVC increased the risk of severe CAD by 158% (Table 2), which demonstrated its independent influence on severe CAD. More importantly, the ROC of our scoring system was reduced to 0.687 in the validation cohort if AVC was excluded. According to these findings, AVC could be helpful for screening of severe CAD in combination analysis.

As compared with the classic scoring system, i.e., the Diamond-Forrester score [8], which is generally applied for predicting CAD risk, our SPS system exhibited similar performance in CAD prediction (C-indices of 0.739 and 0.727, respectively). However, our SPS system was significantly superior to the Diamond-Forrester score for prediction of severe CAD (C-indices of 0.738 vs. 0.639, respectively, shown in Figure 3). This implied that the SPS system was effective for predicting CAD and severe CAD before elective coronary angiography. Moreover, subgroup analysis by different variants, such as age, gender, hypertension, diabetes, and creatinine level, demonstrated the good performance of the SPS system in terms of discrimination and calibration. However, it also revealed that our model was less useful for prediction of severe CAD in patients with relatively higher serum creatinine (0.639 vs. 0.774 in patients with normal kidney function). Early kidney injury may influence the metabolism of lipids and glucose, resulting in poorer performance of our scoring system.

Another interesting point was that our scoring system (which was determined by clinical factors) exhibited a significant positive relationship with Gensini score, which was obtained from the result of invasive coronary angiography examination. Gensini score involves analysis of both coronary artery morphology and percentage of stenosis [1], which is associated with long-term cardiovascular outcomes [3]. Therefore, these data partly indicated that our novel scoring system, using clinical risk factors, may also have the potential to predict the cardiac prognosis. However, further random, prospective clinical studies are needed to document this association.

This study also had several limitations. First, the study population was relatively small, and the study design was cross-sectional, with a lack of follow-up data. Additionally, echocardiography cannot distinguish calcification from fibrosis of the aortic valve; therefore, severe fibrosis may have been misdiagnosed as calcification. Finally, the definition of severe CAD was set according to the results of angiography and Gensini scores. Thus, this system could not explain the association between the occurrence of myocardial ischemia and stenosis. Further prospective studies are needed to clarify the efficacy of our scoring system.

Conclusions

Severe CAD prediction in patients with stable angina was achieved using our novel scoring system, which combined clinical risk factors and echocardiography. This scoring system performed well in patients prior to coronary angiography, which could be helpful for making diagnostic decisions.

Author Contributions

Analyzed the data: Y-HC J-YM. Wrote the paper: Z-WC. Conceived the study: Z-WC. Designed the study: J-BG. Performed the study: J-YQ.

References

1. Gensini GG (1983) A more meaningful scoring system for determining the severity of coronary heart disease. Am J Cardiol 51: 606.
2. Girasis C, Garg S, Raber L, Sarno G, Morel MA, et al (2011) SYNTAX score and Clinical SYNTAX score as predictors of very long-term clinical outcomes in patients undergoing percutaneous coronary interventions: a substudy of SIRolimus-eluting stent compared with pacliTAXel-eluting stent for coronary revascularization (SIRTAX) trial. Eur Heart J 32: 3115–3127.
3. Niccoli G, Giubilato S, Di Vito L, Leo A, Cosentino N, et al (2013) Severity of coronary atherosclerosis in patients with a first acute coronary event: a diabetes paradox. Eur Heart J 34: 729–741.
4. Sinning C, Lillpopp L, Appelbaum S, Ojeda F, Zeller T, et al (2013) Angiographic score assessment improves cardiovascular risk prediction: the clinical value of SYNTAX and Gensini application. Clin Res Cardiol 102: 495–503.
5. de Mulder M, Gitt A, van Domburg R, Hochadel M, Seabra-Gomes R, et al (2011) EuroHeart score for the evaluation of in-hospital mortality in patients undergoing percutaneous coronary intervention. Eur Heart J 32: 1398–1408.
6. Garg S, Sarno G, Garcia-Garcia HM, Girasis C, Wykrzykowska J, et al (2010) A new tool for the risk stratification of patients with complex coronary artery disease: the Clinical SYNTAX Score. Circ Cardiovasc Interv 3: 317–326.
7. Singh M, Gersh BJ, Li S, Rumsfeld JS, Spertus JA, et al (2008) Mayo Clinic Risk Score for percutaneous coronary intervention predicts in-hospital mortality in patients undergoing coronary artery bypass graft surgery. Circulation 117: 356–362.
8. Diamond GA, Forrester JS (1979) Analysis of probability as an aid in the clinical diagnosis of coronary-artery disease. N Engl J Med 300: 1350–1358.
9. Wilson PW, D'Agostino RB, Levy D, Belanger AM, Silbershatz H, et al (1998) Prediction of coronary heart disease using risk factor categories. Circulation 97: 1837–1847.
10. Lee BC, Lee WJ, Hsu HC, Chien KL, Shih TT, et al (2011) Using clinical cardiovascular risk scores to predict coronary artery plaque severity and stenosis detected by CT coronary angiography in asymptomatic Chinese subjects. Int J Cardiovasc Imaging 27: 669–678.
11. Prasad A, Singh M, Lerman A, Lennon RJ, Holmes DR Jr, et al (2006) Isolated elevation in Troponin T after percutaneous coronary intervention is associated with higher long-term mortality. J Am Coll Cardio 48: 1765–1770.
12. Daly C, Norrie J, Murdoch DL, Ford I, Dargie HJ, et al (2003) The value of routine non-invasive tests to predict clinical outcome in stable angina. Eur Heart J 24: 532–540.
13. Adler Y, Vaturi M, Herz I, Iakobishvili Z, Toaf J, et al (2002) Nonobstructive aortic valve calcification: a window to significant coronary artery disease. Atherosclerosis 161: 193–197.
14. Otto CM, Lind BK, Kitzman DW, Gersh BJ, Siscovick DS (1999) Association of aortic-valve sclerosis with cardiovascular mortality and morbidity in the elderly. New Engl J Med 341: 142–147.
15. Hendel RC, Patel MR, Kramer CM, Poon M, Hendel RC, et al (2006) ACCF/ACR/SCCT/SCMR/ASNC/NASCI/SCAI/SIR 2006 appropriateness criteria for cardiac computed tomography and cardiac magnetic resonance imaging: a report of the American College of Cardiology Foundation Quality Strategic Directions Committee Appropriateness Criteria Working Group, American College of Radiology, Society of Cardiovascular Computed Tomography, Society for Cardiovascular Magnetic Resonance, American Society of Nuclear Cardiology, North American Society for Cardiac Imaging, Society for Cardiovascular Angiography and Interventions, and Society of Interventional Radiology. J Am Coll Cardiol 48: 1475–1497.
16. Iung B, Baron G, Butchart EG, Delahaye F, Gohlke-Bärwolf C, et al (2003) A prospective survey of patients with valvular heart disease in Europe: The Euro Heart Survey on Valvular Heart Disease. Eur Heart J 24: 1231–1243.
17. Rajamannan NM, Subramaniam M, Rickard D, Stock SR, Donovan J, et al (2003) Human aortic valve calcification is associated with an osteoblast phenotype. Circulation 107: 2181–2184.
18. Mohler ER 3rd, Gannon F, Reynolds C, Zimmerman R, Keane MG, et al (2001) Bone formation and inflammation in cardiac valves. Circulation 103: 1522–1528.
19. Qian J, Chen Z, Ge J, Ma J, Chang S, et al (2010) Relationship between aortic valve calcification and the severity of coronary atherosclerotic disease. J Heart Valve Dis 19: 466–470.
20. Chen ZW, Qian JY, Jian Y, Ge L, Liu XB, et al (2011) Prevalence and severity of coronary artery disease in diabetic patients with aortic valve calcification. Acta Cardiol 66: 15–20.

Left Ventricular Myocardial Function in Hemodialysis and Nondialysis Uremia Patients: A Three-Dimensional Speckle-Tracking Echocardiography Study

Ran Chen[1], Xia Wu[2], Li-Jun Shen[3], Bei Wang[1], Ming-Ming Ma[1], Yuan Yang[1], Bo-Wen Zhao[1]*

1 Department of Diagnostic Ultrasound and Echocardiography, Sir Run Run Shaw Hospital, Zhejiang University College of Medicine and Sir Run Run Shaw Institute of Clinical Medicine of Zhejiang University, Hangzhou, China, **2** Department of Radiology, Sir Run Run Shaw Hospital, Zhejiang University College of Medicine and Sir Run Run Shaw Institute of Clinical Medicine of Zhejiang University, Hangzhou, China, **3** Department of Ultrasound, The First People's Hospital, Hangzhou Xiao Shan District, Hangzhou, China

Abstract

Background: Several studies have demonstrated that uremic patients who have preserved left ventricular ejection fraction (LVEF) could still have the potential for systolic dysfunction. The aim of this study was to assess the differences between the left ventricular (LV) myocardial function in hemodialysis and nondialysis uremic patients based on three-dimensional speckle-tracking echocardiography.

Methods: The study population consisted of 35 maintenance hemodialysis patients (the hemodialysis group), 30 uremic patients who were hospitalized for the creation of a primary arteriovenous fistula (the nondialysis group), and 32 healthy volunteers. All of the patients had normal left ventricular ejection fractions (i.e., 55% or greater). Three-dimensional speckle tracking echocardiography was performed to assess the left ventricle's global three-dimensional strain, regional longitudinal strain, circumferential strain, and radial strain.

Results: The left ventricular regional longitudinal strain, radial strain, circumferential strain, and global three-dimensional strain were significantly decreased in the nondialysis patients compared with the other two groups (all, $P<0.001$). However, the three-dimensional strain and the regional longitudinal strain were lower in the hemodialysis patients than in the controls ($P<0.01$). In the hemodialysis patients and the control group, the longitudinal strain, circumferential strain, and radial strain were higher at the apical level than they were at the basal level and midlevels. A multivariate linear regression analysis showed that the blood urea nitrogen and creatinine levels were independently associated with the values of the global three-dimensional strain ($\beta=-0.217$, $P=0.000$; $\beta=-0.243$, $P=0.011$, respectively) and the longitudinal strain ($\beta=-0.154$, $P=0.032$; $\beta=-0.188$, $P=0.029$, respectively).

Conclusions: Three-dimensional speckle-tracking echocardiography may detect myocardial dysfunction in patients with uremia who have preserved LVEF. The global three-dimensional strain and the regional longitudinal strain appear to be superior in hemodialysis patients compared with nondialysis patients.

Editor: Xiongwen Chen, Temple University, United States of America

Funding: The research is supported by Specialized Research Fund for the Doctoral Program of Higher Education (20110101120136). The funders had no role in study design, data collection and analysis, decision to publish, or preparation of the manuscript.

Competing Interests: The authors have declared that no competing interests exist.

* Email: zbwcjp@163.com

Introduction

Uremia is associated with an increased risk of cardiovascular diseases, including coronary artery disease, myocardial infarction, and heart failure. Mortality is increased by 10- to 20-fold in dialysis patients compared with healthy individuals [1]. Most studies have used the conventional echocardiographic parameters of cardiac function, such as ejection fraction and fraction shortening, which are frequently normal in uremic patients [2,3]. A previous study showed that the ejection fraction and fraction shortening do not adequately describe the regional systolic function and the loading conditions affecting these parameters [4]. Attention has recently been focused on using Doppler tissue imaging to assess LV regional systolic function through the measurement of tissue velocities, displacement, strain, and strain rate. However, tissue Doppler imaging is limited by Doppler angle dependence, which can identify only the myocardial motion and deformation occurring in the direction of the ultrasound beam [5]. Therefore, it has been used primarily to assess longitudinal strain. However, longitudinal strain is only 1 of the 3 principle components of the regional systolic function [6]. Two-dimensional speckle-tracking echocardiography was also recently adopted to detect the subtle impairment of the LV systolic function in uremic patients who have normal LVEF [7,8]. However, a major limitation of two-dimensional speckle-tracking echocardiography (2D STE) is that it is unable to quantify one of the three components of the local displacement vector because of the three-dimensional (3D) anatomy of the LV and the complex 3D patterns of the wall motion [9].

Three-dimensional speckle-tracking echocardiography (3D STE) is a new and emerging technique. It relies on 3D echocardiographic datasets and tracks the motion of speckles within a scanned volume, irrespective of direction. Yu et al. demonstrated that the 3D strain (3DS), which is best described as the "principle tangential strain," may display the resulting direction's muscle fiber contractions, which are aligned either parallel to or tangential to the myocardial surface [10]. The combination of the three components, 3D optical flow and 3D phase correlation, as well as the 3D intensity correlation, allows the calculation of the 3D motion vector field of the subendocardium. Kleijn et al. confirmed the accuracy of 3D STE for the quantitative assessment of global LV function by using cardiac magnetic resonance imaging as a reference method [11], suggesting that 3D STE has the potential to overcome the limitations of Doppler tissue imaging and 2D STE [12,13]. Therefore, the aim of this study was use 3D STE to investigate the LV global and regional myocardial function in hemodialysis and nondialysis uremic patients who have normal LVEF.

Materials and Methods

Study Participants

Between August 2012 and June 2013, 75 uremic patients with a LVEF of 55% or greater were consecutively enrolled from the nephrology clinic. The cases excluded from the study were 2 patients with arrhythmias, 2 patients with severe valvular disease, 3 patients with uncontrolled hypertension (i.e., systolic blood pressure greater than 140 mmHg and/or diastolic blood pressure greater than 90 mmHg), and 3 patients for whom the 3D STE image quality was inadequate. Finally, 65 patients with uremia were analyzed in this study. The uremia patients included 35 patients on maintenance hemodialysis (the hemodialysis group; 4-hour sessions, 3 times weekly for 3 months or more) who were prescribed a standard dose of dialysis targeting an equilibrated dose (Kt/V of urea) of 1.2 or more and 30 patients who were hospitalized for the creation of a primary arteriovenous fistula (the nondialysis group). We recruited 32 age-matched control volunteers from among individuals who received routine checkups at our hospital who had normal results on electrocardiography, transthoracic echocardiography, multi-slice spiral computed tomography (CT), and coronary angiography and had normal blood pressure. The biochemical indexes of all of the study participants were evaluated at the hospital laboratory. The indexes included total cholesterol, glyceride, hemoglobin, creatinine, and urea nitrogen levels in the blood. Written and informed consent was obtained from all of the study participants. The study was approved by the local ethics committee of the Sir Run Run Shaw Hospital (Hangzhou, China).

Echocardiography Measurements

All of the echocardiographic studies were performed using a commercial scanner (iE33; Philips Medical System, N.A., Bothell, WA, USA). Real-time 3D echocardiographic imaging was performed from the cardiac apex by a fully sampled matrix-array transducer. The full-volume acquisition (which included 6 wedge-shaped volumes) was recorded with 6 consecutive cardiac cycles during a single breath-hold. Moreover, the temporal and spatial resolutions of the images were optimized by decreasing the depth and adjusting the sector width to ensure that the entire LV cavity was included within the pyramidal volume. An experienced echocardiographer obtained all of the echocardiographic images using a standard protocol, and another echocardiographer who was blinded to the clinical data of the study participants analyzed the images. An offline analysis of the data was performed using Tom-Tec 4.0 analysis software (Tom Tec Imaging Systems Gmbh, Unterschleissheim, Bayern, Germany). For the tracing of the endocardium and epicardium, the following five views were displayed: (1) the apical four-chamber view; (2) the apical two-chamber view and the three short-axis views; (3) the apex of the LV; (4) the midlevel of the LV; and (5) the basal level of the LV.

Table 1. Clinical Characteristics of the Uremia and Control Groups.

Parameters	Control (n = 32)	Hemodialysis (n = 35)	Nondialysis (n = 30)
Age (year)	53.05±6.83	52.78±7.65	53.16±5.69
Male/female	20/20	19/21	17/23
Course of disease (year)	-------	5.5±3.3	6.2±2.8
Heart rate (bpm)	75±11	73±10	74±12
Systolic BP (mmHg)	120±15	125±13	128±12
Diastolic BP (mmHg)	75±8	80±9	83±8
Body surface area (m^2)	1.5±0.4	1.6 ±0.3	1.6±0.5
Total cholesterol (mmol/;L)	3.3±0.8	6.8±0.9*	8.0±1.2*
Glyceride (mmol/L)	1.2±0.8	4.8±1.2*	6.3±1.3*
Hb (g/dL)	12.4±0.9	11.3±0.8	8.5±0.6*†
CRE (umol/L)	100.5±26.3	580.5±53.3**	897.8±186.9** ††
BUN (mmol/L)	6.8±1.3	20.6±6.4**	48.6±7.0**††
KT/V	NA	1.3±0.2	NA

BP = blood pressure; BUN = blood urea nitrogen; CRE = creatinine; Hb = hemoglobin; Kt/V = dose of dialysis.
$P<0.01$, compared with the control group.
**$P<0.001$, compared with the control group.
†$P<0.01$, compared with the hemodialysis patient group.
††$P<0.001$, compared with the hemodialysis patient group.

Table 2. Echocardiographic Characteristics of the Uremia and Control Groups.

	Control (n = 32)	Hemodialysis (n = 35)	Nondialysis (n = 30)
LVEDV(mL)	78.9±5.1	95.8±8.1*	109.4±7.2*
LVSDV(mL)	3 5.1±3.5	45.4±2.5*	54.3±2.9*
LVEDD(mm)	49.4±3.5	58.6±3.2*	60.2±2.8*
LVESD(mm)	30.5±4.3	41.3±2.6*	43.5±3.0*
LVEF(%)	62.9±2.4	57.8±1.9	56.7±2.0
IVST(mm)	9.2±0.4	13.8±0.5**	14.5±0.3**
LVPWT(mm)	8.8±0.3	12.8±0.2**	13.3±0.3**
E	85.3± 22.1	83.6±17.8	72.3±10.4*
A	78.61±2.5	85.3±20.1	93.9±19.4*
E/A	1.1±0.5	0.83±0.2	0.8±0.3*
E′	8.3±1.6	7.0±1.0	6.2±0.8*
A′	6.8±1.5	8.0±2.1	9.0±2.2*
E′/A′	1.12±0.3	0.92±0.2	0.71±0.1*
E/E′	10.3±2.7	14.3±2.5**	15.8±3.2**

A = transmitral peak velocity of late-diastole; E = transmitral peak velocity of early-diastole; A′, velocity of late diastole of the mitral annulus; E′ = velocity of early diastole of the mitral annulus; E/A = the ratio of velocity of early and late diastole; E′/A′ = ratio of velocity of early and late diastole of mitral annulus; IVST = interventricular septum thickness; LVEDV, left ventricular end-diastolic volume; LVEDD, left ventricular end-diastolic diameter; LVEF = left ventricular ejection fraction; LVESD, left ventricular end- systolic diameter; LVESV, left ventricular end-systolic volume; LVPWT = left ventricular posterior wall thickness.
*$P<0.01$, compared to the control group.
**$P<0.001$, compared to the control group.

The LV epicardium and endocardium were traced automatically, and the tracings were refined with further adjustment. Thus, in a cardiac cycle, the software was able to perform both global and segmental strain analyses, including the global 3D strain (3DS), regional longitudinal strain (LS), radial strain (RS), and circumferential strain (CS). Meanwhile, the end-systolic and end-diastolic LV volumes and ejection fractions were observed automatically. On the parasternal long-axis view, the thickness of the interventricular septum and LV posterior wall were measured at the end-diastole of the LV. The LV diameters were measured at the end-systole and end-diastole phases. The early (E) and late (A) diastolic peak velocities of the mitral inflow and the early (E′) and late (A′) diastolic peak velocities of the septal mitral annulus were measured by pulse wave Doppler and Doppler tissue imaging. Subsequently, the E/A ratio, E′/A′ ratio, and E/E′ ratio were calculated to evaluate the diastolic function of the LV.

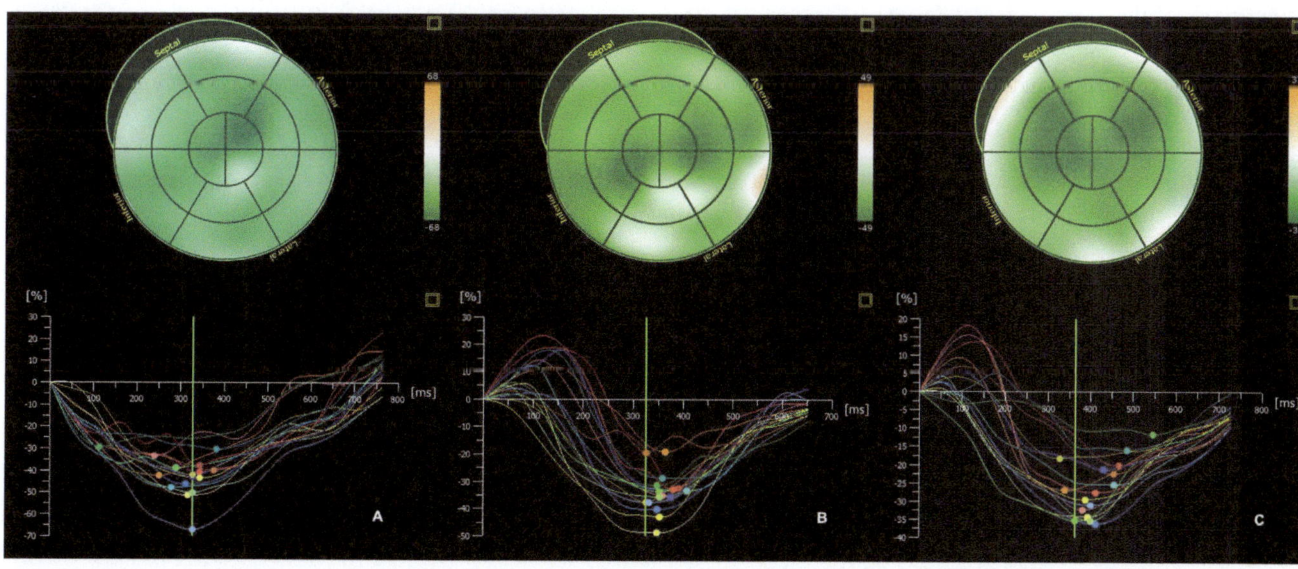

Figure 1. The three-dimensional strain curves of the 16 segments of LV in (A) the controls, (B) the patients in the hemodialysis group, and (C) the nondialysis patients. The color-coded curves indicate the different myocardial segments of the LV. The peak strain values of the different myocardial regions are more decreased in the uremic patients than in the controls. The peak strain is lowest in the nondialysis group.

Table 3. 3D-STE parameters of the Uremia and Control Groups.

		Control (n = 29)	Hemodialysis (n = 30)	Nondialysis (n = 28)
Global	3DS(%)	−38.58±4.25	−25.52±6.81*	−17.75±5.87*,†
Basal	LS	−21.09±3.45	−16.98±2.35*	−10.78±3.08*,†
	CS	−40.63±2.96	−41.69±3.69	−28.58±5.10*,†
	RS	78.08±18.06	77.36±13.37	60.58±12.95*,†
Mid	LS	−22.96±2.65	−15.45±5.23*	−10.39±2.89*,†
	CS	−44.48±5.32	−42.39±4.56	−30.28±2.64*,†
	RS	92.37±8.69	90.78±6.31	64.58±5.87**,††
Apex	LS	−32.43±4.51§,‖	−23.87±3.41*,§,‖	−12.27±2.14*,†
	CS	−50.25±5.68§,‖	−49.24±3.59§,‖	−30.23±3.14**,††
	RS	100.58±10.21§,‖	101.58±16.31§,‖	62.89±7.19**,††

3DS = three-dimensional strain; CS = circumferential strain; LS = longitudinal strain; RS = radial strain; STE = speckle-tracking echocardiography.
*$P<0.01$, compared with the control group.
**$P<0.001$, compared with the control group.
†$P<0.01$, compared with the hemodialysis patient group.
††$P<0.001$, compared with the hemodialysis patient group $P<0.01$, compared with the hemodialysis patient group.
§$P<0.01$, compared with the values at the basal level.
‖$P<0.01$, compared with the values at the midlevel.

Intraobserver Reproducibility and Interobserver Reliability

For the intraobserver reproducibility, 10 subjects were analyzed twice within 4 weeks by one investigator, and the mean values of 16 segments at three levels of LV for RS, CS, LS and 3DS were calculated. The interobserver reliability assessment was performed by analyzing 10 subjects who were chosen randomly by 2 independent investigators. Both observers were blinded to the previous measurements.

Statistical Analysis

All statistical analyses were performed using SPSS version 16.0 software (SPSS, Inc., Chicago, IL, USA). All data were presented as the mean ± the standard deviation (SD). The duration of uremia and hypertension were presented as median values. Differences in the continuous data and categorical data between the patients and the controls were compared using a one-way analysis of variance and χ^2 tests. Independent determinations of subclinical myocardial systolic dysfunction in patients with uremia were examined using multivariate linear regression. The intraclass correlation coefficients (ICCs) method was used to assess the intraobserver reproducibility and the interobserver reliability for the values of the 3D global strain and regional strain. The ICCs were expressed as percentages. The clinical significance was categorized as follows: "excellent," if the ICC was 0.80 or greater; "good," if the ICC was between 0.61 and 0.79; "moderate," if the ICC was between 0.41 and 0.60; and "poor," if the ICC was 0.4 or less [14].

Results

Clinical Parameters

The general clinical indexes and the blood indexes of the hemodialysis group, the nondialysis group, and the control group are summarized in Table 1. Among the three groups, there were no significant differences in sex, age, heart rate, and blood pressure (all, $P>0.05$). However, the total cholesterol and glyceride levels were greater in the hemodialysis and nondialysis groups than in the control group (6.8±0.9 mmol/L and 8.0±1.2 mmol/L vs. 3.3±0.8 mmol/L; 4.8±1.2 mmol/L and 6.3±1.3 mmol/L vs. 1.2±0.8 mmol/L, respectively; $P<0.01$). The total cholesterol and glyceride levels were not significantly different between the hemodialysis and the nondialysis groups. The hemoglobin level was lower in the nondialysis group than in the hemodialysis group and the control group (8.5±0.6 g/dL vs. 11.3±0.8 g/dL and 8.5±0.6 g/dL vs. 12.4±0.9 g/dL, respectively; $P<0.01$). No difference was observed between the hemodialysis group and control group. The creatinine (CRE) and blood urea nitrogen (BUN) levels were significantly greater in the hemodialysis and nondialysis groups than in the control group (580.5±53.3 μmol/L and 897.8±186.9 umol/L vs. 100.5±26.3 umol/L; 20.6±6.4 mmol/L and 48.6±7.0 mmol/L vs. 6.8±1.3 mmol/L, respectively; $P<0.001$). These two levels were significantly decreased in the hemodialysis group compared with the nondialysis group (580.5±53.3 umol/L vs. 897.8±186.9 umol/L and 20.6±6.4 mmol/L vs. 48.6±7.0 mmol/L, respectively; $P<0.001$).

Echocardiographic Characteristics

The echocardiographic parameters of the study groups are shown in Table 2. Compared with the control group, both the nondialysis group and the hemodialysis group demonstrated higher left ventricular end-diastolic volume, left ventricular end-diastolic volume, left ventricular end-diastolic diameter, left ventricular end-systolic diameter, left ventricular septum thickness, left ventricular posterior wall thickness, and E/E′ ratio (all, $P<0.01$). However, there were no significant differences in these factors between the hemodialysis and nondialysis groups. The LVEF was similar in the three groups. Furthermore, the E, A, E/A ratio, E′, A′, and E′/A′ ratio (all, $P<0.01$) were decreased significantly only in the nondialysis group compared with the hemodialysis group and the control group. However, no difference was found between the hemodialysis group and the control group.

Speckle-Tracking Echocardiography Analysis

One hundred and sixty (10%) of 1552 segments were excluded from the 3D STE analysis because of drop-out. The 3D STE analyses of the three groups are shown in Table 3. The LS, CS,

Table 4. Independent factors associated with the systolic functional parameters.

	3DS		LS		RS		CS	
	β	*P*	*β*	*P*	*β*	*P*	*β*	*P*
Duration of Uremia	0.074	.463	0.056	.379	0.021	.089	0.013	.089
Systolic BP	−0.125	.142	−0.074	.284	−0.058	.315	−0.252	.074
LVST	0.062	.326	0.087	.365	0.021	.064	0.700	.125
E/E'	0.004	.245	0.025	.157	0.085	.310	0.018	.584
Total cholesterol	−0.035	.638	−0.042	.793	−0.038	.157	−0.098	.243
Glyceride	−0.041	.548	−0.058	.547	−0.024	.857	−0.035	.142
Hb	0.025	.336	0.102	.970	0.054	.634	0.047	.639
CRE	−0.243	.011	−0.188	.029	−0.116	.213	−0.137	.105
BUN	−0.217	.000	−0.154	.032	−0.128	.122	−0.092	.174

3DS = three-dimensional strain; CS = circumferential strain; LS = longitudinal strain; RS = radial strain; BP = blood pressure; IVST = interventricular septum thickness; E/E' = the ratio of transmitral peak velocity of early-diastole and velocity of early diastole of the mitral annulu; Hb = hemoglobin; BUN = blood urea nitrogen; CRE = creatinine; *β* = *Beta coefficient*

and RS at the three levels of LV and 3DS were decreased in the nondialysis group compared with both the control group and the hemodialysis group (all, $P<0.01$) (Figure 1). In addition, the 3DS and LS at the three levels of LV were lower in the hemodialysis group than in the control group (all, $P<0.01$). In the CS and RS, there was no significant difference between the hemodialysis and the control group. The LS, CS, and RS were higher at the apical level than they were at the basal level and the midlevel in the hemodialysis patients and the control patients. However, these values were not significantly changed in the nondialysis group. Based on the multivariate linear regression analysis, the duration of the uremia, systolic blood pressure, LVST, E/E' ratio, and the levels of the total cholesterol, glyceride, Hb, CRE, and BUN were associated with the 3DS, LS, RS and CS, which were used to examine the risk factors for preclinical myocardial systolic dysfunction. The levels of CRE and BUN were independently associated with the 3DS value ($\beta = -0.217$, $P = 0.000$; $\beta = -0.243$, $P = 0.011$) and the LS value ($\beta = -0.154$, $P = 0.032$; $\beta = -0.188$, $P = 0.029$) (Table 4).

Interobserver and Intraobserver Reproducibility

The ICCs are shown in Table 5. The ICCs were all above 0.8. The mean absolute percentage error of all of the measurements did not exceed 0.1. The intraobserver and interobserver reproducibility for the mean measurements of the LS, CS, and RS in the sixteen segments of the three levels of LV and 3DS were acceptable.

Discussion

Cardiac function is still incompletely characterized in uremia patients. This is the first study to compare the differences in the global and regional myocardial functions in hemodialysis and nondialysis patients based on 3D STE. The primary findings of this study are as follows: (1) the global LV systolic function (EF) was normal in the uremic group; however, the global 3DS and the regional LS, RS, and CS were decreased in the nondialysis group, indicating that the LV regional long-axis, short-axis, and global functions were already impaired; (2) the 3DS and LS were higher in the hemodialysis group than in the nondialysis group, indicating that the LV global and regional long-axis functions were superior in the hemodialysis patients; and (3) the decreased CS and RS were observed only in the nondialysis patients and not in the hemodialysis patients. These results demonstrate that, in myocardial dysfunction, the global LV dysfunction and LV regional long-axis systolic dysfunction appear to be more vulnerable to change compared with the short-axis function.

The LVEF reflects the sum of all of the regional shortening in the left ventricle, and regional wall motion impairment may not reduce the LVEF unless several segments are involved.

In our study, the LVEF was normal in the uremia group; however, the LV regional long-axis, short-axis and global functions were already impaired in the uremia patients as assessed by 3D STE, regardless of whether they were undergoing hemodialysis. The underlying mechanisms of the decreased LV function in uremia patients are complex and not thoroughly understood. We speculated that hypertension, LV hypertrophy, LV remodeling, coronary artery disease, myocardial fibrosis, and apoptosis may contribute to LV dysfunction in uremia patients with preserved LVEF. In addition, we found that the LV global function and regional long-axis function were superior in the hemodialysis patients, as shown by the higher 3DS and LS in the hemodialysis group than in the nondialysis group. We believe that the improvement in the LV function in the hemodialysis patients

Table 5. Reproducibility of interobserver and intraobserver by 3D STE.

		Interobserver		Intraobserver	
		ICC	MAPE	ICC	MAPE
Global	3DS(%)	0.84	0.04	0.85	0.03
Basal	LS	0.85	0.05	0.81	0.05
	CS	0.87	0.07	0.91	0.08
	RS	0.85	0.05	0.89	0.07
Mid	LS	0.83	0.08	0.82	0.04
	CS	0.90	0.04	0.86	0.09
	RS	0.87	0.06	0.85	0.05
Apex	LS	0.81	0.08	0.87	0.07
	CS	0.84	0.07	0.90	0.06
	RS	0.82	0.06	0.84	0.05

3DS = three-dimensional strain; CS = circumferential strain; ICC = intraclass correlation coefficient; LS = longitudinal strain; MAPE = mean absolute percentage error; RS = radial strain.

may have resulted from factors such as improvements in their anemia, malnutrition, calcium-phosphorus metabolism disorder and acid-base balance, etc. These factors may decrease the volume load of the LV and thereby improve the anoxic condition of the tissues and organs. The increase in the myocardial oxygen and blood flow as well as the improvement in the LV remodeling may also promote LV systolic function. Therefore, the results from the current study indicate that the 3DS and LS may be sensitive predictors of preclinical LV dysfunction in patients with uremia, particularly in hemodialysis patients. The detection of subclinical myocardial dysfunction may assist clinical doctors in treating uremia patients earlier (even if the LVEF is normal), and thereby reduce the incidence of cardiovascular disease while improving long-term outcomes.

Yan et al. also demonstrated that the CS and RS decreased only in the nondialysis patients based on the 2D STE [3]. This is similar to the results of our study, showing that the impairment in the short-axis function occurred later than the impairment in the regional long-axis function based on the 3D STE. The possible reasons for this result are (1) the augmented LV wall thickness and cross-fiber shortening, which exert their effects as the interaction between a contraction and a systolic increase in the cross-sectional area of all differently aligned myocardial layers; and (2) the curvature radius of the circumferentially oriented myocardial fibers is smaller than that of the longitudinal fibers, which may entail lower stress and consequently delay the appearance of functional abnormalities [15–17].

In addition, myocardial deformation occurs in three dimensions and can be characterized in the longitudinal direction, as well as in the circumferential and radial directions. Subepicardial fibers play a major role in both the RS and LS [18], and subendocardial fibers are important components in CS [19]. The subepicardium is more susceptible to myocardial ischemia and stiffness than the subendocardium. Maizel et al. reported that myocardial stiffness in the uremic mouse may represent an autonomic nervous dysfunction, cellular calcium, or an energy metabolism disorder, for example [20]. Our study showed that the CS and RS were observed in the nondialysis patients but not in the hemodialysis patients. Therefore, myocardial stiffness may be one factor that causes changes in the LV long-axis function earlier than in the short-axis function in uremia patients.

The LV's contractions travel from the apex to the basal region. Our study also found that the LS, CS, and RS were higher at the apical level than at the basal level and the midlevels in the control and hemodialysis groups. However, this phenomenon did not appear in the nondialysis group. A previous study has shown that myocardial contractility reflects the influence of preload [21]. We postulated that the improvement in water-sodium retention and the removal of fluid decrease the preload in hemodialysis patients compared with the nondialysis patients.

A decreased myocardial strain in uremia patients reportedly results from LV hypertrophy rather than from uremic toxicity [22]. In fact, in this study, the myocardial strain was superior in the hemodialysis patients, and the prevalence of hypertrophy was similar in the hemodialysis and nondialysis groups. Moreover, the multiple linear regression showed that the CRE and BUN levels were independent predictors of the global LV systolic function. The CRE and BUN levels were lower in the hemodialysis group than in the nondialysis group. We therefore assumed that the superior LV systolic function in the hemodialysis patients may result from the removal of uremic toxins. A previous study demonstrated that the injury of the myocardial cell membrane structure could cause cardiac dysfunction in uremic patients that was possibly related to the accumulation of uremic toxins [23]. Mark demonstrated that CRE could inhibit the activity of succinate dehydrogenase (SDH) in myocardial cells, which could lead both to obstacles in ATP production and mitochondrial swelling and fragmentation, and thus imbalance and damage to the nutrition and function of the myocardial cells [24]. Moreover, in some studies, BUN is a powerful predictor of increased mortality in patients hospitalized for heart failure. In older patients hospitalized for heart failure [25], a positive linear relationship was found between the BUN and the occurrence of 1-year mortality. According to our study, both the BUN and the CRE possibly contributed to myocardial dysfunction to a certain degree. In addition, indoxyl sulfate (IS), a uremic toxin, can induce TGF-$\beta$and phospho-NFkB p65 protein expression, and the reactive oxygen species-NF-kB-TGF-β_1 pathway may play a role in cardiac fibrosis. Lekawanvijit et al. showed that cardiac fibrosis is reversible by reducing the serum IS level in uremic rats [26]. Therefore, the reduction in uremic toxins possibly alleviates the injury to the myocardial function in hemodialysis patients.

Study Limitations

The temporal and spatial resolutions are relatively lower in the 3D STE than in the 2D STE. Therefore, several patients had to be excluded because the image quality in 1 or more segments was insufficient for the STE analysis. Moreover, our study included a relatively small number of patients. In addition, the long-term cardiovascular event rates or survival assessment in the patients on maintenance hemodialysis was not presented in this study.

Conclusions

Three-dimensional STE analysis offers a useful tool for predicting the myocardial function of the LV in uremic patients. The global LV systolic function and the short-axis and long-axis regional LV myocardial function may be impaired in nondialysis patients who have preserved ejection fraction. However, the global LV function and regional LV systolic function appeared to be superior in the hemodialysis patients over those in the nondialysis patients. 3DS and LS may be sensitive predictors of LV global and regional systolic dysfunction.

Acknowledgments

The authors wish to thank the study subjects for their participation.

Author Contributions

Conceived and designed the experiments: RC BWZ LJS. Performed the experiments: XW BW MMM. Analyzed the data: RC MMM YY. Wrote the paper: RC XW.

References

1. Foley RN, Parfrey PS, Sarnak MJ (1998) Epidemiology of cardiovascular disease in chronic renal disease. J Am Soc Nephrol 9: S16–23.
2. Hayashi SY, Brodin LA, Alvestrand A, Lind B, Stenvinkel P, et al. (2004) Improvement of cardiac function after haemodialysis. Quantitative evaluation by colour tissue velocity imaging. Nephrol Dial Transplant 19: 1497–1506.
3. Yan P, Li H, Hao C, Shi H, Gu Y, et al. (2011) 2D-speckle tracking echocardiography contributes to early identification of impaired left ventricular myocardial function in patients with chronic kidney disease. Nephron Clin Pract 118: c232–240.
4. Semple D, Smith K, Bhandari S, Seymour AM (2011) Uremic cardiomyopathy and insulin resistance: a critical role for akt? J Am Soc Nephrol 22: 207–215.
5. Aurigemma GP, Gaasch WH, Villegas B, Meyer TE (1995) Noninvasive assessment of left ventricular mass, chamber volume, and contractile function. Curr Probl Cardiol 20: 361–440.
6. Mendes L, Ribeiras R, Adragao T, Lima S, Horta E, et al. (2008) Load-independent parameters of diastolic and systolic function by speckle tracking and tissue doppler in hemodialysis patients. Rev Port Cardiol 27: 1011–1025.
7. Kim HK, Sohn DW, Lee SE, Choi SY, Park JS, et al. (2007) Assessment of left ventricular rotation and torsion with two-dimensional speckle tracking echocardiography. J Am Soc Echocardiogr 20: 45–53.
8. Liu YW, Su CT, Huang YY, Yang CS, Huang JW, et al. (2011) Left ventricular systolic strain in chronic kidney disease and hemodialysis patients. Am J Nephrol 33: 84–90.
9. Saito K, Okura H, Watanabe N, Hayashida A, Obase K, et al. (2009) Comprehensive evaluation of left ventricular strain using speckle tracking echocardiography in normal adults: comparison of three-dimensional and two-dimensional approaches. J Am Soc Echocardiogr 22: 1025–1030.
10. Kang Y, Sun MM, Cui J, Chen HY, Su YG, et al. (2012) Three-dimensional speckle tracking echocardiography for the assessment of left ventricular function and mechanical dyssynchrony. Acta Cardiol 67: 423–430.
11. Kleijn SA, Brouwer WP, Aly MF, Russel IK, de Roest GJ, et al. (2012) Comparison between three-dimensional speckle-tracking echocardiography and cardiac magnetic resonance imaging for quantification of left ventricular volumes and function. Eur Heart J Cardiovasc Imaging 13: 834–839.
12. Perk G, Tunick PA, Kronzon I (2007) Non-Doppler two-dimensional strain imaging by echocardiography—from technical considerations to clinical applications. J Am Soc Echocardiogr 20: 234–243.
13. Ng AC, Tran da T, Newman M, Allman C, Vidaic J, et al. (2008) Comparison of myocardial tissue velocities measured by two-dimensional speckle tracking and tissue Doppler imaging. Am J Cardiol 102: 784–789.
14. Fleiss JL (1986) The design and analysis of clinical experiments. New York: Wiley. xiv, 432 p. p..
15. Rakhit DJ, Zhang XH, Leano R, Armstrong KA, Isbel NM, et al. (2007) Prognostic role of subclinical left ventricular abnormalities and impact of transplantation in chronic kidney disease. Am Heart J 153: 656–664.
16. Fagugli RM, Reboldi G, Quintaliani G, Pasini P, Ciao G, et al. (2001) Short daily hemodialysis: blood pressure control and left ventricular mass reduction in hypertensive hemodialysis patients. Am J Kidney Dis 38: 371–376.
17. Serri K, Reant P, Lafitte M, Berhouet M, Le Bouffos V, et al. (2006) Global and regional myocardial function quantification by two-dimensional strain: application in hypertrophic cardiomyopathy. J Am Coll Cardiol 47: 1175–1181.
18. Buckberg GD, Coghlan HC, Hoffman JI, Torrent-Guasp F (2001) The structure and function of the helical heart and its buttress wrapping. VII. Critical importance of septum for right ventricular function. Semin Thorac Cardiovasc Surg 13: 402–416.
19. Gotte MJ, Germans T, Russel IK, Zwanenburg JJ, Marcus JT, et al. (2006) Myocardial strain and torsion quantified by cardiovascular magnetic resonance tissue tagging: studies in normal and impaired left ventricular function. J Am Coll Cardiol 48: 2002–2011.
20. Maizel J, Six I, Slama M, Tribouilloy C, Sevestre H, et al. (2009) Mechanisms of aortic and cardiac dysfunction in uremic mice with aortic calcification. Circulation 119: 306–313.
21. Bogaert J, Rademakers FE (2001) Regional nonuniformity of normal adult human left ventricle. Am J Physiol Heart Circ Physiol 280: H610–620.
22. Popovic ZB, Kwon DH, Mishra M, Buakhamsri A, Greenberg NL, et al. (2008) Association between regional ventricular function and myocardial fibrosis in hypertrophic cardiomyopathy assessed by speckle tracking echocardiography and delayed hyperenhancement magnetic resonance imaging. J Am Soc Echocardiogr 21: 1299–1305.
23. Sarnak MJ, Levey AS, Schoolwerth AC, Coresh J, Culleton B, et al. (2003) Kidney disease as a risk factor for development of cardiovascular disease: a statement from the American Heart Association Councils on Kidney in Cardiovascular Disease, High Blood Pressure Research, Clinical Cardiology, and Epidemiology and Prevention. Circulation 108: 2154–2169.
24. Marks AR (1997) Intracellular calcium-release channels: regulators of cell life and death. Am J Physiol 272: H597–605.
25. Smith GL, Shlipak MG, Havranek EP, Foody JM, Masoudi FA, et al. (2006) Serum urea nitrogen, creatinine, and estimators of renal function: mortality in older patients with cardiovascular disease. Arch Intern Med 166: 1134–1142.
26. Lekawanvijit S, Kompa AR, Manabe M, Wang BH, Langham RG, et al. (2012) Chronic kidney disease-induced cardiac fibrosis is ameliorated by reducing circulating levels of a non-dialysable uremic toxin, indoxyl sulfate. PLoS One 7: e41281.

Association of Renal Biochemical Parameters with Left Ventricular Diastolic Dysfunction in a Community-Based Elderly Population in China

Jingmin Zhou[1]ʖ, Xiaotong Cui[1]ʖ, Xuejuan Jin[1]ʖ, Jun Zhou[1], Hanying Zhang[2], Bixiao Tang[2], Michael Fu[3], Hans Herlitz[4], Jie Cui[1], Hongmin Zhu[1], Aijun Sun[1], Kai Hu[1], Junbo Ge[1]*

1 Shanghai Institute of Cardiovascular Diseases, Zhongshan Hospital, Fudan University, Shanghai, China, **2** Fengjing Community Health Center, Jinshan District, Shanghai, China, **3** Section of Cardiology, Department of Medicine, Sahlgrenska University Hospital/Östra Hospital, University of Gothenburg, Gothenburg, Sweden, **4** Section of Nephrology, Department of Medicine, Sahlgrenska University Hospital/Östra Hospital, University of Gothenburg, Gothenburg, Sweden

Abstract

Background: Relationship of left ventricular diastolic dysfunction (LVDD) with parameters that could provide more information than hemodynamic renal indexes has not been clarified. We aimed to explore the association of comprehensive renal parameters with LVDD in a community-based elderly population.

Methods: 1,166 community residents (aged ≥ 65 years, 694 females) participating in the Shanghai Heart Health Study with complete data of renal parameters were investigated. Echocardiography was used to evaluate diastolic function with conventional and tissue Doppler imaging techniques. Serum urea, creatinine, urea-to-creatinine ratio, estimated glomerular filtration rate (eGFR) and urinary albumin-to-creatinine ratio (UACR) were analyzed on their associations with LVDD.

Results: The prevalence of LVDD increased in proportion to increasing serum urea, urea-to-creatinine ratio and UACR. These three renal parameters were found negatively correlated to peak early (E) to late (A) diastolic velocities ratio (E/A), and positively to left atrial volume index; UACR also positively correlated with E to peak early (E′) diastolic mitral annular velocity ratio (E/E′). Serum urea, urea-to-creatinine ratio and UACR correlated with LVDD in logistic univariate regression analysis, and urea-to-creatinine ratio remained independently correlated to LVDD [Odds ratio (OR) 2.82, 95% confidence interval (CI) 1.34–5.95] after adjustment. Serum urea (OR 1.18, 95%CI 1.03–1.34), creatinine (OR 6.53, 95%CI 1.70-–25.02), eGFR (OR 0.22, 95%CI 0.07–0.65) and UACR (OR 2.15, 95%CI 1.42–3.24) were revealed independent correlates of advanced (moderate and severe) LVDD.

Conclusions: Biochemical parameters of renal function were closely linked with LVDD. This finding described new cardio-renal relationship in the elderly population.

Editor: Antonio Carlos Seguro, University of São Paulo School of Medicine, Brazil

Funding: This study is funded by grants from the Key Projects in the National Science & Technology Pillar Program in the Eleventh (2006BAI01A04) and Twelfth (2011BAI11B10) Five-year Plan Period of China, and the Exchange Program Fund of Doctoral Student under the Fudan University Graduate School. The funders had no role in study design, data collection and analysis, decision to publish, or preparation of the manuscript.

Competing Interests: The authors have declared that no competing interests exist.

* E-mail: jbge@zs-hospital.sh.cn

ʖ These authors contributed equally to this work.

Introduction

Heart failure (HF) with preserved ejection fraction (HFPEF) has increasingly attracted attention for its high prevalence and poor prognosis [1]. Left ventricular diastolic dysfunction (LVDD) has been considered as one of the principal pathophysiologic mechanisms [2] and part of essential diagnostic indexes [3] of HFPEF. Both HFPEF and LVDD have been commonly demonstrated in aged population [4,5]. Of note, the prevalence of chronic kidney disease (CKD) [6] and the CKD-associated mortality [7] were also significantly higher in HFPEF than HF with reduced ejection fraction (HFREF) among the elderly patients. However, the association between renal function and LVDD in elderly population has not been fully clarified. It was observed that renal insufficiency was associated with LVDD in patients with [8] or without [9] symptomatic HF. But so far, studies have mainly focused on the relationship between LVDD and dynamic renal parameters including estimated glomerular filtration rate (eGFR) and creatinine clearance [6–10]. However, renal biochemical parameters such as serum urea, urea-to-creatinine ratio and urinary albumin-to-creatinine ratio (UACR) that could provide additional information than dynamic renal indexes have not yet been reported in LVDD and HFPEF. Furthermore, most former studies were carried out in hospitalized patients while little is known about general population. In the present study, we aimed to explore the association of comprehensive renal parameters including serum urea, creatinine, urea-to-creatinine ratio, eGFR and UACR with LVDD in a community-based elderly population in China.

Methods

Ethics statement

The present study conforms to the ethical guidelines of the 1975 Declaration of Helsinki and was approved by the Ethics Committee of Zhongshan hospital affiliated to Fudan University. Written informed consent was obtained from each participant during recruitment.

Study design and population

This study was part of Shanghai Heart Health Study (SHHS) [11], which is an ongoing large population study to investigate the incidence, prevalence, morbidity and mortality of cardiovascular diseases in community adults of Jinshan District of Shanghai, China. From January 2007 to June 2008, 1955 community residents older than 65 years were recruited and underwent a baseline survey including general information by self-administered questionnaire, standard 12-leads electrocardiogram (ECG), chest X-ray, and serum and urine biochemical parameters examination. The sample was followed up every 2 years. The biochemical parameters we used were measured in the first follow-up in 2009-2010. During the second follow-up in 2011, participants were invited to undergo an echocardiography examination. Finally 1166 participants with completed renal function and echocardiographic data were included in the present study. Those who did not have complete data from biochemical or echocardiographic analyses were excluded.

Clinical, demographic and biochemical parameters

Clinical and demographic data were obtained from questionnaires at recruitment including age, gender, smoking and education status, and previous diseases and drug therapies. Blood pressure was measured with the manual mercury sphygmomanometer after a 5-min rest in a sitting position using phases 1 and 5 of the Korotkoff sounds for systolic and diastolic blood pressure (SBP and DBP), respectively. Height and body weight were measured simultaneously. Waist circumference was measured in midway between the lower limit of the rib cage and the iliac crest with the subject standing using a flexible and non-distensible tape. Heart rate (HR) was read out from standard 12-leads ECG measured after 5 minutes in supine position.

Coronary heart disease (CHD) was defined as a history of myocardial infarction or angina pectoris, or angiography confirmed coronary stenosis > 70%. Atrial fibrillation was documented by either medical history or the ECG examination, both paroxysmal and persistent atrial fibrillation were included. Stroke was diagnosed by past cranial computed tomography or magnetic resonance imaging. Those who had smoked more than three cigarettes a day for at least one year were defined as smokers, both former and current smokers were included. Diabetes mellitus was diagnosed by definite disease history, or using of oral hypoglycemic drugs or insulin, or fasting blood glucose (FBG) ≥ 7 mmol/l. Hypertension was diagnosed by persistent resting blood pressure greater than 140/90 mmHg, or a definite disease history. Body mass index (BMI) was calculated as weight (kg)/height $(m)^2$. Obesity was a BMI of 28 kg/m^2 or higher, or a waist circumference of at least 85 cm in men or 80 cm in women. Dyslipidemia was considered present if the subject had a definite disease history or met any of the following: total cholesterol (TC) ≥ 6.22 mmol/l, triglycerides > 2.26 mmol/l, low-density lipoprotein cholesterol (LDL-C) ≥ 4.14 mmol/l, or high-density lipoprotein cholesterol (HDL-C) < 1.04 mmol/l.

Venous blood sample was obtained after a 12-hour-overnight fast and transferred every day to the central laboratory of Zhongshan hospital. After centrifugation and routine blood test, the serum was stored at −80°C until measurement of N-terminal pro-B type natriuretic peptide (NT-proBNP) using a fully automated electrochemiluminescence sandwich immunoassay on an Elecsys 1010 (Roche Diagnostics, Basel, Switzerland). Renal function parameters, and serum glucose and lipids were assessed by standard methods. The eGFR was calculated using the modified Modification of Diet in Renal Disease (MDRD) equations recommended by the Chinese eGFR Investigation Collaboration [eGFR (ml/min/1.73 m^2) = 175 × (Serum creatinine)$^{-1.234}$ × age$^{-0.179}$ × 0.79 (if female) (Serum creatinine: mg/dl, age: years)] [12]. An overnight morning urine sample was also collected to measure the urinary albumin using the immune turbidimetric method (DiaSys Diagnostic Systems, Shanghai) and the urinary creatinine using the enzymatic colorimetric method (Roche/Hitachi). The UACR was calculated with these two parameters [UACR = urinary albumin × 1000/(urinary creatinine × 0.113)].

Echocardiography

Echocardiograms were performed by using a commercially available echocardiography (Acuson Sequoia 218, Siemens, Germany) with a 2.5 or 3.5 MHz transducer according to the recommendations of the American Society of Echocardiography [13,14]. Two-dimensional and Doppler images were obtained in the parasternal long and short axes and the apical 4- and 2-chamber long-axis views. M-mode echocardiograms of the left ventricle (LV) were recorded from the parasternal long-axis view. All recordings included at least 3 cardiac cycles and were digitally stored for off-line analysis. Left ventricular end-diastolic diameter (LVEDD), left ventricular end-systolic diameter (LVESD), interventricular septal thickness (IVST) and posterior wall thickness (PWT) were measured by M-mode or 2-dimensional echocardiography from the parasternal long axis view. Left ventricular mass (grams) was calculated as 0.80 × (1.04 × $(IVST + LVEDD + PWT)^3$ − $(LVEDD)^3$) + 0.6 according to Devereux et al [15], which was further divided by body surface area (BSA) as left ventricular mass index (LVMI). Left ventricular ejection fraction (LVEF) was calculated from LV end-systolic and end-diastolic volumes (LVESV and LVEDV) measured from the apical 4- and 2-chambers views, using the modified biplane Simpson's method. Left atrial (LA) volume was measured with the same method, and was indexed to BSA as the LA volume index (LAVI). Doppler echocardiographic recordings were performed by pulsed wave Doppler with the sample volume at the tips of the mitral valve in the apical 4-chamber view. Peak early (E) and late (A) diastolic velocities, the E/A ratio, and the deceleration time (DT) of early diastolic velocity were measured as indicators of LV end-diastolic pressure. Assessment of peak early (E') and late (A') diastolic mitral annular velocity was performed by pulsed wave tissue Doppler imaging (TDI) of the lateral wall in the apical 4-chamber view.

Criteria for diagnosis of LVDD

As recommended by the Heart Failure and Echocardiography Associations of European Society of Cardiology (ESC), both conventional and TDI echocardiographic techniques were used for diagnosis of LVDD [3]. In the present study, the LVDD diagnosis was made according to the criteria proposed by ESC [3] and to those adopted by Zhang et al in their study [16] with minor modifications. LVDD was considered to be present if any of the following criteria were met: (1) E/E' > 8; (2) E/A < 0.5 and DT > 280ms; (3) LVMI > 149 g/m^2 (male) or LVMI > 122 g/m^2 (female); or (4) LAVI > 40 ml/m^2.

Classification of severity of LVDD

There are not uniformly recommended classifications for different degrees of LVDD. ESC guidelines in 2012 recommended 125 pg/ml of NT-proBNP as exclusion criteria of heart failure [5], while 220 pg/ml of NT-proBNP was previously shown to have positive predictive value of LVDD in diagnosis of HFPEF [3]. Therefore we chose 125 and 220 pg/ml as cut-off values to define mild LVDD with NT-proBNP < 125 pg/ml, moderate LVDD with NT-proBNP between 125 and 220 pg/ml, and severe LVDD with NT-proBNP ≥ 220 pg/ml, respectively.

Statistical analysis

Participants were divided into two groups according to left ventricular diastolic function: normal diastolic function group and subjects with LVDD. Comparisons between the two groups were performed using *t* tests or Wilcoxon rank sum tests for continuous variables and chi-square tests for categorical variables. Comparisons of LVDD prevalence among tertiles of the renal parameter were analyzed by Pearson chi-square tests. Further pairwise comparisons used chi-square tests and Bonferroni method to judge the significance of differences. Considering that the parameters do not obey the bivariate normal distribution, we analyzed the relationship of renal parameters with echocardiographic indexes by Spearman correlation analysis and scatter plot. Logistic multivariate regression analysis was used to further investigate the relationship of renal parameters with LVDD and its severity. Variables adjusted in the models of logistic analysis included demographic variables (age, gender), clinical measures (BMI, heart rate, SBP), risk factors (hypertension, diabetes, dyslipidemia, smoking), cardiac co-morbidities (CHD, atrial fibrillation), biochemical parameters (FBG, NT-proBNP), and LVEF. All analyses were performed with Stata version 11.0 (College Station, TX, USA). *P* values less than 0.05 were considered to represent significance.

Results

Characteristics of participants

LVDD was diagnosed in 464 (39.8%) subjects out of the 1166 participants. Compared to participants without LVDD, subjects with it were more often female, more likely to have CHD, atrial fibrillation and hypertension, while less likely to smoke. Lower heart rate but higher levels of urea, urea-to-creatinine ratio, UACR and NT-proBNP were found in subjects with LVDD. Age, BMI, SBP, creatinine, eGFR and LVEF were similar between subjects with or without LVDD (**Table 1**).

Prevalence of LVDD in relation to different renal parameters

The prevalence of LVDD increased in proportion to increasing values of serum urea (P= 0.05), urea-to-creatinine ratio (P= 0.005) and UACR (P= 0.029) (**Figure 1**). The prevalence of LVDD was significantly higher in subjects with serum urea (P= 0.029), urea-to-creatinine ratio (P= 0.001) and UACR (P= 0.008) located in the top tertile than in the bottom. This trend was not observed with respect to creatinine and eGFR (Data not shown).

Relationship of renal parameters with echocardiographic indexes

Serum urea (**Figure 2**), urea-to-creatinine ratio (**Figure 3**) and UACR (**Figure 4**) were negatively correlated to E/A ratio and positively correlated to LAVI. Besides, UACR was positively correlated to E/E' ratio (**Figure 4**).

Association of renal parameters with presence and severity of LVDD

Logistic univariate analysis showed that serum urea [odds ratio (OR) 1.12, 95% confidence interval (CI) 1.04–1.20], urea-to-creatinine ratio (OR 3.02, 95% CI 1.56–5.86) and UACR (OR 1.30, 95% CI 1.05–1.60) were associated with LVDD in this cohort. After adjusted for confounders, urea-to-creatinine ratio remained as an independent correlate of LVDD (**Table 2**). Neither serum creatinine nor eGFR correlated with LVDD before or after adjustment. **Table 2** also showed that serum urea, creatinine, eGFR and UACR were all independently correlated to the advanced LVDD in the multivariate logistic analysis. Parallely, these parameters were correlated to NT-proBNP level (**Table 3**).

Subgroup analysis in participants with normal renal function

Most participants in community have normal renal function. So further analysis was made in a subgroup with eGFR > 60 ml/min/1.73 m^2. In this subgroup, urea-to-creatinine ratio was still independently correlated to LVDD. While creatinine was negatively and eGFR was positively correlated to LVDD (**Table 4**).

Discussion

In the present study, we found for the first time in our knowledge that higher levels of serum urea, urea-to-creatinine ratio and UACR were correlated to increasing prevalence of LVDD in a community-based elderly population of China, and this was supported by their negative correlations to E/A ratio and positive correlations to LAVI and E/E'. Moreover, urea-to-creatinine ratio was an independent correlate of LVDD. Thus, renal function has proved to be closely linked with LVDD in this community-based elderly population.

Although serum urea has been demonstrated to be predictive of adverse outcome in HFPEF patients [17,18], to the best of our knowledge, its relationship with LVDD in conjunction with other measures of renal function has not been investigated in the general elderly population. Traditionally, serum urea has been considered as a less specific marker of renal function than GFR, since it is affected by extra-renal factors like protein intake and catabolism [19]. However, serum urea may rise independently of changes in GFR because of enhanced proximal and distal tubular reabsorption by the effect of arginine-vasopressin (AVP) on the urea transporter under neurohormonal activation [19–21]. Recently, McKie et al reported that patients with preclinical diastolic dysfunction showed impaired renal cyclic guanosine monophosphate (cGMP) activation which contributed to impaired natriuresis in response to volume expansion [22]. The impaired natriuresis indicates higher reabsorption of urea and increasing serum urea concentration. These previous findings about the cardio-renal response suggest a possible explanation for the association between higher urea levels and LVDD observed in the present study. Furthermore, in the work by McKie et al [22], impaired cGMP activation and natriuresis were not paralleled by increased E/E', which is consistent with our finding that serum urea was related with E/A and LAVI but not E/E'.

Table 1. Characteristics of participants according to presence and absence of LVDD.

	Total	Without LVDD	With LVDD	*P* value*
Demographics				
n	1166	702	464	
Age (yrs)	72.7±4.8	72.7±4.7	72.9±4.9	0.658
Female (%)	59.5	55.7	65.3	0.001
Heart rate (bpm)	74±14	75±14	72±15	<0.001
BMI (kg/m^2)	22.3±2.6	22.2±2.7	22.3±2.6	0.717
SBP (mmHg)	131±14	130±13	131±14	0.184
DBP (mmHg)	80±9	80±8	80±9	0.268
Co-morbidities				
CHD (%)	3.5	2.6	5.0	0.030
Atrial fibrillation (%)	4.6	2.1	8.4	<0.001
Stroke (%)	2.6	3.0	1.9	0.267
Hypertension (%)	44.4	41.7	48.5	0.023
Diabetes (%)	12.0	12.3	11.6	0.753
Dyslipidemia (%)	43.1	43.2	42.9	0.926
Smoking (%)	30.2	33.6	25.0	0.002
Obesity (%)	32.6	31.5	34.3	0.321
Laboratory variables				
Urea (mmol/l)	6.3±1.7	6.2±1.6	6.5±1.8	0.003
Creatinine (μmol/l)	64 (48–80)	64 (50–81)	62 (47–80)	0.098
Urea-to-creatinine ratio	96 (73–126)	92 (72–122)	102 (77–135)	<0.001
Uric acid (μmol/l)	339.8±94.9	338.7±94.5	341.5±95.5	0.762
eGFR (ml/min/1.73 m^2)	108 (79–144)	106 (78–142)	111 (80–147)	0.320
UACR (μg/mg Cr)	14.0 (6.1–33.3)	12.8 (5.7-–30.6)	16.5 (7.0–39.2)	0.008
FBG (mmol/l)	5.9±1.5	5.9±1.6	5.9±1.4	0.500
TC (mmol/l)	4.9±1.0	4.9±1.0	4.9±1.0	0.479
TG (mmol/l)	1.7±1.0	1.7±1.1	1.6±1.0	0.110
LDL-C (mmol/l)	3.2±1.2	3.2±1.2	3.2±1.3	0.885
HDL-C (mmol/l)	1.4±0.4	1.4±0.4	1.4±0.3	0.884
NT-proBNP (pg/ml)	110.6 (65.2–193.7)	96.3 (57.8–173.6)	130.4 (77.1–232.8)	<0.001
LVEF (%)	64±9	65±8	64±10	0.660

Values of creatinine, urea-to-creatinine ratio, eGFR, UACR and NT-proBNP are median (interquartile), other values are mean ± SD or %.
HR, heart rate; BMI, body mass index; SBP, systolic blood pressure; DBP, diastolic blood pressure; CHD, coronary heart disease; eGFR, estimated glomerular filtration rate; UACR, urinary albumin-to-creatininie ratio; FBG, fasting blood glucose; TC, total cholesterol; TG, triglycerides; LDL-C, low density lipoprotein cholesterol; HDL-C, high density lipoprotein cholesterol; NT-proBNP, N-terminal pro-B type natriuretic peptide; LVEF, left ventricular ejection fraction.
*Compared between subjects with and without LVDD.

The serum urea-to-creatinine ratio has been extensively used for the differentiation of "pre-renal" dysfunction from intrinsic renal parenchymal disease [23], and has been suggested positively correlated with poor outcomes in patients with acute or chronic HF [24–26]. Neuroendocrine activation might also serve as one of the potential reasons for urea-to-creatinine ratio elevation in pre-renal ischemia [20,21]. Therefore, the aforementioned mechanism with regard to urea and LVDD could also interpret the independent relation of urea-to-creatinine ratio with LVDD. Our findings about a positive relation of urea and urea-to-creatinine ratio with LVDD but lack of relation of creatinine and eGFR with LVDD may suggest a neuroendocrine activation status in LVDD subjects. We hypothesize that serum urea and urea-to-creatinine ratio are more sensitive than eGFR and creatinine to represent the early neuroendocrine activation in LVDD, when the cardiac output has not reduced yet and glomerular filtration is still normal. Further studies are warranted to test these relationships and the hypothesis.

Available findings about urinary albumin excretion (UAE) and its relation with diastolic function remain conflicting [27–30]. The CHARM study found that the prevalence of increased UACR, a convenient method for detection of UAE [27], was similar in HFPEF (41%) and HFREF patients [28], whereas HARVEST study reported that UAE was unrelated to LV mass in subjects with stage 1 hypertension [29]. Furthermore, Post et al found that elevated random spot UACR was a marker of increased LV mass [30]. In the present study, we found 1) the prevalence of LVDD increased with the increasing UACR, 2) UACR was related to echocardiographic indexes like E/E', E/A and LAVI, and 3) UACR was independently associated with the severity of LVDD. Therefore our findings not only extend previous studies by Post et al but also suggest LVDD as pathophysiologic link between UAE

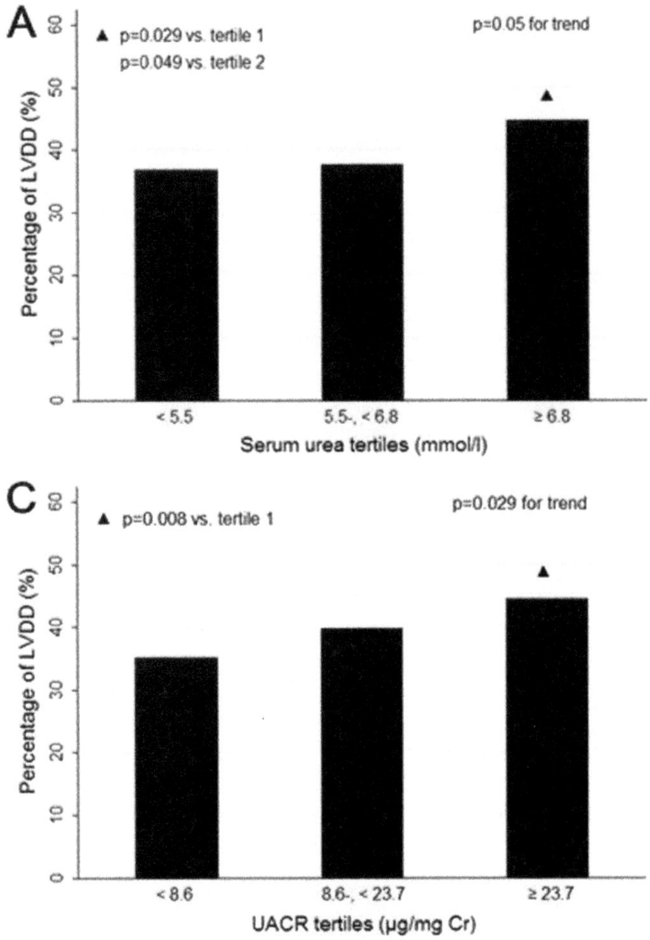

Figure 1. Prevalence of LVDD according to serum urea, urea-to-creatinine ratio, and UACR. The prevalence of LVDD is 36.9%, 37.6% and 44.6% in tertile 1, 2 and 3 of serum urea respectively. It is 33.8%, 40.5% and 45.1% for urea-to-creatinine ratio and 35.1%, 39.7% and 44.5% for UACR, respectively. LVDD, left ventricular diastolic dysfunction; UACR, urinary albumin-to-creatinine ratio.

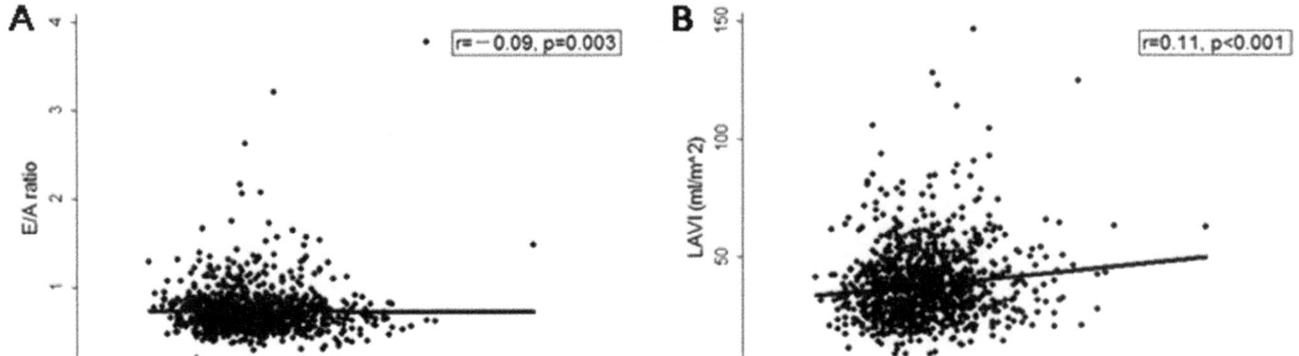

Figure 2. Relationship between serum urea and echocardiographic indexes (E/A and LAVI). A) Serum urea was negatively correlated to E/A ratio. **B**) Serum urea was positively correlated to LAVI. LAVI, left atrial volume index.

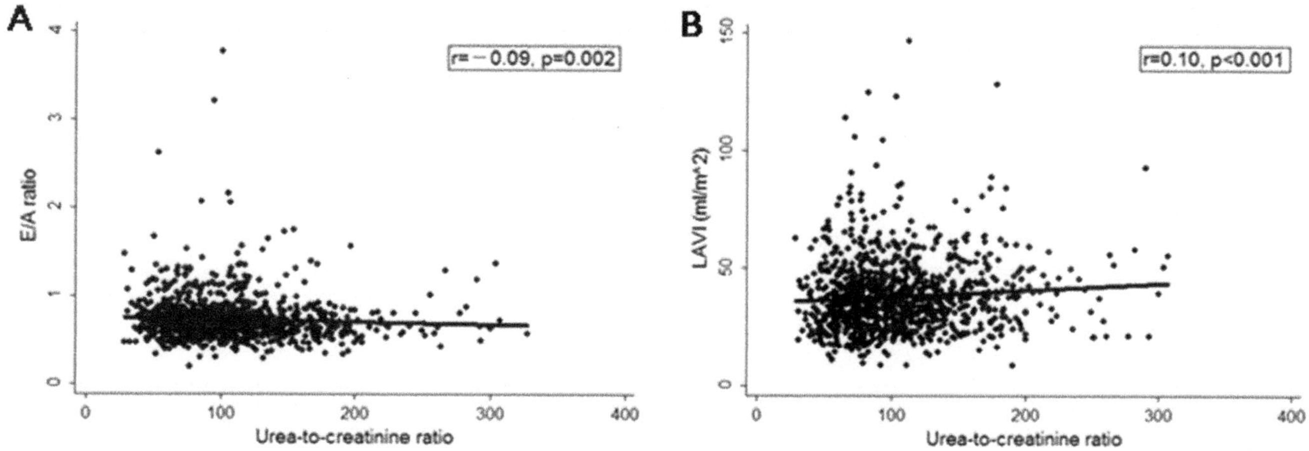

Figure 3. Relationship between urea-to-creatinine ratio and echocardiographic indexes (E/A and LAVI). A) Urea-to-creatinine ratio was negatively correlated to E/A ratio. **B)** Urea-to-creatinine ratio was positively correlated to LAVI. LAVI, left atrial volume index.

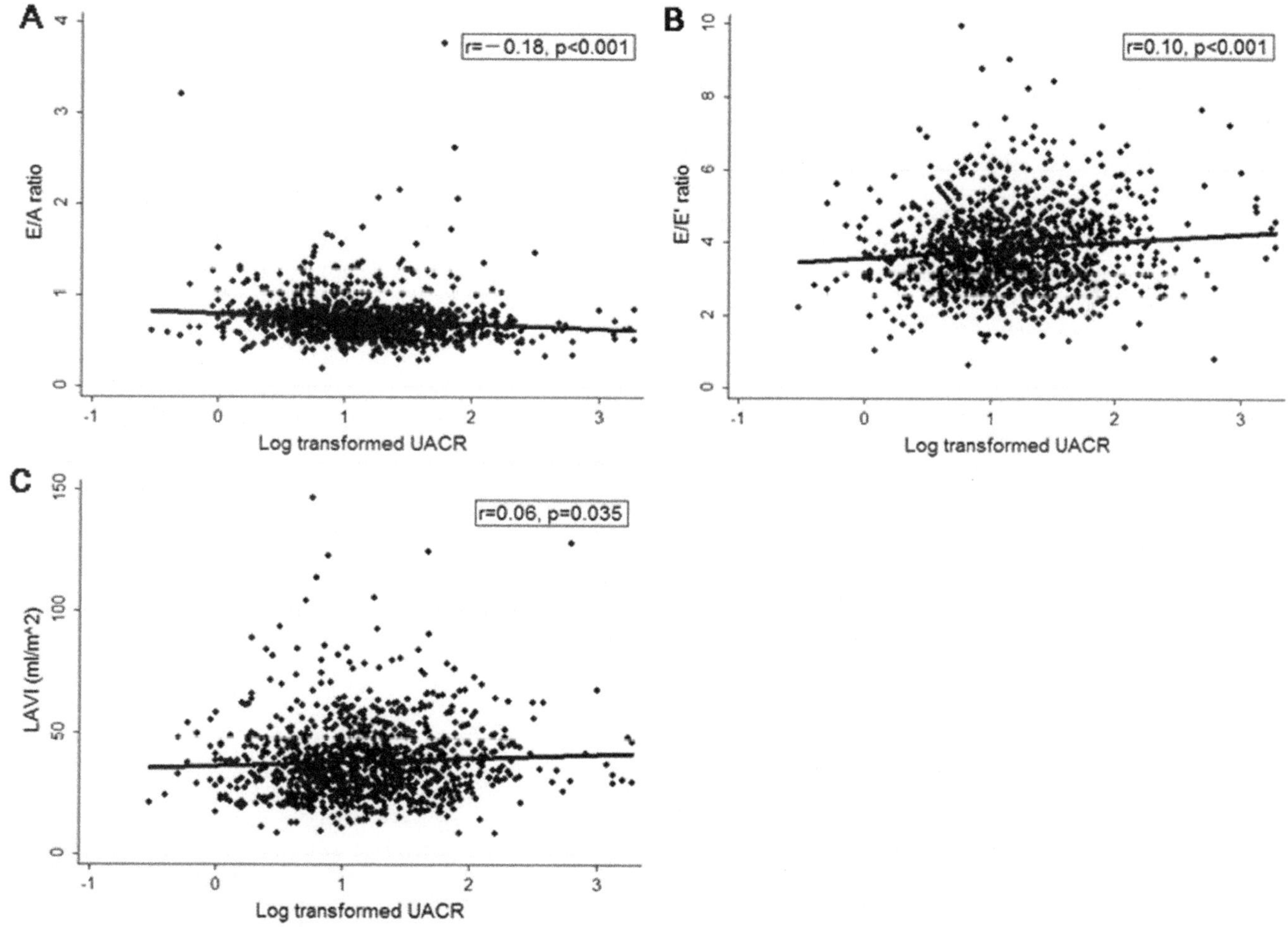

Figure 4. Relationship between UACR and echocardiographic indexes (E/A, E/E′ and LAVI). A) UACR was negatively correlated to E/A ratio. **B)** UACR was positively correlated to LAVI. **C)** UACR was also positively correlated to E/E′ ratio. UACR, urinary albumin-to-creatinine ratio; LAVI, left atrial volume index.

Table 2. The association of biochemical renal parameters with LVDD and severity of LVDD.

Variable***	LVDD*			Advanced LVDD**		
	OR	95% CI	*P* value	OR	95% CI	*P* value
Urea (mmol/l)	1.07	0.99–1.16	0.087	1.18	1.03–1.34	0.013
Creatinine (μmol/l)	0.47	0.21–1.06	0.070	6.53	1.70–25.02	0.006
Urea-to-creatinine ratio	2.82	1.34–5.95	0.006	0.58	0.18–1.94	0.379
eGFR (ml/min/ 1.73 m^2)	1.85	0.95–3.60	0.070	0.22	0.07–0.65	0.006
UACR (μg/mg Cr)	1.10	0.86–1.40	0.451	2.15	1.42–3.24	<0.001

OR, odds ratio; CI, confidence interval. Other abbreviations as in Table 1.
*Adjusted for age, gender, heart rate, BMI, SBP, smoking status, presence or absence of hypertension, diabetes mellitus, CHD, and atrial fibrillation; FBG, NT-proBNP and LVEF. NT-proBNP is log transformed before entering models.
**Adjusted the same parameters except NT-proBNP.
***Per 1 unit increase in urea values; per 1 log unit increase in creatinine, urea-to-creatinine ratio, eGFR and UACR values.

Table 4. The association of renal parameters with LVDD in subpopulation with eGFR > 60 ml/min/1.73 m^2.

Variable	Unadjusted			Adjusted*		
	OR**	95% CI	*P* value	OR**	95% CI	*P* value
Urea (mmol/l)	1.10	1.01-1.19	0.021	1.07	0.98-1.16	0.138
Creatinine (μmol/l)	0.28	0.11-0.69	0.006	0.33	0.12-0.90	0.031
Urea-to-creatinine ratio	3.93	1.89-8.15	<0.001	3.06	1.35-6.92	0.007
eGFR (ml/min/ 1.73 m^2)	2.18	1.00-4.72	0.049	2.48	1.09-5.64	0.031
UACR (μg/mg Cr)	1.26	1.01-1.59	0.045	1.10	0.84-1.43	0.491

OR, odds ratio; CI, confidence interval.
*Adjusted for age, gender, heart rate, BMI, SBP, smoking status, presence or absence of hypertension, diabetes mellitus, CHD, and atrial fibrillation; FBG, NT-proBNP and LVEF. NT-proBNP is log transformed before entering models. Abbreviations as in Table 1.
**OR is per 1 unit increase in urea values; per 1 log unit increase in creatinine, urea-to-creatinine ratio, eGFR and UACR values.

and mortality [31]. Endothelial dysfunction might represent a contributory mechanism to this association since it has been proved to be associated with both UAE [32,33] and LVDD [34–36].

UACR is suggested not specific for kidney disease but a marker of systemic inflammation and microvascular damage including endothelial dysfunction [37,38], which is an predominant early step in the process of clinical overt cardiovascular disease [39]. Nevertheless, eGFR mainly reflects the hemodynamic status of the kidney. Since isolated LVDD was found associated with endothelial dysfunction [34–36] but unlikely to cause decline of cardiac output and renal macrovascular perfusion in the early stage, it could be understood why LVDD was correlated with UACR but not with eGFR in the present study.

Both population-based studies [40,41] and studies on hospitalized HFPEF patients [42,43] support our choice of NT-proBNP as tool to grade LVDD since in both settings NT-proBNP was found to be directly associated with LVDD severity. The relationship of renal parameters with NT-proBNP uncovered in our study, together with other studies demonstrating that NT-proBNP levels are affected by declining renal function [44–46], are in keeping with the theory that the clearance of NT-proBNP occurs solely in the kidney [47]. This finding also indicates that when NT-proBNP is employed to evaluate the presence or severity of LVDD, renal function should be considered because both decreased clearance of kidney and increased production due to LVDD could lead to the rise of NT-proBNP.

Table 3. The association of biochemical renal parameters with NT-proBNP.

Variable	NT-proBNP	
	*r**	*P* value
Urea (mmol/l)	0.12	<0.001
Creatinine (μmol/l)	0.07	0.021
Urea-to-creatinine ratio	0.01	0.667
eGFR (ml/min/1.73 m^2)	−0.13	<0.001
UACR (μg/mg Cr)	0.18	<0.001

Abbreviations as in Table 1.
*r, Spearman correlation coefficient.

The subgroup analysis in subjects with normal renal function (eGFR > 60 ml/min/1.73 m^2) revealed, for the first time, an interesting result that eGFR was independently and positively correlated to LVDD. It has been demonstrated that there is a significant and positive correlation between GFR and LV mass in non-diabetic patients with mild to moderate hypertension [48], concurring with our result to some extent. Considering these findings, we assume that glomerular hyperfiltration may be linked to LVDD. Nevertheless, more studies are still needed to confirm this assumption.

The present study has some limitations. First, specific data on symptoms or signs related to HF were not available. Additionally, we did not assess Ar_d–A_d because of constraints in echocardiographic examination time per participant. Ar_d–A_d was still kept in the latest European Consensus document as a second-line criteria of LVDD [3]. However, studies suggested that Ar_d–A_d was often obtained less successfully (49%–84%) in clinic than other diastolic measures [49,50], and pulmonary venous inflow had more inter-reader variability than mitral valve inflow and annular tissue Doppler [50]. Emery et al also found that even in hospitalized patients, very few of them presented Ar_d–A_d > 30ms, and the measure had minimal sensitivity [49]. All of these indicated that Ar_d–A_d probably contribute little to overall diastolic function assessment.

Conclusions

In summary, the present study suggests that higher levels of serum urea, urea-to-creatinine ratio and UACR are linked with increasing prevalence of LVDD, and urea-to-creatinine ratio is an independent correlate of LVDD. Although serum creatinine and eGFR are not associated with LVDD in the whole community cohort, they, together with serum urea and UACR, are independently associated with advanced LVDD in parallel with increased NT-proBNP level. Our findings contribute to further understanding of the cardio-renal relationship in the elderly population.

Acknowledgments

We thank all the community residents participating in the study, and staffs providing help from the Fengjing Community Health Center.

Author Contributions

Conceived and designed the experiments: JMZ XTC XJJ KH MF JBG. Performed the experiments: XTC XJJ JZ HYZ BXT JC HMZ AJS. Analyzed the data: XTC XJJ JZ KH MF HH. Contributed reagents/materials/analysis tools: HYZ BXT HH AJS . Wrote the paper: XTC JMZ KH MF HH JBG.

References

1. Owan TE, Hodge DO, Herges RM, Jacobsen SJ, Roger VL, et al. (2006) Trends in prevalence and outcome of heart failure with preserved ejection fraction. N Engl J Med 355: 251–259.
2. Zile MR, Baicu CF, Gaasch WH. (2004) Diastolic heart failure-abnormalities in active relaxation and passive stiffness of the left ventricle. N Engl J Med 350: 1953–1959.
3. Paulus WJ, Tschöpe C, Sanderson JE, Rusconi C, Flachskampf FA, et al. (2007) How to diagnose diastolic heart failure: a consensus statement on the diagnosis of heart failure with normal left ventricular ejection fraction by the Heart Failure and Echocardiography Associations of the European Society of Cardiology. Eur Heart J 28: 2539–2550.
4. Owan TE, Redfield MM. (2005) Epidemiology of diastolic heart failure. Prog Cardiovasc Dis 47: 320–332.
5. McMurray JJ, Adamopoulos S, Anker SD, Auricchio A, Böhm M, et al. (2012) ESC Guidelines for the diagnosis and treatment of acute and chronic heart failure 2012: The Task Force for the Diagnosis and Treatment of Acute and Chronic Heart Failure 2012 of the European Society of Cardiology. Developed in collaboration with the Heart Failure Association (HFA) of the ESC. Eur Heart J 33: 1787–1847.
6. Kerzner R, Gage BF, Freedland KE, Rich MW. (2003) Predictors of mortality in younger and older patients with heart failure and preserved or reduced left ventricular ejection fraction. Am Heart J 146: 286–290.
7. Ahmed A, Rich MW, Sanders PW, Perry GJ, Bakris GL, et al. (2007) Chronic kidney disease associated mortality in diastolic versus systolic heart failure: a propensity matched study. Am J Cardiol 99: 393–398.
8. Bruch C, Rothenburger M, Gotzmann M, Wichter T, Scheld HH, et al. (2007) Chronic kidney disease in patients with chronic heart failure-impact on intracardiac conduction, diastolic function and prognosis. Int J Cardiol 118: 375–380.
9. Sato B, Yoshikawa D, Ishii H, Suzuki S, Inoue Y, et al. (2013) Relation of plasma indoxyl sulfate levels and estimated glomerular filtration rate to left ventricular diastolic dysfunction. Am J Cardiol 111: 712–716.
10. Nishio M, Sakata Y, Mano T, Ohtani T, Takeda Y, et al. (2008) Difference of clinical characteristics between hypertensive patients with and without diastolic heart failure: the roles of diastolic dysfunction and renal insufficiency. Hypertens Res 31: 1865–1872.
11. Ge JB, Zhou JM, Jin XJ. (2012) Shanghai Heart Health Study: design and objectives. Shanghai Medical Journal 35: 1–6.
12. Ma YC, Zuo L, Chen JH, Luo Q, Yu XQ, et al. (2006) Modified glomerular filtration rate estimating equation for Chinese patients with chronic kidney disease. J Am Soc Nephrol 17: 2937–2944.
13. Gottdiener JS, Bednarz J, Devereux R, Gardin J, Klein A, et al. (2004) American Society of Echocardiography recommendations for use of echocardiography in clinical trials. J Am Soc Echocardiogr 17: 1086–1119.
14. Nagueh SF, Appleton CP, Gillebert TC, Marino PN, Oh JK, et al. (2009) Recommendations for the evaluation of left ventricular diastolic function by echocardiography. J Am Soc Echocardiogr 22: 107–133.
15. Devereux RB, Alonso DR, Lutas EM, Gottlieb GJ, Campo E, et al. (1986) Echocardiographic assessment of left ventricular hypertrophy: comparison to necropsy findings. Am J Cardiol 57: 450–458.
16. Zhang Y, Safar ME, Iaria P, Agnoletti D, Protogerou AD, et al. (2010) Prevalence and prognosis of left ventricular diastolic dysfunction in the elderly: The PROTEGER Study. Am Heart J 160: 471–478.
17. Feola M, Aspromonte N, Canali C, Ceci V, Giovinazzo P, et al. (2005) Prognostic value of plasma brain natriuretic peptide, urea nitrogen, and creatinine in outpatients > 70 years of age with heart failure. Am J Cardiol 96: 705–709.
18. Shenkman HJ, Zareba W, Bisognano JD. (2007) Comparison of prognostic significance of amino-terminal pro-brain natriuretic Peptide versus blood urea nitrogen for predicting events in patients hospitalized for heart failure. Am J Cardiol 99: 1143–1145.
19. Schrier RW. (2008) Blood urea nitrogen and serum creatinine: not married in heart failure. Circ Heart Fail 1: 2–5.
20. Schrier RW, Abraham WT. (1999) Hormones and hemodynamics in heart failure. N Engl J Med 341: 577–585.
21. Schrier RW. (2006) Role of diminished renal function in cardiovascular mortality: marker or pathogenetic factor? J Am Coll Cardiol 47: 1–8.
22. McKie PM, Schirger JA, Costello-Boerrigter LC, Benike SL, Harstad LK, et al. (2011) Impaired natriuretic and renal endocrine response to acute volume expansion in pre-clinical systolic and diastolic dysfunction. J Am Coll Cardiol 58: 2095–2103.
23. Cecil RL, Goldman L, Ausiello DA. (2008) Cecil medicine. Philadelphia: Saunders Elsevier.
24. Aronson D, Mittleman MA, Burger AJ. (2004) Elevated blood urea nitrogen level as a predictor of mortality in patients admitted for decompensated heart failure. Am J Med 116: 466–473.
25. Smith GL, Shlipak MG, Havranek EP, Foody JM, Masoudi FA, et al. (2006) Serum urea nitrogen, creatinine, and estimators of renal function-mortality in older patients with cardiovascular disease. Arch Intern Med 166: 1134–1142.
26. Lin HJ, Chao CL, Chien KL, Ho YL, Lee CM, et al. (2009) Elevated blood urea nitrogen-to-creatinine ratio increased the risk of hospitalization and all-cause death in patients with chronic heart failure. Clin Res Cardiol 98: 487–492.
27. National Kidney Foundation. (2002) K/DOQI clinical practice guidelines for chronic kidney disease: evaluation classification and stratification. Am J Kidney Dis 39: S1–S266.
28. Jackson CE, Solomon SD, Gerstein HC, Zetterstrand S, Olofsson B, et al; CHARM Investigators and Committees. (2009) Albuminuria in chronic heart failure: prevalence and prognostic importance. Lancet 374: 543–550.
29. Palatini P, Graniero GR, Mormino P, Mattarei M, Sanzuol F, et al. (1996) Prevalence and clinical correlates of microalbuminuria in stage I hypertension. Results from the Hypertension and Ambulatory Recording Venetia Study (HARVEST Study). Am J Hypertens 9: 334–341.
30. Post WS, Blumenthal RS, Weiss JL, Levine DM, Thiemann DR, et al. (2000) Spot urinary albumin-creatinine ratio predicts left ventricular hypertrophy in young hypertensive African-American men. Am J Hypertens 13: 1168–1172.
31. Redfield MM, Jacobsen SJ, Burnett JC Jr, Mahoney DW, Bailey KR, et al. (2003) Burden of systolic and diastolic ventricular dysfunction in the community:appreciating the scope of the heart failure epidemic. JAMA 289: 194–202.
32. Stehouwer CD, Nauta JJ, Zeldenrust GC, Hackeng WH, Donker AJ, et al. (1992) Urinary albumin excretion, cardiovascular disease, and endothelial dysfunction in non-insulin-dependent diabetes mellitus. Lancet 340: 319–323.
33. Stehouwer CD, Gall MA, Twisk JW, Knudsen E, Emeis JJ, et al. (2002) Increased urinary albumin excretion, endothelial dysfunction, and chronic low-grade inflammation in type 2 diabetes: progressive, interrelated, and independently associated with risk of death. Diabetes 51: 1157–1165.
34. Ma LN, Zhao SP, Gao M, Zhou QC, Fan P. (2000) Endothelial dysfunction associated with left ventricular diastolic dysfunction in patients with coronary heart disease. Int J Cardiol 72: 275–279.
35. Zizek B, Poredos P. (2007) Increased left ventricular mass and diastolic dysfunction are associated with endothelial dysfunction in normotensive offspring of subjects with essential hypertension. Blood Press 16: 36–44.
36. Elesber AA, Redfield MM, Rihal CS, Prasad A, Lavi S, et al. (2007) Coronary endothelial dysfunction and hyperlipidemia are independently associated with diastolic dysfunction in humans. Am Heart J 153: 1081–1087.
37. El Nahas M. (2010) Cardio-Kidney-Damage: a unifying concept. Kidney Int 78: 14–18.
38. Malik AR, Sultan S, Turner ST, Kullo IJ. (2007) Urinary albumin excretion is associated with impaired flow- and nitroglycerin-mediated brachial artery dilatation in hypertensive adults. J Hum Hypertens 21: 231–238.
39. Abdelhafiz AH, Ahmed S, El Nahas M. (2011) Microalbuminuria: marker or maker of cardiovascular disease. Nephron Exp Nephrol 119 Suppl 1: e6–e10.
40. Kloch-Badelek M, Kuznetsova T, Sakiewicz W, Tikhonoff V, Ryabikov A, et al; European Project On Genes in Hypertension (EPOGH) Investigators. (2012) Prevalence of left ventricular diastolic dysfunction in European populations based on cross-validated diagnostic thresholds. Cardiovasc Ultrasound 10:10.
41. Abhayaratna WP, Marwick TH, Becker NG, Jeffery IM, McGill DA, et al. (2006) Population-based detection of systolic and diastolic dysfunction with amino-terminal pro-B-type natriuretic peptide. Am Heart J 152: 941–948.
42. Tschöpe C, Kasner M, Westermann D, Gaub R, Poller WC, et al. (2005) The role of NT-proBNP in the diagnostics of isolated diastolic dysfunction: correlation with echocardiographic and invasive measurements. Eur Heart J 26: 2277–2284.
43. Grewal J, McKelvie R, Lonn E, Tait P, Carlsson J, et al. (2008) BNP and NT-proBNP predict echocardiographic severity of diastolic dysfunction. Eur J Heart Fail 10: 252–259.
44. Vickery S, Price CP, John RI, Abbas NA, Webb MC, et al. (2005) B-type natriuretic peptide (BNP) and amino-terminal proBNP in patients with CKD: relationship to renal function and left ventricular hypertrophy. Am J Kidney Dis 46: 610–620.
45. DeFilippi C, van Kimmenade RR, Pinto YM. (2008) Amino-terminal pro-B-type natriuretic peptide testing in renal disease. Am J Cardiol 101: 82–88.
46. van Kimmenade RR, Januzzi JL Jr, Bakker JA, Houben AJ, Rennenberg R, et al. (2009) Renal clearance of B-type natriuretic peptide and amino terminal pro-B-type natriuretic peptide: a mechanistic study in hypertensive subjects. J Am Coll Cardiol 53: 884–890.

47. Panteghini M, Clerico A. (2004) Understanding the clinical biochemistry of N-terminal pro-B-type natriuretic peptide: The prerequisite for its optimal clinical use. Clin Lab 50: 325–331.
48. Schmieder RE, Messerli FH, Garavaglia G, Nunez B. (1990) Glomerular hyperfiltration indicates early target organ damage in essential hypertension. JAMA 264: 2775–2780.
49. Emery WT, Jadavji I, Choy JB, Lawrance RA. (2008) Investigating the European Society of Cardiology Diastology Guidelines in a practical scenario. Eur J Echocardiogr 9: 685–691.
50. Bess RL, Khan S, Rosman HS, Cohen GI, Allebban Z, et al. (2006) Technical aspects of diastology: why mitral inflow and tissue Doppler imaging are the preferred parameters? Echocardiography 23: 332-–339.

11

Cardiovascular Effects of Dietary Salt Intake in Aged Healthy Cats: A 2-Year Prospective Randomized, Blinded, and Controlled Study

Valérie Chetboul[1,2]*, Brice Stéphane Reynolds[3], Emilie Trehiou-Sechi[1], Patrick Nguyen[4], Didier Concordet[5], Carolina Carlos Sampedrano[1], Isabelle Testault[6], Jonathan Elliott[7], Jérôme Abadie[8], Vincent Biourge[9], Hervé Pierre Lefebvre[3]

1 Unité de Cardiologie d'Alfort, Centre Hospitalier Universitaire Vétérinaire d'Alfort, Université Paris-Est, Ecole Nationale Vétérinaire d'Alfort, Maisons-Alfort, France, **2** INSERM, U955, Equipe 03, Créteil, France, **3** Unité de Recherche Clinique, Université de Toulouse, INP, Ecole Nationale Vétérinaire de Toulouse, Toulouse, France, **4** Nutrition and Endocrinology Unit, LUNAM Université, Oniris, National College of Veterinary Medicine, Food Science and Engineering, Nantes, France, **5** UMR 1331 Toxalim, INRA, Université de Toulouse, INP, Ecole Nationale Vétérinaire de Toulouse, Toulouse, France, **6** Atlantia Veterinary Hospital, Nantes, France, **7** Department of Comparative Biomedical Sciences, Royal Veterinary College, Royal College Street, Camden, London, United Kingdom, **8** Department of Pathology LUNAM Université, Oniris, National College of Veterinary Medicine, Food Science and Engineering, Nantes, France, **9** Centre de Recherches, Royal Canin SAS, Aimargues, France

Abstract

High salt dry expanded diets are commercially available for cats to increase water intake and urine volume, as part of the prevention or treatment of naturally occurring urinary stone formation (calcium oxalates and struvites). However, chronic high salt intake may have potential cardiovascular adverse effects in both humans, especially in aging individuals, and several animal models. The objective of this prospective, randomized, blinded, and controlled study was to assess the long-term cardiovascular effects of high salt intake in healthy aged cats. Twenty healthy neutered cats (10.1±2.4 years) were randomly allocated into 2 matched groups. One group was fed a high salt diet (3.1 g/Mcal sodium, 5.5 g/Mcal chloride) and the other group a control diet of same composition except for salt content (1.0 g/Mcal sodium, 2.2 g/Mcal chloride). Clinical examination, systolic and diastolic arterial blood pressure measurements, standard transthoracic echocardiography and conventional Doppler examinations were repeatedly performed on non-sedated cats by trained observers before and over 24 months after diet implementation. Radial and longitudinal velocities of the left ventricular free wall and the interventricular septum were also assessed in systole and diastole using 2-dimensional color tissue Doppler imaging. Statistics were performed using a general linear model. No significant effect of dietary salt intake was observed on systolic and diastolic arterial blood pressure values. Out of the 33 tested imaging variables, the only one affected by dietary salt intake was the radial early on late diastolic velocity ratio assessed in the endocardium of the left ventricular free wall, statistically lower in the high salt diet group at 12 months only (P = 0.044). In conclusion, in this study involving healthy aged cats, chronic high dietary salt intake was not associated with an increased risk of systemic arterial hypertension and myocardial dysfunction, as observed in some elderly people, salt-sensitive patients and animal models.

Editor: Rudolf Kirchmair, Medical University Innsbruck, Austria

Funding: Royal Canin SAS, a petfood company, has sponsored financially this study. Vincent Biourge is a full time employee of Royal Canin, SAS. Vincent Biourge was involved in the study design, in designing and providing the diets, in the preparation of the manuscript and in the decision to publish. He was not involved in data collection and all other investigators were blinded to the dietary treatments.

Competing Interests: Royal Canin SAS, a petfood company, has sponsored financially this study. Vincent Biourge is a full time employee of Royal Canin, SAS.

* E-mail: vchetboul@vet-alfort.fr

Introduction

On one hand, salt is a vital element for physiologic functions, including extra cellular fluid volume and blood pressure (BP) homeostasis, but on the other hand salt in excess may have potential deleterious cardiovascular effects [1]. Various experimental animal models, as well as human clinical trials and epidemiological studies, including the standardized worldwide INTERSALT Study, have provided evidence for a causal association between salt consumption and increase in BP values. However the results of these studies have been inconsistent and a marked variable individual salt sensitivity is evident, related in part to a genetic basis [2–5]. A high salt intake has also been demonstrated to be associated with myocardial function changes [6,7] as well as increased left ventricular (LV) mass in both animal models [8,9] and humans [10–12], independent of effects on BP.

Lower urinary tract diseases, such as urolithiasis and idiopathic cystitis, are common in the feline species [13]. One aspect of their long-term management is to increase water intake in order to subsequently increase urine volume and reduce urine solute concentration, which can be achieved by increasing dietary sodium [14–16]. Previous studies have shown the efficacy of appropriately designed high-salt dry diets to reduce struvite and calcium oxalate supersaturation (the most common minerals found in feline uroliths) and to dissolve naturally occurring feline struvite urinary stones [17,18]. Therapeutic diets for cats with lower urinary tract diseases, characterized by a high salt content, are hence currently commercially available in order to enhance water intake and urine output. Several studies have already focused on the renal and cardiovascular safety of these high salt diets, and all reported the absence of significant adverse effect on systemic arterial BP, while significantly increasing water intake and decreasing urine specific gravity in comparison with cats fed a control diet [15,16,19,20]. Nevertheless, none of the latter studies specifically focused on the potential deleterious effects of high-salt diets on global and regional myocardial function using sensitive imaging techniques such as tissue Doppler imaging (TDI). Additionally, these studies were all short- or medium-term feeding trials of 1-week to 6-month duration, performed on young (mean age 1 to 2.5 years old) to middle-aged adult cats (mean age of 7 years) only [15,19,20]. However aged cats are known to be at risk for both systemic arterial hypertension [21,22] and chronic kidney diseases [23], two conditions that can be worsened by high-sodium diets in salt-sensitive humans and laboratory animals [24–27].

The objective of the present prospective, randomized, blinded, and controlled study was therefore to assess the long-term cardiovascular effects of dietary salt intake in healthy aged cats, using systemic arterial BP measurement, standard 2-dimensional (2D) and M-mode transthoracic echocardiography, conventional Doppler examination, and also 2D color TDI.

Materials and Methods

Animals

The present cardiovascular prospective study was performed concomitantly to another protocol, whose aim was to assess the effect of dietary salt intake on renal function using glomerular filtration rate (GFR) measurement, kidney ultrasonography, including renal resistive index assessment, and urinalysis [28]. Both inclusion and exclusion criteria used in the present study were identical to those of the latter protocol [28]. Briefly, 26 Domestic Shorthair neutered aged cats (10.1±2.4 years [5.3–14.5], 4.8±0.7 kg [3.6–6.5]) from a research colony housed in an indoor research facility with a 12 h light/dark cycle, controlled temperature (18–21°C) and ventilation (250 m^3/h, 12 h/day) were screened for suitability for entry to the study. After baseline evaluations, cats were included in the study only if they were compliant for all scheduled procedures and if they were healthy on the basis of physical examination, BP measurement, routine urine and blood analyses, kidney ultrasonography, standard echocardiography, and conventional Doppler examination. According to the above-mentioned inclusion criteria, 20/26 healthy cats (10 males and 10 females; 10.1±2.4 years [5.5–11.7]; 4.8±0.7 kg [3.6–6.5]) were included in the study. Five out of the 26 cats from the research colony could not be included because of hyperthyroidism and chronic kidney disease (n = 1), chronic kidney disease (n = 1), hypertrophic cardiomyopathy (n = 1), chronic kidney disease and hypertrophic cardiomyopathy (n = 1), chronic liver disease (n = 1), and marked uncooperative behavior (n = 1). After group allocation, the 20 recruited healthy cats were allowed to acclimate with the other cats of their group for a 2 week-period, and were then regularly monitored over 2 years.

Randomization procedure

To control the potential confounding effect of renal dysfunction on cardiac function and *vice versa*, a stratified randomization was performed. The 20 recruited healthy cats were first stratified in 3 subsets according to 2D color TDI results at baseline: normal (n = 8/20), subnormal (i.e., presence of regional post-systolic contraction waves for the left ventricular free wall (LVFW) and/or the interventricular septum (IVS) without any other alteration; n = 6/20), and abnormal (i.e., mild to moderate regional diastolic alterations characterized by an early on late diastolic velocity ratio (E/A ratio) <1; n = 6/20) [29]. The following randomization procedure was then performed separately within each subset (Table 1): cats were ranked according to their GFR and paired. In each pair of cats, the first was randomly assigned to one diet group and the second was assigned to the other diet group. This ensured that the cats in each diet group were well matched with regard to both renal and cardiac function. In addition, comparability of the 2 groups for all the variables of interest at baseline was assessed by use of Student's t-test. Any condition that could interfere with the study objective (occurrence of disease, need for treatment) or for which continuation of the study raised ethical concerns led to exclusion of affected cats.

Diets

During screening, inclusion, group allocation and acclimation, cats were fed a maintenance dry expanded diet (*Veterinary Diet, Neutered Cats, Young Male, Royal Canin S.A.S., Aimargues, France*) with a sodium content of 0.7% as fed basis. After the acclimation period, cats were then monitored over 2 years while fed 70 g/day of either the high-salt diet (HSD, *Veterinary Diet, Feline Urinary High Dilution, Royal Canin S.A.S., Aimargues, France*, 1.3% sodium content and 2.27% chloride as fed basis) or the control diet (CD) of the same composition except for the level of sodium and chloride (0.35% sodium, 0.70% chloride) that was replaced with corn flour (Table 2). The level of salt chosen for the control diet is that commonly found in commercial dry cat foods. The food amount (70 g/day) was arbitrarily selected to be greater than the usual consumption of these cats. Food leftovers were weighed and each cat's exact food intake recorded daily. Cats had also free access to water.

Experimental design

The protocol was reviewed and approved by the animal care and use committee of "Pays-de-la-Loire" (file n°CEEA.2012.152) local as well as the Royal Canin ethic committee. This study was conducted according to conditions approved by the French Ministry of Agriculture and to the guidelines of the Guide for Care and Use of Laboratory Animals [30]. Physical examination, systolic and diastolic arterial BP, standard echocardiography, and conventional Doppler examination as well as 2D color TDI were performed at baseline and at 6, 12, and 24 months. Physical examination and BP measurements were also performed at 3 months, and body weight was assessed weekly throughout the study. Investigators were blinded to the treatment groups and cats were randomly ranked for iterative measurements (i.e., physical examination, BP measurements, conventional ultrasound examinations, and TDI) at each follow-up point.

Blood pressure measurement

Systolic and diastolic systemic arterial BP was measured indirectly in awake cats by the same trained observers (CCS, ET) by use of a Doppler system (*811-BL Parks Medical Electronics Inc, ALOHA, OR*), as previously described [31] and according to the guidelines currently recommended for the feline species [22]. Systemic arterial hypertension was defined as BP >160 (systolic) and/or >100 (diastolic) mmHg [22].

Standard echocardiography and conventional Doppler examination

Standard transthoracic echocardiography and conventional Doppler examination were performed by a single trained observer

Table 1. Final Group allocation for the 20 healthy cats included in the study.

Cat ID Code	TDI results	Gender	GFR (mL/min/kg)	Group
16	Normal	M	1.2	C
18	Normal	M	1.8	HS
7	Normal	M	1.8	C
13	Normal	F	1.8	HS
25	Normal	M	2.1	HS
23	Normal	F	2.1	C
14	Normal	F	2.5	HS
5	Normal	F	2.5	C
9	Subnormal	F	1.7	HS
21	Subnormal	F	1.9	C
4	Subnormal	M	1.9	C
6	Subnormal	F	2.0	HS
19	Subnormal	M	2.2	C
10	Subnormal	F	2.3	HS
8	Abnormal	M	1.6	C
17	Abnormal	M	1.6	HS
12	Abnormal	M	1.7	HS
24	Abnormal	F	1.8	C
11	Abnormal	M	1.9	HS
22	Abnormal	F	2.1	C

GFR, glomerular filtration rate; M, male; F, female; C, control group; HS, high salt group; TDI, tissue Doppler imaging.
Normal: normal systolic and diastolic radial and longitudinal myocardial function assessed by TDI.
Subnormal: normal systolic and diastolic radial and longitudinal myocardial function, except for the presence of regional post-systolic contraction waves for the longitudinal motion of the left ventricular free wall and/or the interventricular septum.
Abnormal: regional diastolic dysfunction (as assessed by an E/A ratio <1; E and A: early and late diastolic TDI waves).

(VC) using an ultrasound unit (*Vivid 7 dimension, General Electric medical system, Waukesha, Wis, USA*) equipped with 2 phased-array transducers 7S (3.5–8 MHz) and 10S (4.5–11.5 MHz). All ultrasound examinations were carried out with continuous electrocardiogram (ECG) monitoring in awake cats, gently restrained in the standing position as already described and validated by our group [32]. A mean of 3 measurements was obtained for each M-mode parameter on 3 consecutive cardiac cycles on the same frame. Left ventricular (LV) diameters, LVFW and IVS thicknesses were measured at end-diastole and end-systole from the right parasternal short-axis view [33] by use of the 2D-guided M-mode according to the recommendations of the American Society of Echocardiography [34], and the LV shortening fraction was then calculated. Measurements of the aorta (Ao) and the left atrial (LA) diameter were obtained by a 2D method at end-diastole, and the LA/Ao ratio was then calculated [32]. The end-diastolic subaortic IVS thickness was also measured using a 2D method from the right parasternal 5-chamber view at the level of the attachments of the left *chordae tendineae* to the mitral valve leaflets, as previously described [31]. The presence of a systolic anterior motion of the mitral valve, defined as a motion of the anterior mitral valve leaflet towards the LV outflow tract, was also assessed using both 2D and M-modes. Lastly, maximal systolic aortic velocity and maximal early and late diastolic mitral flow velocities (mitral E and A waves, respectively) were determined using the pulsed-wave Doppler mode from the left apical 5- and 4-chamber views, respectively, and the mitral E/A ratio was then calculated. The isovolumic relaxation time (IVRT, time interval between end of aortic flow velocity and onset of transmitral flow) was also calculated from the left apical 5-chamber view using the pulsed-wave Doppler mode. Echocardiographic and Doppler examinations were considered as normal if the latter 2D, M-mode, and Doppler variables were within the reference ranges published by our group [29].

Table 2. Nutrient composition of the diets used in the study.

Nutrient (g/Mcal ME)	HSD	CD
Moisture	13.6±0.8	16.0±1.5
Proteins	87.0±3.8	84.0±2.8
Fat	39.2±1.8	39.5±1.5
Minerals	21.1±1.3	15.3±0.3
Total Dietary Fiber	16.1±2.0	18.0±2.3
Sodium	3.1±0.1	1.0±0.1
Chloride	5.5±0.3	2.2±0.3
ME (kcal/kg, NRC 2006)	3976±55	4000±32

CD: control diet; HSD: High salt diet (Veterinary Diet Urinary High Dilution, Royal Canin, Aimargues, France); ME: Metabolizable energy; NRC: National Research Council.

Tissue Doppler imaging examination

All 2D color TDI examinations were performed and interpreted in awake standing cats with continuous ECG monitoring by the same single observer (VC) and using the same ultrasound unit as for standard echocardiography, as previously described and validated [35]. Real-time color Doppler was superimposed on the gray scale with a high frame rate (between 180 and 280 frames/s). The Doppler receive gain was adjusted to maintain optimal coloring of the myocardium (i.e., without any black spots), and the Doppler velocity range was set as low as possible to avoid aliasing. All digital images were stored and analyzed using specific software (*Echopac Dimension, General Electric Medical System, Waukesha, Wisc, USA*). A 1×1 mm sample was used and a tissue velocity profile displayed in each sample location. Peak myocardial velocities resulting from radial LVFW motion were measured in systole, early and late diastole (S, E and A waves) using the right parasternal ventricular short-axis view, and measurements were made between the 2 papillary muscles in sub-endocardial and sub-epicardial segments of the LVFW (Figure 1). Peak systolic (S), early (E) and late (A) diastolic longitudinal velocities were also measured using the standard left apical 4-chamber view in 3 myocardial segments, i.e., 2 from the LVFW (at the base and the apex, Figure 2) and 1 from the IVS (at the base). The TDI diastolic E/A ratio was calculated for each of these 5 myocardial segments. Radial systolic myocardial velocity gradients (MVG, defined as the difference between sub-endocardial and sub-epicardial systolic velocities) and longitudinal systolic MVG (defined as the difference between basal and apical systolic LVFW velocities) were also calculated for each phase of the cardiac cycle. Lastly, mean heart rate was calculated by ECG monitoring during each radial and longitudinal TDI examination from the same 3 cardiac cycles used for velocity measurements.

Statistical analysis

Data are expressed as mean ± standard deviation. Time course of body weight was analyzed by a linear mixed effects model incorporating diet, time and diet by time interaction as fixed effects, cats within diet and cats by time interaction as random effects with a software (*R Development Core Team (2009). R: A language and environment for statistical computing. R Foundation for Statistical Computing, Vienna, Austria. ISBN 3-900051-07-0, URL* http://www.R-project.org). For other variables, standard repeated measures analyses were performed with another software package (*Systat version 8.0, SPSS Inc, Chicago, IL, USA*) by use of the following generalized linear model:

$$Y_{i,j,k} = \mu + diet_i + period_j + diet * period_{i,j} + cat(diet)_{j,k} + \varepsilon_{i,j,k}$$

With:

$Y_{i,j,k}$ being the value of variable Y for Cat k with diet i in Period j

μ being the general mean effect

$diet_i$ being the effect of diet (i = HSD or CD)

$period_j$ being the effect of period (j = 0, 3, 6, 12 or 24 months)

$diet*period_{i,j}$ being the diet by period interaction term of the model

$cat(diet)_{j,k}$ being the effect of cat nested in its diet group

$\varepsilon_{i,j,k}$ being the error of the model.

Effect of dietary salt intake on tested variables was primarily assessed through the diet by period interaction term of the model. Whenever a significant diet by period interaction was detected, results of cats from the HSD group were compared to those from the CD group at each period by use of a Student's t-test. A value of $P<0.05$ was considered significant.

Results

Study feline population and follow-up

All recruited cats (n = 20) completed the first 12-month period and 16/20 the 24-month follow-up, as 4 cats were removed from the study between 12 and 24 months (2 from each diet group, i.e., cats #11, #16, #18 and #24, see Table 1). Cats #11 and #18 from the HSD group died suddenly at 13 and 21 months from no obvious cause and intracranial meningioma at full necropsy, respectively. Cat #24 from the CD group was euthanized at 13 months because of cancer (fibrosarcoma) and cat #16 from the same group was removed from the study at 17 months because of occurrence of diabetes mellitus. Analysis of the diets confirmed that, apart from salt content, differences between the 2 diets were negligible and could not interfere with the study objective. Mean caloric intake over the study period was 46±11 kcal ME/kg/day for the HSD group and 48±6 kcal ME/kg/day for the CD group, representing a dietary sodium intake of 144±36 and 45±5 mg/kg/day, respectively.

Diet effects on physical examination

All cats that completed the study remained healthy throughout the first 12-month period (n = 20) and between 12 and 24 months (n = 16), without any sign of congestive heart failure. Cardiac auscultation did not reveal any arrhythmia. Heart rate was comparable at baseline between the 2 groups (167±18 bpm and 186±25 bpm for the CD and HSD groups, respectively), and remained stable over the 24-month period. A mild but significant (P = 0.043) decrease in body weight of approximately 120 g/year was similarly observed in both diet groups during the study period (from 4.8±0.7 kg on the first day of the diet test period to 4.5±0.8 kg after 2 years in the whole study population).

Diet effects on systolic and diastolic BP

Systolic as well as diastolic BP values were comparable at baseline between the CD and HSD groups (i.e., 149±6 mmHg and 153±3 mmHg in systole, 78±8 mmHg and 78±11 mmHg in diastole, respectively). No systemic arterial hypertension was found in any cat throughout the 24-month study period, and no significant effect of the diet composition was found during the whole study period.

Diet effects on 2D and M-mode echocardiographic variables

All 2D and M-mode echocardiographic variables (n = 9) assessed at baseline were similar between the two groups (Table 3) and remained within reference intervals throughout the study for all cats [29]. No systolic anterior motion of the mitral valve, leading to LV outflow tract obstruction, was detected in any cat using both 2D and M-modes. No significant statistical effect of diet composition was found on any of the tested echocardiographic variables.

Diet effects on conventional Doppler variables

The 3 tested conventional Doppler variables assessed at baseline were comparable between the CD and HSD groups (Table 3), and remained within reference intervals throughout the 24-month study period for all cats [29]. None of them was affected by the diet.

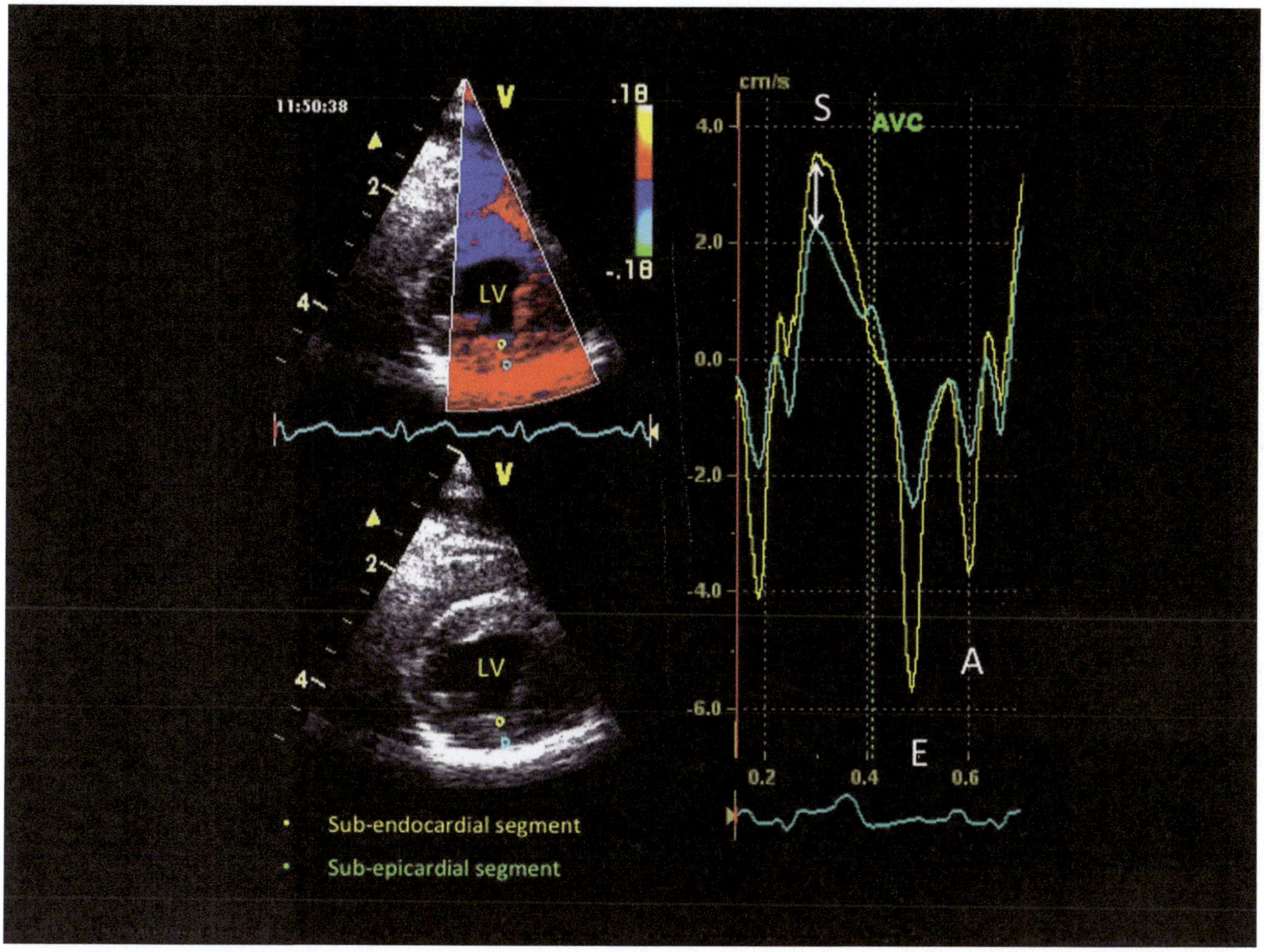

Figure 1. Radial velocity profiles obtained in a healthy recruited cat by two-dimensional color tissue Doppler imaging from the right parasternal transventricular short-axis view, simultaneously in a sub-endocardial (yellow) and a sub-epicardial (green) segment of the left ventricular free wall. *S, E and A: peak myocardial velocity during systole, early diastole and late diastole, respectively. AVC: aortic valve closure. Double arrow: systolic myocardial velocity gradient. LV: left ventricle.*

Diet effects on radial and longitudinal systolic and diastolic 2D color TDI variables

Radial and longitudinal 2D color TDI variables (n = 11) were comparable at baseline between the CD and HSD groups (Table 4). A significant diet by period interaction over the study period was observed for the TDI E/A ratio measured in the sub-endocardial segment (P = 0.009). When compared at each period, this ratio was significantly different between groups at 12 months only (1.7±0.3 and 1.4±0.4 for the CD and HSD groups, respectively; P = 0.044). Other TDI variables were not affected by the diet.

Discussion

In the present prospective study, BP, heart rate, cardiac morphology as well as myocardial function remained unaffected in healthy aged cats fed a HSD (1.3% sodium content and 2.27% chloride as fed) for 24 months, as compared with those fed a CD similar in all respects except for the salt content (0.35% sodium, 0.70% chloride).

The present protocol has several major key features: the study was prospective, controlled, blinded, randomized, and performed over a long-term period (24 months *versus* maximum 6 months in other feline studies on the topic [15,16,19,20]). Moreover, for conventional echocardiography and TDI examinations, only one single trained experienced observer was involved, thus limiting the variability for the assessed imaging measurements to intra-operator variation [32,35]. Additionally, cats in each diet group were deliberately matched with regard to both renal and cardiac function, as respectively assessed by GFR and TDI examination. This was of particular importance as, on the one hand, renal function can be altered in feline heart diseases [36] and, on the other hand, cats with chronic kidney diseases can undergo changes in cardiac morphology and function, partly due to systemic arterial hypertension that is commonly associated with chronic kidney disease in this species [22,31]. Lastly, aged cats with a mean age of 10 years (only 1 cats/group were less than 7 *(i.e:5.3 yr)* years of age) were deliberately recruited, as old cats are likely to be at higher risk than younger cats for spontaneous systemic arterial hypertension and chronic kidney diseases [21–23], both of which are known to be worsened by high salt intake in human patients and laboratory animals [24–27]. Additionally, 1) BP has been shown in some studies to increase with age in the feline species [22], 2) a significant positive relationship between salt intake and the slope of

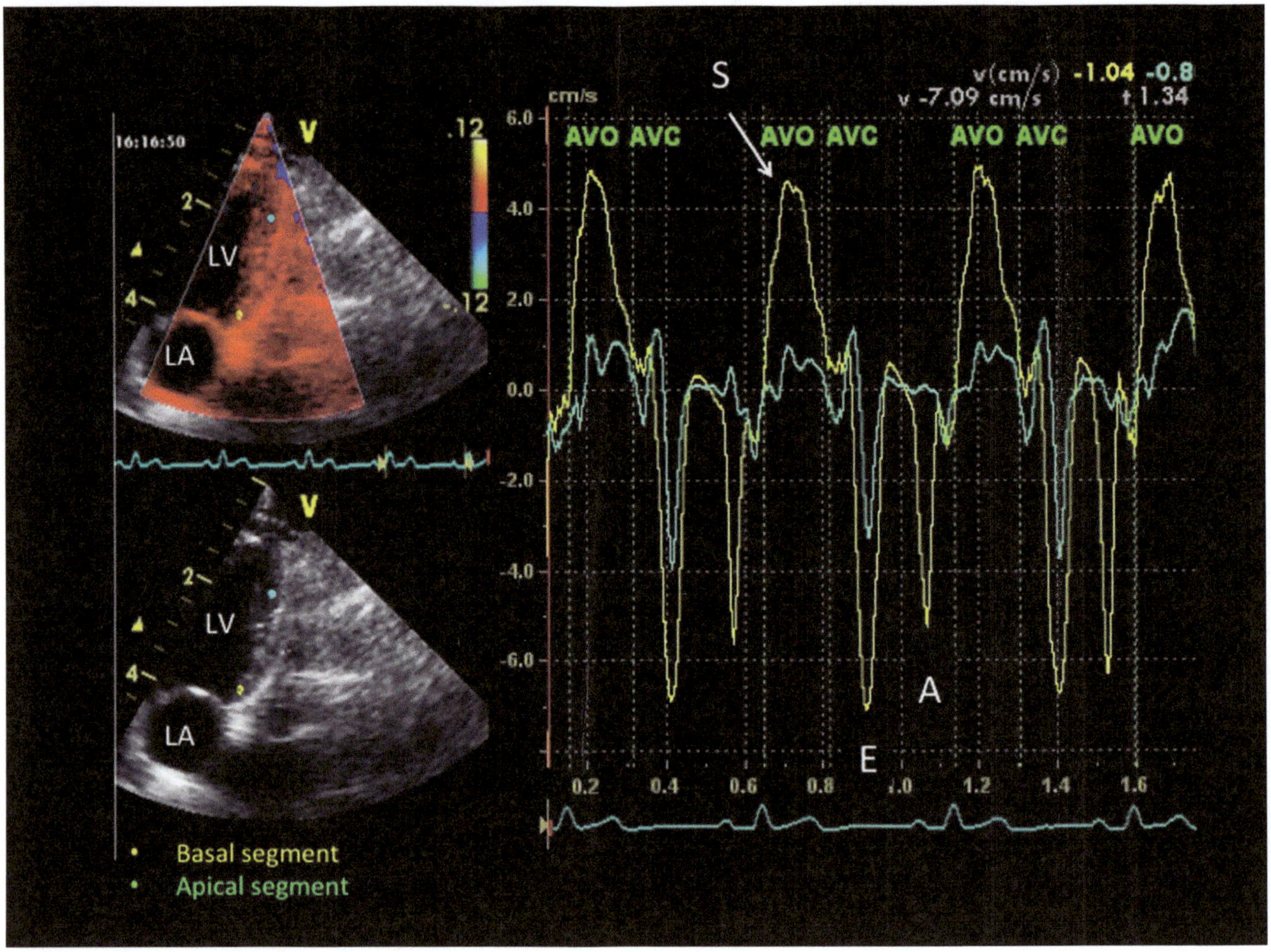

Figure 2. Longitudinal velocity profiles obtained in a healthy recruited cat by two-dimensional color tissue Doppler imaging from the left apical 4-chamber view, simultaneously in a basal (yellow) and apical (green) segment of the left ventricular free wall. *S, E and A: peak myocardial velocity during systole, early diastole and late diastole, respectively. AVO and AVC: aortic valve opening and aortic valve closure, respectively. LA: left atrium. LV: left ventricle.*

the rise in BP with age has been reported in humans [27], and lastly, 3) age-related increase in salt sensitivity, although not demonstrated in the cat, is well recognized in humans, resulting at least in part, from the impairment of several mechanisms involved in sodium regulation, including a reduced ability to appropriately excrete a salt load owing to a decline in renal function and reduced generation of natriuretic substances, such as prostaglandin E2 and dopamine [27,37].

Although the topic still remains debated and controversial in human medicine [38–41], there is substantial evidence supporting the deleterious effects of high consumption of salt on health, particularly regarding the cardiovascular system. For example, many studies showed a significant causal relationship between high salt intake and the development of systemic arterial hypertension in salt-sensitive patients and laboratory animals, and raised BP is known to be a major independent risk factor of cardiovascular diseases [1–3,25–27,37,42]. Conversely, as recently shown by high quality evidence, a reduction in salt intake decreases BP in both hypertensive and normotensive individuals, and is associated with a reduced risk of stroke and fatal coronary heart disease [43–46]. Most international guidelines recommend therefore restricting salt intake in people [26,27,47,48]. Several mechanisms by which high sodium intake diets can promote the development of hypertension have been reported, including changes in vascular reactivity, the renin-angiotensin-aldosterone system, and sympathetic reflexes [25,49,50,51]. All these data led us to measure BP in all animals throughout the study period at Day 0 and then at 3, 6, 12, and 24 months in the present study, in order to assess the cardiovascular safety of one of the HS diets commercially available for cats with lower urinary tract diseases. No systemic arterial hypertension was found in any cat throughout the 24-month study period. No significant effect of the diet was detected either. The positive above-mentioned relationship between salt intake and the slope of the rise in BP with age reported in humans [27] was hence not found in these aged cats, which do not seem therefore to be sensitive to the deleterious vascular effects of excess dietary salt intake as observed in elderly people. These results are in accordance with those reported in this species in short- and medium-term feeding trials, showing that high salt feeding (2.9 to 3.2 g Na/Mcal) does not affect BP in healthy cats [15,16,19,20].

In addition to its influence on BP, dietary sodium may exert several non-blood pressure-related effects, which result in direct target-organ damage, including myocardial hypertrophy and fibrosis as well as alteration of myocardial function, thus

Table 3. Effects of dietary salt content on conventional echocardiographic and standard Doppler variables (means ± SD) assessed in healthy aged cats fed a high salt diet (HSD, n = 10) or a control diet (CD, n = 10) over 24 months.

Imaging variables	0		6 months		12 months		24 months	
	CD	HSD	CD	HSD	CD	HSD	CD	HSD
M-mode variables								
LVDd (mm)	14.5±1.3	13.8±1.2	14.4±2.1	13.9±0.7	15.0±1.1	14.2±1.4	13.9±1.4	13.7±1.0
LVDs (mm)	6.7±0.9	6.7±1.3	6.7±1.3	6.6±1.1	6.9±1.4	6.1±1.0	5.9±1.3	6.0±1.0
LVFWd (mm)	4.6±0.3	4.3±0.4	4.5±0.3	4.3±0.4	4.5±0.3	4.5±0.4	4.5±0.5	4.2±0.4
LVFWs (mm)	7.9±0.7	7.5±0.8	7.9±0.8	7.7±0.9	8.2±0.6	8.0±0.9	8.6±1.0	7.9±1.0
IVSd (mm)	4.8±0.4	4.8±0.5	4.8±0.4	4.7±0.4	4.8±0.4	4.8±0.5	4.6±0.4	4.3±0.4
IVSs (mm)	7.8±0.9	7.7±0.7	8.1±1.1	7.8±0.7	8.1±0.7	8.0±0.7	8.3±0.8	7.7±0.7
Fractional shortening (%)	53.9±6.2	51.5±7.3	53.6±6.0	52.7±7.3	54.6±7.3	57.3±5.1	57.9±7.0	56.3±7.7
Two-dimensional variables								
Left atrium/aorta	0.84±0.08	0.83±0.07	0.81±0.09	0.75±0.12	0.87±0.14	0.82±0.14	0.78±0.09	0.75±0.12
Subaortic IVSd (mm)	4.4±0.6	4.5±0.5	4.5±0.6	4.5±0.5	4.6±0.5	4.5±0.5	4.6±0.5	4.4±0.3
Doppler variables								
Peak aortic flow velocity (m/s)	1.2±0.3	1.2±0.2	1.1±0.2	1.1±0.1	1.2±0.2	1.2±0.2	1.0±0.2	1.1±0.2
Mitral E wave/A wave ratio	1.5±0.3	1.5±0.7	1.5±0.3	1.6±0.9	1.3±0.2	1.4±1.0	1.2±0.2	1.3±0.5
Isovolumic relaxation time (ms)	49±7	48±12	46±4	45±7	47±6	51±5	50±8	52±6

LVDd: Left ventricular end-diastolic diameter. LVDs: Left ventricular end-systolic diameter. LVFWd: left ventricular free wall at end-diastole. LVFWs: left ventricular free wall at end-systole. IVSd: interventricular septum at end-diastole. IVSs: interventricular septum at end-systole.

Table 4. Effects of dietary salt content on radial and longitudinal tissue Doppler imaging (TDI) variables (means ± SD) assessed in healthy aged cats fed a high salt diet (HSD, n = 10) or a control diet (CD, n = 10) over 24 months.

TDI variables	0		6 months		12 months		24 months	
	CD	HSD	CD	HSD	CD	HSD	CD	HSD
Radial motion of the left ventricular free wall								
Heart rate (beats/min)	177±18	170±12	181±22	180±15	166±18	178±12	167±13	176±17
Systolic radial MVG (cm/s)	2.4±0.7	2.1±0.6	2.7±0.7	2.1±0.7	2.5±0.6	2.5±0.6	2.7±0.6	2.7±0.8
E/A ratio endocardium	1.4±0.4	1.7±0.5	1.8±0.4	2.0±0.6	**1.7±0.3**	**1.4±0.4***	1.7±0.7	1.3±0.6
E/A ratio epicardium	1.6±0.7	2.0±1.4	2.5±1.3	2.4±1.2	2.4±1.2	1.7±0.6	2.9±2.3	1.7±1.2
Longitudinal motion of the left ventricular free wall								
Heart rate (beats/min)	178±19	165±23	183±23	187±20	170±16	180±16	174±31	177±17
Systolic MVG base-apex (cm/s)	2.2±0.9	2.5±1.3	2.4±0.7	2.3±1.2	2.3±0.7	2.5±1.1	2.4±0.6	2.6±0.8
E/A ratio at the base	1.8±1.5	1.5±0.5	1.4±0.5	1.7±0.9	1.5±0.7	1.6±0.8	1.2±0.5	1.2±0.5
E/A ratio at the apex	2.8±2.7	4.3±6.6	2.1±1.5	2.9±1.8	2.5±2.3	3.0±1.7	5.2±7.6	2.3±1.6
Longitudinal motion of the interventricular septum								
Heart rate (beats/min)	176±34	175±16	186±26	185±17	180±25	184±19	174±24	189±15
S wave at the base (cm/s)	5.5±2.0	5.8±1.6	5.7±1.8	6.0±1.5	6.0±1.8	6.4±1.4	6.1±1.7	6.5±1.1
E/A ratio at the base (cm/s)	1.0±0.5	1.2±0.6	1.2±0.5	1.3±0.7	1.1±0.5	1.1±0.4	1.1±0.5	0.9±0.5

S, E and A: peak myocardial velocity during systole, early diastole and late diastole, respectively. MVG: myocardial velocity gradient.
*P = 0.044 versus CD group.

amplifying the effect of BP on the LV. These BP-independent cardiac adverse effects have been demonstrated in animal models [8,9] and in both normotensive people and patients with essential hypertension [10–12,24,52,53]. For example, in normal mice, chronic excess salt intake has been shown to induce a IVS-predominant LV hypertrophy, associated with an increase in collagen density, angiotensin converting enzyme activity, angiotensin II type 1 receptor density, and extracellular signal regulated kinase phosphorylation. All the latter data regarding the BP-independent cardiac adverse effects led us to perform a conventional echocardiographic examination on all animals throughout the present study (at Day 0 and then at 6, 12, and 24 months). Nevertheless, no significant statistical effect of diet composition was found on either 2D or M-mode echocardiographic variables, including myocardial wall thicknesses and LV diameters. Additionally, neither obstruction of the LV outflow tract (as confirmed by maximal systolic aortic velocity measurement) nor systolic anterior motion of the mitral valve (a common cause of dynamic obstruction of the LV outflow tract in cats with hypertrophic cardiomyopathy [54]) were detected, and the LA/Ao ratio remained unchanged over the whole study period. In other words, the 24-month diet was not associated with diffuse or localized myocardial hypertrophy, changes in LV diameters, and left atrial dilation.

As high salt diets have also been shown to modulate and affect myocardial function, particularly during the diastolic time [6,7,55], and as feline systemic arterial hypertension is associated with myocardial dysfunction occurring independently of the presence of myocardial hypertrophy [56], another aim of the present study was to assess the effect of high salt intake on myocardial function in the recruited aged cats. For this purpose, 2D color TDI, which has been shown by our group to be repeatable and reproducible in the awake cat [35], was chosen to complement the conventional echocardiographic and Doppler data and accurately analyze the effect of HSD on segmental myocardial function. We have previously demonstrated that 2D color TDI is more sensitive than conventional ultrasound techniques in detecting myocardial dysfunction in the feline species, even in the absence of overt myocardial changes [56–58]. As feline spontaneous hypertrophic cardiomyopathy and chronic systemic hypertension (SHT) can both lead to radial and longitudinal diastolic myocardial alteration and can both induce a longitudinal-predominant systolic LVFW dysfunction [56–58], both radial and longitudinal LV motions were assessed using 2D color TDI in the present study. Nevertheless, the 24-month HSD diet was not associated with overt systolic and diastolic dysfunction, as respectively the shortening fraction and both mitral E/A ratio and IVRT remained unchanged throughout the study. Similarly, regional radial and longitudinal systolic myocardial function, as assessed by TDI systolic velocity gradients (respectively, between sub-endocardial and sub-epicardial segments, and between basal and apical segments) remained unaltered throughout the 24-month study period. The 24-month HS diet had no effect either on the longitudinal diastolic function, as assessed by the longitudinal TDI E/A ratio in basal and apical segments of the LVFW as well as at the base of the IVS. Similarly, no difference according to dietary salt intake in the radial TDI E/A ratio repeatedly measured in the sub-endocardial and sub-epicardial segments of the LVFW over 24 months was found in the cats of the present study, except for the sub-endocardial TDI E/A ratio that was significantly lower in the HSD group (1.4 ± 0.4) than in the CD group (1.7 ± 0.3) at 12 months. Nevertheless, this 0.3 mean difference can be considered as biologically negligible [29,35], and was detected only one time (at 12 months), and therefore cannot be interpreted as a long-term consistent adverse effect of HSD on sub-endocardial radial diastolic function. Additionally, given the number of TDI measurements that were compared during the whole study period, it is highly likely that this sole difference was detected just by chance.

In conclusion, in the present study, high dietary salt intake (3.1 g Na/Mcal) over 24 months had no adverse effects on BP, heart rate, cardiac morphology as well as global and regional myocardial function as assessed by 2D and M-mode echocardiography, conventional Doppler examination, and 2D color TDI in healthy aged cats. However, these results cannot be generalized to diseased cats suffering from spontaneous systemic arterial hypertension, cardiomyopathies, or chronic kidney disease. Additionally, further studies are needed to confirm this lack of salt-sensitivity in larger healthy populations of various feline breeds and mixed-breeds (Domestic short and long haired cats), and to understand the underlying mechanisms of this potential species specificity.

Acknowledgments

The authors would like to sincerely thank Samuel Ninet, Thérèse Frégier and Philippe Bleis (Oniris), Thomas Daste and Amélie Dutech (National Veterinary School of Toulouse) for their technical assistance during the animal phase, Claude Germain (National Veterinary School of Toulouse) and Joëlle Ribaut (National Veterinary School of Toulouse) for administrative and logistical support.

Author Contributions

Conceived and designed the experiments: VC BSR PN DC JE IT JA VB HPL. Performed the experiments: VC BSR ET-S CCS IT. Analyzed the data: VC BSR DC HPL. Contributed reagents/materials/analysis tools: BSR JE VB HPL. Wrote the paper: VC BSR PN JE JA VB HPL.

References

1. Ely DL (1997) Overview of dietary sodium effects on and interactions with cardiovascular and neuroendocrine functions. Am J Clin Nutr 65: 594S–605S.
2. Elliott P (1989) The INTERSALT study: an addition to the evidence on salt and blood pressure, and some implications. J Hum Hypertens 3: 289–298.
3. Stamler J (1997) The INTERSALT Study: background, methods, findings, and implications. Am J Clin Nutr 65(2 Suppl): 626S–642S.
4. Hu G, Qiao Q, Tuomilehto J (2002) Nonhypertensive cardiac effects of a high salt diet. Curr Hypertens Rep 4: 13–17.
5. He FJ, Burnier M, Macgregor GA (2011) Nutrition in cardiovascular disease: salt in hypertension and heart failure. Eur Heart J 32: 3073–3080.
6. Williams JS, Solomon SD, Crivaro M, Conlin PR (2006) Dietary sodium intake modulates myocardial relaxation responsiveness to angiotensin II. Transl Res 148: 49–54.
7. Tzemos N, Lim PO, Wong S, Struthers AD, MacDonald TM (2008) Adverse cardiovascular effects of acute salt loading in young normotensive individuals. Hypertension 51: 1525–30.
8. Lal A, Veinot JP, Leenen FH (2003) Prevention of high salt diet-induced cardiac hypertrophy and fibrosis by spironolactone. Am J Hypertens 16: 319–323.
9. Le Corvoisier P, Adamy C, Sambin L, Crozatier B, Berdeaux A, et al. (2010) The cardiac renin-angiotensin system is responsible for high-salt diet-induced left ventricular hypertrophy in mice. Eur J Heart Fail 12: 1171–1178.
10. Rodriguez CJ, Bibbins-Domingo K, Jin Z, Daviglus ML, Goff DC Jr, et al (2011) Association of sodium and potassium intake with left ventricular mass: coronary artery risk development in young adults. Hypertension 58: 410–416.
11. de la Sierra A, Lluch MM, Paré JC, Coca A, Aguilera MT, et al. (1996) Increased left ventricular mass in salt-sensitive hypertensive patients. J Hum Hypertens 10: 795–799.
12. Beil AH, Schmieder RE, Messerli FH (1994) Salt intake, blood pressure, and cardiovascular structure. Cardiovasc Drugs Ther 8: 425–432.
13. Gerber B, Boretti FS, Kley S, Laluha P, Müller C, et al (2005) Evaluation of clinical signs and causes of lower urinary tract disease in European cats. J Small Anim Pract 46: 571–577.
14. Hawthorne AJ, Markwell PJ (2004) Dietary sodium promotes increased water intake and urine volume in cats. J Nutr 34: 2128S–2129S.
15. Luckschander N, Iben C, Hosgood G, Gabler C, Biourge V (2004) Dietary NaCl does not affect blood pressure in healthy cats. J Vet Intern Med 18: 463–467.

16. Kirk CA, Jewell DE, Lowry SR (2006) Effects of sodium chloride on selected parameters in cats. Vet Ther 7: 333–346.
17. Houston DM, Rinkardt NE, Hilton J (2004) Evaluation of the efficacy of a commercial diet in the dissolution of feline struvite bladder uroliths. Vet Ther 5: 187–201.
18. Houston DM, Weese HE, Evason MD, Biourge V, van Hoek I (2011) A diet with a struvite relative supersaturation less than 1 is effective in dissolving struvite stones in vivo. Br J Nutr 106: S90–S92.
19. Buranakarl C, Mathur S, Brown SA (2004) Effects of dietary sodium chloride intake on renal function and blood pressure in cats with normal and reduced renal function Am J Vet Res 65: 620–626.
20. Xu H, Laflamme DPL, Long GL (2009) Effects of dietary sodium chloride on health parameters in mature cats. J Feline Med Surg 11: 435–441.
21. Jepson RE (2011) Feline systemic hypertension: Classification and pathogenesis. J Feline Med Surg 13: 25–34.
22. Brown S, Atkins C, Bagley R, Carr A, Cowgill L, et al. (2007) American College of Veterinary Internal Medicine. Guidelines for the identification, evaluation, and management of systemic hypertension in dogs and cats. J Vet Intern Med 21: 542–558.
23. Syme HM, Markwell PJ, Pfeiffer D, Elliott J (2006) Survival of cats with naturally occurring chronic renal failure is related to severity of proteinuria. J Vet Intern Med 20: 528–535.
24. du Cailar G, Ribstein J, Mimran A (2002) Dietary sodium and target organ damage in essential hypertension. Am J Hypertens 15: 222–229.
25. dos Santos L, Gonçalves MV, Vassallo DV, Oliveira EM, Rossoni LV (2006) Effects of high sodium intake diet on the vascular reactivity to phenylephrine on rat isolated caudal and renal vascular beds: Endothelial modulation. Life Sci 78: 2272–2279.
26. Mohan S, Campbell NR (2009) Salt and high blood pressure. Clin Sci 117: 1–11.
27. He FJ, MacGregor GA (2010) Reducing population salt intake worldwide: from evidence to implementation. Prog Cardiovasc Dis 52: 363–382.
28. Reynolds BS, Chetboul V, Nguyen P, Testault I, Concordet DV, et al. (2013) Effects of dietary salt intake on renal function: a 2-year study in healthy aged cats. J Vet Intern Med 27: 507–15.
29. Chetboul V, Carlos Sampedrano C, Tissier R, Gouni V, Saponaro V, et al (2006) Quantitative assessment of velocities of the annulus of the left atrioventricular valve and left ventricular free wall in healthy cats by use of two-dimensional color tissue Doppler imaging. Am J Vet Res 67: 250–8.
30. Guide for Care and Use of Laboratory Animals, Institute of Laboratory Animals Resources, Commission on Life Sciences, National Research Council, Washington, D.C.: The National Academy Press; 1996.
31. Chetboul V, Lefebvre HP, Pinhas C, Clerc B, Boussouf M, et al. (2003) Spontaneous feline hypertension: clinical and echocardiographic abnormalities, and survival rate. J Vet Intern Med 17: 89–95.
32. Chetboul V, Concordet D, Pouchelon JL, Athanassiadis N, Muller C, et al. (2003) Effects of inter- and intra-observer variability on echocardiographic measurements in awake cats. J Vet Med A Physiol Pathol Clin Med 50: 326–331.
33. Thomas WP, Gaber CE, Jacobs GJ, Kaplan PM, Lombard CW, et al. (1993) Recommendations for standards in transthoracic two-dimensional echocardiography in the dog and cat. Echocardiography Committee of the Specialty of Cardiology, American College of Veterinary Internal Medicine. J Vet Intern Med 7: 247–252.
34. Sahn DJ, DeMaria A, Kisslo J, Weyman A (1978) Recommendations regarding quantitation in M-mode echocardiography: Results of a survey of echocardiographic measurements. Circulation 58: 1072–1083.
35. Chetboul V, Athanassiadis N, Carlos C, Nicolle AP, Tissier R, et al. (2004) Quantification, repeatability, and reproducibility of feline radial and longitudinal left ventricular velocities by tissue Doppler imaging. Am J Vet Res 65: 566–72.
36. Gouni V, Chetboul V, Pouchelon JL, Carlos Sampedrano C, Maurey C, et al. (2008) Azotemia in cats with feline hypertrophic cardiomyopathy: prevalence and relationships with echocardiographic variables. J Vet Cardiol 10: 117–123.
37. Zemel MB, Sowers JR (1988) Salt sensitivity and systemic hypertension in the elderly. Am J Cardiol 61: 7H–12H.
38. Walker J, MacKenzie AD, Dunning J (2007) Does reducing your salt intake make you live longer? Interact Cardiovasc Thorac Surg 6: 793–798.
39. Dumler F (2009) Dietary sodium intake and arterial blood pressure. J Ren Nutr 19: 57–60.
40. Taylor RS, Ashton KE, Moxham T, Hooper L, Ebrahim S (2011) Reduced dietary salt for the prevention of cardiovascular disease: a meta-analysis of randomized controlled trials (Cochrane review). Am J Hypertens 24: 843–53.
41. Borke JA, Wyer PC (2013) Eating a larger number of high-salt foods is not associated with short-term risk of acute decompensation in patients with chronic heart failure. J Emerg Med 44: 36–45.
42. Kassab S, Miller MT, Novak J, Reckelhoff J, Clower B, et al. (1998). Endothelin-A receptor antagonism attenuates the hypertension and renal injury in Dahl salt-sensitive rats. Hypertension 31 (1 Pt 2): 397–402.
43. Aburto NJ, Ziolkovska A, Hooper L, Elliott P, Cappuccio FP, et al. (2013) Effect of lower sodium intake on health: systematic review and meta-analyses. BMJ 346: f1326.
44. He FJ, Li J, Macgregor GA (2013) Effect of longer term modest salt reduction on blood pressure: Cochrane systematic review and meta-analysis of randomised trials. BMJ. 2013 Apr 3;346:f1325.
45. Salehi-Abargouei A, Maghsoudi Z, Shirani F, Azadbakht L (2013) Effects of Dietary Approaches to Stop Hypertension (DASH)-style diet on fatal or nonfatal cardiovascular diseases—incidence: a systematic review and meta-analysis on observational prospective studies. Nutrition 29: 611–618.
46. Penz ED, Joffres MR, Campbell NR (2008) Reducing dietary sodium and decreases in cardiovascular disease in Canada. Can J Cardiol. 24: 497–491.
47. Pearson TA, Blair SN, Daniels SR, Eckel RH, Ockene JM, et al. (2002) AHA Guidelines for primary prevention of cardiovascular disease and stroke: 2002 Update: Consensus panel guide to comprehensive risk reduction for adult patients without coronary or other atherosclerotic vascular diseases. Circulation 106: 388–391.
48. Morrison AC, Ness RB (2011) Sodium intake and cardiovascular disease. Annu Rev Public Health 32: 71–90.
49. Nishida Y, Ding J, Zhou M, Chen Q, Murakami H, et al. (1998) Role of nitric oxide in vascular hyperresponsiveness to norepinephrine in hypertensive Dahl rats. J Hypertens 16: 1611–1618.
50. Ferrari AU, Mark AL (1987). Sensitization of aortic baroreceptors by high salt diet in Dahl salt-resistant rats. Hypertension 10: 55–60.
51. Simchon S, Manger WM, Brown TW (1991) Dual hemodynamic mechanisms for salt-induced hypertension in Dahl salt-sensitive rats. Hypertension 17 (6 Pt 2): 1063–1071.
52. Kupari M, Koskinen P, Virolainen J (1994) Correlates of left ventricular mass in a population sample aged 36 to 37 years. Focus on lifestyle and salt intake. Circulation 89: 1041–1050.
53. Perry IJ, Beevers DG (1992) Salt intake and stroke: a possible direct effect. J Hum Hypertens 6: 23–25.
54. Schöber K, Todd A (2010) Echocardiographic assessment of left ventricular geometry and the mitral valve apparatus in cats with hypertrophic cardiomyopathy. J Vet Cardiol 12: 1–16.
55. Mak GS, Sawaya H, Khan AM, Arora P, Martinez A, et al. (2013) Effects of subacute dietary salt intake and acute volume expansion on diastolic function in young normotensive individuals. Eur Heart J Cardiovasc Imaging 14: 1092–1098.
56. Carlos Sampedrano C, Chetboul V, Gouni V, Nicolle AP, Pouchelon JL, et al. (2006) Systolic and diastolic myocardial dysfunction in cats with hypertrophic cardiomyopathy or systemic hypertension. J Vet Intern Med 20: 1106–1115.
57. Chetboul V, Blot S, Carlos Sampedrano C, Thibaud JL, Granger N, et al. (2006) Tissue Doppler imaging for detection of radial and longitudinal myocardial dysfunction in a family of cats affected by dystrophin-deficient hypertrophic muscular dystrophy. J Vet Intern Med 20: 640–647.
58. Carlos Sampedrano C, Chetboul V, Mary J, Tissier R, Abitbol M, et al. (2009) Prospective echocardiographic and tissue Doppler imaging screening of a population of Maine Coon cats tested for the A31P mutation in the myosin-binding protein C gene: a specific analysis of the heterozygous status. J Vet Intern Med 23: 91–99.

Echocardiographic Evidence of Innate Aortopathy in the Human Intracranial Aneurysm

Yong-Won Shin[1], Keun-Hwa Jung[1,2]*, Jeong-Min Kim[3], Young Dae Cho[4], Soon-Tae Lee[1,2], Kon Chu[1,2]*, Manho Kim[1,2], Sang Kun Lee[1,2], Moon Hee Han[4], Jae-Kyu Roh[1,5]

1 Department of Neurology, Laboratory for Neurotherapeutics, Biomedical Research Institute, Seoul National University Hospital, Seoul, South Korea, **2** Program in Neuroscience, Neuroscience Research Institute of SNUMRC, College of Medicine, Seoul National University, Seoul, South Korea, **3** Department of Neurology, Chung-Ang University Medical Center, College of Medicine, Chung-Ang University, Seoul, South Korea, **4** Department of Radiology, Seoul National University Hospital, Seoul, South Korea, **5** Department of Neurology, Armed Forces Capital Hospital, Seongnam, Gyeunggido, South Korea

Abstract

Background: Intracranial aneurysm (IA) is significantly more prevalent in patients with coarctation of the aorta or bicuspid aortic valve than in the general population, suggesting a common pathophysiology connecting IA and aortopathy. Here, we analyzed echocardiographic aortic root dimension (ARD) in patients with IA to confirm this possibility.

Methods: From January 2008 to December 2010, 260 consecutive patients with IA who were admitted to our institution for coil embolization or for acute stroke management and who also underwent echocardiography were enrolled. We hypothesized that patients with large, ruptured, or multiple IAs are more likely to harbor co-prevalent aortopathy as measured by ARD compared to patients with small, isolated, unruptured IAs. Eccentric group was defined as patients aged <55 years with at least one ruptured aneurysm, an aneurysm ≥7 mm in size, or multiple aneurysms; the remainder was classified into a non-eccentric group. Clinical, angiographic, and echocardiographic findings of the two groups were compared.

Results: ARD was significantly larger in the eccentric group than in the non-eccentric group ($P = 0.049$), and the difference was confirmed by multivariable analysis ($P = 0.02$). Subgroup analysis of patients aged <55 years showed similar result for ARD ($P = 0.03$), whereas hypertension was more associated with the non-eccentric group ($P = 0.01$). In addition, height was inversely related to aneurysm size after adjustment for age, sex, weight, ARD, smoking status, and number of aneurysms ($P = 0.004$).

Conclusions: A certain group of IA patients share a common intrinsic wall defect with aortopathy. Shared neural crest cell origin may give rise to this phenomenon.

Editor: Jean-Claude Baron, INSERM U894, Centre de Psychiatrie et Neurosciences, Hopital Sainte-Anne and Université Paris 5, France

Funding: This study was supported by a grant from the Korean Health Technology R&D Project, Ministry of Health & Welfare, Republic of Korea (HI12C0421). Dr. Keun-Hwa Jung was supported by the Seoul National University Hospital Research Fund (04201311120). The funders had no role in study design, data collection and analysis, decision to publish, or preparation of the manuscript.

Competing Interests: The authors have declared that no competing interests exist.

* Email: jungkh@gmail.com (KHJ); stemcell.snu@gmail.com (KC)

Introduction

Intracranial aneurysms (IAs), outpouches of weakened arterial walls, occur in 2–5% of the general population [1], [2]. IAs are usually asymptomatic, but rupture can have devastating consequences [3]. The pathophysiology of aneurysm formation, growth, and rupture is poorly understood. Local shear stress and inflammatory processes may explain vulnerable locations and the pathogenic process of IAs but have limited value for identifying potentially susceptible patients [4], [5]. Major risk factors such as hypertension, smoking, and female sex are insufficient to explain high interpersonal vulnerability differences [6]. Multiple aneurysms are found in 15–45% of patients with IA [7], [8], suggesting that a substantial number of patients are naturally aneurysm-prone. Epidemiological studies have shown that a developmental defect may be involved in the formation of multiple IAs [9], [10]. The contribution of innate arterial wall fragility to aneurysmal pathogenesis is supported by genetic, experimental, and clinical studies [9–21]. Therefore, characterization of intrinsic wall defects is important for improving our understanding of the nature of IAs.

Bicuspid aortic valve (BAV) and coarctation of the aorta (CoA) are congenital conditions that frequently occur with dilated aortic root and aortic or cervical dissection [11]. Intracranial aneurysms are also more prevalent in patients with BAV [12] or CoA [13], implying that IA and aortic pathologies share a common developmental defect. However, the rarity of patients presenting with these conditions makes it hard to extend the relationship to the general population. We postulated that a significant proportion of patients with IA have innate cerebral arteriopathy and aortopathy concomitantly, irrespective of BAV and CoA, and we designed the current study to uncover evidence of innate aortopathy in IA using aortic root dimension (ARD), a common echocardiographic marker.

Methods

Study population

Consecutive patients who were admitted to our institute between January 2008 and December 2010 for coil embolization for IA (hereafter "coiled patients," $n = 871$) were initially screened. Of 871 coiled patients, 238 underwent transthoracic echocardiography. Indications for echocardiographic evaluation were not predefined owing to retrospective nature of this study, but in general, old age and/or cardiovascular risk factors underwent the echocardiography. For the same period, we also screened the existence of IA in patients who were admitted for acute ischemic stroke (hereafter "stroke patients," $n = 852$). Stroke patients were selected because almost all patients underwent echocardiography, which is advantageous for getting echocardiographic data and mitigating selection bias in the retrospective study design. IAs were found in 59 stroke patients and all underwent transthoracic echocardiography during the same period. Three of 297 patients screened were excluded because of overlap between the two groups.

Patients with dissecting aneurysm ($n = 9$), fusiform aneurysm ($n = 2$), or extracranial carotid artery aneurysm ($n = 1$) were excluded because these aneurysm types have different pathologic characteristics. Patients with autosomal dominant polycystic kidney disease ($n = 7$), Ehler-Danlos syndrome type IV ($n = 1$), or granulomatous arteritis with multiple aneurysms ($n = 1$) were excluded because these conditions are associated with aneurysm formation. Patients with missing height information ($n = 13$) were excluded because height is a principal determinant of ARD [22]. A total of 260 patients were finally included in the analysis.

Clinical information about the coiled patients was retrieved from the database prospectively maintained by trained interventionists using a standardized case registration form. Data from stroke patients were collected from the nationwide Korean Stroke Registry, which was started in 1999 to investigate the characteristics, mechanisms, risk factors, and neurological outcomes of stroke in Korea [23]. The stroke registry is based on a predefined registration form filled out by trained physicians or research nurses, and data fidelity was confirmed by experienced vascular neurologists. The study was approved by the Human Subject Research Committee of the Seoul National University Hospital. Written informed consent was obtained from all patients or their next of kin.

Data acquisition and interpretation

The following clinical information was collected from each patient at admission: demographic characteristics (age at admission, sex, height, and weight), atherosclerotic risk factors (hypertension [HTN], diabetes mellitus [DM], hyperlipidemia, and smoking status), and history of atrial fibrillation, coronary artery disease (CAD; angina pectoris or myocardial infarction), or cerebrovascular accident (stroke or transient ischemic attack). HTN was identified when the blood pressure was repeatedly measured at >140 mm Hg systolic or >90 mm Hg diastolic or when the patients were on antihypertensive medication. Hyperlipidemia was defined as an elevated LDL cholesterol (≥160 mg/dl) or total cholesterol (≥240 mg/dl) or treatment with a lipid-lowering agent. DM diagnosis was based on a previous history of DM or the diagnostic guidelines of the American Diabetes Association [24]. Body mass index was calculated as weight/(height)^2 (kg/m^2), and body surface area (BSA) was calculated with the Mosteller formula [25]. We also searched medical records and available computed tomography data to determine whether patients had CoA.

Echocardiographic data included ARD, left atrial (LA) dimension, interventricular septal end diastolic dimension (IVSd), left ventricular end diastolic posterior wall dimension (LVPWd), and presence of aortic valve pathology such as aortic regurgitation, aortic stenosis, or BAV. Given that ARD is frequently associated with aortic pathology such as ascending aortic aneurysm, dissection, and coarctation of aorta [11], ARD was selected as a potential marker for aortopathy. Other routine markers, LA dimension, IVSd, and LVPWd were selected for comparisons. ARD was measured by the leading-edge-to-leading-edge technique, at end diastole or at the widest dimension best visualized regardless of the cardiac cycle [26]. LA dimension, LVPWd, and IVSd were also measured according to the recommendations of the American Society of Echocardiography [26]. All echocardiographic findings were double checked by two experienced cardiologists at the time of evaluation.

IAs were diagnosed and characterized on the basis of conventional angiography or magnetic resonance angiography. Maximal diameter of IA was determined, and the largest aneurysm was used in the analysis if the patient had multiple aneurysms. Aneurysms of ≥7 mm were considered large according to previous studies [27], [28]. All imaging studies were evaluated by two experienced neuroradiologists.

Statistical analysis

Patient demographics and clinical features were analyzed using descriptive statistics. Data are expressed as means ± standard deviations or numbers (percentages). Echocardiographic markers were analyzed as absolute measures or as indexed to either BSA or height. For comparisons between two groups, the Pearson χ^2 test or the Fisher two-tailed exact test was used for categorical variables, and the Student t test or the Mann-Whitney U test was used for continuous variables. One-way ANOVA was used for multiple comparisons. Bivariate correlations were performed with Pearson coefficients. Variables with clinical importance or with P values of <0.10 in univariable analysis were included in multivariable analysis. For subgroup analysis of patients aged < 55, we performed backward stepwise logistic regression analysis with a P value for entry of 0.05 and a P value for removal of 0.1. For multiple linear regression analysis, independent variables were selected according to the result of correlation analysis. Statistical significance was set at $P<0.05$, and SPSS (ver. 18.0 SPSS Inc., Chicago, IL) was used for the analyses.

Results

Age distribution of study population

The age distribution of the study group showed heterogeneity but skewed towards older ages (64.1±10.3 years, Figure 1A). Stroke patients with IA consisted mainly of an old age population (70.4±9.1 years, Figure 1B), whereas coiled patients had an additional population with younger ages (Figure 1C). The age distribution of patients with IAs with eccentric characteristics (large, multiple, and rupture) were bimodal (Figure. 1D–F).

Characteristics of eccentric and non-eccentric groups

To separate patients with potential intrinsic arterial wall defects, we selected an eccentric group consisting of patients aged <55 years with at least one of the following features: aneurysm size ≥ 7 mm, multiple aneurysms, or rupture presentation; all other patients were categorized as non-eccentric. As owing to the group

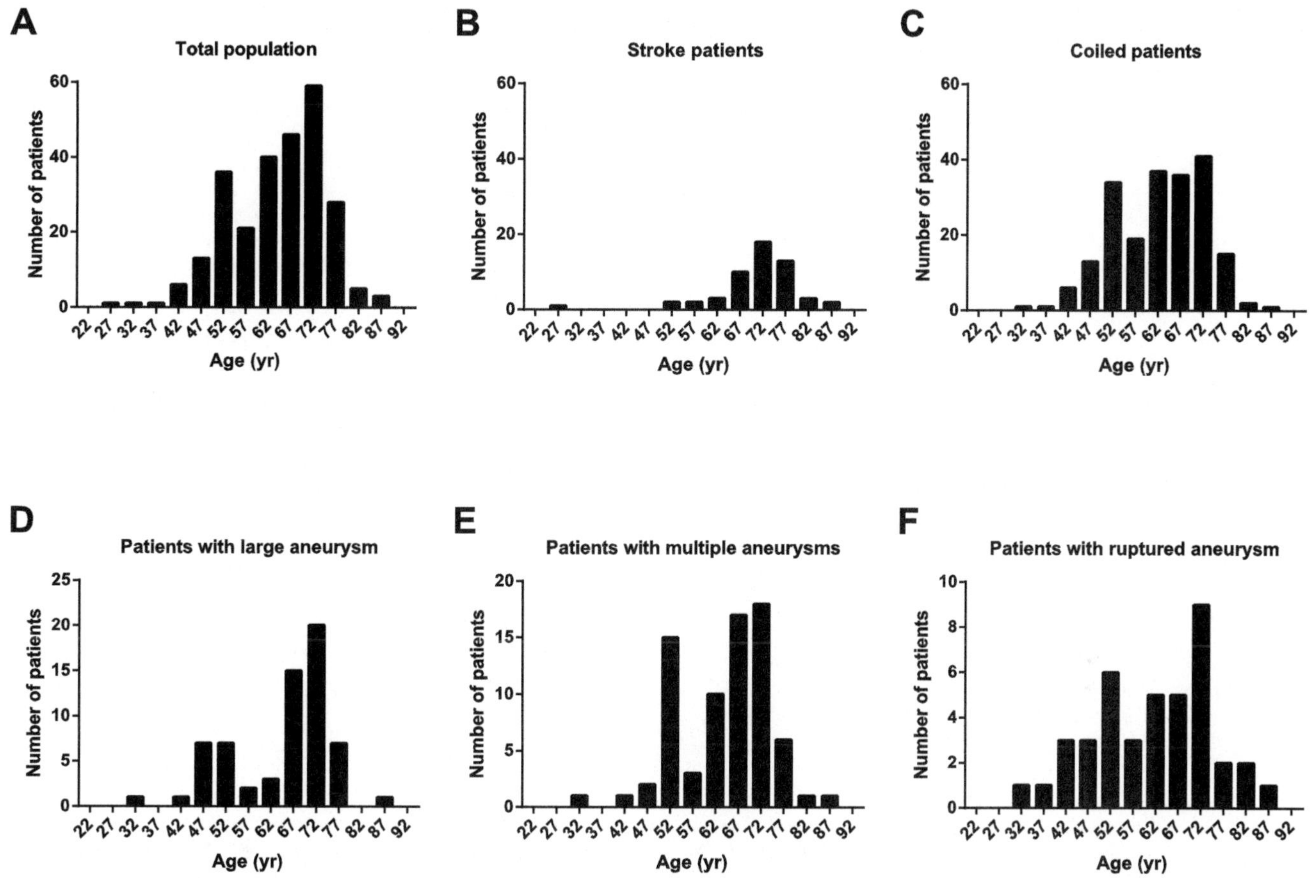

Figure 1. Age distribution of the study population. (a) Age distribution of the total population ($n = 260$) was bimodal; there were a large number of patients aged 50–54 years. (b) The stroke patients ($n = 57$) were relatively old, and the distribution was unimodal. (c) Age distribution of the coiled patients ($n = 206$) demonstrate another peak which contributed to the bimodality of the total population. Patients with (d) large IAs (≥7, $n = 64$), (e) multiple aneurysms ($n = 75$), and (f) a ruptured aneurysm ($n = 41$) also showed bimodal age distributions. The labels on the x-axis indicate mean ages of 5-year age groups starting at age 20.

definitions, age and the number of aneurysms and ruptured aneurysms differed between the groups (Table S1). Aneurysms tended to be larger in the eccentric group with a borderline significance. The non-eccentric group was shorter than the eccentric group, perhaps because of age differences. Cerebrovascular risk factors (HTN, DM, and hyperlipidemia) and history of stroke or CAD were significantly higher in the non-eccentric group than in the eccentric group. Absolute values of ARD of the eccentric group was significantly larger than that of the non-eccentric group. The ARDs indexed to BSA or to height showed no significant differences. LA dimension was significantly smaller in eccentric group when indexed to BSA and height but not as absolute measures. IVSd and LVPWd were not significantly different between the groups. BAV and CoA were not found in the study population.

Independent association of ARD with eccentricity

Multivariable analysis showed that only ARD and age differed significantly between the two groups (Table 1). Female sex was included in the model because of its significant effect on aneurysm characteristics [6], but it was not significant after adjustment. Atherosclerotic risk factors (HTN, DM, hyperlipidemia, smoking status, and history of stroke or CAD) were not associated with eccentricity. LA dimension did not differ between the groups. Additional logistic regression analysis with other echocardiographic findings (e.g., IVSd and LVPWd) also showed no difference between the groups (Table S2). The results were not different when only the coiled patients were analyzed (Table S2 and S3). All of the results were reconfirmed by the analyses using indexed echocardiographic measures. Because of the significant age discrepancy between the two groups, we also performed subgroup analysis with only patients who were aged <55 years (eccentric group, $n = 33$; non-eccentric group, $n = 25$). Univariable analysis showed no significant difference in age between the groups ($P = 0.61$). Atherosclerotic risk factors and echocardiographic markers were also not different between the groups except for HTN ($P = 0.03$). Logistic regression analysis by a backward stepwise selection method selected three variables in the final model: HTN, ARD, and height (Table 2); ARD remained significantly different, while age differences were eliminated. HTN was more frequently associated with non-eccentricity, suggesting that some mechanism other than hypertension is implicated in eccentricity. Patients in the eccentric group tended to be short, although the statistical significance was marginal. Analyses using indexed values also showed similar trend except for height which did not show independent relationship with eccentricity.

Table 1. Results of multivariable logistic regression analysis of determinants of eccentricity.

	Using absolute echocardiographic measurement		Indexed to BSA		Indexed to height	
	OR (95% CI)	*P* value	OR (95% CI)	*P* value	OR (95% CI)	*P* value
Age	0.78 (0.70–0.86)	<0.001	0.82 (0.76–0.88)	<0.001	0.81 (0.75–0.87)	<0.001
Female	1.87 (0.29–12.10)	0.51	1.27 (0.23–6.98)	0.78	1.38 (0.25–7.60)	0.71
Height	0.98 (0.90–1.07)	0.62	1.01 (0.93–1.10)	0.83	1.00 (0.93–1.08)	0.96
ARD	1.19 (1.03–1.36)	0.02	1.22 (1.00–1.49)	0.048	1.26 (1.04–1.53)	0.02
LA dimension	0.99 (0.91–1.07)	0.75	0.98 (0.86–1.12)	0.78	1.00 (0.88–1.12)	0.94
Hypertension	0.40 (0.12–1.37)	0.15	0.44 (0.14–1.34)	0.15	0.40 (0.13–1.24)	0.11
Diabetes mellitus	0.70 (0.07–7.23)	0.77	0.60 (0.06–5.69)	0.66	0.61 (0.06–5.86)	0.67
Hyperlipidemia	0.44 (0.10–2.02)	0.29	0.51 (0.13–2.05)	0.34	0.48 (0.12–1.95)	0.30
Former or current smoking	1.97 (0.34–11.46)	0.45	1.65 (0.33–8.26)	0.54	1.90 (0.39–9.28)	0.43
History of stroke or CAD*	0.34 (0.05–2.29)	0.27	0.41 (0.07–2.37)	0.32	0.38 (0.06–2.32)	0.29

*Patients with ischemic stroke, transient ischemic attack, or coronary artery disease (angina pectoris or myocardial infarction) were included.
BSA: body surface area; OR: odds ratio; CI: confidence interval; CAD: coronary artery disease; ARD: aortic root dimension; LA: left atrial.

Relationship between height and other variables

The initial unadjusted data indicated that patients in the eccentric group were taller than those in the non-eccentric group, but the difference was not significant after adjustment for age and other factors. The relationship between height and eccentricity was reversed when the analysis was restricted to patients aged <55 years, however this relationship was not statistically significant and no relationship was found when using indexed data. Owing to the unclear relationship between height and eccentricity, further analysis to find an association between height and IA was conducted. Correlation analysis showed that age, sex, weight, ARD, smoking status, and size and number of aneurysms were correlated with height ($P \leq 0.001$, except for the number of aneurysms, $P = 0.003$). Linear regression with all these variables showed that age, sex, weight, and aneurysm size were independently associated with height (Table 3). Height and aneurysm size were negatively correlated, and patients with a large aneurysm tended to congregate in the low-height group (Figure 2).

Discussion

In this study, we tried to identify a pathological interrelationship between intracranial arteries and the ascending aorta in patients with IA. The tunica media of both arteries have a common embryological origin (neural crest cells) and a similar structure of cross-linked elastin and collagen [4], [11], [29–32], but data supporting a pathological relationship between diseases involving the two structures is limited [12], [13]. Moreover, these studies involved patients with rare disease conditions. Some genetic variation associated with both IA and aortic aneurysm has been reported [19], but investigations under routine clinical practice are lacking. Here, we assessed for a pathogenic link between the two diseases by evaluating ARD without restriction to specific disorders.

The age distribution of the study population was bimodal. Although old age and known risk factors for IA may have some contribution to the older-age peak, the younger-age peak suggests that other mechanisms operate. Intrinsic arterial wall defects could affect aneurysm formation, growth, and rupture, leading to early detection. However, there are several factors that affect the age distribution. Patients with multiple risk factors at middle and advanced age tend to have further diagnostic evaluation including angiography. Moreover, patients who underwent screening brain imaging in midlife might contribute to the bimodal age distribution, considering that most IAs are asymptomatic. The markedly high prevalence of IA among patients aged 50–54 years in our data supports this possibility. However, this age distribution likely indicates that a significant number of IAs form before age 55 or before vascular risk factors sufficiently affect IA generation.

ARD tends to increase with age and height [22]. However, we found that the ARD in the eccentric group was significantly larger than that in the non-eccentric group, despite the younger age of the former. Subgroup analysis intended to eliminate the effect of the age distribution difference reconfirm this difference. The large ARD in the eccentric group may have been affected by height; however, multivariable analysis confirmed that the association between large ARD and eccentricity was independent of height,

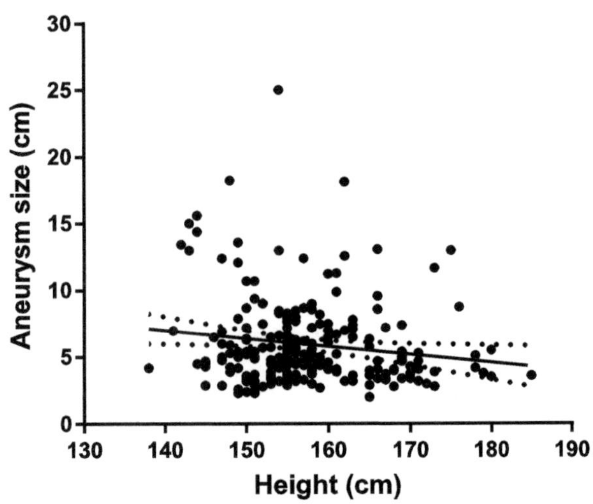

Figure 2. Scatter plot of aneurysm size versus height. Aneurysm size tended to decrease with increasing height. The fitted regression line for the association is shown as a solid line with the 95% confidence intervals shown as dotted lines ($R^2 = 0.046$).

Table 2. Subgroup analysis of patients aged <55 years.

	Using absolute echocardiographic measurement		Indexed to BSA		Indexed to height	
	OR (95% CI)	*P* value	OR (95% CI)	*P* value	OR (95% CI)	*P* value
Hypertension	0.16 (0.04–0.58)	0.005	0.162 (0.04–0.60)	0.006	0.18 (0.05–0.62)	0.007
ARD	1.18 (1.02–1.37)	0.03	1.39 (1.05–1.85)	0.02	1.31 (1.03–1.66)	0.03
Height	0.93 (0.86–1.00)	0.06	-		-	

OR: odds ratio; CI: confidence interval; ARD: aortic root dimension.

and subgroup analysis with absolute values of echocardiographic markers, but not with indexed values, even showed a trend toward short stature in the eccentric group. Furthermore, HTN, known to be associated with an increase in ARD, was more related to non-eccentricity in the subgroup analysis. The difference was independent of aortic valve pathology (BAV, aortic stenosis and aortic regurgitation).

A previous study by Curtis et al. [33] showed that fewer patients with both CoA and IA had BAV or ascending aortopathy than patients with CoA and without IA. However, the difference was not statistically significant ($P = 0.36$), was not adjusted for other factors, and have different demographics. Another study by Schievink et al. [12] found no relationship between thoracic aortic dilatation and the presence of IA in a bicuspid valve group. But only 6 of patients with BAV had IA in this subgroup analysis. More to the point, we focused on the eccentricity, not the presence, of IA and its relationship with ARD. The above-mentioned studies only consider the presence of IA and do not specifically consider the nature of IA in their analysis. Considering the pathophysiological heterogeneity in IA, we hypothesized that a certain group, not all, of IA patients have concomitant aortopathy and defined the eccentric group as accordingly.

A plausible explanation for the link between IA and ascending aortic pathology is neurocristopathy arising from the embryonic neural crest. The neural crest is a key structure in the vertebrate embryo and plays a major role in the development of head structures, the aortic arch and cervicocephalic arteries, skin melanocytes, much of the peripheral nervous system, some endocrine cells, and various other structures [29–32]. Combinations of BAV, CoA, aortic root dilatation, aortic and cervical arterial dissection, and histologically, cystic medial wall degeneration are considered as phenotypes of neurocristopathy because the aortic valve, the medial wall of the aortic arch, and the cervicocephalic arteries derive from neural crest cells [11], [29–31], and abnormal development of these cells can result in vascular fragility [31]. Neural crest cells make smooth muscle cells and pericytes in the medial wall of intracranial arteries [32]. Phenotypic modulations of vascular smooth cells in the medial layer disrupt the structural integrity of the vessel walls and contribute to IA formation [4]. There are also anecdotal reports of an association between IA and Parry-Romberg syndrome [14], [15] and congenital heart diseases [16], suggesting neurocristopathy as a common factor. A higher detection rate of IA in neurofibromatosis type 1, a neurocristopathy spectrum disease, was reported in a case-control study [17]. Southerland et al. recently suggested that the association between IA, Moyamoya disease, fibromuscular dysplasia, and cervical dissection, which share common pathological features of transformation of smooth muscle cells and degraded elastic laminae [18], is reminiscent of neurocristopathy. These studies, taken together with our findings on the relationship between IA and ARD, imply that some intrinsic intracranial arterial wall defects may also affect the ascending aorta, and, conclusively, could be regarded as one part of neurocristopathy.

Other echocardiographic values analyzed in our study support this perspective. During cardiogenesis, neural crest cells play a role in aorticopulmonary septation and aortic valve and left ventricular outflow tract development [29–31] but are apparently not involved in the formation of the atrial chambers and most of the ventricular wall structures, which are derived mainly from cardiac mesenchyme [30]. Unlike ARD, LVPWd, IVSd, and LA dimension did not differ significantly between the two groups. The differential contributions of these echocardiographic measurements to eccentricity support the different embryological origins of these structures.

Recent genetic evidence supports the implication of neurocristopathy in IA. A genome-wide association study identified several loci variants associated with IA; specifically, single-nucleotide polymorphisms in chromosome 9p21.3 are associated with various arterial disorders including CAD and aortic aneurysm [19]. Underexpression of ANRIL, a large noncoding RNA in the 9p21.3 locus, seems to mediate neural crest-derived tumors

Table 3. Results of multiple linear regression analysis of association between height and other variables.

	β± SE	*P* value
Age	−0.10±0.03	0.002
Female	−10.83±0.79	<0.001
Weight	0.21±0.04	<0.001
Aneurysm size	−0.29±0.10	0.004

Stepwise selection method was used for multiple regression analysis. Body surface area and body mass index were excluded from the model owing to their multicollinearity with weight.
β: non-standardized regression coefficient; SE: standard error.

including melanomas and plexiform neurofibroma [34–36] along with IA and CAD [19], [34–36]. A recent ablation study that revealed the heterogeneous origin of coronary artery smooth muscle cells also investigated the role of endothelin receptor type-A (EDNRA) in craniofacial and cardiovascular development from neural crest cells [37]. An association between IA and single-nucleotide polymorphisms in or near the EDNRA gene [19–21] also supports our concept. Taken together, the results of genetic, embryological, and clinical studies suggest that neurocristopathy is a unifying pathogenesis of these seemingly unrelated disorders, but additional studies are required to solidify the involvement of neural crest in the disorders.

In our study, patients with large aneurysms tended to be short, which provides additional evidence of systemic or developmental involvement in IA. Neural crest cells differentiate into bone and cartilage and into thyroid parafollicular cells, which secrete calcitonin, and can affect the development of the adenohypophysis, which produces growth-related hormones [29], [38]. Neurofibromatosis type 1 is a representative disorder in which neurocristopathy can accompany short stature and osteoporosis [39]. However, in our study, the height difference between the eccentric and non-eccentric groups was not statistically significant, and other developmental and systemic diseases may affect both IA and height. Further investigation is needed to explain this phenomenon.

Cardiovascular risk factors were more prevalent in our cohort than in the general population, owing to retrospective inclusion of subjects with available echocardiography data. Known racial/ethnic differences in IA phenotype also limit generalization of our result to other ethnic populations. The possibility of undiagnosed monogenic connective tissue diseases should be considered as well because these were retrospectively excluded from the analysis. Lastly, the small sample size and the use of only one marker, ARD, for aortopathy are another limitation of this study. A population-based study and the use of other markers of aortic pathology would be needed to validate the findings.

ARD, a novel indicator for a shared pathogenesis of IA and aortopathy, and embryological implication as neurocristopathy sheds a new light on future work to understand the pathophysiology of IAs. Additional intrinsic properties of IA should be characterized for better diagnosis and treatment of IA.

Supporting Information

Table S1 Demographic and clinical features of the study population.

Table S2 P-values for other echocardiographic markers.

Table S3 Results of multivariable logistic regression analysis of determinants of eccentricity in coiled patients.

Author Contributions

Conceived and designed the experiments: YWS KHJ. Performed the experiments: YWS KHJ JMK YDC MHH. Analyzed the data: YWS KHJ JMK YDC STL KC MK SKL JKR MHH. Contributed reagents/materials/analysis tools: STL KC MK SKL JKR. Wrote the paper: YWS KHJ.

References

1. Vlak MH, Algra A, Brandenburg R, Rinkel GJ (2011) Prevalence of unruptured intracranial aneurysms, with emphasis on sex, age, comorbidity, country, and time period: a systematic review and meta-analysis. Lancet Neurol 10: 626–636.
2. Rinkel GJ, Djibuti M, Algra A, van Gijn J (1998) Prevalence and risk of rupture of intracranial aneurysms: a systematic review. Stroke 29: 251–256.
3. Rinkel GJ, Algra A (2011) Long-term outcomes of patients with aneurysmal subarachnoid haemorrhage. Lancet Neurol 10: 349–356.
4. Chalouhi N, Ali MS, Jabbour PM, Tjoumakaris SI, Gonzalez LF, et al. (2012) Biology of intracranial aneurysms: role of inflammation. J Cereb Blood Flow Metab 32: 1659–1676.
5. Meng H, Tutino VM, Xiang J, Siddiqui A (2013) High WSS or Low WSS? Complex Interactions of Hemodynamics with Intracranial Aneurysm Initiation, Growth, and Rupture: Toward a Unifying Hypothesis. AJNR Am J Neuroradiol. Published Online First: 4 July 2013. doi: 10.3174/ajnr.A3558.
6. Nguyen TV, Chandrashekar K, Qin Z, Parent AD, Zhang J (2009) Epidemiology of intracranial aneurysms of Mississippi: a 10-year (1997–2007) retrospective study. J Stroke Cerebrovasc Dis 18: 374–380.
7. Rinne J, Hernesniemi J, Puranen M, Saari T (1994) Multiple intracranial aneurysms in a defined population: prospective angiographic and clinical study. Neurosurgery 35: 803–808.
8. Nehls DG, Flom RA, Carter LP, Spetzler RF (1985) Multiple intracranial aneurysms: determining the site of rupture. J Neurosurg 63: 342–348.
9. Campos C, Churojana A, Rodesch G, Alvarez H, Lasjaunias P (1998) Multiple Intracranial Arterial Aneurysms: A Congenital Metameric Disease? Review of 113 Consecutive Patients with 280 AA. Interv Neuroradiol 4: 293–299.
10. Casimiro MV, McEvoy AW, Watkins LD, Kitchen ND (2004) A comparison of risk factors in the etiology of mirror and nonmirror multiple intracranial aneurysms. Surg Neurol 61: 541–545.
11. Schievink WI, Mokri B (1995) Familial aorto-cervicocephalic arterial dissections and congenitally bicuspid aortic valve. Stroke 26: 1935–1940.
12. Schievink WI, Raissi SS, Maya MM, Velebir A (2010) Screening for intracranial aneurysms in patients with bicuspid aortic valve. Neurology 74: 1430–1433.
13. Connolly HM, Huston J, 3rd, Brown RD, Jr., Warnes CA, Ammash NM, et al. (2003) Intracranial aneurysms in patients with coarctation of the aorta: a prospective magnetic resonance angiographic study of 100 patients. Mayo Clin Proc 78: 1491–1499.
14. Pichiecchio A, Uggetti C, Grazia Egitto M, Zappoli F (2002) Parry-Romberg syndrome with migraine and intracranial aneurysm. Neurology 59: 606–608.
15. Schievink WI, Mellinger JF, Atkinson JL (1996) Progressive intracranial aneurysmal disease in a child with progressive hemifacial atrophy (Parry-Romberg disease): case report. Neurosurgery 38: 1237–1241.
16. Schievink WI, Mokri B, Piepgras DG, Gittenberger-de Groot AC (1996) Intracranial aneurysms and cervicocephalic arterial dissections associated with congenital heart disease. Neurosurgery 39: 685–689.
17. Schievink WI, Riedinger M, Maya MM (2005) Frequency of incidental intracranial aneurysms in neurofibromatosis type 1. Am J Med Genet A 134A: 45–48.
18. Southerland AM, Meschia JF, Worrall BB (2013) Shared associations of nonatherosclerotic, large-vessel, cerebrovascular arteriopathies: considering intracranial aneurysms, cervical artery dissection, moyamoya disease and fibromuscular dysplasia. Curr Opin Neurol 26: 13–28.
19. Alg VS, Sofat R, Houlden H, Werring DJ (2013) Genetic risk factors for intracranial aneurysms: a meta-analysis in more than 116,000 individuals. Neurology 80: 2154–2165.
20. Yasuno K, Bakircioglu M, Low SK, Bilguvar K, Gaal E, et al. (2011) Common variant near the endothelin receptor type A (EDNRA) gene is associated with intracranial aneurysm risk. Proc Natl Acad Sci U S A 108: 19707–19712.
21. Low SK, Takahashi A, Cha PC, Zembutsu H, Kamatani N, et al. (2012) Genome-wide association study for intracranial aneurysm in the Japanese population identifies three candidate susceptible loci and a functional genetic variant at EDNRA. Hum Mol Genet 21: 2102–2110.
22. Vasan RS, Larson MG, Levy D (1995) Determinants of echocardiographic aortic root size. The Framingham Heart Study. Circulation 91: 734–740.
23. Lee BC, Roh JK, Korean Stroke R (2006) International experience in stroke registries: Korean Stroke Registry. Am J Prev Med 31: S243–245.
24. American Diabetes A (2010) Diagnosis and classification of diabetes mellitus. Diabetes Care 33 Suppl 1: S62–69.
25. Mosteller RD (1987) Simplified calculation of body-surface area. N Engl J Med 317: 1098.
26. Lang RM, Bierig M, Devereux RB, Flachskampf FA, Foster E, et al. (2005) Recommendations for chamber quantification: a report from the American Society of Echocardiography's Guidelines and Standards Committee and the Chamber Quantification Writing Group, developed in conjunction with the European Association of Echocardiography, a branch of the European Society of Cardiology. J Am Soc Echocardiogr 18: 1440–1463.

27. Investigators UJ, Morita A, Kirino T, Hashi K, Aoki N, et al. (2012) The natural course of unruptured cerebral aneurysms in a Japanese cohort. N Engl J Med 366: 2474–2482.
28. Wiebers DO, Whisnant JP, Huston J, 3rd, Meissner I, Brown RD, Jr., et al. (2003) Unruptured intracranial aneurysms: natural history, clinical outcome, and risks of surgical and endovascular treatment. Lancet 362: 103–110.
29. Dupin E, Sommer L (2012) Neural crest progenitors and stem cells: from early development to adulthood. Dev Biol 366: 83–95.
30. Noden DM, Poelmann RE, Gittenberger-de Groot AC (1995) Cell origins and tissue boundaries during outflow tract development. Trends Cardiovasc Med 5: 69–75.
31. Rosenquist TH, Beall AC, Modis L, Fishman R (1990) Impaired elastic matrix development in the great arteries after ablation of the cardiac neural crest. Anat Rec 226: 347–359.
32. Etchevers HC, Vincent C, Le Douarin NM, Couly GF (2001) The cephalic neural crest provides pericytes and smooth muscle cells to all blood vessels of the face and forebrain. Development 128: 1059–1068.
33. Curtis SL, Bradley M, Wilde P, Aw J, Chakrabarti S, et al. (2012) Results of screening for intracranial aneurysms in patients with coarctation of the aorta. AJNR Am J Neuroradiol 33: 1182–1186.
34. Pasmant E, Sabbagh A, Masliah-Planchon J, Ortonne N, Laurendeau I, et al. (2011) Role of noncoding RNA ANRIL in genesis of plexiform neurofibromas in neurofibromatosis type 1. J Natl Cancer Inst 103: 1713–1722.
35. Bishop DT, Demenais F, Iles MM, Harland M, Taylor JC, et al. (2009) Genome-wide association study identifies three loci associated with melanoma risk. Nat Genet 41: 920–925.
36. Cunnington MS, Santibanez Koref M, Mayosi BM, Burn J, Keavney B (2010) Chromosome 9p21 SNPs Associated with Multiple Disease Phenotypes Correlate with ANRIL Expression. PLoS Genet 6: e1000899.
37. Arima Y, Miyagawa-Tomita S, Maeda K, Asai R, Seya D, et al. (2012) Preotic neural crest cells contribute to coronary artery smooth muscle involving endothelin signalling. Nat Commun 3: 1267.
38. Etchevers HC, Vincent C, Couly G (2001) Neural crest and pituitary development. In: Rappaport R, Amselem S, editors. Hypothalamic–Pituitary Development: Genetic and Clinical Aspects. Basel: Karger. pp. 13–29.
39. Elefteriou F, Kolanczyk M, Schindeler A, Viskochil DH, Hock JM, et al. (2009) Skeletal abnormalities in neurofibromatosis type 1: approaches to therapeutic options. Am J Med Genet A 149A: 2327–2338.

13

Association of Serum Periostin with Cardiac Function and Short-Term Prognosis in Acute Myocardial Infarction Patients

Lin Ling[1], Yan Cheng[2], Liucheng Ding[3], Xiangjun Yang[1]*

1 Department of Cardiology, the First Affiliated Hospital of Soochow University, Suzhou, China, 2 Department of Cardiology, The Affiliated Wuxi People's Hospital of Nanjing Medical University, Wuxi, China, 3 The Second Affiliated Hospital of Nanjing Medical University, Nanjing, China

Abstract

Background: Periostin was proved to play an important role in extra-cellular matrix remodeling after acute myocardial infarction (AMI). Myocardial periostin was markedly up-regulated after AMI and participated in the maladaptive process of cardiac remodeling. However, few researches focused on the circulating periostin and its significance. This study aims to investigate the association of serum periostin level with cardiac function and short-term prognosis in AMI patients.

Methodology/Principal Findings: We totally recruited 50 patients diagnosed as ST-elevation myocardial infarction. Blood samples were taken within 12 hours after the onset of AMI before emergency coronary revascularization procedures. Serum periostin was measured using enzyme-linked immunosorbent assay. All patients received echocardiography examination within one week after hospitalization. Correlations of serum periostin with echocardiography parameters, Killip class and myocardium injury biomarkers (CK-MB/troponin T) were investigated. AMI patients were divided into two groups by serum periostin level (higher/lower periostin group) and followed up for six months. Primary endpoints included cardiovascular mortality, nonfatal stroke/transient ischemic attack, chest pain occurrence and re-hospitalization. Secondary endpoint referred to composite cardiovascular events including all the primary endpoints.

Result: Serum periostin was in negative association with left ventricular ejection fraction (LVEF) ($r = -0.472$, $*p<0.01$) and left atrium diameter (LAD) ($r = -0.328$, $*p<0.05$). Positive correlation was found between serum periostin level and Killip class ($r = 0.395$, $*p<0.01$). There was no association between serum periostin and CK-MB or troponin T ($p>0.05$). After six months follow up, patients in higher periostin group showed increased composite cardiovascular events ($*p<0.05$). Patients showed no significant difference in primary endpoints between the two groups.

Conclusions/Significance: Serum periostin was in negative correlation with LVEF and LAD, in positive association with Killip class and higher serum periostin level may be predictive for worse short-term disease prognosis indicated as more composite cardiovascular events six months post AMI.

Editor: Tianqing Peng, University of Western Ontario, Canada

Funding: This work was supported by the Youth Science and Technology of Suzhou Science and Education Project, Grant No. KJXW2013004. The funders had no role in study design, data collection and analysis, decision to publish, or preparation of the manuscript.

Competing Interests: The authors have declared that no competing interests exist.

* E-mail: xiangjun_yang@126.com

Introduction

Acute myocardial infarction (AMI) remains as a worldwide public health problem with an increasing rate of incidence and causes irreversible cardiomyocytes impairment [1]. Ventricular remodeling due to persistent ischemia and hypoxia after myocardial infarction leads to the development of heart failure [2]. The interaction between myocytes and myocardial fibroblasts in the extra-cellular matrix (ECM) was proved to play a critical role in all stages of cardiac remodeling and subsequent heart failure. Activation of myocardial fibroblasts through both stretch-related signaling and neuron-endocrine effectors led to the secretion of various ECM proteins. These proteins conducted molecular signals, regulated cell kinetics and finally altered the structure of extra-cellular matrix [3,4].

Periostin was a 90-kDa extra-cellular matrix protein secreted by fibroblasts, which acted as an important regulator in ventricular remodeling process such as pathological hypertrophy or fibrosis after myocardial injury. Periostin was proved to be related closely to the onset and development of coronary artery disease [5,6]. Elevated expression of periostin protein was found in the infracted myocardium of AMI rat [7]. Exogenously over-expression of periostin gene in the heart led to impaired cardiac function, including left ventricle dilation, cardiac myocytes decrease and collagen deposition increase, which suggested a correlation between elevated periostin with deteriorated cardiac function. Furthermore, inhibition the expression of periostin was able to improve cardiac systolic ejection function and animal survival rate [8]. These researches demonstrated a detrimental effect of periostin in cardiovascular system. However, other researches have drawn opposite conclusions about the effect of periostin on myocardium remodeling. Dennis Ladage et al found that delivery of periostin peptide into the pericardial space of MI swine exerted beneficial effects on myocardium repair, reducing infarct myocardium size, attenuating left ventricular systolic function and increasing capillary density post MI. Another research group demonstrated that periostin was able to induce reentry of differentiated mammalian cardiomyocytes into the cell cycle both *in vitro* and *in vivo*. Delivery of recombinant periostin into the heart of MI rat improved cardiac systolic function, reduced fibrosis and hypertrophy as well as enhanced myocardium repair [9–10].

Although the net effect of periostin on ventricular remodeling after acute myocardial infarction has not reached a consensus, there is no doubt that this molecule acts as an important regulator in this process. Myocardial periostin was significantly up-regulated after AMI and participated actively in cardiac remodeling. However, few researches focused on the change in circulating periostin after AMI. This study was designed to investigate the association of serum periostin level with cardiac function and short term disease prognosis in acute myocardial infarction patients. Our study found that serum periostin was in negative association with left ventricular ejection fraction and left atrium diameter as well as in positive association with Killip class in acute myocardial infarction patients. Higher serum periostin level was related to increased composite cardiovascular events after six months follow up post AMI.

Materials and Methods

Ethics Statement

Clinical researches were approved by the Ethics Review Board for Clinical Studies of the First Affiliated Hospital of Soochow University (Suzhou, China, Approval Number: SZC10582). All clinical studies confirmed to ethics guidelines of the 1975 Declaration of Helsinki. All patients were informed with and signed written consent of this study. We did not conduct research outside of our country of residence.

Study Subjects

We totally enrolled 50 patients of acute myocardial infarction (ST elevation) in our study. All patients were in consistent with the following diagnostic standards for ST elevated acute myocardial infarction: i Clinical history of ischemic type chest pain; ii ECG changes. New ST elevation at the J point in at least 2 contiguous leads of 0.2 mV in men or 0.15 mV in women in leads V2–V3 and/or of 0.1 mV in other contiguous chest leads or the limb leads; New or presumably new left-bundle branch block; iii Evidence of myocardial injury or necrosis indicated by elevated serum cardiac biomarker, especially troponin T (Clinical Practice Guidelines on Management of STEMI, 2013). All patients received coronary revascularization procedures and standard drug therapy for coronary artery disease after hospitalization. Basic clinical characteristics including gender, age, coronary heart disease history, hypertension history, diabetes history, smoking history were collected and fasting blood sample were taken for measurement of glucose, cholesterol, high-density lipoprotein cholesterol (HDLc), low-density lipoprotein cholesterol (LDLc), triglyceride and renal function. Blood sample for periostin and myocardial injury biomarkers evaluation was taken within 12 hours after the onset of AMI before emergent coronary revascularization procedures. All blood tests were performed in the hospital's laboratory.

Determination of Serum Periostin Level

Serum periostin was measured using the DuoSet® ELISA kits (R&D Systems) according to manufacture's instructions. Briefly, plates were coated with 100 μl of capture antibody and incubated overnight. After blocking with PBS containing 1%BSA overnight, 100 μl of diluted serum samples or recombinant periostin standards at different concentrations were added and incubated for 2 h at 37°C. Then 100 μl of detection antibody was incubated for 2 h at 37°C and streptavidin-HRP for 20 min. Plate washing were performed with 400 μl of washing buffer (0.05% Tween-20 in PBS) after every incubation for at least three times. Wells were incubated with 100 μl substrate solution for 20 min and stopped by adding 50 μl stop solution (2 N H_2SO_4). The optical density was measured at 450 nm and 570 nm using a micro-plate reader (Bio-Rad Laboratories, CA, USA) and the absorbance at 570 nm was subtracted from the absorbance at 450 nm. Each experiment was performed in duplicate wells and averaged for statistical analysis.

Evaluation of Patients Cardiac Function

Trans-thoracic echocardiography was performed to assess cardiac function of acute myocardial infarction patients. All patients finished echocardiography examination within one week after hospitalization. A trained echo-cardiologist blinded to the experiment performed all the measurements with GE Vivid 7 system (GE Health Care, Netherlands). Left ventricular M-mode spectrum was performed in standard parasternal long-axis view to measure LV diameter at end cardiac diastole (LVDd) and systole (LVDs). The Teicholz method was used to calculate left-ventricular volumes and left-ventricular ejection fraction. Index including left ventricular posterior wall thickness (LVPWT), inter-ventricular septal thickness at diastole (IVSTd), left atrial diameter (LAD) and aorta dimension (AoD) were measured. All measurements were repeated for three consecutive pulsation cycles and averaged for statistical analysis.

Patients Follow up Visit

Patients involved in this study were followed up for major cardiovascular events six months after the onset of acute myocardial infarction. We set primary and secondary clinical endpoints for evaluation of major cardiovascular events. Primary endpoints included cardiovascular mortality, nonfatal stroke or transient ischemic attack, typical chest pain occurrence and re-hospitalization due to unstable angina pectoris, re-infarction or heart failure. Cardiovascular mortality was defined as death due to fatal myocardial infarction, coronary intervention procedure, congestive heart failure, stroke, sudden cardiac death or other cardiovascular causes. Secondary endpoint was defined as composite cardiovascular events including all the four primary endpoints.

Statistical Analysis

All continuous variables were expressed as mean ± SD. Comparisons between two groups were performed with unpaired Student's t-test and comparisons among three or more groups were assessed by one-way ANOVA with Dunnett's post-test. Categorical variables were expressed as percentages. Chi-square test was used for comparisons of categorical variables. Spearman correlation was used to analyze the relationship between serum periostin level and other parameters. A p value of <0.05 (two-tailed) was considered significance. All analyses were performed using SPSS 17.0 software (SPSS, Inc.).

The authors have full access to the data and take responsibility for its integrity. All authors have read and agreed to the manuscript as written.

Results

Correlation of Periostin Level with Clinical Characteristics in AMI Patients

The average age of patients was 63.30±12.78 years. AMI patients showed an average serum periositn level of 203.35±16.90 ng/ml. We analyzed the relationships of serum periostin level with patients' clinical characteristics by spearman correlation. Baseline characteristics including gender, CHD history, hypertension, diabetes mellitus, smoking history, age, heart rate, triglyceride, cholesterol, HDLc, LDLc, venous glucose, creatinine and blood urea nitrogen (BUN) showed no correlations with serum periostin level (Table 1).

Association of Periostin Level with Coronary/ Echocardiography Parameters and Myocardium Injury Biomarkers in AMI Patients

Coronary and echocardiography parameters as well as myocardium injury biomarkers were assessed in AMI patients and their relationship with serum periostin level were analyzed. Number of diseased coronary vessels or implanted stents showed no correlation with periostin level. Among the echocardiography parameters, serum periostin was in negative correlation with left ventricular ejection fraction (r = −0.472, $p<0.01$) and left atrium diameter (r = −0.328, $p<0.05$) (Figure 1 A–B). Furthermore, serum periostin was in positive correlation with Killip class after AMI (r = 0.395, $p<0.01$) (Figure 1C). Patients classified as Killip I showed lower serum periostin level compared with those classified as Killip class III or higher ($p<0.05$). Correlation of periostin with coronary and echocardiography parameters was shown in Table 2. We also measured myocardial injury biomarkers in AMI patients. Serum troponin T and CK-MB showed good correlation with each other (r = 0.728, $p<0.01$) but neither of them showed significant correlation with serum periositn (Figure 2). Detailed parameters of echocardiography were presented in Table S1.

Patients with Higher Periostin Level Showed more Composite Cardiovascular Events after Six Months Follow up

In order to assess the effect of serum periositn on short-term prognosis, we followed up patients for major cardiovascular events six months after the onset of AMI. All patients were divided into two groups based on median periostin level (188 ng/ml), named as higher periostin group (N = 25) and lower periostin group (N = 25).

Table 1. Relationship between Clinical Characteristics and Serum Periostin Level in AMI Patients.

Parameters	Periostin (ng/ml) or Pearson correlation coefficient	P value
Categorical variables		
Gender		
Male	200.55±18.72	0.783
Female	211.33±38.56	
CHD history		
+	146.97±45.33	0.501
−	205.70±17.48	
Hypertension		
+	185.31±16.11	0.138
−	238.37±38.08	
Diabetes mellitus		
+	217.86±20.77	0.489
−	193.68±24.66	
Smoking		
+	197.41±25.69	0.768
−	207.65±22.78	
Continuous variables	r	
Age (yr)	−0.138	0.341
Heart Rate (bmp)	0.109	0.450
Triglycerid (mmol/L)	0.031	0.829
Cholesterol (mmol/L)	0.043	0.769
HDLc (mmol/L)	−0.190	0.186
LDLc (mmol/L)	0.126	0.382
Glucose (mmol/L)	0.124	0.393
Creatinine (umol/L)	−0.021	0.882
BUN (umol/L)	−0.186	0.195

All determinations were performed in the fasting state. CHD: coronary heart disease; HDLc: high density lipoprotein cholesterol; LDLc: low density lipoprotein cholesterol; BUN: blood urea nitrogen; Date presented as mean±SD; Spearman correlation was used to analyze the relationship between periostin level and variables.

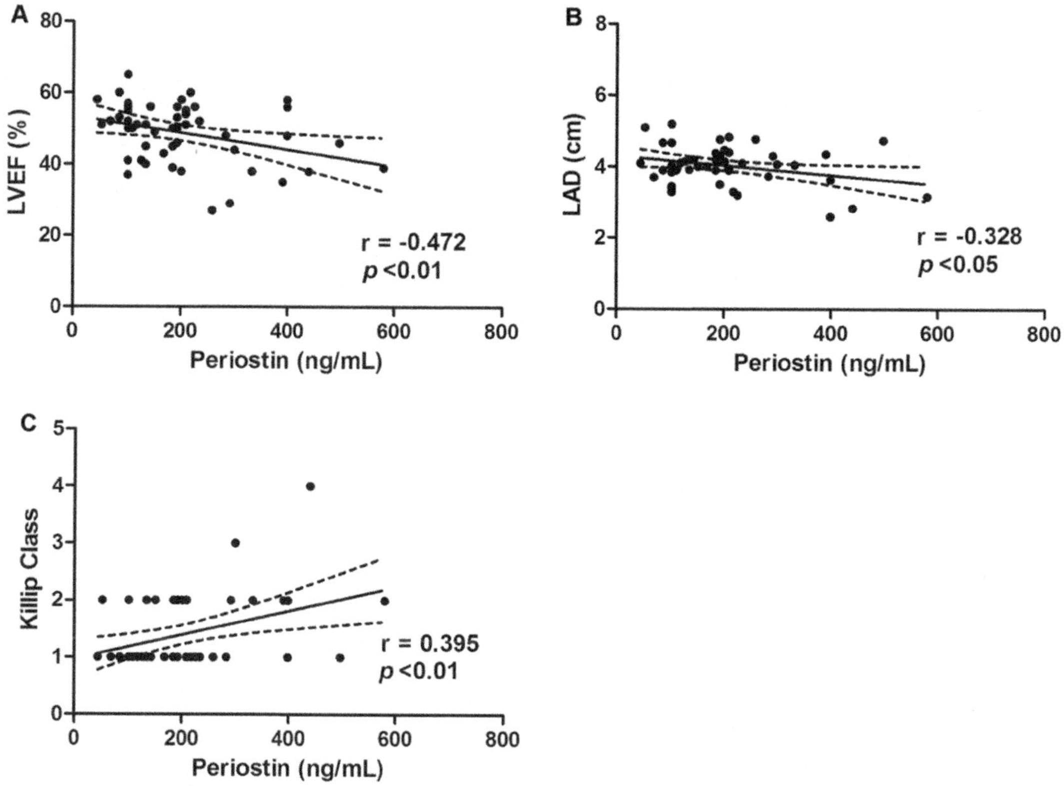

Figure 1. Association of periostin level with echocardiography parameters and Killip class. (A) Serum periostin level was in negative correlation with left ventricle ejection fraction in AMI patients ($r = -0.472$, $p<0.01$). (B) Serum periostin level was in negative correlation with left atrium diameter in AMI patients ($r = -0.328$, $p<0.05$). (C) Serum periostin level was in positive correlation with Killip class in AMI patients ($r = 0.395$, $p<0.01$).

Basic clinical characteristics including gender, age, hypertension, diabetes, smoking history, blood glucose, cholesterol, HDLc, LDLc, triglyceride and renal function showed no difference between the two groups (Table 3). There was no difference in primary endpoints including cardiovascular mortality, nonfatal stroke or transient ischemic attacks, chest pain occurrence and re-hospitalization between the two groups. Patients with higher serum periostin showed increased composite cardiovascular events after six months follow up ($p<0.05$, Table 4). The net effect of perisotin on six month cardiovascular outcomes post-AMI was shown in Figure 3.

Discussion

Acute myocardial infarction is one of the lethal diseases in the world, with an increasing morbidity and threatens the public

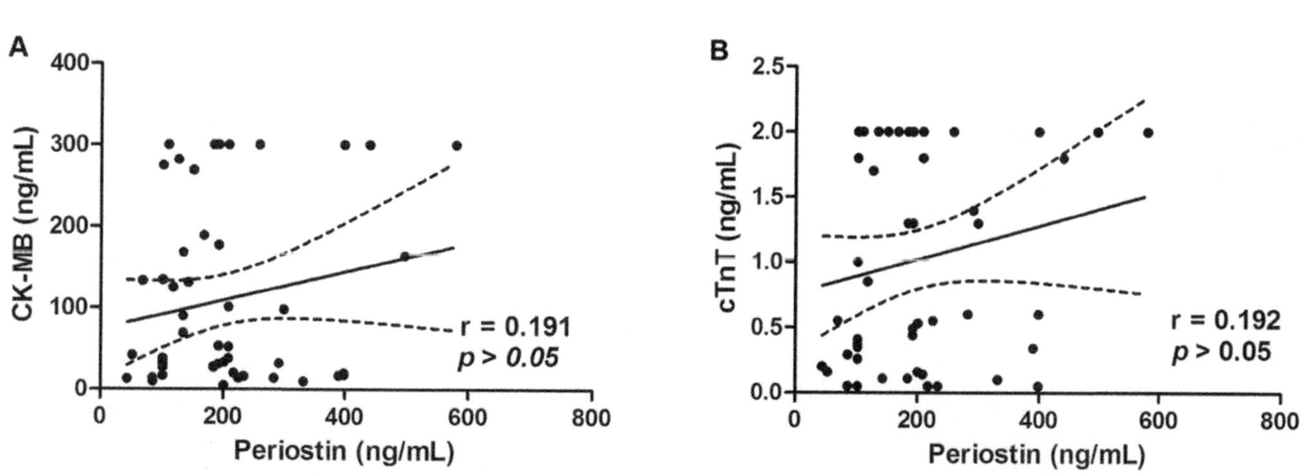

Figure 2. Serum periostin showed no correlation with myocardium injury biomarkers CK-MB (A) ($r = 0.191$, $p>0.05$) or Troponin T (B) ($r = 0.192$, $p>0.05$) in AMI patients.

Table 2. Correlation of Periostin with Coronary/Echocardiography Parameters after AMI.

Parameters	Periostin (ng/ml) or Pearson correlation coefficient	P value
Number of Stents		
0 (n = 7)	173.47±35.64	0.947
1 (n = 23)	208.43±24.83	
2 (n = 12)	218.41±41.35	
3 (n = 5)	198.90±35.78	
CABG (n = 3)	181.32±109.80	
Number of Coronary Artery with Stenosis		
1 (n = 15)	196.15±34.74	0.552
2 (n = 17)	228.67±25.09	
≥3 (n = 18)	185.44±29.03	
Killip Class		
1	175.82±17.67	0.024*
2	241.76±35.05	
≥3	369.52±70.06	
Echocardiography parameters	r	
LVEF	−0.472	0.002*
LVDd	−0.163	0.285
LVPWT	−0.092	0.550
IVSTd	0.090	0.557
LAD	−0.328	0.028*
AoD	−0.114	0.456

LVEF: left ventricular systolic ejection fraction; LVDd: left ventricular end diastolic diameter; LVPWT: left ventricular posterior wall thickness; IVSTd: inter-ventricular septal thickness in diastole; LAD: left atrium diameter; AoD: aorta dimension. Date presented as mean±SD; Spearman correlation was used to analyze the relationship between periostin level and variables. *$p<0.05$.

health. The local ischemia and hypoxia conditions after AMI caused irreversible cardiomyocytes death or apoptosis and these cardiomyotes were gradually replaced by interstitial fibrosis through ventricular remodeling process. As scar and fibrosis structure lacked the ability of contractility and electric activity, systolic function and electric coupling of the heart were impaired and these finally led to deteriorated cardiac function [11,12]. Activated fibroblasts in the extra-cellular matrix secreted various ECM proteins that contributed to ventricular remodeling after AMI. Through binding to targeted receptors and conducting cell signaling, these proteins played an important role in regulation of

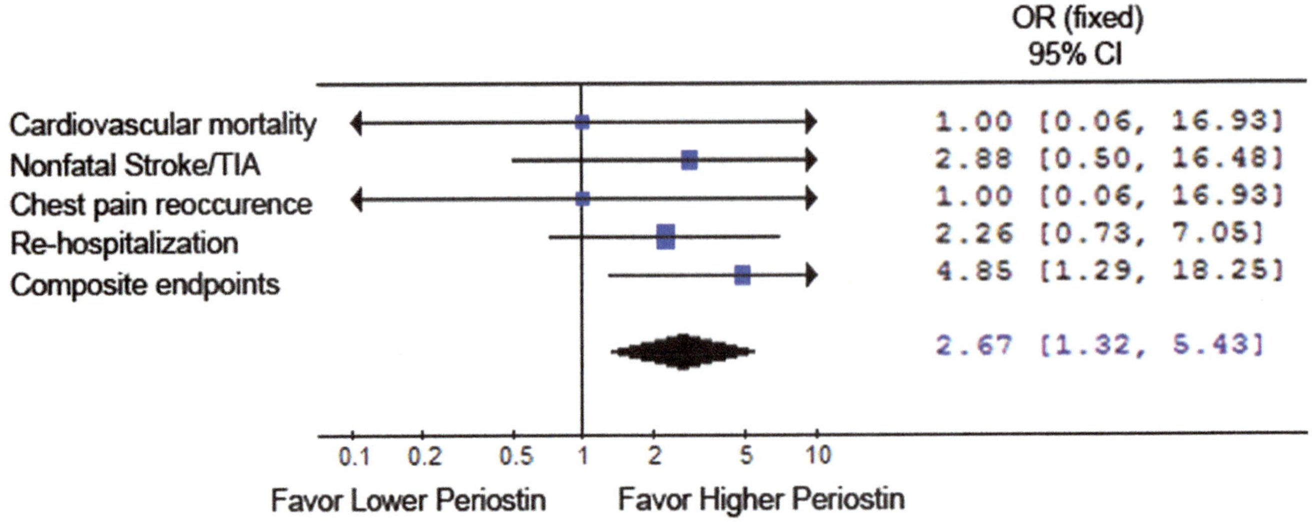

Figure 3. Effect of serum periostin on cardiovascular outcomes six months post AMI.

Table 3. Clinical Characteristics of AMI Patients at follow up.

Basic characteristics	Higher Periostin group	Low Periostin group	P value
N	25	25	–
Age (year)	64.2±12.02	62.4±13.69	0.624
Male (%)	80%	68%	0.333
Hypertension (%)	56%	76%	0.136
Diabetes mellitus (%)	36%	44%	0.546
Smoking (%)	52%	36%	0.254
Drugs	–	–	–
Aspirin	100%	100%	–
Clopidogrel	100%	100%	–
ACEI or ARB	100%	100%	–
Statins	100%	100%	–
triglyceride (mmol/L)	1.91±1.22	1.53±1.02	0.246
cholesterol (mmol/L)	4.58±1.07	4.14±0.97	0.139
HDLc (mmol/L)	0.87±0.2	0.98±0.41	0.230
LDLc (mmol/L)	2.50±0.76	2.08±0.79	0.065
Glucose (mmol/L)	7.21±3.13	6.96±2.41	0.751
Cr (umol/L)	67.79±15.75	71.14±22.26	0.542
BUN (umol/L)	6.01±1.71	6.46±2.21	0.414

All determinations were performed in the fasting state.
ACEI: Angiotensin-converting enzyme inhibitor; ARB: Angiotensin II receptor antagonists; HDLc: high density lipoprotein cholesterol; LDLc: low density lipoprotein cholesterol; Cr: creatinine; BUN: blood urea nitrogen.
Date presented as mean±SD.

cardiomyoctes kinetics such as proliferation, migration and apoptosis [13–17].

Periostin is an extra-cellular protein proved to play an important role in cardiovascular development and disease [18]. Periostin is expressed at very early stages of embryogenesis but is not detectable in the normal adult heart. However, after cardiac injury such as myocardial infarction, pump failure or pressure overload, the mRNA and protein expression of periostin were greatly elevated in the heart [19]. Periostin showed close relationship with pressure overload induced maladaptive left ventricular hypertrophy, which was highly associated with end-stage heart failure [20]. In periostin knockout mice, cardiac healing after AMI was impaired and more cardiac ruptures were found. Smaller and less abundant collagen was also seen in periostin knockout mice, suggesting impaired collagen fibril formation in the lack of periostin gene [21]. Periostin over-expressed mensechymal stem cells implantation into the myocardium after AMI led to significantly histological and functional improvement, including decreased infarct size, reduced apoptotic myocardial cells and increased micro vessel density, indicating a cardio-protective role of periostin combined with stem cell transplantation [22]. Gene polymorphisms analysis in Chinese population showed that rs3829365 of the periostin gene was associated with susceptibility to, and severity of heart failure, suggesting a role of periostin in disease prediction and severity assessment [23]. Acute myocardial infarction patients showed decreased circulating level of periostin compared with control volunteers and periostin level was in negative correlation with patients' cardiac function three months after AMI [24]. All these studies demonstrated that periostin acted as an important factor in the process of extracellular matrix remodeling under cardiac adverse conditions such as damage and pressure overload.

This study investigated the association of serum periostin level with cardiac function, coronary situation, biomarkers and clinical characteristics in acute myocardial infarction patients. The six month prognosis was also assessed. We found that serum periostin level was in negative association with left ventricular ejection fraction and left atrium diameter, in positive correlation with Killip class and showed no relationship with serum CK-MB or troponin T. Patients with higher serum periostin level exhibited increased composite cardiovascular events after six months follow up.

In our study, serum periositn level showed negative correlation with LVEF, suggesting that patients with lower left systolic function had higher circulating periostin level. Killip class represented left ventricular failure degree in the acute period after AMI. Serum periositn level was in positive correlation with Killip class. This was in consistent with the results of periostin and LVEF, suggesting a relationship of higher periostin level with worse left ventricular function. CK-MB and troponin T are well documented serum biomarkers for myocardial infarction and reflected myocardium injury [25]. We found no correlation between serum periositn and these two biomarkers, indicating that periositn was less likely an index related to myocardial injury. Whether higher circulating periostin level led to lower systolic function or resulted from worse heart function was not known. A lot of researches focused on the direct effect of periostin on cardiomyocytes and myocardium but had not reached a similar conclusion yet. Some showed that periostin was able to induce cardiomyocytes proliferation *in vitro* and acted as a cardio-protective factor [9]. Others found that over expression of periostin did not stimulate DNA synthesis, mitosis, or cytokinesis of cardiomyocytes in vitro or in vivo [26]. The actual effect of

Table 4. Cardiovascular Events of AMI Patients after Six Months Follow Up.

Cardiovascular Events	Higher Periostin group (N = 25)	Lower Periostin group (N = 25)	P value
Primary endpoints			
-Cardiovascular mortality	1	1	1.0
-Nonfatal Stroke/TIA	5	2	0.337
-Chest pain occurrence	14	9	0.156
-Re-hospitalization	1	1	1.0
Secondary endpoints			
-Composite endpoints	21	13	0.015*

TIA: transient ischemic attack; *$p<0.05$.

periostin, no matter it is protective, detrimental or neutral needs further confirmation.

According to our results, we concluded that periostin showed good correlation with cardiac systolic function and short term prognosis in ST elevation acute myocardial infarction patients. Higher serum periostin level was associated with worse left ventricular function and deteriorated short term prognosis. In the present study, we visited patients for six months and this was a relatively short period for myocardial infarction patients. Long term observation for cardiovascular major events and clinical prognosis would be needed in the further study. Our present study enrolled myocardial infarction patients with ST elevation and did not include non-ST elevation myocardial infarction patients or unstable angina patients. As these patients shared the similar pathological process as unstable plaque, the serum periostin level in these patients would better be analyzed in further experiments.

Supporting Information

Table S1 Echocardiography Parameters of AMI Patients. LVEF: left ventricular systolic ejection fraction; LVDd: left ventricular end diastolic diameter; LVPWT: left ventricular posterior wall thickness; IVSTd: inter-ventricular septal thickness in diastole; LAD: left atrium diameter; AoD: aorta dimension. Date presented as mean±SD.

Author Contributions

Conceived and designed the experiments: LL XY. Performed the experiments: LL YC LD. Analyzed the data: LL YC LD XY. Wrote the paper: LL XY.

References

1. Ho KK, Anderson KM, Kannel WB, Grossman W, Levy D (1993) Survival after the onset of congestive heart failure in Framingham Heart Study subjects. Circulation 88(1): 107–115.
2. Go AS, Mozaffarian D, Roger VL, Benjamin EJ, Berry JD, et al. (2013) Heart disease and stroke statistics–2013 update: a report from the American Heart Association. Circulation 127(1): e6–e245.
3. Snider P, Hinton RB, Moreno-Rodriguez RA, Wang J, Rogers R, et al. (2008) Periostin is required for maturation and extracellular matrix stabilization of noncardiomyocyte lineages of the heart. Circ Res 102(7): 752–760.
4. Oka T, Xu J, Kaiser RA, Melendez J, Hambleton M, et al. (2007) Genetic Manipulation of Periostin Expression Reveals a Role in Cardiac Hypertrophy and Ventricular Remodeling. Circ Res 101: 313–321.
5. Dorn GW (2007) Periostin and myocardial repair, regeneration, and recovery. N Engl J Med 357(15): 1552–1554.
6. Wang D, Oparil S, Feng JA, Li P, Perry G, et al. (2003) Effects of pressure overload on extracellular matrix expression in the heart of the atrial natriuretic peptide-null mouse. Hypertension 42(1): 88–95.
7. Iekushi K, Taniyama Y, Azuma J, Katsuragi N, Dosaka N, et al. (2007) Novel mechanisms of valsartan on the treatment of acute myocardial infarction through inhibition of the antiadhesion molecule periostin. Hypertension 49(6): 1409–1414.
8. Katsuragi N, Morishita R, Nakamura N, Ochiai T, Taniyama Y, et al. (2004) Periostin as a novel factor responsible for ventricular dilation. Circulation 110: 1806–1813.
9. Kuhn B, del Monte F, Hajjar RJ, Chang YS, Lebeche D, et al. (2007) Periostin induces proliferation of differentiated cardiomyocytes and promotes cardiac repair. Nat Med 13(8): 962–969.
10. Ladage D, Yaniz-Galende E, Rapti K, Ishikawa K, Tilemann L, et al. (2013) Stimulating myocardial regeneration with periostin Peptide in large mammals improves function post-myocardial infarction but increases myocardial fibrosis. PLoS One 8(5): e59656.
11. Jin J, Wang H, Song YM, Li AM, Qin J, et al. (2010) Clinical outcome and left ventricular remodeling in AMI patients with insufficient myocardial reperfusion after recanalization. Clin Invest Med 33(5): E304–312.
12. Taniguchi N, Nakamura T, Sawada T, Matsubara K, Furukawa K, et al. (2010) Erythropoietin prevention trial of coronary restenosis and cardiac remodeling after ST-elevated acute myocardial infarction (EPOC-AMI): a pilot, randomized, placebo-controlled study. Circ J 74(11): 2365–2371.
13. Chatila K, Ren G, Xia Y, Huebener P, Bujak M, et al. (2007) The role of the thrombospondins in healing myocardial infarcts. Cardiovasc Hematol Agents Med Chem 5(1): 21–27.
14. Dobaczewski M, Gonzalez-Quesada C, Frangogiannis NG (2010) The extracellular matrix as a modulator of the inflammatory and reparative response following myocardial infarction. J Mol Cell Cardiol 48(3): 504–511.
15. Okamoto H, Imanaka-Yoshida K (2012) Matricellular proteins: new molecular targets to prevent heart failure. Cardiovasc Ther 30(4): e198–209.
16. Schellings MW, Pinto YM, Heymans S (2004) Matricellular proteins in the heart: possible role during stress and remodeling. Cardiovasc Res 64(1): 24–31.
17. Jugdutt BI, Palaniyappan A, Uwiera RR, Idikio H (2009) Role of healing specific matricellular proteins and matrix metalloproteinases in age-related enhanced early remodeling after reperfused STEMI in dogs. Mol Cell Biochem 322(1–2): 25–36.
18. Litvin J, Zhu S, Norris R, Markwald R (2005) Periostin family of proteins: therapeutic targets for heart disease. Anat Rec A Discov Mol Cell Evol Biol 287(2): 1205–1212.
19. Roy R, Brodarac A, Kukucka M, Kurtz A, Becher PM, et al. (2013) Cardioprotection by placenta-derived stromal cells in a murine myocardial infarction model. J Surg Res 185(1): 70–83.
20. Stansfield WE, Andersen NM, Tang RH, Selzman CH (2009) Periostin is a novel factor in cardiac remodeling after experimental and clinical unloading of the failing heart. Ann Thorac Surg 88(6): 1916–1921.
21. Shimazaki M, Nakamura K, Kii I, Kashima T, Amizuka N, et al. (2008) Periostin is essential for cardiac healing after acute myocardial infarction. J Exp Med 205(2): 295–303.
22. Cho YH, Cha MJ, Song BW, Kim IK, Song H, et al. (2012) Enhancement of MSC adhesion and therapeutic efficiency in ischemic heart using lentivirus delivery with periostin. Biomaterials 33(5): 1376–1385.
23. Wang F, Song Y, Jiang Y, Yang C, Ding Z (2011) Associations among periostin gene polymorphisms, clinical parameters and heart failure: a case-control study in 1104 Chinese individuals. J Cardiovasc Med (Hagerstown) 12(7): 469–474.
24. Cheng CW, Wang CH, Lee JF, Kuo LT, Cherng WJ (2012) Levels of blood periostin decrease after acute myocardial infarction and are negatively associated with ventricular function after 3 months. J Investig Med 60(2): 523–528.
25. O'Gara PT, Kushner FG, Ascheim DD, Casey Jr DE, Chung MK, et al. (2013) 2013 ACCF/AHA guideline for the management of ST-elevation myocardial infarction: executive summary: a report of the American College of Cardiology

Foundation/American Heart Association Task Force on Practice Guidelines. J Am Coll Cardiol 61(4): 485–510.

26. Lorts A, Schwanekamp JA, Elrod JW, Sargent MA, Molkentin JD (2009) Genetic manipulation of periostin expression in the heart does not affect myocyte content, cell cycle activity, or cardiac repair. Circ Res 104(1): e1–7.

14

Characteristics of Myocardial Postsystolic Shortening in Patients with Symptomatic Hypertrophic Obstructive Cardiomyopathy before and Half a Year after Alcohol Septal Ablation Assessed by Speckle Tracking Echocardiography

Jiansong Yuan[1]ᵍ, Shi Chen[2]ᵍ, Shubin Qiao[1]*, Fujian Duan[3], Jiafen Zhang[3], Hao Wang[3]

1 Department of Cardiology, State Key Laboratory of Cardiovascular Disease, Fuwai Hospital, National Center for Cardiovascular Disease, Peking Union Medical College and Chinese Academy of Medical Sciences, Beijing, China, **2** Department of Cardiology, West China Hospital, Sichuan University, Chengdu, Sichuan, China, **3** Department of Echocardiography, State Key Laboratory of Cardiovascular Disease, Fuwai Hospital, National Center for Cardiovascular Disease, Peking Union Medical College and Chinese Academy of Medical Sciences, Beijing, China

Abstract

Objectives: Postsystolic shortening (PSS) has been proposed as a marker of myocardial dysfunction. Percutaneous transluminal septal myocardial ablation (PTSMA) is an alternative therapy for patients with hypertrophic obstructive cardiomyopathy (HOCM) that results in sustained improvements in atrial structure and function. We investigated the effects of PTSMA on PSS in HOCM patients using speckle tracking imaging.

Methods: Conventional echocardiographic and PSS parameters were obtained in 18 healthy controls and 30 HOCM patients before and half a year after PTSMA.

Results: Compared with the healthy controls, the number of segments having PSS and the average value of PSS were significantly increased in the HOCM patients. At 6 months after PTSMA, both the number of segments having PSS (10.5 ± 2.8 vs. 13.2 ± 2.6; $P<0.001$) and the average value of PSS (-1.24 ± 0.57 vs. -1.55 ± 0.56; $P=0.009$) were significantly reduced. Moreover, the reductions in the average value of PSS correlated well with the reductions in the E-to-Ea ratio ($r=0.705$, $P<0.001$).

Conclusions: Both the number of segments having PSS and the average value of PSS were significantly increased in the HOCM patients. PTSMA has a favourable effect on PSS, which may partly account for the persistent improvement in LV diastolic function in HOCM patients after PTSMA.

Editor: Yiru Guo, University of Louisville, United States of America

Funding: The authors have no support or funding to report.

Competing Interests: The authors have declared that no competing interests exist.

* E-mail: yuanjs100@sina.com

ᵍ These authors contributed equally to this work.

Introduction

Postsystolic shortening (PSS) is considered myocardial shortening after the point of aortic valve closure, which has been known for years. PSS is found in one-third of normal myocardium [1]; however, it is increased by different cardiovascular diseases [2–4]. The presence and degree of PSS has been found to be associated with severe cardiac abnormalities [5]. PSS has been suggested as a marker of myocardial ischemia and fibrosis [6–7]. A previous study observed that patients with hypertrophic cardiomyopathy (HCM) had more PSS than normal controls [4]. Percutaneous transluminal septal myocardial ablation (PTSMA) is an alternative type of therapy for patients with hypertrophic obstructive cardiomyopathy (HOCM) that may result in the long-term improvement of symptoms and partly reverse myocardial ischemia and fibrosis [8–11]. However, it is unclear whether PTSMA can decrease PSS in HOCM patients. Speckle tracking echocardiography (STE) is a novel ultrasonic technique, which can be used for measuring myocardium deformation during the cardiac cycle and is well suited for the quantification of PSS. This study was designed to quantitatively analyse and compare myocardial longitudinal PSS by STE in HOCM patients before and half a year after PTSMA to determine the effect of PTSMA on PSS.

Methods

This study was reviewed and proved by the Ethics Committee of Beijing Fuwai Hospital. Written informed consents were obtained from all patients and control subjects.

Study population

The study population consisted of 38 patients with symptomatic obstructive HCM (HOCM) who were referred for PTSMA to our centre between May 2012 and December 2012. However, 5 patients underwent surgical myectomy and mitral-valve replacement, and 3 patients failed to return for the follow-up examination. The final cohort included 30 patients. The diagnoses of HCM were obtained by means of 2-dimensional echocardiography in patients with interventricular septal thicknesses ≥1.5 cm who had no other causes attributed to their left ventricular (LV) hypertrophy. The selection criteria for PTSMA were as follows: the persistence of symptoms despite being administered the maximum tolerated dosage of medication; a left ventricular outflow tract (LVOT) gradient >50 mmHg at rest or > 100 mmHg after provocation; accessible septal branches, particularly of the left anterior descending coronary artery; the absence of a significant intrinsic abnormality of the mitral valve; and other conditions for which cardiac surgery was indicated. PTSMA were performed as previously described [12–13]. PTSMA success was defined as an improvement in the New York Heart Association (NYHA) class and a reduction in the LVOT pressure gradient of 50% of the baseline. Eighteen age- and gender-matched healthy controls were included from the subjects who visited our hospital for annual routine medical examinations.

Echocardiography

Each subject underwent an echocardiographic evaluation using a commercially available echocardiographic scanner (IE33, Philips Medical Systems, Best, Netherlands) that was equipped with an S5-1 transducer (frequency transmitted, 1.7 MHz; frequency received, 3.4 MHz) before and half a year after the PTSMA procedure. One lead electrocardiogram was recorded continuously. A 2-dimensionally guided M-mode echocardiography was performed to measure the thicknesses of the interventricular septum and left ventricular posterior wall (LVPW). The wall thickness was measured at the level of the mitral valve and papillary muscles in each of the four myocardial segments and at the apical level in the anterior and posterior segments using parasternal short-axis views. The maximum LV wall thickness was defined as the greatest thickness in any single segment. The left ventricular ejection fraction (LVEF) and the left atrial end-systolic volume (LAV) were calculated using a modified Simpson's biplane method in the apical 4- and 2-chamber views. The maximal early and late diastolic inflow velocities (E and A waves), E-to-A ratio, and deceleration time (DT) of the E wave were obtained using a pulsed wave Doppler. The sample volume was placed immediately below the level of the mitral leaflet tips in the apical 4-chamber view. The LV outflow tract (LVOT) gradient was measured using a continuous-wave Doppler in the apical 5-chamber view. The TDI of the mitral annulus movement was performed using the apical 4-chamber view. A 1.5-mm sample volume was placed at the lateral side of mitral annular. The velocity of mitral annular was measured in early diastole (Ea) and with atrial contraction (Aa). Analyses of the isovolumic relaxation time (IVRT) were performed.

Strain Data Acquisition and Analysis

Three cardiac cycles were recorded in apical 4-, 2-, and 3-chamber views using grey-scale acquisition at a frame rate over 80 s^{-1}. The off-line longitudinal strain data analysis was performed with QLAB 6.0 software (Philips Medical Systems, Andover, Massachusetts, USA). Eighteen segments from 6 LV walls were assessed, namely, the basal, mid, and apical segments for the inferior and anterior septum, and the anterior, anterolateral, inferolateral and inferior wall. The peak negative systolic strain was recorded to assess segmental myocardial systolic function. PSS was defined as the segmental shortening in the diastole beyond the minimum systolic segment length (the peak negative strain in the diastole minus the peak negative strain in the systole). If the minimum segment length was within the systole, PSS was set to zero (Figure 1). The average values of PSS from all 18 segments were then calculated and were considered to be the global PSS.

The reproducibility of measurements of PSS was assessed by inter- and intra-observer agreement. Intra-observer agreement was determined by having one observer repeating the measurements of these variables in all 30 patients. Inter-observer agreement was determined by having a second observer measuring these variables in the same patients. We used the Cohen kappa coefficient to determine inter- and intra-observer agreement of the presence of PSS in different myocardial segments. Spearman, coefficient was performed to assess inter- and intra-observer agreement of average value of PSS in each subjects.

Statistical analyses

The data are presented as the mean±SD for the continuous variables or as percentages for the categorical variables. The clinical characteristics were compared using the *t*-test for the continuous variables and the chi-square test for the categorical variables. The correlations between changes in the number of myocardial segments with PSS and average values of PSS and the improvement of the E/Ea ratio at half a year after the PTSMA procedure were examined using the Pearson's test. All probability values were for 2-tailed tests. A value of $P<0.05$ was considered indicative of a statistically significant result. Data processing and statistical analyses were performed using SPSS 17.0 software (SPSS, Chicago, IL, USA).

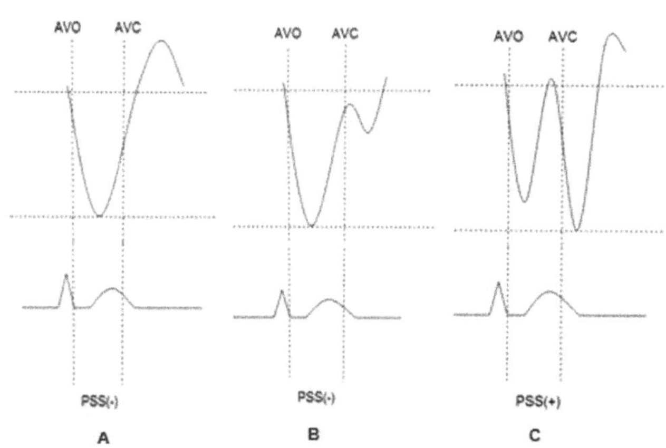

Figure 1. Strain curves during cardiac cycle with (C) and without (A,B) postsystolic shortening (PSS). AVO, timing of aortic valve opening; AVC, timing of aortic valve closure.

Results

The basic clinical characteristics of the HOCM patients and healthy controls are summarised in Table 1. There were no significant differences between the two groups in terms of age, gender, height, weight, heart rate, systolic blood pressure or diastolic blood pressure. Most of the patients experienced severe symptoms of heart failure. The mean NYHA functional class was 2.7±0.3, and 73.3% of the patients were in the NYHA functional class III despite optimal medical therapy that consisted of beta-blockers in 23 (76.7%) patients and calcium-channel blockers in 7 (26.7%) patients. Because of serious side effects or contraindications, 3 patients received neither beta-blockers nor calcium-channel blockers.

The conventional echocardiographic parameters in HOCM patients before PTSMA and the control group are shown in Table 2. According to disease characteristics, patients with HOCM exhibited higher LVEF, greater LAV, and thicker LV walls for both the ventricular septum and the posterior wall. The mean baseline resting LVOT gradient for the HOCM patients was 92.4±32.2 mmHg. All of the HOCM patients had abnormal diastolic function before the PTSMA procedure. The transmitral E-wave velocities, A-wave velocities and E/A ratios were similar between the two groups, whereas the DT and IVRT were significantly prolonged in patients with HOCM. The TDI parameters from the lateral mitral annulus showed that the early diastolic peak velocities were significantly lower in HOCM patients. Additionally, the E/Ea ratio in HOCM patients was more than twice as high in healthy controls.

Figure 2 shows the comparison of the number of myocardial segments having PSS and the average value of PSS between the two groups. As shown, patients with HOCM had a greater number of segments with PSS and greater PSS values than healthy controls(13.20±2.62 vs 5.74±2.05,P<0.001; −1.55±0.57 vs −1.05±0.64,P = 0.012). In HOCM patients group, the inter- and intra-observer agreement is very high in both the presence of PSS in different myocardial segments (Kappa = 0.911,p< 0.001;Kappa = 0.831,p<0.001) and the average value of PSS(r = 0.871,p<0.001;r = 0.810,p<0.001).

During the ablation procedure, the mean amount of alcohol that was injected was 2.37±0.90 ml. Right-bundle branch blocks occurred at a rate of 36.7% (11 patients). Transitory trifascicular blocks occurred at a rate of 23.3% (7 patients). No patient underwent a permanent pacemaker implantation following the procedure. There was no peri-interventional mortality during the observational period.

Changes in the conventional echocardiographic parameters in the patients with HOCM at half a year following the PTSMA procedure are shown in Table 2. Patients exhibited an obvious decrease in the LVOT gradient. The PTSMA produced a significant reduction in the interventricular septal thickness. The left ventricular posterior wall also decreased in size, but this change was not statistically significance. The left atrial volume indexed to body surface area was significantly reduced following PTSMA at half a year. There were no significant changes in the E-wave velocity, A-wave velocity, or the E/A ratio. However, the reduction in DT and IVRT were indicative of the amelioration of the LV diastolic dysfunction. Similar trends in the DTI parameters of the diastolic function were also observed. There was an obvious increase in the Ea velocities, resulting in a significant reduction in the E-to-Ea ratio.

As shown in Figures 3, 4 and 5, both the number of myocardial segments having PSS and the average value of PSS were significantly reduced(13.20±2.62 vs 10.53±2.83,P<0.001; −1.55±0.57 vs −1.24±0.57,P = 0.009). In addition, a significant correlation between the reduction of the average value of PSS and the reduction of the E-to-Ea ratio was observed (r = 0.705, P< 0.001; Figure 5).

Table 1. Clinical characteristics of study participants.

	Control subjects (n = 18)	HOCM patients (n = 30)	P value
Age,(years)	43.4±11.5	45.6±11.2	0.532
Male, *n* (%)	13 (72.2)	20 (66.7)	0.757
Height,(cm)	166.9±5.5	167.3±5.7	0.833
Weight,(kg)	64.4±8.4	69.3±9.8	0.084
Family history of hypertrophic cardiomyopathy, *n* (%)	0 (0)	5 (16.7)	—
Previous syncope, *n* (%)	0 (0)	8 (26.7)	—
Previous dyspnea, *n* (%)	0 (0)	20 (64.5)	—
Heart rate, (bpm)	69.1±7.2	69.8±9.4	0.781
SBP, (mmHg)	118.7±6.5	113.3±14.4	0.083
DBP, (mmHg)	70.8±5.6	71.5±9.6	0.783
NYHA classes	—	2.7±0.4	—
β-blocker	0 (0)	23(76.7)	—
Ca channel blocker	0 (0)	8 (26.7)	—

HOCM, hypertrophic obstructive cardiomyopathy; HR, heart rate; SBP, systolic blood pressure; DBP, diastolic blood pressure; NYHA, New York Heart Association.

Table 2. Conventional echocardiographic characteristics of healthy controls and HOCM patients at baseline and half a year after PTSMA.

Characteristics	Healthy controls (n = 18)	HOCM patients at baseline (n = 30)	P value*	HOCM patients half a year after PTSMA (n = 30)	P value&
Septum thickness (mm)	8.5±1.1	21.3±5.7	<0.001	18.9±6.2	0.122
LVPW thickness (mm)	8.7±1.5	12.9±3.4	<0.001	12.4±3.2	0.580
maxLVT (mm)	—	23.6±4.9	—	21.1±5.9	0.080
LAV index (ml/m^2)	19.1±3.4	44.7±10.7	<0.001	35.3±11.1	<0.001
LVEF (%)	63.9±5.5	74.8±8.4	<0.001	74.1±6.0	0.712
LVOT gradient (mmHg)	—	92.4±32.2	—	27.2±17.6	<0.001
Mitral E velocity (cm/s)	80.7±15.9	84.2±23.8	0.582	86.4±20.8	0.711
Mitral A velocity (cm/s)	65.8±21.8	83.0±37.4	0.083	90.8±33.9	0.401
E/A ratio	1.4±0.5	1.2±0.5	0.224	1.1±0.5	0.589
DT (ms)	175.2±8.0	231.1±46.4	<0.001	193.3±18.7	<0.001
IVRT (ms)	76.5±7.0	122.5±22.5	<0.001	100Ð 9±18.1	<0.001
Lateral Ea (cm/s)	12.2±4.0	5.5±1.6	<0.001	7.1±1.3	<0.001
Lateral Aa (cm/s)	8.5±2.4	7.9±1.7	0.322	8.1±1.8	0.723
E/Ea ratio	7.2±2.4	16.3±6.5	<0.001	12.5±4.2	<0.001

*, P value of comparing between control subjects and HOCM patients at baseline; &, P value of comparing between HOCM patients at baseline and HOCM patients at half a year after PTSMA; HOCM, hypertrophic obstructive cardiomyopathy; LVPW, left ventricular posterior wall; maxLVT,maximal left ventricular thickness;LAV, left atrial volume; LVEF, left ventricular ejection fraction; LVOT, left ventricular outflow tract; DT, E deceleration time; IVRT, isovolumic relaxation time.

Discussion

Our study provides unprecedented data regarding the PSS parameters in HOCM patients before and half a year after a PTSMA procedure. We found that compared with healthy controls, both the number of myocardial segments having PSS and the average value of PSS were significantly increased in the HOCM patients. At half a year following PTSMA, both parameters of PSS were significantly improved. Moreover, the reduction of the average value of PSS in the patients was significantly correlated with the reduction of the E-to-Ea ratio.

In 1986, Bertha and colleagues observed myocardial segments shorting after the point of the aortic valve closure into the early diastole using the sonomicrometry technique; they named the phenomenon "postsystolic shortening" [14]. Subsequent studies demonstrated that PSS is a nonspecific feature that occurs in both healthy hearts and in different heart diseases [2–4]. However, PSS is observed more frequently and with greater amplitude in the ischemia myocardium than in a normal myocardial [3]. Previous studies showed that PSS could distinguish the ischemia myocardial and reflect the severity of myocardial ischemia [8–11]. Myocardial fibrosis is another major reason for an increasing PSS. Plaksej and colleagues observed that with the progression of NYHA functional

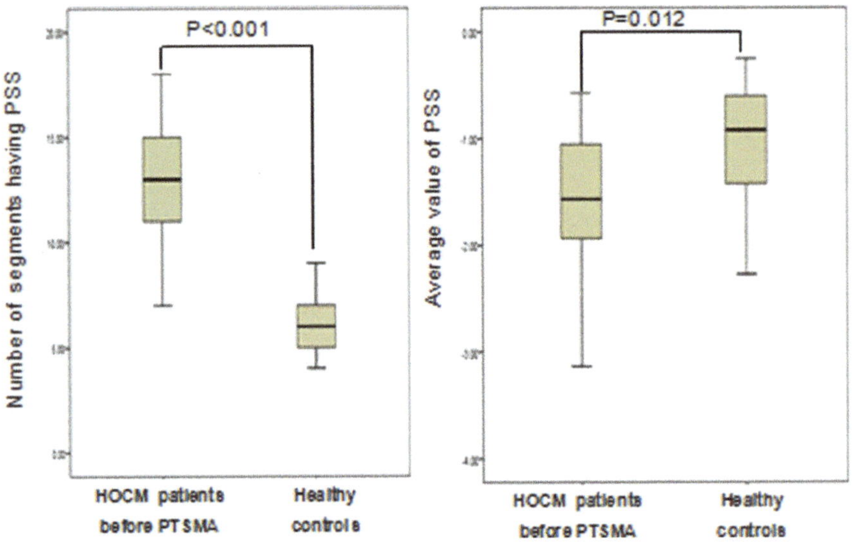

Figure 2. Comparison of the number of segments having PSS (left) and the average value of PSS (right) between obstructive hypertrophic cardiomyopathy (HOCM) patients before septal ablation and healthy controls. PTSMA, percutaneous transluminal septal myocardial ablation.

classes in heart failure patients, the concentration of circulating markers of myocardial fibrosis increased and the PSS index also increased [15]. Tsai further found that in hypertension patients, increased serum procollagen type I carboxyterminal propeptide (PICP), which is considered a circulating maker for myocardial fibrosis, was correlated with increased PSS [16]. Currently, a precise explanation for the association between myocardial fibrosis and PSS is difficult. However, previous studies found that myocardial fibrosis can hinder the unfolding of the left ventricle [17] and delay the myocardial relaxation that may partly contribute to the delayed myocardial shortening into the early diastole.

Hypertrophic cardiomyopathy (HCM) is a genetically transmitted myocardial disease characterised by varying degrees of myocardial hypertrophy. Microvascular dysfunction, characterised by a blunted vasodilator reserve in the absence of an epicardial coronary stenosis, is very common in patients with HCM [18–19]. It is mostly a result of the intimal and medial hyperplasia of the

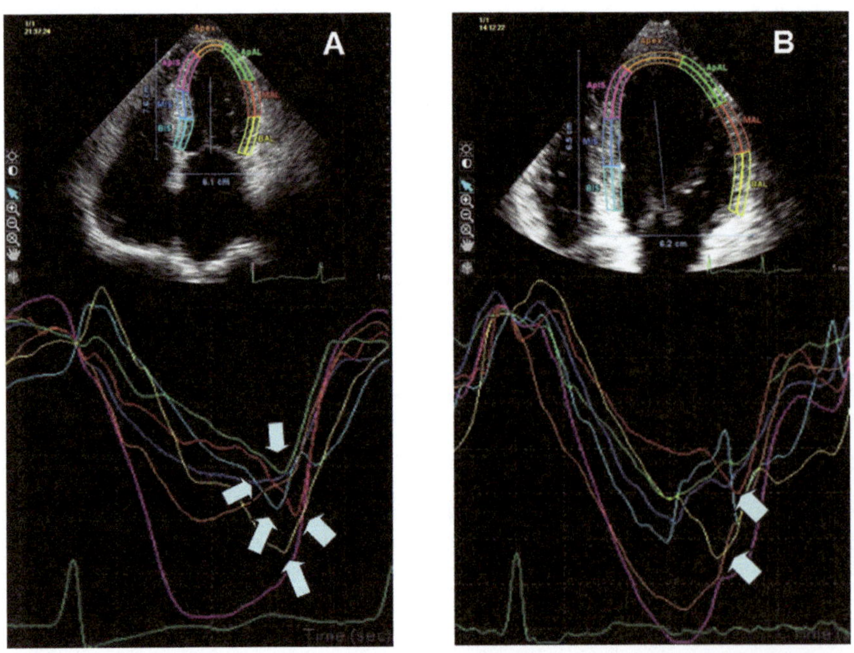

Figure 3. Strain curves from the apical 4-chamber view at baseline (A) and half a year after successful septal ablation (B) in a HOCM patient. The number of segments having PSS was significantly reduced at half a year after PTSMA. ***Arrows,*** Strain curves showing postsystolic shortening (PSS).

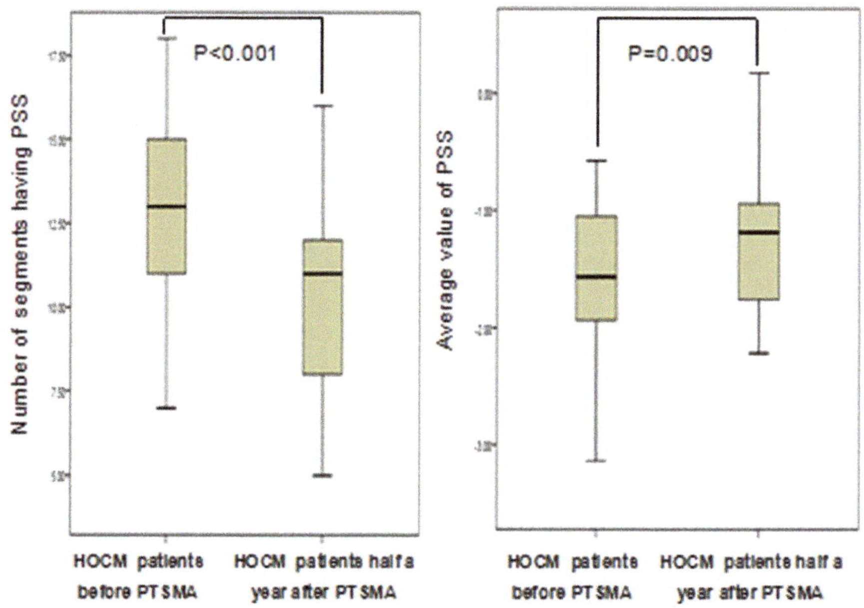

Figure 4. Comparison of the number of segments having PSS (left) and the average value of PSS (right) between HOCM patients before and half a year after septal ablation.

intramural coronary arteries and subsequent lumen reduction [20]. Extravascular compression following hypertrophy of the LV wall and the elevated LV end-diastolic pressure is another major reason [21]. Microvascular dysfunction, in turn, can lead to myocardial ischemia because of hypoperfusion in the corresponding area. Myocardial fibrosis is a prominent pathological feature of HCM. Myocardial fibrosis is closely related with the symptoms in HCM patients and is an independent marker of an unfavourable prognosis in this disease [22–23]. Thus, it is reasonable to consider whether PSS increases in patients with HCM. However, few studies have focused on PSS in HCM patients. In 2003, Stoylen described PSS in a patient with apical HCM in a case study [24]. In 2006, Ito and colleagues investigated PSS in 30 HCM patients

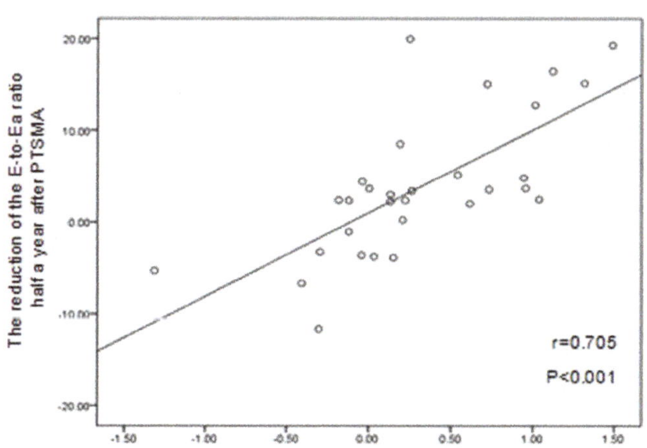

Figure 5. The relationship between the reductions in the average value of PSS and the changes in the E-to-Ea ratio in HOCM patients at half a year after a PTSMA procedure.

and 30 healthy controls using strain imaging based on tissue Doppler [4]. They found that compared with the healthy controls, the incidence of PSS was noticeably more frequent, and the postsystolic index used to assess the severity of PSS was higher in HCM patients. In our study, we assessed PSS in HCM patients using speckle tracking imaging, which is angle independent and less susceptible to signal noise compared with Doppler strain. However, our results were similar with previous studies. We found that both the number of myocardial segments having PSS and the average value of PSS were significantly increased in the HCM patients.

Currently, PTSMA is considered to be an alternative therapy to surgical myomectomy for patients with HOCM that results in the immediate relief of a LVOT obstruction, the regression of LV hypertrophy and the sustained improvement in LV diastolic function [8–9,25]. Thus, it is reasonable to hypothesise that PTSMA can improve microvascular dysfunction by relieving the extravascular compression in HOCM patients. Recent evidence supports that PTSMA has a favourable effect on microvascular dysfunction. Soliman evaluated the intramyocardial flow dynamics with an adenosine myocardial contrast echocardiography in healthy volunteers and 14 HOCM patients before and 6 months after PTSMA. Soliman found that 6 months after PTSMA, both the myocardial flow reserve and the septal hyperemic endo-to-epi myocardial blood flow ratio were significantly improved [21]. In another study [26], Timmer performed a ^{15}O-water PET study to obtain the resting myocardial blood flow and the coronary vasodilator reserve in 15 HOCM patients before and half a year after the PTSMA. In the study, Timmer observed similar results as Soliman, and he further proved that with the improvement of microvascular dysfunction, myocardial energy was restored in the HOCM patients after PTSMA. Furthermore, some studies have suggested that PTSMA can also partly reverse myocardial fibrosis in HOCM patients [11,27–28]. Thus, it is reasonable to consider whether PTSMA can reduce PSS in HOCM patients. However, to our knowledge, there is no study that focuses on the effect of PTSMA on PSS in HOCM patients. Our study showed that

PTSMA can significantly reduce PSS in patients with HOCM and may result in improvements in microvascular dysfunction and myocardial fibrosis.

Impaired LV diastolic function is the most common pathophysiological feature of HCM, which has been implicated as the primary determinant of symptoms related to heart failure in HCM patients [29–30]. PSS can delay myocardial relaxation resulting in an increased LV filling pressure. Ito reported that the number of segments having PSS correlated significantly with the isovolumic relaxation time in patients with HCM [4]. Ito's results indicated that PSS might contribute to the impaired LV diastolic function in patients with HCM. Significant and sustained improvement in the LV diastolic function has been observed in the short- and long-term following a PTSMA [25]. However, the mechanism of improvement in the LV diastolic function is still unclear. In this study, we found that the decrease in the average value of PSS correlated well with the reduction of the E-to-Ea ratio, which is widely used to estimate the LV filling pressure. Our results indicated that the reduction in PSS might partly account for the sustained improvement of the LV diastolic function in HOCM patients after a successful PTSMA.

This study had several limitations. In addition to the relatively small sample size and the retrospective study design, the invasive measurements of the LV diastolic function were not performed during the course of this study. Instead, we used the E-to-Ea ratio to reflect the LV filling pressure. However, Geske reported that there was only a modest correlation between the estimated LV filling pressure with the use of the E-to-Ea ratio and the directly measured pressure in HCM patients [31].

Conclusions

In conclusion, compared with the healthy controls, the number of segments having PSS and the average value of PSS were significantly increased in the HOCM patients prior to the septal ablation. PTSMA was found to have a favourable effect on PSS, which may partly account for the persistent improvement in the LV diastolic function in HOCM patients after PTSMA. A larger, prospective study with invasive catheters to evaluate the LV filling pressure is necessary to confirm our results.

Author Contributions

Conceived and designed the experiments: JY SC SQ HW. Performed the experiments: JY FD JZ. Analyzed the data: JY SC. Contributed reagents/materials/analysis tools: JY SC. Wrote the paper: JY SC.

References

1. Voigt JU, Lindenmeier G, Exner B, Regenfus M, Werner D, et al.(2003) Incidence and characteristics of segmental postsystolic longitudinal shortening in normal, acutely ischemic and scarred myocardium. J Am Soc Echocardiogr 16:415–23.
2. Nakai H, Takeuchi M, Nishikage T, Lang RM, Otsuji Y (2009) Subclinical left ventricular dysfunction in asymptomatic diabetic patients assessed by two-dimensional speckle tracking echocardiography: correlation with diabetic duration. Eur J Echocardiogr 10:926–932.
3. Yang L, Qiu Q, Zhang HZ, Xia JX (2007) Characteristics of myocardial postsystolic shortening in patients with coronary artery disease assessed by strain rate imaging. Chin Med J (Engl) 120:1894–7.
4. Ito T, Suwa M, Tonari S, Okuda N, Kitaura Y (2006) Regional postsystolic shortening in patients with hypertrophic cardiomyopathy: its incidence and characteristics assessed by strain imaging. J Am Soc Echocardiogr 19:987–93.
5. Carlhäll C, Wranne B, Jurkevicius R (2003) Is left ventricular postsystolic longaxis shortening a marker for severity of hypertensive heart disease? Am J Cardiol 91:1490–93.
6. Kukulski T, Jamal F, D'Hooge J, Bijnens B, De Scheerder I,et al. (2002) Acute changes in systolic and diastolic events during clinical coronary angioplasty: a comparison of regional velocity, strain rate and strain measurement. J Am Soc Echocardiogr 15: 1–12.
7. Voigt JU, Exner B, Schmiedehausen K, Huchzermeyer C, Reulbach U, et al. (2003) Strain rate imaging during dobutamine stress echocardiography provides objective evidence of inducible ischemia. Circulation 107:2120–26.
8. Jensen MK, Almaas VM, Jacobsson L, Hansen PR, Havndrup O, et al.(2011) Long-term outcome of percutaneous transluminal septal myocardial ablation in hypertrophic obstructive cardiomyopathy: a Scandinavian multicenter study. Circ Cardiovasc Interv 4:256–65.
9. Malek LA, Chojnowska L, Klopotowski M, Maczynska R, Demkow M, et al. (2008) Long term exercise capacity in patients with hypertrophic cardiomyopathy treated with percutaneous transluminal septal myocardial ablation. Eur J Heart Fail 10:1123–6.
10. Soliman OI, Geleijnse ML, Michels M, Dijkmans PA, Nemes A, et al. (2008) Effect of successful alcohol septal ablation on microvascular function in patients with obstructive hypertrophic cardiomyopathy. Am J Cardiol 101:1321–7.
11. Stroud RE, Deschamps AM, Lowry AS, Hardin AE, Mukherjee R, et al.(2005) Plasma monitoring of the myocardial specific tissue inhibitor of metalloproteinase-4 after alcohol septal ablation in hypertrophic obstructive cardiomyopathy. J Card Fail 11: 124–30.
12. Chen S, Duan F, Yuan J, Qiao S, Lv X, et al.(2013) Effect of septal ablation on regional diastolic dysfunction and diastolic asynchrony in patients with hypertrophic obstructive cardiomyopathy: a follow-up study using speckle tracking echocardiography. Echocardiography 30:564–71.
13. Yuan J, Qiao S, Zhang Y, You S, Duan F, et al. (2010) Follow-up by cardiac magnetic resonance imaging in patients with hypertrophic cardiomyopathy who underwent percutaneous ventricular septal ablation. Am J Cardiol 106:1487–91.
14. Bertha BG, Folts JD (1986) Phasic mitral blood flow and regional left ventricular dimensions: possible mechanism of active assist to ventricular filling. Circulation 74:901–11.
15. Plaksej R, Kosmala W, Frantz S, Herrmann S, Niemann M, et al.(2009) Relation of circulating markers of fibrosis and progression of left and right ventricular dysfunction in hypertensive patients with heart failure. J Hypertens 27:2483–91.
16. Tsai WC, Liu YW, Chen JY, Huang YY, Shih JY, et al.(2012) Postsystolic strain index is associated with delayed diastolic lengthening and diastolic dysfunction of the left ventricle in untreated hypertension. J Hypertens 30:787–93.
17. Ellims AH, Iles LM, Ling LH, Hare JL, Kaye DM, et al.(2012) Diffuse myocardial fibrosis in hypertrophic cardiomyopathy can be identified by cardiovascular magnetic resonance, and is associated with left ventricular diastolic dysfunction. J Cardiovasc Magn Reson 14:76.
18. Olivotto I, Girolami F, Sciagrà R, Ackerman MJ, Sotgia B, et al.(2011) Microvascular function is selectively impaired in patients with hypertrophic cardiomyopathy and sarcomere myofilament gene mutations. J Am Coll Cardiol 58:839–48.
19. Huang L, Han R, Ai T, Sun Z, Bai Y, et al.(2013) Assessment of coronary microvascular dysfunction in hypertrophic cardiomyopathy: first-pass myocardial perfusion cardiovascular magnetic resonance imaging at 1.5 T. Clin Radiol 68:676–82.
20. Dai Z1, Aoki T, Fukumoto Y, Shimokawa H (2013) Coronary perivascular fibrosis is associated with impairment of coronary blood flow in patients with non-ischemic heart failure. J Cardiol 60:416–21.
21. Soliman OI, Geleijnse ML, Michels M, Dijkmans PA, Nemes A, et al.(2008) Effect of successful alcohol septal ablation on microvascular function in patients with obstructive hypertrophic cardiomyopathy. Am J Cardiol 101:1321–7.
22. Prinz C, Van Buuren F, Bogunovic N, Bitter T, Faber L, et al.(2012) In patients with hypertrophic cardiomyopathy myocardial fibrosis is associated with both left ventricular and left atrial dysfunction. Acta Cardiol 67:187–93.
23. Green JJ, Berger JS, Kramer CM, Salerno M (2012) Prognostic value of late gadolinium enhancement in clinical outcomes for hypertrophic cardiomyopathy. JACC Cardiovasc Imaging 5:370–7.
24. Stoylen A, Sletvold O, Skjaerpe T (2003) Post systolic shortening in nonobstructive hypertrophic cardiomyopathy with delayed emptying of the apex: a Doppler flow, tissue Doppler and strain rate imaging case study. Echocardiography 20:167–71.
25. Jassal DS, Neilan TG, Fifer MA, Palacios IF, Lowry PA, et al.(2006) Sustained improvement in left ventricular diastolic function after alcohol septal ablation for hypertrophic obstructive cardiomyopathy. Eur Heart J 27:1805–10.
26. Timmer SA, Knaapen P, Germans T, Dijkmans PA, Lubberink M, et al.(2011) Effects of alcohol septal ablation on coronary microvascular function and myocardial energetics in hypertrophic obstructive cardiomyopathy. Am J Physiol Heart Circ Physiol 301:H129–37.
27. Bradham WS, Gunasinghe H, Holder JR, Multani M, Killip D, et al. Release of matrix metalloproteinases following alcohol septal ablation in hypertrophic obstructive cardiomyopathy. J Am Coll Cardiol 40:2165–73.
28. Nagueh SF, Stetson SJ, Lakkis NM, Killip D, Perez-Verdia A, et al.(2001) Decreased expression of tumor necrosis factor-a and regression of hypertrophy after nonsurgical septal reduction therapy for patients with hypertrophic obstructive cardiomyopathy. Circulation 103:1844–50.

29. Biagini E, Spirito P, Rocchi G, Ferlito M, Rosmini S, et al.(2009) Prognostic implications of the Doppler restrictive filling pattern in hypertrophic cardiomyopathy. Am J Cardiol 104:1727–31.
30. Matsumura Y, Elliott PM, Virdee MS, Sorajja P, Doi Y, et al. (2002) Left ventricular diastolic function assessed using Doppler tissue imaging in patients with hypertrophic cardiomyopathy: relation to symptoms and exercise capacity. Heart 87:247–51.
31. Geske JB, Sorajja P, Nishimura RA, Ommen SR (2007) Evaluation of left ventricular filling pressures by Doppler echocardiography in patients with hypertrophic cardiomyopathy: correlation with direct left atrial pressure measurement at cardiac catheterization. Circulation 116:2702–8.

15

miR-181c Regulates the Mitochondrial Genome, Bioenergetics, and Propensity for Heart Failure *In Vivo*

Samarjit Das[1], Djahida Bedja[2,3], Nathaniel Campbell[1], Brittany Dunkerly[1,4], Venugopal Chenna[5], Anirban Maitra[1,5,6], Charles Steenbergen[1]*

1 Department of Pathology, Johns Hopkins University, Baltimore, Maryland, United States of America, **2** Department of Cardiology, Johns Hopkins University, Baltimore, Maryland, United States of America, **3** Australian School of Advanced Medicine, Macquarie University, Sydney, Australia, **4** Notre Dame of Maryland University, Baltimore, Maryland, United States of America, **5** Departments of Pathology and Translational Molecular Pathology, Houston, Texas, United States of America, **6** Department of Oncology, Johns Hopkins University, Baltimore, Maryland, United States of America

Abstract

MicroRNAs (miRNAs) are small non-coding RNAs, which inhibit the stability and/or translation of a mRNA. miRNAs have been found to play a powerful role in various cardiovascular diseases. Recently, we have demonstrated that a microRNA (miR-181c) can be encoded in the nucleus, processed to the mature form in the cytosol, translocated into the mitochondria, and ultimately can regulate mitochondrial gene expression. However the *in vivo* impact of miR-181c is unknown. Here we report an *in-vivo* method for administration of miR-181c in rats, which leads to reduced exercise capacity and signs of heart failure, by targeting the 3′-end of mt-COX1 (cytochrome c oxidase subunit 1). We cloned miR-181c and packaged it in lipid-based nanoparticles for systemic delivery. The plasmid DNA complexed nanovector shows no apparent toxicity. We find that the mRNA levels of mitochondrial complex IV genes in the heart, but not any other mitochondrial genes, are significantly altered with miR-181c overexpression, suggesting selective mitochondrial complex IV remodeling due to miR-181c targeting mt-COX1. Isolated heart mitochondrial studies showed significantly altered O_2-consumption, ROS production, matrix calcium, and mitochondrial membrane potential in miR-181c-treated animals. For the first time, this study shows that miRNA delivered to the heart *in-vivo* can lead to cardiac dysfunction by regulating mitochondrial genes.

Editor: Yibin Wang, David Geffen School of Medicine at UCLA, United States of America

Funding: This work was supported by grants from the National Institutes of Health, R01HL39752 (CS) and U54CA151838 (AM), and a Scientist Development Grant from the American Heart Association 14SDG18890049 (SD). BD gratefully acknowledges her support from the Sister Alma McNicholas Fund from the Notre Dame of Maryland University. The funders had no role in study design, data collection and analysis, decision to publish, or preparation of the manuscript.

Competing Interests: The authors have declared that no competing interests exist.

* E-mail: csteenb1@jhmi.edu

Introduction

Mitochondria, which contain their own DNA, mRNA, tRNA and ribosomes [1], are semi-autonomous organelles, but they import many critical proteins, which are encoded by nuclear genes [1,2]. Critical to mitochondrial function are five respiratory chain complexes in the inner mitochondrial membrane that generate a proton gradient across the membrane, which produces ATP [1–4]. Most of the respiratory chain complex subunits are encoded by nuclear genes, except for some subunits of complex I, III, and IV, which are encoded by mitochondrial DNA and synthesized on mitochondrial ribosomes [1].

MicroRNAs (miRNAs) are small (~19–22 nt), stable non-coding RNAs that critically modulate post-transcriptional gene regulation by binding at the 3′-UTR of corresponding mRNAs [5]. Because of this binding at the 3′-UTR of mRNAs, miRNA either block translation or cause message degradation through RNA Induced Silencing Complex (RISC) mediated events [5]. Several groups suggested that miRNA exist in mitochondria [6–10], but recent work from our group demonstrate that miRNA exist in heart mitochondria and are functionally important [11,12]. We showed that miR-181c, derived from the nuclear genome, translocates to the mitochondria, and more importantly, regulates mitochondrial gene expression and affects mitochondrial function [11]. Coordination of nuclear gene expression and mitochondrial gene expression is thus essential. Our work shows that miRNA can regulate mitochondrial gene expression, specifically that miR-181c binds to the 3′-end of the mRNA of a mitochondrial gene, mt-COX1, a subunit of complex IV of the respiratory chain, and initially results in a decrease in mt-COX1 protein, complex IV remodeling, and increased production of reactive oxygen species [11].

In the present study, we examined whether this *in vitro* finding is applicable *in vivo*, using a novel miR-181c delivery system using lipid based cationic nanoparticles [13].

Results

In vivo characterization of nanovectors for systemic miR-181c delivery

The nanovector is an electrostatic complex of positively charged liposomal nanoparticles and negatively charged plasmid DNA (in this case, expressing miR-181c) [13]. After pilot *in vivo* studies using several doses and different time-points, we optimized a 4 mg/kg dose of plasmid DNA, which increases miR-181c levels in heart tissue ~2 fold with 6 injections over 3 weeks. Thereafter, we evaluated the potential for adverse effects from systemic nanovector therapy by evaluating both hematologic and histologic samples (Fig. 1) from rats that had received either sham (empty vector) or miR-181c nanovector. No detectable amounts of serum pro-inflammatory cytokines, TNF-α, IL-2, or IFN-γ, were found in either group, 8 hours after I.V. administration. We also monitored the blood pressure of the animals during the treatment period, and did not observe any difference between the two groups (Fig. 2A). We observed that miR-181c overexpression groups are more physically active and gain less weight during the first 2 weeks of the treatment (Fig. 2B); we measured serum and urine glucose and found no evidence that the animals were diabetic. We also observed that the miR-181c-treated group develops fatigue much earlier during exercise than the sham group. Using a forced swimming test [14], we have found that the miR-181c-treated animals could only swim for 7–9 minutes on the 20th day of the treatment, whereas the sham group could swim the entire 20 minutes without any sign of fatigue (Fig. 2C).

Systemic miR-181c delivery with nanovectors shows signs of heart failure

We measured the expression of miR-181c in the heart, and found a ~2 fold increase (Fig. 3A). We had previously found that endogenous miR-181c localizes to mitochondria [11], so we isolated RNA from the mitochondria [11] of the hearts treated with nanovector *in vivo*, and the miR-181c-treated group shows a significantly higher level of miR-181c in the heart-derived mitochondria (Fig. 3B). Although we did not find any sign of hypertrophy (Fig. 3C), using echocardiography, we find that miR-181c overexpression causes a significant decrease in left ventricular fractional shortening (FS) and markedly lower ejection fraction (EF) (Fig. 4A–C).

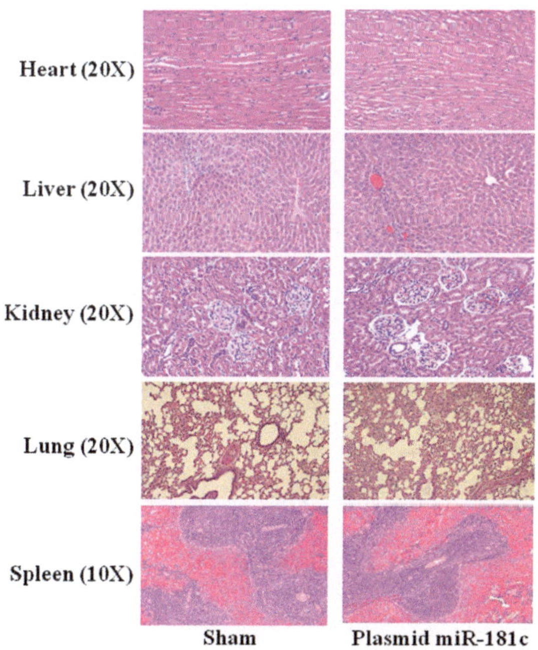

Figure 1. Effect of miR-181c in different organs by systemic delivery. 3 weeks after treating the rats with nanoparticles with/without miR-181c expression vector, we stained sections of five different organs with hematoxylin and eosin (H&E). Image magnification was 20× for heart, liver, kidney, and lung, and 10× for spleen.

Systemic miR-181c delivery target mitochondrial gene in the heart

We next assessed the functional consequences of translocation of miR-181c into the mitochondria. We have previously found that miR-181c can regulate the mt-COX1 gene and causes mitochondrial complex IV remodeling [11]; therefore, we measured each of the mitochondrial genome components of complex IV. Indeed, we found a significant decrease of both mRNA (Fig. 5A) and total protein content (Fig. 5B) of mt-COX1 in the miR-181c overexpressing hearts, confirming our *in-vitro* observation that miR-181c regulates mt-COX1 expression [5]. We also observed a significant decrease in mRNA levels of both mt-COX2 and mt-COX3 but not any other mitochondrial genes, such as complex I or V components, ND1 or ATPase 8 (Fig. 5A); there was also no effect on TFAM level (Fig. 5C). This further confirms our *in-vitro* observation of mitochondrial complex IV remodeling [11]. Unlike our acute *in-vitro* study, at Day 20 of the nanovector treatment, we found a significant decrease of mt-COX2 protein (Fig. 5B), suggesting that a decrease in the expression of mt-COX1 over time results in a reduction in the amount of other Complex IV components. This differs from our earlier *in-vitro* [11] work, in which, after 48 hr of miR-181c overexpression, we observed a significant decrease in mt-COX1 protein levels, but a significant increase in mt-COX2 protein levels. This likely reflects the longer duration of miR-181c overexpression in our *in vivo* protocol. We suggested that complex IV remodeling was occurring and that as a result of lower mt-COX1 levels, an adaptive response was activated, resulting in higher mt-COX2 levels. Unlike our *in-vitro* data, this *in vivo* (day 22) data suggests that miR-181c significantly decreases the mRNA and protein content of multiple complex IV mitochondrial genes (mt-COX1, mt-COX2 and mt-COX3) (Fig. 5A, 5B). Figure S1 in File S1 shows that a shorter (2 week) treatment causes changes in mRNA expression levels of mitochondrial complex IV subunits in a manner that more closely resembles what we have observed *in-vitro*. *In vivo*, we did not see a significant change either in miR-181c expression (Fig. S2 in File S1), or in mRNA levels of mt-COX1 or mt-COX2 in the heart at 2 weeks; however, we did observe a significantly higher level of mt-COX3. These data suggest that miR-181c overexpression *in vivo* has progressive effects on mitochondrial complex IV. It appears that only complex IV is altered since we have measured ND2 and ATPase 8 mRNA levels and have not found any changes with miR-181c overexpression (Fig. S1 in File S1). However, changes occur not just in COX subunits that are products of the mitochondrial genome, but also in COX subunits that are derived from the nuclear genome such as COX VIIa (Fig. 5D). On the other hand, not all COX subunits are downregulated. We found that COX 5A and COX 5B are not significantly altered by chronic miR-181c overexpression *in vivo*. The effect of miR-181c overexpression using nanovector delivery is transient. We observed that miR-181c expression was not increased in several animals that were followed for 3 weeks after the completion of treatment, and the transient nature of miR overexpression with nanovector treatment has been reported previously [13].

Systemic miR-181c delivery regulates Mitochondrial Function

To determine whether miR-181c regulates mitochondrial energy metabolism, we measured O_2 consumption [15]. To focus specifically on complex IV, we used the complex IV substrates, TMPD and ascorbate. Complete inhibition of Complex IV would lead to metabolic inhibition and loss of oxidative phosphorylation (OXPHOS) as a means of energy generation. However, partial

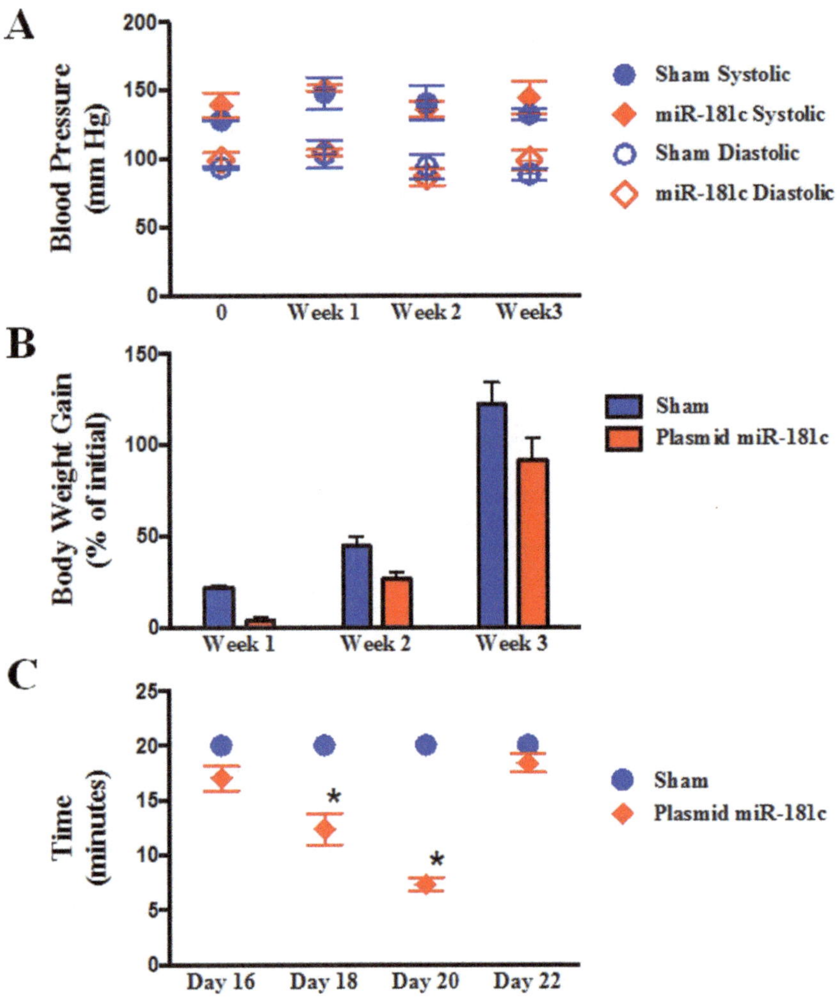

Figure 2. Physical Properties of the rats during the Treatment Protocols. (A) **Blood Pressure.** We used a non-invasive, tail cuff method, to measure diastolic blood pressure (DBP) and systolic blood pressure (SBP). We did not observe any significant difference between the two groups, either in DBP or SBP. The red color indicates the plasmid miR-181c treated group, and the blue color indicates the sham group. n = 3. (B) **Body weight.** Rats were weighed during the treatment period, and we found that the weight gain of miR-181c-treated rat group is significantly lower than the sham group, up to day 11. This is not a toxic reaction, but it is due to the high activity of these animals. These animals are not diabetic (dipstick and blood glucose tests were performed). But after day 13, miR-181c-treated animals become lethargic. The red bar indicates the plasmid miR-181c treated group, and the blue bar indicates the sham group. n = 12.(C) **Forced Swimming Test.** miR-181c overexpression shows a significant difference in exercise capacity compared to the sham group after the 18th day of treatment. Together with the echocardiography data we optimized day 20 for assessment.

inhibition through reduced expression of Complex IV subunits has a more complex effect on mitochondrial function. As we saw in our *in-vitro* study [11], the rate of O_2 consumption is significantly increased in miR-181c overexpressing mitochondria compared to the sham after adding complex IV substrate (Fig. 6A). To further evaluate the mechanism by which miR-181c alters mitochondrial respiration, we measured ROS production in isolated mitochondria. Overexpression of miR-181c significantly increased the rate of ROS generation in the miR-181c-treated group (Fig. 6B). We used two different substrates, glutamate/malate for complex I and succinate for complex II. We could not use TMPD/ascorbate because TMPD interferes with the amplex red signal. The increase in ROS production in isolated heart mitochondria from the miR-181c-treated group provides a partial explanation for the increase in O_2 consumption.

To further characterize the effect of miR-181c overexpression on mitochondrial function, we measured mitochondrial membrane potential ($\Delta\Psi_m$). We used TMRE [16,17] to measure $\Delta\Psi_m$ in isolated mitochondria and found that the miR-181c-treated group shows a markedly higher level of TMRE fluorescence compared to the sham group, suggesting a significantly higher $\Delta\Psi_m$ with miR-181c overexpression (Fig 7A). $\Delta\Psi_m$ dissipates completely upon addition of 20 μM CCCP, as is observed in the end of the TMRE fluorescence graph in Figure 7A.

One explanation for this high $\Delta\Psi_m$ would be if miR-181c overexpression causes mitochondrial matrix Ca^{2+} concentration to increase [18,19] and this activates calcium-sensitive mitochondrial dehydrogenases [19,20]. To assess whether mitochondrial matrix Ca^{2+} concentration is increased, we examined direct targets of Ca^{2+} in the mitochondrial matrix such as α-ketoglutarate dehydrogenase (αKGDH) and pyruvate dehydrogenase (PDH), which is regulated by a calcium-sensitive dephosphorylation mechanism. Activity of both of αKGDH and PDH are increased in the presence of calcium and we measured an increase in activity

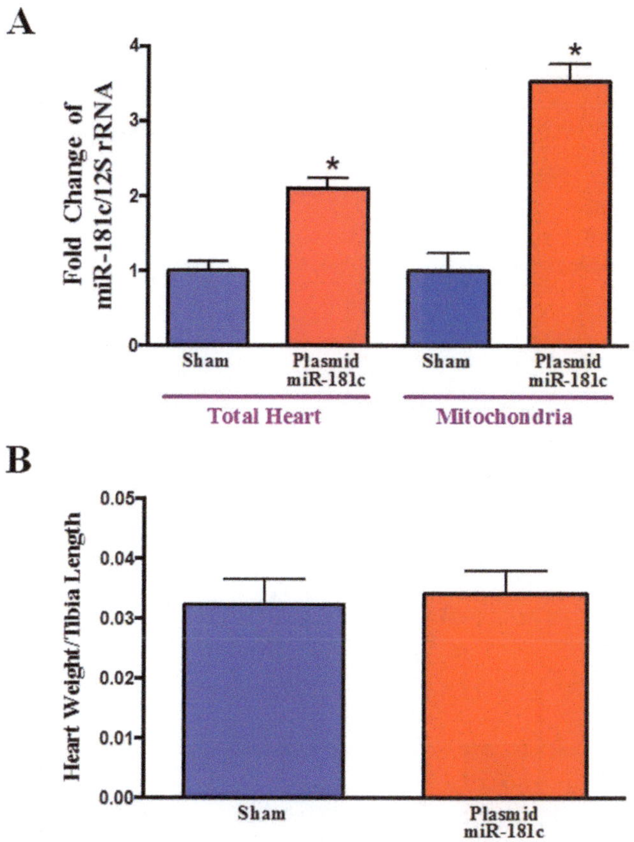

Figure 3. Effect of 3 weeks of nanovector delivery (i.v). (A) **miR-181c expression in the Heart and in the Heart-derived Mitochondrial Fraction.** qPCR shows that miR-181c expression in the whole heart homogenate is almost 1.5 times higher in the plasmid miR-181c group compared to its sham group. We isolated mitochondrial miRNA enriched total RNA, using our published protocol [5]. We also monitored the quality and integrity of the isolated RNAs, as described previously[5]. qPCR shows that miR-181c expression is almost 2.5 times higher in the miR-181c-treated group compared to its sham group. We used the mitochondrial gene product, 12S rRNA, as a normalization control [5]. *$p<0.05$ vs. sham (n = 6 for whole heart, and n = 4 for the mitochondrial fraction). (B) **Heart Weight.** We measured the wet weight of the whole heart and measured the corresponding tibial length of each rat. The ratio of heart weight to tibial length is not different among the groups, suggesting no sign of hypertrophy in the miR-181c-treated rats. (n = 12).

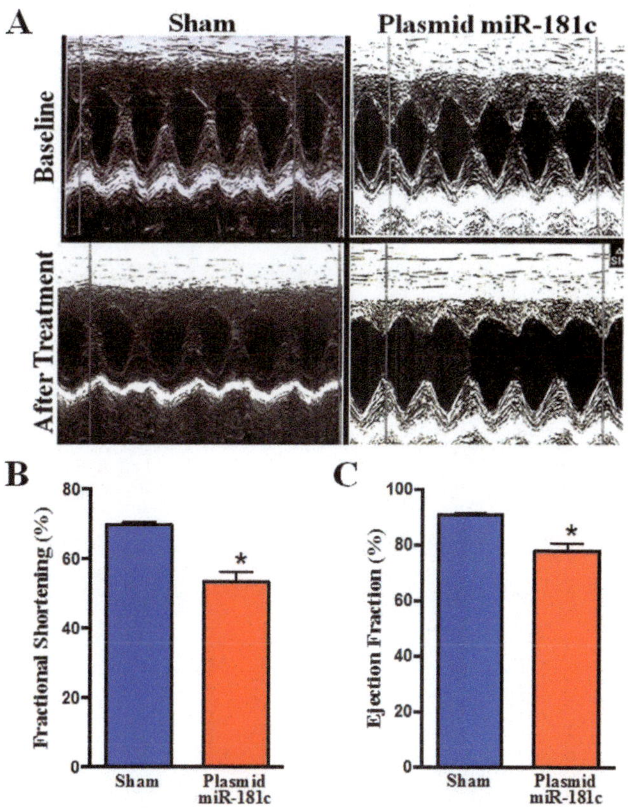

Figure 4. Echocardiography. (A) 2D M-mode and Doppler echocardiography was performed on non-anesthetized rats, before (top) and after (lower) the sham (left) or the miR-181c expression vector (right) treatment. (B) Percent fractional shortening, and (C) ejection fraction, were calculated using the software of the echocardiography instrument (n = 10).

of both PDH (Fig. 7E) and αKGDH (Fig. 7F) in the miR-181c-treated mitochondria. To investigate possible mechanisms to explain the increase in matrix calcium, we examined the expression of the mitochondrial calcium uniporter (MCU), and found that MCU expression was increased in the miR-181c treatment group (Fig. 7D). Although the miR-181c-treated mitochondria are fully energized, an increase in matrix Ca^{2+} may have detrimental effects on the ability of mitochondria to take up and retain additional Ca^{2+}, and may make the mitochondria more susceptible to opening of the mitochondrial permeability transition pore. To assess the mitochondrial calcium retention capacity, Ca^{2+} was added to mitochondria in small increments. As shown in Figure 7B-C, mitochondria derived from miR-181c-treated hearts have a reduced ability to accumulate and retain Ca^{2+} and are very susceptible to mPTP opening with Ca^{2+} addition. After addition of sufficient calcium to complex the EGTA in the buffer (40 μM), we added 10 μM Ca^{2+} every 2 min. After only 2 boluses of Ca^{2+}, the mitochondria released the accumulated Ca^{2+} in the miR-181c overexpression group, indicating mPTP opening, whereas it took the sham group 8 additional Ca^{2+} pulses before Ca^{2+} release occurred. Thus there are potential detrimental effects of the increase in matrix calcium, and the increase in ROS, that occurs with miR-181c overexpression.

Discussion

Over the past few years, there have been numerous studies that have pointed to the significant role of miRNAs in heart diseases by regulating nuclear genes [21,22]. We have shown that miRNA can also target the mitochondrial genome in myocytes [11]. There are multiple novel aspects of this study, which further reveal mechanistic insights concerning the pathophysiologic effects of prolonged miR-181c overexpression, involving mitochondrial gene regulation, *in-vivo*.

To our knowledge, this is the first study to address the functional consequences of a MitomiR (viz., miR-181c) in the heart and its physiologic relevance *in-vivo*. Secondly, although nanovector delivery of a miRNA is a well established approach in oncology, our study is the first demonstration that a miRNA can be manipulated in non-neoplastic tissue using a plasmid-containing nanovector. We find that reduced expression of mitochondrial complex IV subunits leads to increased matrix calcium and

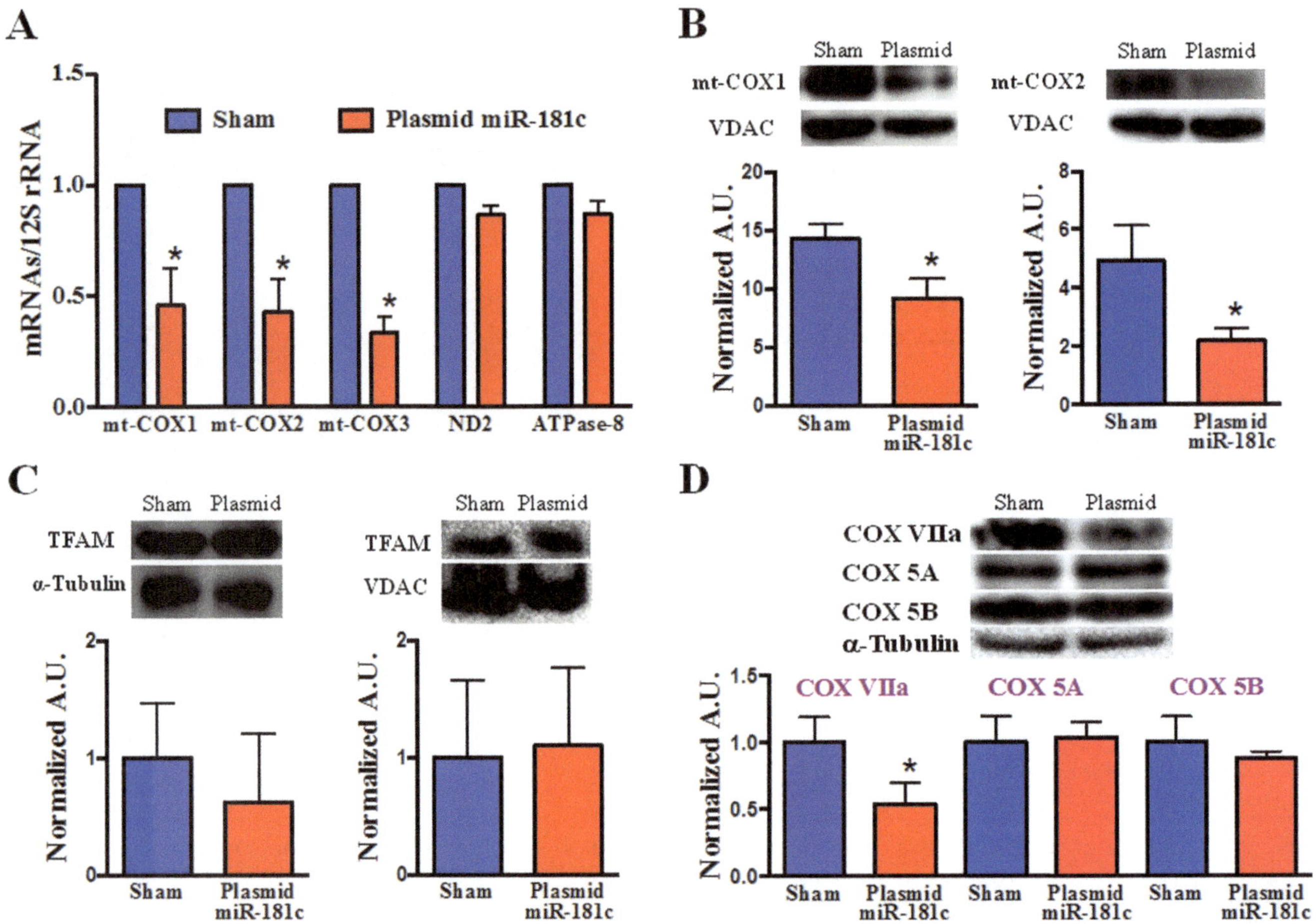

Figure 5. Mitochondrial Complex IV Remodeling after miR-181c Treatment. (A) qPCR data show that overexpression of miR-181c significantly reduces the mRNA levels of all mitochondrial complex IV genes with 3 weeks treatment. The treatment protocol has no effect on other mitochondrial genes, such as ND2 (complex I) and ATPase 8 (complex V). Content of mRNA was first normalized to 12S rRNA, a mitochondrial gene, as 12S rRNA expression did not change with miR-181c overexpresssion. Then we normalized the data to the sham group. *$p<0.05$ vs. sham ($n=6$). (B) Western blot shows that miR-181c overexpression significantly reduces the protein content of both mt-COX1 and mt-COX2. VDAC was used as a loading control. The data were normalized to the sham group. *$p<0.05$ vs. sham ($n=6$). (C) Western blot shows that miR-181c overexpression has no effect on Transcription Factor A, Mitochondria (TFAM), either in the total heart homogenate (left panel) or the heart-derived mitochondrial fraction (right panel). TFAM plays an important role in mitochondrial gene transcription, by activating 3 different promoter regions in the D-loop area of the mitochondrial genome. TFAM also translocates from the cytosol to the mitochondria as part of the mitochondrial gene transcription process. α-tubulin (for total heart homogenate) and VDAC (mitochondrial fraction) were used as loading controls. The data were normalized to the sham group ($n=3$). (D) Western blot shows the changes of other isoforms of mitochondrial respiratory chain complex IV. We have observed a significant decrease in the protein content of COX VIIa in the miR-181c overexpression groups, but no effect on COX 5A and COX 5B. α-tubulin was used as the loading control. The data were normalized to the sham group ($n=3$).

activation of citric acid cycle dehydrogenases that increase the flow of protons and electrons into the electron transport chain, resulting in an increase in $\Delta\Psi_m$, while there is a decrease in complex IV activity, which shunts electrons into alternate pathways, culminating in increased ROS production. The high $\Delta\Psi_m$ indicates that mitochondrial function is preserved and provides a thermodynamic basis for high matrix [Ca^{2+}]. Thus despite reduced activity of complex IV, respiration is overall higher in the miR-181c-treated group (Fig 6A).

One of the key findings of this study is that overexpression of miR-181c leads to dysfunction of complex IV, which activates ROS generation and O_2 consumption; involving increased matrix [Ca^{2+}]. Increased matrix [Ca^{2+}] activates Complex III and several dehydrogenases, leading to an increase in $\Delta\Psi_m$ [18,19]. Concurrently there is an increase in ROS generation, perhaps related to both the increase in membrane potential and the increase in citric acid cycle activity, while the transfer of electrons and protons to molecular oxygen through Complex IV is inhibited. Despite the increase in ROS generation, $\Delta\Psi_m$ remains high and the mitochondria are fully energized. There are numerous studies explaining the potential role of complex III in ROS generation [1], and there is also abundant evidence that complex I can generate ROS, particularly in the context of high $\Delta\Psi_m$ and partial inhibition of complex IV [1]. Others have found that partial inhibition of complex IV can markedly increase ROS production without necessarily decreasing ATP synthesis [23]. An increase in matrix Ca^{2+} concentration, by increasing the activity of several citric acid cycle dehydrogenases [19,20], would increase the flow of electrons and protons into the electron transport chain, increasing $\Delta\Psi_m$ [18,19]. $\Delta\Psi_m$ is the driving force for Ca^{2+} uptake [23], and furthermore, this increase in $\Delta\Psi_m$ could explain the increase in ROS, as the flow of electrons and protons into the

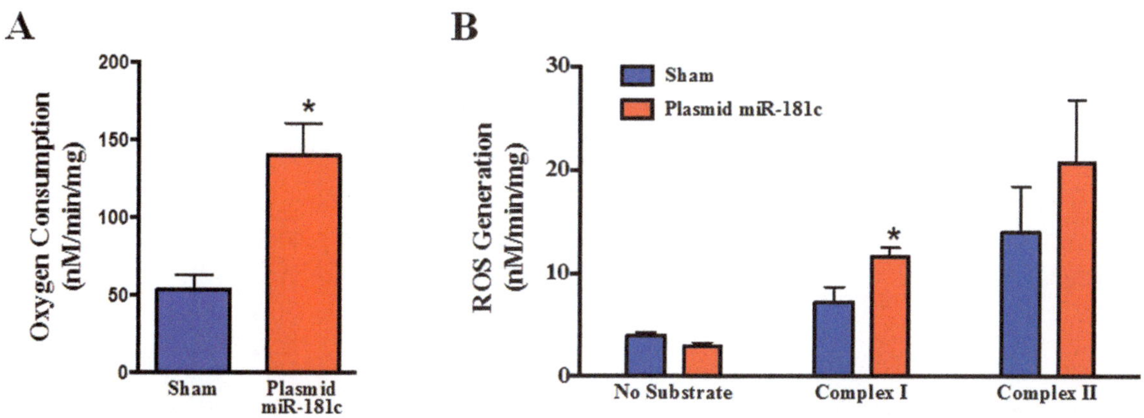

Figure 6. Mitochondrial function. Effect of 3 weeks of nanovector treatment on isolated mitochondria. (A) O_2 consumption was measured after adding the substrate for complex IV, TMPD/ascorbate. Overexpression of miR-181c markedly increases respiration compared to the sham, after adding TMPD/Ascorbate. These data show the role of miR-181c on mitochondrial energy metabolism by altering complex IV. $^{*}P<0.05$ vs sham, n = 6. (B) Rate of ROS generation from heart-mitochondria overexpressing miR-181c. Without any substrate the rate of ROS production is not different between the two treatment groups. But, using glutamate/malate (complex I) and succinate (complex II), ROS production is significantly higher in the miR-181c overexpression groups. $^{*}p<0.05$ vs. sham, n = 4.

electron transport chain increases while the terminal step is partially inhibited. This study highlights an unusual aspect of mitochondrial biology, involving complex IV remodeling and ROS generation.

The heart gets most of its energy from electron transport, coupled to oxidative phosphorylation. O_2 is the ultimate electron acceptor for the mitochondrial respiratory chain, and the addition of electrons and protons to O_2 to form water is catalyzed by cytochrome c oxidase, the terminal complex in the respiratory chain. mt-COX1 is a core component of cytochrome oxidase in the inner membrane of the mitochondria. Loss of cytochrome oxidase activity would be expected to affect mitochondrial energy metabolism, and mitochondrial dysfunction is important in many diseases [24–27]. Even though complex IV plays a critical role in the electron transport chain and in OXPHOS, the consequences of altered complex IV function are poorly understood. In a yeast model, it has been shown that mt-COX1 binds to mt-COX2 with the help of Mg^{2+} or Mn^{2+} ions, and this forms the catalytic core of complex IV [28]. In this study we have shown that chronic overexpression of miR-181c in the rat heart leads to significant down-regulation of mt-COX1 and mt-COX2 (Fig. 5A–B). Despite complex IV remodeling and reduction in the expression of key subunits following miR-181c overexpression, overall mitochondrial function and membrane potential are well maintained because of an increase in matrix $[Ca^{2+}]$, which increases the activity of other electron transport components. Although mitochondrial function is maintained, the high membrane potential and partial inhibition of complex IV leads to increased ROS production. Increased ROS production could eventually lead to impaired mitochondrial function which ultimately could be associated with decreased $\Delta\Psi_m$, and ROS production in the setting of high matrix $[Ca^{2+}]$ could lead to opening of a non-specific pore in the mitochondrial membrane known as the mitochondrial permeability transition pore (mPTP) [3,4,15]. Increased ROS production could have other consequences as well, including reduced contractile function, as has been observed with postischemic stunning [31,32]. In fact, like our miR-181c overexpressor model, the role of ROS and Ca^{2+} in the pathogenesis of myocardial stunning is well documented [31,33]; including mitochondrial matrix $[Ca^{2+}]$ overload [34].

Our data suggest that complex IV remodeling affects more than just the subunits that are products of the mitochondrial genome and subject to direct regulation by miR-181c within the mitochondrial matrix. There are also changes to peripheral complex IV subunits that are products of the nuclear genome such as COX VIIa, but not to all of the subunits derived from the nuclear genome such as COX 5A and COX 5B. The loss of COX VIIa protein over time, as well as mt-COX2, may be related to increased degradation. A role for LON-mediated degradation of COX subunits in regulation of complex IV subunit composition has been reported previously [35].

Taken together, the results demonstrate that chronic overexpression of miR-181c has a role in heart failure by targeting the mitochondrial gene, mt-COX1, which ultimately leads to dysfunctional complex IV, altered mitochondrial metabolism, and ROS generation. We have also identified an underlying mechanism by which complex IV inhibition can activate ROS production in the mitochondria, by increasing matrix $[Ca^{2+}]$, which activates mitochondrial dehydrogenases. Our study used a novel systemic miRNA delivery system, using cationic nanovectors, in the heart. This technology may lead to innovative new therapeutic interventions for heart disease.

Materials And Methods

Animals

Male Sprague-Dawley rats (150–175 g, Harlan Sprague-Dawley) were used in this study. They were provided with food and water *ad libitum*. We tested glucose levels in both the blood and urine, using a blood glucose meter (OneTouch Basic, Milpitas, CA) and dipsticks. Rats were treated humanely and all experimental procedures were approved by the Institutional Animal Care and Use Committee of Johns Hopkins University.

miR-181c expression constructs

miR-181c and 361 bp of flanking sequence was amplified from rat genomic DNA using polymerase, and cloned into the EcoRI and XhoI sites of the MSCV-Neo vector (Clontech Laboratories). The sequences of the amplified products were confirmed by both PCR and sequencing [29,30]. Primer sequences are provided in Table 1.

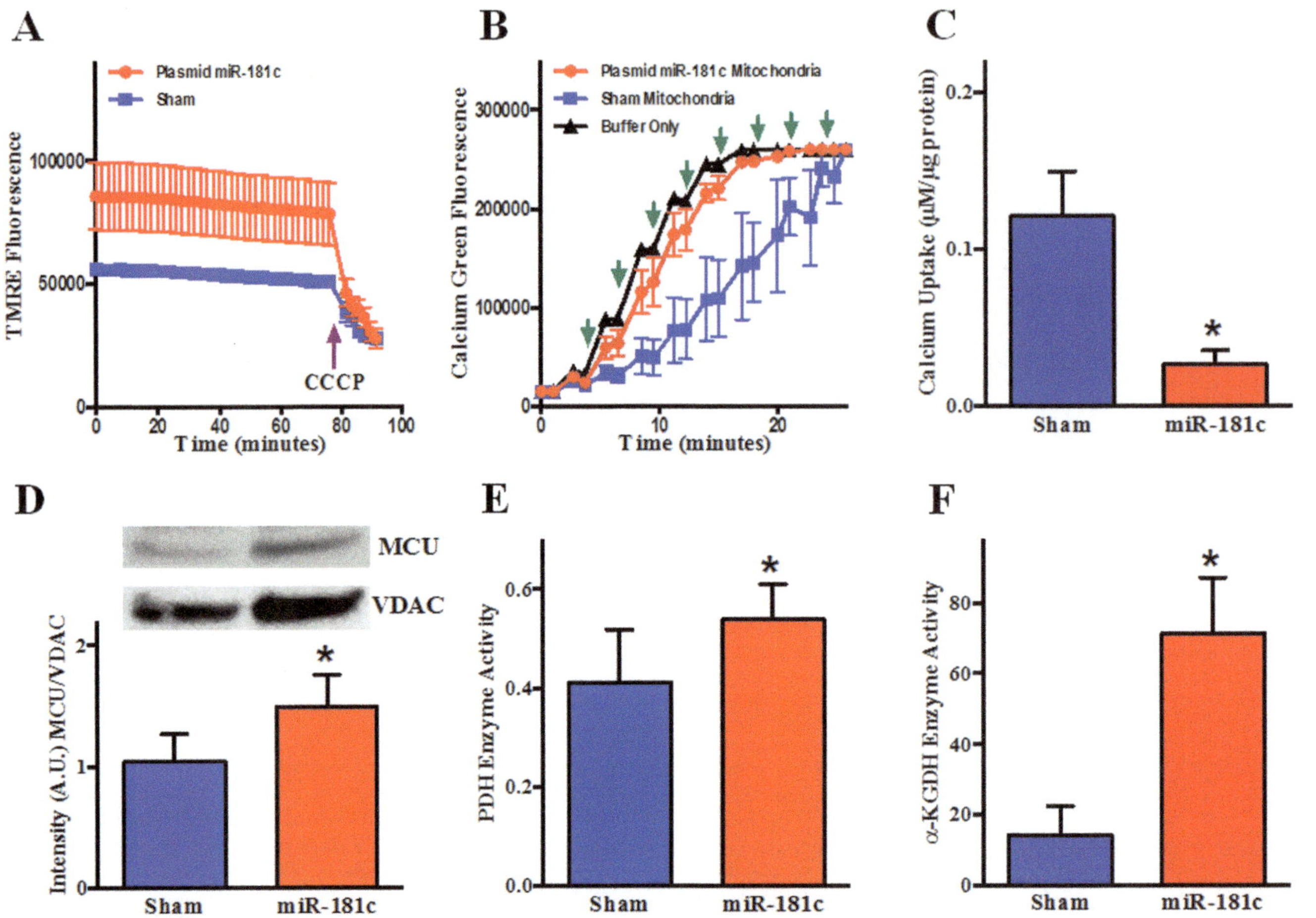

Figure 7. Effect of miR-181c on Mitochondrial Function. Heart-derived mitochondria were isolated from the two groups of rats after 3 weeks of treatment. (A) TMRE (tetramethylrhodamine methyl ester) fluorescence was measured from mitochondria supplied with glutamate/malate from two different treatment groups for 25 min, followed by the addition of the uncoupler, CCCP (Carbonyl cyanide m-chlorophenyl hydrazone). The miR-181c treatment group showed a higher level of TMRE intensity before the CCCP addition. n = 3. (B) Isolated mitochondria were incubated with Calcium Green 5N and fluorescence intensity was monitored after adding Ca^{2+}. Following a Ca^{2+} pulse, fluorescence increases initially, but reverts back towards baseline as mitochondria take up Ca^{2+}. When mitochondria take up enough Ca^{2+}, the mPTP opens. This results in Ca^{2+} release and a decrease in fluorescence. (↑) indicates addition of 10 μM Ca^{2+}. n = 3. (C) Western blot shows that miR-181c overexpression significantly increases the protein content of the mitochondrial calcium uniporter (MCU) both from total heart homogenate and mitochondrial fraction. VDAC was used as a loading control. The data were normalized to the sham group. *$p<0.05$ vs. sham (n = 4). (D) pyruvate dehydrogenase (PDH) and (E) α-ketoglutarate dehydrogenase (αKGDH) activities were significantly higher in the isolated mitochondria from the miR-181c treated hearts compared to sham, suggesting that the mitochondrial matrix Ca^{2+} concentration is increased in the miR-181c treated animals.

Preparation of nanovector for systemic miR-181c delivery in the rats

Liposomal nanoparticles were prepared by dissolving cationic amphiphile (DOTAP) and co-lipids (cholesterol and DSPE-PEG-OMe) in a 5:5:0.1 mM ratio, respectively, in a mixture of chloroform and methanol. The organic solvent was removed at 44–45°C, under vacuum by using a rotary evaporator, followed by a gentle flow of moisture-free nitrogen and the remaining dried film of lipid was then kept under high vacuum for 8 hours. 5% glucose was added to the vacuum-dried lipid film and the mixture was allowed to hydrate overnight. The vial was vortexed for 2 to 3 minutes at room temperature and occasionally shaken in a 45°C water bath to produce multilamellar vesicles. Small unilamellar vesicles were prepared by sonication of the multilamellar vesicles in an ice bath for 3 to 4 minutes until clarity, using a Branson 450 sonifier (Danbury) at 100% duty cycle and 25-W output power. The nanovector is an electrostatic complex of positively-charged liposomal nanoparticles and negatively-charged plasmid Nucleotide, and was prepared by mixing pMSCV-Neo vectors expressing miR-181c and liposome on a 1:3 Nucleotide/lipid charge ratio basis. This nanovector is administered i.v. to rats through the tail vein, as described previously [13,29].

Table 1. Primer Sequences for PCR and Sequencing.

Forward:	5′- TCTCCTGGGTGTCCAAAAAG-3′
Reverse:	5′- ACCCACCGACAACAATGAAT -3′

a) miR-181c.

Experimental Protocol

We used a dose of 4 mg of nanovector/Kg body weight, and have optimized a regimen of 6 injections into the tail vein over 2 weeks. There is also a 1 week period (days 15–21) to allow expression of the vector *in vivo*. We optimized this protocol by monitoring cardiac function by echocardiography and forced swimming before, during, and after nanovector delivery.

Echocardiography

Sequoia C256 ultrasound system, (Siemens, Mountain View, CA) equipped with 15-MHz linear array transducer was used. 2 Dimensional, M-mode, and Doppler echocardiography were performed to assess cardiac function and morphology in treated and sham treated rats, without anaesthesia [30].

Forced Swim Test

The Forced Swim test or Porsolt swim test is a standard assay to assess exercise tolerance in rats [14]. Rats were placed in a cylinder (20 cm diameter, 45 cm height) filled with 25°C water to a level of 40 cm. Rats were monitored for changes in exercise tolerance after nanovector treatment for 2 weeks, with iv injection 3 times a week and then evaluated on day 16, 18, 20, and 22 following initiation of the treatment protocol. The rats remain in the water for a maximum of 20 minutes. The swim test was terminated if the rat showed signs of exhaustion. All sessions are videotaped and scored offline for time spent swimming. After each session, rats were removed and placed in a clean cage under a heating lamp to dry before being returned to the home cage or performing echocardiography [31].

Langendorff Rat Heart Preparation

After sufficient anesthesia was achieved with ketamine (19 mg/Kg body wt.) - Xylazine (10 mg/Kg body wt.) cocktail, i.p., rats were anticoagulated with heparin sodium (500 IU/kg body weight, i.v. injection) (Elkin-Sinn Inc., Cherry Hill, NJ). Hearts were excised, cannulated, and perfused with Krebs-Henseleit buffer containing (in mmol/L) NaCl 120, KCl 5.9, $MgSO_4$ 1.2, $CaCl_2$ 1.25, $NaHCO_3$ 25, and glucose 11. The buffer was aerated with 95% O_2 and 5% CO_2, to give a pH of 7.4 at 37°C as described previously [15]. All hearts are perfused to wash out blood and stabilize for 15 minutes, followed by perfusion with RNAlater (Qiagen, Valencia, CA), 10 ml diluted in Krebs-Henseleit buffer, for another minute [11].

Isolated Mitochondria Protocols

Freshly isolated mitochondria were prepared from hearts after perfusion with RNAlater, by differential centrifugation [11]. Briefly, at the end of perfusion, the left ventricle was dissected out and placed in Buffer A (in mM: 180 KCl, 2 EGTA, 5 MOPS; 0.2% BSA; pH: 7.25). The tissue was then digested with trypsin (0.0001 g/0.1 g tissue) in 0.7 ml of ice-cold Buffer B (in mM: 225 Mannitol, 75 sucrose, 5 MOPS, 0.5 EGTA, 2 Taurine; pH: 7.25) and finally homogenized with Buffer B with a protease inhibitor cocktail (Roche Applied Science, Indianapolis, IN) using a Polytron. To further separate the heart mitochondria from other cellular components and tissue debris, a series of differential centrifugations were performed in a Microfuge 22R centrifuge (Beckman Coulter, Fullerton, CA) at 4°C. The crude pellet was then lysed with QIAzol (Qiagen, Valencia, CA) [11].

RNA isolation

Total RNA were isolated, from whole hearts, mitochondrial fraction of the hearts, as described above, using a miRNeasy kit (Qiagen, Valencia, CA) and RNase free DNase kit (Qiagen, Valencia, CA) [11]. To characterize the integrity of the isolated RNA, spectrophotometric evaluation was performed, using Nanodrop (Thermo Scientific, Wilmington, DE). All the samples whose A_{260} (absorbance at 260 nm) value is more than 0.15 is used for further experiments. As the $A_{260}<0.15$ suggest poor quality of RNA. The ratio of the readings at 260 nm and 280 nm (A_{260}/A_{280}) was also measured in order to check the purity of the isolated RNA.

qRT-PCR

After performing the purity and integrity test, the RNA was reverse transcribed using a miScript Reverse Transcription Kit (Qiagen, Valencia, CA). PCR was performed using a miScript SYBR green PCR kit (Qiagen, Valencia, CA) and detected with a CFX96 detector (Bio-Rad, Hercules, CA). The primer sequences have been previously described [7]. All reactions were performed in triplicate.

Mitochondrial Respiration Assay

The ADP-dependence of mitochondrial respiration was assessed at 25°C in a chamber containing respiration buffer (in mM) KCl 140, EGTA 10, HEPES 20, Oxalic Acid 5, K2HPO4 5 and pH 7.25 and connected with a Clark-type O2 electrode (Instech) and O2 monitor (Model 5300, YSI, Inc) [11]. After injecting the mitochondria (200 µg) into the air sealed chamber, Complex IV activity was measured by addition of TMPD/Ascorbate (0.2 mM and 5 mM) and the respiratory rate was determined [11].

Reactive Oxygen Species (ROS) Production Assay

Hydrogen peroxide (H_2O_2) production from isolated mitochondria was measured fluorimetrically by measurement of oxidation of Amplex Red to fluorescent resorufin (Life Technologies, Carlsbad, CA). Isolated heart-mitochondria was incubated in buffer containing 120 mM KCl, 1 mM EGTA, 5 mM MOPS, and 5 mM K_2HPO_4 (pH 7.25). All incubations also contained 50 µM Amplex Red and 5 U/ml of horseradish peroxidase. The increase in fluorescence at an excitation of 544 nm and an emission of 590 nm was monitored. Standard curves were generated using known amounts of hydrogen peroxide [11].

Mitochondrial Calcium Retention Capacity Assays

After the 3 week nanovector treatment protocol, we isolated the heart mitochondria, and the extra-mitochondrial calcium concentration was measured at room temperature in Costar 96-well plate reader by Fluostar (BMG Labtech Inc., Durham, NC) using 2 µM fluorescent Ca^{2+} indicator Calcium Green-5N (Molecular Probes, Eugene, OR). The fluorescence was excited at 485 nm and recorded at 520 nm. The concentration of isolated heart-mitochondria was 250 µg in a buffer containing 125 mM KCl, 10 mM MOPS, 1 mM KH_2PO_4, 2.5 mM $MgCl_2$, and 20 µM EGTA; the pH was adjusted at 7.4. We added sufficient Ca^{2+} to chelate the EGTA, followed by 10 µM Ca^{2+} pulses to assess calcium retention capacity [17]. Two measurements were made after each pulse to demonstrate that a stable value had been obtained. In the buffer only group, there are no mitochondria and therefore the difference in fluorescence is a measure of how much Ca^{2+} was taken up by the mitochondria.

Whole Hearts or Isolated Mitochondrial Fraction Preparation for Western Blot

Whole heart or isolated mitochondrial samples were lysed with RIPA buffer and protein content was measured using a Bradford assay [6]. Protein samples and molecular weight standards were separated by 1D gel electrophoresis. After transfer to a PVDF membrane, the membrane was incubated with antibody that recognizes proteins such as mt-COX-1 (Cat#sc-58347) (Santa Cruz Biotechnologies Inc., Santa Cruz), mt-COX2 (Cat#A-6404) (Life Technologies, Carlsbad, CA), MCU (Cat#ab121499), TFAM (Cat#ab131607), COX 5A (Cat#ab180129), COX 5B (Cat#ab110263) and COX VIIa (Cat#ab110268) (Abcam, Cambridge, MA) and VDAC (Cat#4866) (Cell Signaling Technologies, Danvers, MA) in Tris-Buffered Saline (pH 7.4) with 1% TWEEN 20 (TBS-T) with 5% BSA or nonfat dry milk at 4°C overnight. Membranes were incubated with the secondary antibody, appropriate horseradish peroxidase–conjugated IgG in TBS-T with 5% nonfat dry milk for 1 hour at room temperature. Immunoreactive protein was visualized using an enhanced chemiluminescence analysis kit (GE HealthCare, Piscataway, NJ).

Statistics

All the data are presented as Means ±SEM. Statistical significance ($p<0.05$) was determined between groups using ANOVA for multiple groups or Student *t*-test for two groups.

Supporting Information

File S1

Author Contributions

Conceived and designed the experiments: SD AM CS. Performed the experiments: SD DB NC VC BD. Analyzed the data: SD DB AM CS. Wrote the paper: SD AM CS.

References

1. Chen JQ, Cammarata PR, Baines CP, Yager JD (2009) Regulation of mitochondrial respiratory chain biogenesis by estrogens/estrogen receptors and physiological, pathological and pharmacological implications. Biochim. Biophys. Acta. 1793: 1540–1570.
2. Lam MP, Scruggs SB, Kim TY, Zong C, Lau E, et al. (2012) An MRM-based workflow for quantifying cardiac mitochondrial protein phosphorylation in murine and human tissue. J. Proteomics 75: 4602–4609.
3. Das S, Steenbergen C (2012) Mitochondrial Adenine Nucleotide Transport and Cardioprotection. J. Mol. Cell. Cardiol. 52: 448–453.
4. Steenbergen C, Das S, Su J, Wong R, Murphy E (2009) Cardioprotection and altered mitochondrial adenine nucleotide transport. Basic Res. Cardiol. 104: 149–156.
5. Ambros V (2004) The functions of animal microRNAs. Nature 431: 350–355.
6. Bandiera S, Rüberg S, Girard M, Cagnard N, Hanein S, et al. (2011) Nuclear outsourcing of RNA to human mitochondria. PLoS One 6: e20746.
7. Barrey E, Saint-Auret G, Bonnamy B, Damas D, Boyer O, et al. (2011) Pre-microRNA and mature microRNA in human mitochondria. PLoS One 6: e20220.
8. Bian Z, Li LM, Tang R, Hou DX, Chen X, et al. (2010) Identification of mouse liver mitochondria-associated miRNAs and their potential biological functions. Cell Res. 20: 1076–1078.
9. Kren BT, Wong PY, Sarver A, Zhang X, Zeng Y, et al. (2009) MicroRNAs identified in highly purified liver-derived mitochondria may play a role in apoptosis. RNA Biol. 6: 65–72.
10. Sripada L, Tomar D, Prajapati P, Singh R, Singh AK, et al. (2012) Systematic analysis of small RNAs associated with human mitochondria by deep sequencing: detailed analysis of mitochondrial associated miRNA. PLoS On. 7: e44873.
11. Das S, Ferlito M, Kent OA, Fox-Talbot K, Wang R, et al. (2012) Nuclear miRNA Regulates the Mitochondrial Genome in the Heart. Circ. Res. 110: 1596–1603.
12. Latronico MV, Condorelli G (2012) The might of microRNA in mitochondria. Circ. Res. 110: 1540–1542.
13. Pramanik D, Campbell NR, Karikari C, Chivukula R, Kent OA, et al. (2011) Restitution of Tumor Suppressor MicroRNAs Using a Systemic Nanovector Inhibits Pancreatic Cancer Growth in Mice. Mol. Cancer Ther. 10: 1470–1480.
14. Abel EI (1993) Physiological correlates of the forced swim test in rats. Physiology & Behavior 54: 309–317.
15. Das S, Wong R, Rajapakse N, Murphy E, Steenbergen C (2008) Glycogen synthase kinase 3 inhibition slows mitochondrial adenine nucleotide transport and regulates voltage-dependent anion channel phosphorylation. Circ. Res. 103: 983–991.
16. Wong R, Steenbergen C, Murphy E (2012) Mitochondrial permeability transition pore and calcium handling. Methods Mol. Biol. 810: 235–242.
17. Nguyen TT, Stevens MV, Kohr M, Steenbergen C, Sack MN, et al. (2011) Cysteine 203 of cyclophilin D is critical for cyclophilin D activation of the mitochondrial permeability transition pore. J. Biol. Chem. 286: 40184–40192.
18. Komary Z, Tretter L, Adam-Vizi V (2010) Membrane potential-related effect of calcium on reactive oxygen species generation in isolated brain mitochondria. Biochim. Biophys Acta. 1797: 922–928.
19. Glancy B, Balaban RS (2012) Role of mitochondrial Ca^{2+} in the regulation of cellular energetics. Biochemistry 51: 2959–2973.
20. Balaban RS (2009) The role of Ca(2+) signaling in the coordination of mitochondrial ATP production with cardiac work. Biochim. Biophys. Acta. 1787: 1334–1341.
21. van Rooij E, Marshall WS, Olson EN (2008) Toward microRNA-based therapeutics for heart disease: the sense in antisense. Circ. Res. 103: 919–928.
22. Dorn GW 2nd, Matkovich SJ, Eschenbacher WH, Zhang Y (2012) A human 3′ miR-499 mutation alters cardiac mRNA targeting and function. Circ. Res. 110: 958–967.
23. Brookes P, Darley-Usmar VM (2002) Hypothesis: the mitochondrial NO(*) signaling pathway, and the transduction of nitrosative to oxidative cell signals: an alternative function for cytochrome C oxidase. Free Radic. Biol. Med. 32: 370–374.
24. Begriche K, Massart J, Robin MA, Bonnet F, Fromenty B (2013) Mitochondrial adaptations and dysfunctions in nonalcoholic fatty liver disease. Hepatology 58: 1497–1507.
25. Mick DU, Fox TD, Rehling P (2011) Inventory control: cytochrome c oxidase assembly regulates mitochondrial translation. Nat. Rev. Mol. Cell Biol. 12: 14–20.
26. Lesnefsky EJ, Moghaddas S, Tandler B, Kerner J, Hoppel CL (2001) Mitochondrial dysfunction in cardiac disease: ischemia—reperfusion, aging, and heart failure. J. Mol. Cell. Cardiol. 33: 1065–1089.
27. Ambrosio G, Zweier JL, Duilio C, Kuppusamy P, Santoro G, et al. (1993) Evidence that mitochondrial respiration is a source of potentially toxic oxygen free radicals in intact rabbit hearts subjected to ischemia and reflow. J. Biol. Chem. 268: 18532–18541.
28. Florens L, Schmidt B, McCracken J, Ferguson-Miller S (2001) Fast deuterium access to the buried magnesium/manganese site in cytochrome c oxidase. Biochemistry 40: 7491–7497.
29. Chang TC, Wentzel EA, Kent OA, Ramachandran K, Mullendore M, et al. (2007) Transactivation of miR-34a by p53 broadly influences gene expression and promotes apoptosis. Mol. Cell. 26: 745–752.
30. Moens AL, Champion HC, Claeys MJ, Tavazzi B, Kaminski PM, et al. (2008) High-dose folic acid pretreatment blunts cardiac dysfunction during ischemia coupled to maintenance of high-energy phosphates and reduces postreperfusion injury. Circulation 117: 1810–1819.
31. Bolli R, Marbán E (1999) Molecular and cellular mechanisms of myocardial stunning. Physiol Rev. 79: 609–634.
32. Bolli R, Zughaib M, Li XY, Tang XL, Sun JZ, et al. (1995) Recurrent ischemia in the canine heart causes recurrent bursts of free radical production that have a cumulative effect on contractile function. A pathophysiological basis for chronic myocardial "stunning". J. Clin. Invest. 96: 1066–1084.
33. Kitakaze M, Weisman HF, Marban E (1988) Contractile dysfunction and ATP depletion after transient calcium overload in perfused ferret hearts. Circulation 77: 685–695.
34. Ragone MI, Consolini AE (2009) CARDIAC role of the mitochondrial Ca2+ transporters in the high-$[K+]_o$ cardioprotection of rat hearts under ischemia and reperfusion: a mechano-energetic study. J. Cardiovasc. Pharmacol. 54: 213–222.
35. Fukuda R, Zhang H, Kim JW, Shimoda L, Dang CV, et al. (2007) HIF-1 regulates cytochrome oxidase subunits to optimize efficiency of respiration in hypoxic cells. Cell 129: 111–122.

Longitudinal Strain Is a Marker of Microvascular Obstruction and Infarct Size in Patients with Acute ST-Segment Elevation Myocardial Infarction

Loïc Bière[1,2], Erwan Donal[3], Gwenola Terrien[1,2], Gaëlle Kervio[3], Serge Willoteaux[1,4], Alain Furber[1,2], Fabrice Prunier[1,2]*

1 L'UNAM Université, Angers, France, **2** Université Angers, UPRES EA3860, Laboratoire Cardioprotection, Remodelage et Thrombose, CHU Angers, Service de Cardiologie, Angers, France, **3** Service de Cardiologie et CIC-IT 804, CHU de Rennes & Laboratoire Traitement du Signal et de l'Image, INSERM U1099, Rennes, France, **4** Université Angers, UPRES EA3860, Laboratoire Cardioprotection, Remodelage et Thrombose, CHU Angers, Service de Radiologie, Angers, France

Abstract

Objectives: We assessed the value of speckle tracking imaging performed early after a first ST-segment elevation myocardial infarction (STEMI) in order to predict infarct size and functional recovery at 3-month follow-up.

Methods: 44 patients with STEMI who underwent revascularization within 12 h of symptom onset were prospectively enrolled. Echocardiography was performed 3.9±1.2 days after myocardial reperfusion, assessing circumferential (CGS), radial (RGS), and longitudinal global (GLS) strains. Late gadolinium-enhanced cardiac magnetic imaging (CMR), for assessing cardiac function, infarct size, and microvascular obstruction (MVO), was conducted 5.6±2.5 days and 99.4±4.6 days after myocardial reperfusion.

Results: GLS was evaluable in 97% of the patients, while CGS and RGS could be assessed in 85%. Infarct size significantly correlated with GLS ($R = 0.601$, $p < 0.001$), RGS ($R = -0.405$, $p = 0.010$), CGS ($R = 0.526$, $p = 0.001$), ejection fraction ($R = -0.699$, $p < 0.001$), wall motion score index (WMSI) ($R = 0.539$, $p = 0.001$), and left atrial volume ($R = 0.510$, $p < 0.001$). Baseline ejection fraction and GLS were independent predictors of 3-month infarct size. MVO mass significantly correlated with GLS ($R = 0.376$, $p = 0.010$), WMSI ($R = 0.387$, $p = 0.011$), and ejection fraction ($R = -0.389$, $p = 0.011$). In multivariate analysis, GLS was the only independent predictor of MVO mass ($p = 0.015$). Longitudinal strain $> -6.0\%$ within the infarcted area exhibited 96% specificity and 61% sensitivity for predicting the persistence of akinesia (≥3 segments) at 3-month follow-up.

Conclusions: Speckle-tracking strain imaging performed early after a STEMI is easy-to-use as a marker for persistent akinetic territories at 3 months. In addition, GLS correlated significantly with MVO and final infarct size, both parameters being relevant post-MI prognostic factors, usually obtained via CMR.

Editor: Vincenzo Lionetti, Scuola Superiore Sant'Anna, Italy

Funding: No current external funding sources for this study. The funders had no role in study design, data collection and analysis, decision to publish, or preparation of the manuscript.

Competing Interests: The authors have declared that no competing interests exist.

* E-mail: FaPrunier@chu-angers.fr

Introduction

Echocardiography is a useful tool for risk stratification and prognosis assessment following acute myocardial infarction (AMI). Several echocardiographic parameters, such as left ventricular (LV) volume, ejection fraction (EF), wall motion score index (WMSI), presence of mitral regurgitation, and left atrial volume, have been shown to provide prognostic information [1–4]. LV volume and EF are the primary means for assessing myocardial systolic function and myocardial damage after AMI. Nevertheless, it must be taken into account that these indices are global and load-dependent. The development of cardiac magnetic resonance imaging (CMR) with the tagging approach and echocardiography with the speckle-tracking strain imaging has provided additional tools to assess global and regional functions according to myocardial fiber orientation and position within the myocardial thickness [5–7]. As a result, longitudinal, radial, and circumferential functions can be distinctively assessed. Using speckle-tracking imaging, several studies have demonstrated the usefulness of longitudinal and circumferential strains in differentiating between sub-endocardial and transmural AMI, and assessing post-AMI prognosis [7–9].

CMR is currently considered to be the most reliable method for determining microvascular obstruction (MVO) in the first days after reperfusion [10] and for measuring accurately infarct size a few weeks later [11,12], both parameters being well-established prognosticators [11,13,14]. However, CMR accessibility is limited, whereas echocardiography is readily available.

In the present study, we sought to prospectively assess the value of speckle tracking imaging performed within the first days after successful reperfusion in ST-segment elevation myocardial infarc-

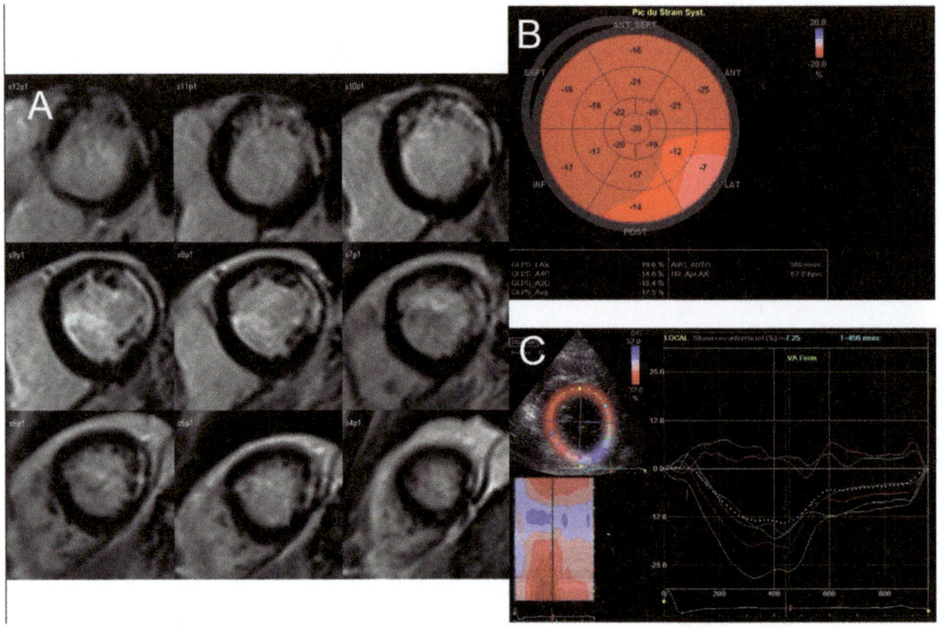

Figure 1. A case of lateral infarction related to the occlusion of the proximal circumflex coronary artery. A, CMR late gadolinium hyperenhancement slices of left ventricular short axis showing non transmural extension of myocardial infarct in the lateral zone; B, longitudinal global strain reprensented on bull's eye view; it illustrates the correspondance between the late gadolimium enhancement (A) and the blunted longitudinal strain of the basal segments of the antero-lateral and infero-lateral left ventricular walls; C, the same blunted strain of the basal antero-lateral and infero-lateral left ventricular walls is observed in parasternal view when considering the circumferential function.

tion (STEMI) patients in order to predict initial microvascular obstruction (MVO) and infarct size at a later time point.

Method

Patients with STEMI admitted to the Angers university hospital were prospectively enrolled. Inclusion criteria were as follows:

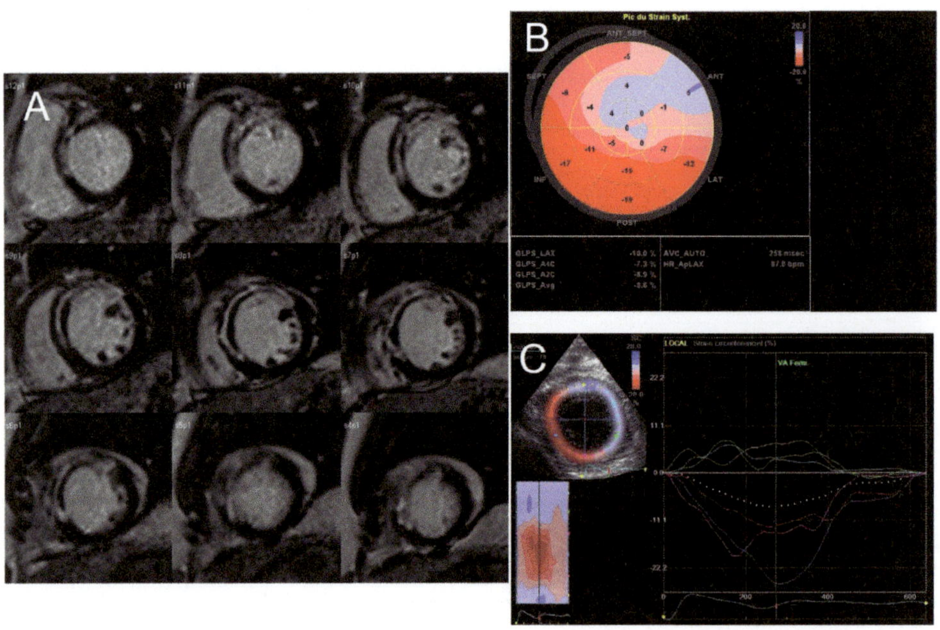

Figure 2. A case of anterior infarction related to the occlusion of the proximal left anterior descending coronary artery. A, CMR late gadolinium hyperenhancement slices of left ventricular short axis showing transmural extension of myocardial infarct in anterior and antero-septal zones and central hypoenhancement defining microvascular obstruction; B, longitudinal global strain represented on bull's eye view; there is a severe dyskinesia (blue color) of the anterior wall; C, dyskinesia is also observed in parasternal view when considering the circumferential deformation of this severe transmural infarction.

primary or rescue percutaneous coronary intervention (PCI) for first STEMI within 12 hours of symptom onset; age above 18 years; culprit coronary artery with proximal occlusion, *i.e.*, proximal or mid-left anterior descending coronary artery, proximal dominant circumflex coronary artery, or proximal right coronary artery; thrombosis in myocardial infarction (TIMI)-flow Grade 0 or 1 prior to PCI, and successful revascularisation with TIMI-flow Grade 2 or 3 after stenting. Diagnosis of STEMI was defined by chest pain for at least 30 minutes, ST-segment elevation ≥0.1 mV in at least two or more limb leads, or ST-segment elevation ≥0.2 mV in two or more contiguous precordial leads. Exclusion criteria were cardiogenic shock, history of myocardial infarction or aorto-coronary bypass surgery, contraindication to CMR and cardiac arrest before PCI.

Baseline echocardiography was performed within 5 days after myocardial reperfusion. CMR was performed at baseline, within 10 days after myocardial reperfusion in order to assess MVO, with the examination repeated at 3-month follow-up in order to quantify infarct size and infarct transmurality.

The protocol was approved by the Institutional ethics committee at the University Hospital of Angers (France), and the study was conducted in accordance with the Declaration of Helsinki and French regulatory requirements. Prior to being included into the study, the patients gave their written informed consent.

Echocardiography

Images were obtained in the left lateral decubitus position with a commercially available VIVID 7 system (GE Healthcare, Horten, Norway) using a 2.5 MHz transducer at a depth of 14 to 16 cm. Standard data on bi-dimensional echocardiography was collected according to American Society of Echocardiography (ASE) guidelines [15], with LV size evaluated by M-mode on a parasternal long axis view, and wall motion scored using a 16-segment LV model as follows: 1 = normokinetic, 2 = hypokinetic, 3 = akinetic, and 4 = dyskinetic. LV and left atrial volumes were estimated using the biplane Simpson's method from apical four-chamber and two-chamber views. Aortic stenosis and mitral regurgitation were quantified [15].

For 2D-strain analysis, apical four-, three-, and two-chamber views, and parasternal short axis view at papillary muscle level were stored in cine-loop format, triggered to the QRS complex during one heart cycle with frame rates between 55 and 70 frames/sec. These cine loops were then analyzed off-line on the EchoPAC (GE healthcare, Horten, Norway) system, based on frame-by-frame tracking of natural acoustic markers [16]. Peak systolic longitudinal strain (LS) was determined for each of the 16 segments, and longitudinal global strain was then calculated. Peak radial and circumferential systolic strains were determined from papillary muscle level short axis view, with mean values computed. All acquisitions and analyses were carried out by a single experienced cardiologist blinded to the CMR results (Figures 1 & 2).

For 2D-strain analysis, inter-observer and intra-observer agreements were determined based on recordings obtained from twenty random patients.

Cardiac Magnetic Resonance Imaging

CMR scans were performed with 1.5-T imager (Avanto, Siemens, Erlangen, Germany) using an 8-element phased-array cardiac receiver coil. Localization was carried out using breath-hold real-time and steady-state free precession images of true anatomical axes of the heart.

LV function was assessed by means of cine imaging using a segmented steady-state free precession pulse sequence in multiple short-axis, long-axis, and four-chamber views covering the entire LV. Typical in-plane resolution was 1.6×1.9 mm, with a 7.0 mm section thickness and the following parameters: repetition time (TR)/echo time (TE): 2.6 ms/1.3 ms; flip angle: 80°; matrix: 256×208; temporal resolution: 35–50 ms. Receiver bandwidth was set to 930 Hz/px and adapted to the shorter echo spacing (3.1 ms).

Late gadolinium enhancement (LGE) was performed 10–12 minutes following initiation of gadoterate meglumine (DOTAREM, Guerbet, Aulnay-sous-Bois, France), administered in cumulative dose calculated at 0.2 mmol/kg of body weight, along with a two-dimensional segmented inversion-recovery gradient-echo pulse sequence. Typical in-plane resolution was 1.68×1.68 mm, with a 7.0 mm section thickness and the following parameters: TE: 4.66 ms; flip angle: 30°; image acquisition triggered at every other heartbeat; matrix: 256×208. Inversion

Table 1. Characteristics of the patient population (n = 41).

Variable	
Age , y	57±12
Male, % (n)	82 (34)
Smoking, % (n)	56 (23)
Diabetes, % (n)	19 (8)
Hypertension, % (n)	39(16)
Family history of CAD, % (n)	41 (17)
Dyslipidemia, % (n)	56 (23)
Primary PCI, % (n)	80 (33)
Time onset of symptoms to PCI (min)	226 (176.5;303.7)
Culprit coronary artery: LAD/LCx/RCA (%)	66/17/17
Peak CPK, UI/L	1845 (1196;3149)
Medications at 3 months including aspirin, statins, clopidogrel, angiotensin-renin system inhibitors, and beta-blockers, %	95

CAD: coronary artery disease; PCI: percutaneous coronary intervention; LAD: left anterior descending coronary artery; LCx: left circumflex coronary artery; RCA: right coronary artery; CPK: creatinin phosphokinase.

Table 2. Echocardiography and CMR data.

	Baseline	3-months follow-up
Parameter	**Mean±SD**	**Mean±SD**
Echocardiographic data		
LVEDV index (mL/m^2)	75.3 (60.7;90.4)†	
LVESV index (mL/m^2)	34.9 (24.9;46.4)†	
WMSI	1.4±0.2	
LVEF (%)	51.2±7.3	
E/E′	10 (8;13)	
Deceleration time of E (ms)	207±43	
LA volume (mL)	40 (26.6;49.8)	
Sphericity index	1.6±0.2	
MR grade 1/ 2 /3/4 (%)	24/2/0/0	
GLS (%)	−13.9±3.4	
CGS (%)	−14.5±3.6	
RGS (%)	32.7±11.7	
CMR data		
LGE mass (g)	17.5 (12.0;35.0)	14.0 (7.5;24.5)*
Transmural Infarction % (n)	63 (26)	34 (14)*
LVEDV index (mL/m^2)	83.4 (72.9;96.3)	80.6 (69.2;93.9)
LVESV index (mL/m^2)	38.6 (34.1;54.5)	34.0 (27.0;51.0)*
LVEF (%)	50 (45.0;55.5)	57.0 (47.5;62.0)*
LVM index (gr/m^2)	62.9±10.9	56.0±11.0*
MVO mass (g)	2.4±2.5	

LV: left ventricular; LVEDV: LV end-diastolic volume; LVESV: LV end-systolic volume; WMSI: wall motion score index; LVEF: LV ejection fraction; LVM: LV mass; E: E peak velocity on trans-mitral Doppler; E′: E peak velocity on tissue Doppler at the mitral annulus; LA: left atrium; MR: mitral regurgitation; GLS: longitudinal global strain; CGS: circumferential global strain; RGS: radial global strain; LGE: late gadolinium enhancement.
*signifies $p<0.05$ when comparing baseline and 3-month CMR results (McNemar or Wilcoxon test).
†signifies $p<0.05$ when comparing baseline global functional parameters as assessed by TTE and CMR (Wilcoxon test).

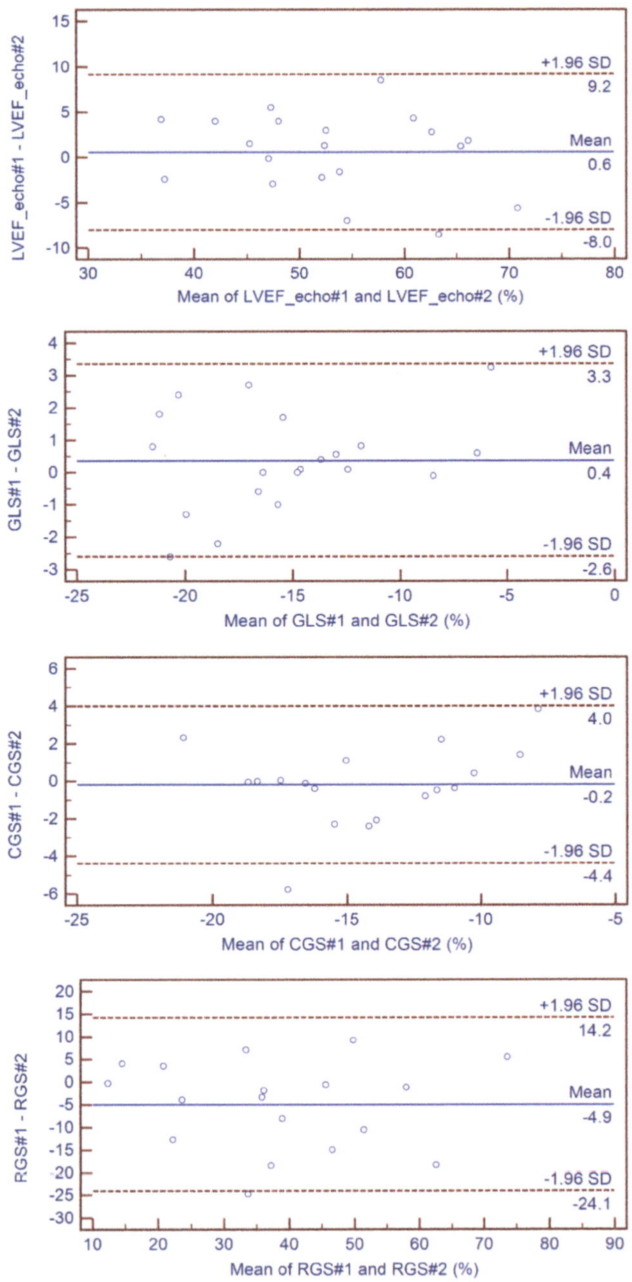

Figure 3. Interobserver Bland and Altman plots. Echo: echocardiography; LVEF: left ventricular ejection fraction; GLS: global longitudinal strain; RGS: radial global strain; CGS: circumferential global strain; #1 for observer 1 and #2 for observer 2; SD: standard deviation.

time was set to null the normal viable myocardium signal and typically ranged from 240 ms to 300 ms.

All deidentified images were analyzed at the central core laboratory by two experienced observers who were blinded to the patient data. Commercially available software (QmassMR 7.1, the Netherlands) was used for the analysis. Endocardial and epicardial borders were outlined manually on all end-diastolic and end-systolic short-axis cine slices. LV end-systolic and end-diastolic volumes, EF, and LV myocardial mass were then calculated in a standard manner.

The recommended 17-segment system was employed [17], with the two blinded observers' consensus required.

LV segmental motion was assessed visually using a three-grade scale: 0 = normal; 1 = hypokinesia; 2 = akinesia, dyskinesia, or systolic expansion.

Transmural myocardial LGE extension was assessed visually. The segmental extent of LGE was assessed as follows: 0 = 0%; 1 = 1%–25%; 2 = 26%–50%; 3 = 51%–75%; 4 = 76%–100% hyperenhancement. We considered myocardium non viable if LGE exceeded 75% of mural extent. LGE area was manually defined on all segments, and infarct size was defined as the total LGE mass. Microvascular obstruction (MVO) was identified by the presence of a central hypoenhancement within the bright signal [10], and the MVO area was manually traced on all segments. In cases where no MVO was present, MVO mass was set at zero. For CMR parameter analysis, including LV volumes, EF, mass, LGE mass, and MVO mass, inter-observer agreements were determined based on data gathered from 20 random patients.

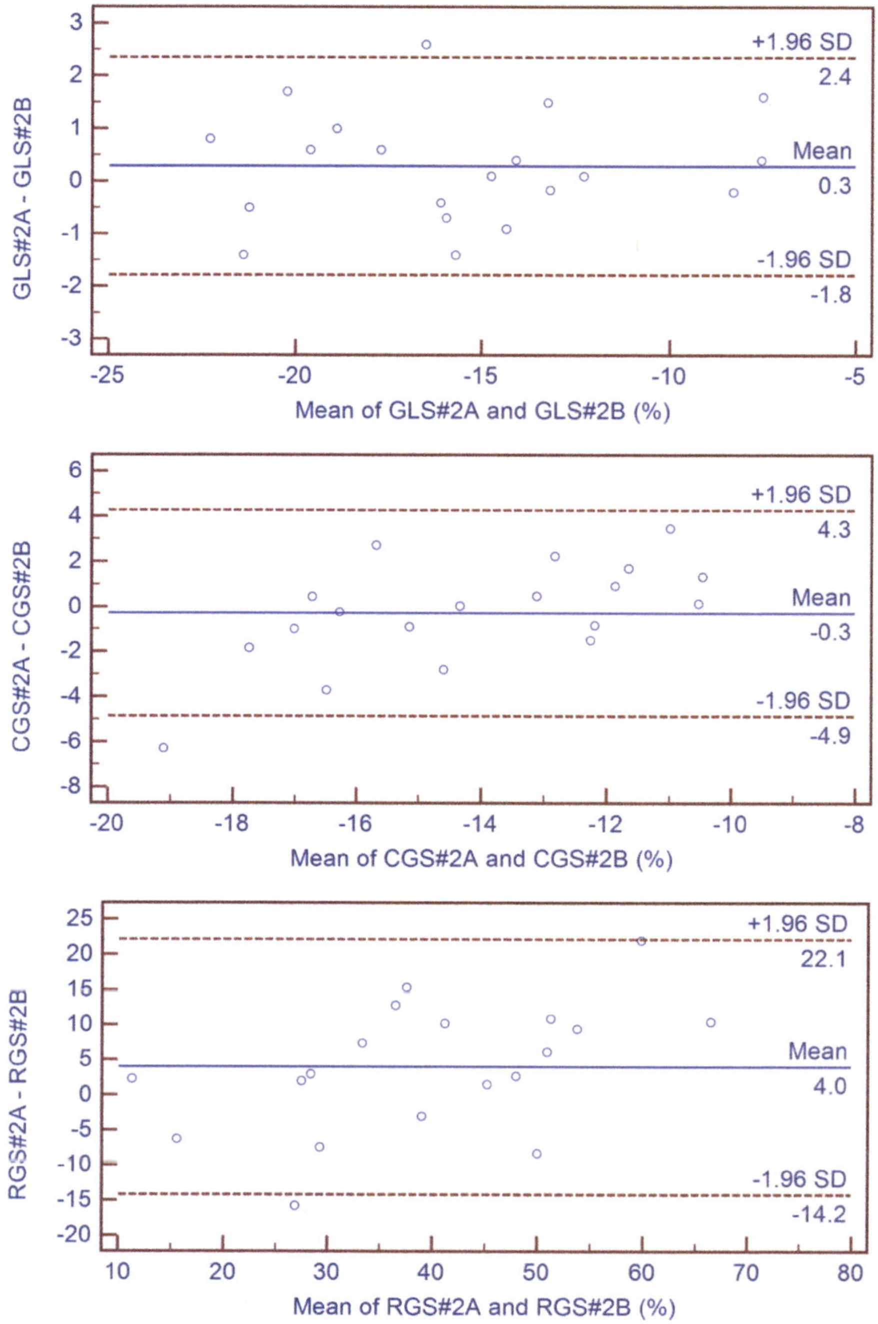

Figure 4. Intra-observer Bland and Altman plots. GLS: global longitudinal strain; RGS: radial global strain; CGS: circumferential global strain; #2A for first measurement and #2B for second measurement; SD: standard deviation.

Infarcted Area Analysis

A segment was considered as part of the infarcted area if LGE was present in more than 50% of the circumferential extent for that segment [18]. Mean LGE segmental extent in the infarcted area was calculated, with a value >75% required for the diagnosis of transmural infarction.

The mean value of longitudinal strain was calculated within the infarcted area (infarct LS) so as in the remote myocardium area.

Statistical Analysis

Data was presented as mean±standard deviation or median (25th;75th percentiles) in cases of non-normal distribution, with categorical data expressed as frequencies and percentages. We compared baseline with 3-month CMR data using McNemar test or a Chi-squared test, as appropriate. Baseline echocardiographic and CMR data obtained at 3-month follow-up was compared using Pearson's correlation test. P-values <0.05 were considered statistically significant.

For multivariate analyses, echocardiographic data was tested by a descending step-by-step linear regression analysis, including

Table 3. Multivariate analysis of echographic data for predicting CMR-derived infarct size (n = 35).

variable	Linear correlation coefficient	P value	Linear regression coefficient ß	Confidence Intervals	P value
GLS	0.601	<0.001	0.877	0.078 −1.679	0.033
RGS	−0.405	0.010			
CGS	0.526	0.001			
LVEF echo	−0.699	<0.001	−0.653	−1.077 - −0.229	0.004
WMSI	0.539	0.001			
LA volume	0.510	0.001	0.195	−0.015–0.405	0.068

GLS: global longitudinal strain; RGS: radial global strain; CGS: circumferential global strain; LVEF echo: LVEF obtained with echocardiography; WMSI: wall motion score; LA: left atrium.

variables with p values <0.05. The linear relation between dependent and independent variables was tested, as was the normal distribution of the residuals on PP plots. Analysis was performed using SPSS version 15.0 for Windows (SPPS, Inc, Chicago, IL).

We calculated the specificity, sensitivity, as well as positive and negative values of different parameters for predicting myocardial contractility recovery at 3-months (absence of recovery was defined by ≥3 akinetic segments at 3 month). ROC curves were generated.

Inter-observer agreement was studied in a blinded fashion using echocardiographic and CMR scans randomly selected from 20 patients, which were analyzed on EchoPac and QmassMR software by two different observers. Intra-observer agreement was also tested in a blinded fashion using 20 speckle tracking examinations, which were analyzed at two different times on EchoPac. Inter-and intra-observer agreements were assessed using the Bland and Altman method [19], and intraclass correlation coefficients (ICC) [20] were calculated. For radial and circumferential strain reproducibility analysis, two examinations were not evaluable due to lack of echogenicity on parasternal view.

Results

In total, 44 patients were included in the study between February 2009 and March 2010. Of these, three were excluded from analysis, one because of surgically treated significant ischemic mitral regurgitation at 1-month follow-up, another because of significant aortic stenosis, and the remaining patient because of pace-maker implantation prior to the second CMR. Characteristics of the remaining 41 patients are summarized in Table 1. Of note, two patients with acute anterior STEMI presented small inferobasal, previously unknown infarctions. Echocardiographies were conducted 3.9±1.2 days and CMR 5.6±2.5 days and 99.4±4.6 days following myocardial reperfusion, with echocardiographic and CMR data summarized in Table 2.

Feasibility and Reproducibility of 2D Strain Analysis

No patient was excluded from analysis due to insufficient apical acoustic windows. Longitudinal global strain data was assessed in 40 (97%) patients, and radial and circumferencial strain data in 35 (85%).

Bland and Altman tests for longitudinal, radial, and circumferential global strains and LVEF are illustrated in Figures 3 and 4. While longitudinal strain was the most reproducible method (ICC 0.97 [0.93;0.99]), circumferential (ICC 0.92 [0.78;0.97]), and (ICC 0.90 [0.71;0.96]) radial strains were sufficiently reproducible to be integrated in the afterward analysis. Excellent inter-observer agreements for CMR parameters were achieved with the corresponding ICC coefficients as follows: LVEF (0.99 [0.98;1.00]), LVEDV index (0.99 [0.99;1.00]), LVESV index (0.99 [0.98;1.00]), LGE mass (0.99 [0.98;1.00]), and MVO mass (0.99 [0.98;1.00]).

Correlations between Early Echocardiographic Assessment and Infarct Size as Measured by CMR at 3-month Follow-up

LGE mass evaluated at 3 months significantly correlated with the following echocardiographic data: longitudinal global strain (GLS) (R = 0.601, p<0.001), radial global strain (RGS) (R = −0.405, p = 0.010), circumferential global strain (CGS) (R = 0.526, p = 0.001), LV EF (R = −0.699, p<0.001), WMSI (R = 0.539, p = 0.001), and left atrial volume (R = 0.510, p<0.001).

In multivariate analyses, as illustrated in Table 3, baseline LVEF and GLS were independent predictors of LGE mass at 3 months (respectively, p = 0.004 and p = 0.033).

Table 4. Multivariate analysis for predicting MVO mass (n = 35).

variable	Linear correlation coefficient	p value	Linear regression coefficient ß	Confidence Interval	P value
GLS	0.376	0.01	0.403	0.071–0.605	0.015
RGS	−0.259	0.06			
WMSI	0.387	0.011			
LVEF echo	−0.389	0.011			

GLS: global longitudinal strain; RGS: radial global strain; WMSI: wall motion score; LVEF echo: LVEF obtained with echocardiography.

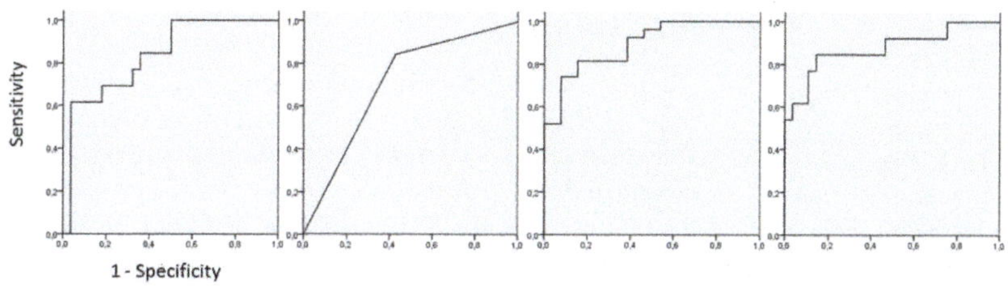

	Mean LS in the infarcted area	Microvascular obstruction	LVEF	Infarct size
ROC auc	0.835	0.709	0.892	0.876

Figure 5. Nonparametric ROC plots of several imaging baseline parameters to the presence of a 3 segment akinesia at follow-up.

When studying transmural extension of LGE at 3 months, LVEF and CGS were related to LGE above 75% of transmural extension (respectively, $p = 0.002$ and $p = 0.037$).

Echocardiographic Assessment of MVO Measured by CMR at Baseline

MVO was reported in 24 patients (58.5%), and MVO mass significantly correlated with the following echocardiographic data: GLS ($R = 0.376$, $p = 0.010$), WMSI ($R = 0.387$, $p = 0.011$), and EF ($R = -0.389$, $p = 0.011$).

In multivariate analyses, GLS was the only independent predictor of MVO mass (Table 4).

Segmental Analysis and Follow-up Functional Prognosis

Mean GLS was $-13.9 \pm 3.4\%$. Mean LS in the remote and infarcted segments was $-15.7 \pm 3.7\%$ and $-10.5 \pm 4.6\%$, respectively. Concerning the infarcted myocardium, mean LS of viable and non viable segments was $-14.8 \pm 4.6\%$ and $-9.1 \pm 4.7\%$, respectively.

Overall, 23 patients presented an akinesia affecting at least three segments at baseline, 10 having recovered at 3-month follow-up.

ROC curves for predicting akinesia ≥ 3 segments at follow-up are displayed in Figure 5. A cut-off of infarct LS $> -6.0\%$ exhibited a 96% specificity for this prediction (Figure 5 & Table 5). The association of infarct LS $> -6.0\%$ with a MVO extending over two segments increased sensitivity and specificity (Table 5).

Discussion

In the present study, 2D-strain echocardiography conducted within the first days after successful reperfusion in STEMI patients was feasible and provided relevant prognostic information. GLS was a marker of 1) MVO mass assessed a few days after reperfusion and 2) infarct size at 3-month follow-up, while 3) infarct LS $> -6.0\%$ measured at the acute phase showed good specificity for diagnosis of a persistent akinesia (≥ 3 segments) at 3-month follow-up but a poor sensitivity (61%).

Cardiac imaging techniques at the acute myocardial infarction phase mainly aim to provide prognostic factors. Infarct size is well-recognised as a strong outcome predictor following myocardial infarction [21,22], while the evaluation of transmural myocardial infarct extension is predictive of myocardial viability [23]. CMR performed a few weeks after AMI occurrence allows for quantifying these two prognostic factors using LGE [12,24]. When LGE-CMR is performed earlier, *i.e.,* a few days after reperfusion, the examination is instrumental in detecting and quantifying MVO [10,14]. All these factors are predictive of LV remodeling, which is associated with poorer outcome [25]. Echocardiography, as a bedside tool, is able to provide prognostic information at the acute myocardial infarction phase [2,26], and LVEF and WMSI are the main echocardiographic parameters strongly predictive of all-cause mortality following AMI [27,28]. In the majority of cases, LVEF is assessed using the Simpson's biplane method [29]. However, this measurement is a global LV function evaluation using a volumetric approach, and its reproducibility requires training and experience. In contrast, WMSI is rather a regional function parameter, and its evaluation is subjective. Cardiac mechanics are complex, and these two parameters do not allow us to study the spatial organization of myocardial fibers [30]. While longitudinal or long-axis function is mainly accounted for by sub-endocardial layers organized in an oblique clockwise orientation, short-axis function, reflecting the thickening of the myocardium visible in 2D-echocardiography, is mainly due to circumferentially oriented mid-layers and an outer layer arranged in an oblique anticlockwise direction.

New echocardiographic modalities, such as strain imaging, provide new insights into cardiac mechanics, with 2D-strain echocardiography being a highly promising tool [16]. This angle-

Table 5. Imaging parameters for the prediction of an akinesia affecting at least 3 segments at follow-up.

	Sensitivity (%)	Specificity (%)	PPV (%)	NPV (%)
Infarct LS>−6.0%	61	96	89	84
MVO	57	85	48	89
MVO over 2 segments	54	100	100	82
Infarct LS>−6.0% AND/OR MVO over 2 segments	85	96	92	93

LS: longitudinal strain; MVO: microvascular obstruction.

independent echocardiographic method has been validated against sonomicrometry in animals and tagged-CMR in humans for measuring myocardial deformation [31]. Longitudinal, radial, and circumferential strain can be quantified, reflecting these different deformations. Longitudinal strain has been shown to be the first altered function in AMI due to early necrosis of sub-endocardial layers of myocardial fibers [32], while radial function is still preserved. It has been demonstrated that circumferential strain allows investigators to differentiate between sub-endocardial and trans-mural infarction [9,33]. Thus, though load-dependent, these parameters provide a more accurate insight into regional myocardial function and its impact on global function.

GLS has recently been studied in AMI, being shown to exhibit a predictive value for infarct size and LVEF recovery [6,34–38]. Several studies have demonstrated the feasibility of measuring these parameters in the AMI setting [5,39]. Our study confirmed GLS's value as a marker of infarct size in AMI patients, as evaluated by CMR at 3 months. We studied strain parameters in the three main axes (radial, longitudinal, and circumferential), whereas most other published studies were chiefly focused on longitudinal strain alone [36]. Reproducibility and feasibility of GLS have been well-established in the AMI setting [5,6,34,35,39], which underlines the parameter's value as a prognostic tool. However, it appears crucial to also assess radial and circumferential strains on account of the complex organisation and interaction between these deformation parameters [7]. Therefore, in our prospective study comparing CMR and echocardiography, baseline circumferential strain provided information on the transmural extension of infarction. This clinically relevant observation is concordant with results obtained in chronic ischemic cardiomyopathy [9,15,33]. In the infarction setting, radial strain is conserved and has thus less usefullness. In the recent VALIANT echocardiographic sub-study, both longitudinal and circumferential strains were predictors of outcomes, whereas only circumferential strain was predictive of remodeling, suggesting that preserved circumferential function might help restrain ventricular enlargement after AMI. [7].

Our CMR study provided additive information on MVO, another post-MI prognostic factor, as GLS was shown to significantly correlate with MVO mass. To the best of our knowledge, MVO's influence on myocardial strain is still unclear, although MVO was shown to exhibit a significantly negative impact on regional function at the segmental level [40].

Limitations

This was a prospective, monocentric study, with echocardiography and CMR required to be performed within the first days after reperfusion. Therefore, including a large patient number proved difficult, and the main limitation of our study is its small sample size, essentially due to limited CMR accessibility. As a consequence, we were not able to assess initial strain imaging values so as to predict later LV remodeling, although encouraging results were obtained with surrogate markers, notably myocardial infarct size and MVO.

Our study was exclusively based on 2D strain analysis, itself limited to the quality of view acquisition and to its 2D nature. In-plane and out-of-plane motion may, in fact, pose a problem for strain analysis, which not encountered when using the 3D or MR-tagging approach [41].

It is worth mentioning that although the cut-offs and corresponding sensitivity, specificity, and predictive negative and positive values were specific to our dataset, they were nevertheless of particular interest in terms of defining how GLS relates to akinetic territory. However, when computing the limits of agreements for GLS (see figure 3) and the differences in GLS between viable and not viable segments in infracted myocardium, it should be cautioned that this thresholds may be insufficiently precise for an individual assessment.

Conclusion

2D-strain echocardiography carried out as a bedside test within a few days after reperfusion in STEMI patients provides indices similar to those obtained using CMR. Further studies involving larger patient series and registries are needed to confirm the parameters' prognostic value in terms of LV remodeling and clinical patient outcome.

Author Contributions

Conceived and designed the experiments: LB ED FP. Performed the experiments: LB ED GK GT SW. Analyzed the data: LB ED SW AF FP. Contributed reagents/materials/analysis tools: SW AF. Wrote the paper: LB ED.

References

1. Gibbons RJ, Valeti US, Araoz PA, Jaffe AS (2004) The quantification of infarct size. J Am Coll Cardiol 44: 1533–1542.
2. Moller JE, Hillis GS, Oh JK, Reeder GS, Gersh BJ, et al. (2006) Wall motion score index and ejection fraction for risk stratification after acute myocardial infarction. Am Heart J 151: 419–425.
3. Solomon SD, Skali H, Anavekar NS, Bourgoun M, Barvik S, et al. (2005) Changes in ventricular size and function in patients treated with valsartan, captopril, or both after myocardial infarction. Circulation 111: 3411–3419.
4. Mollema SA, Nucifora G, Bax JJ (2009) Prognostic value of echocardiography after acute myocardial infarction. Heart 95: 1732–1745.
5. Vartdal T, Brunvand H, Pettersen E, Smith HJ, Lyseggen E, et al. (2007) Early prediction of infarct size by strain Doppler echocardiography after coronary reperfusion. J Am Coll Cardiol 49: 1715–1721.
6. Park YH, Kang SJ, Song JK, Lee EY, Song JM, et al. (2008) Prognostic value of longitudinal strain after primary reperfusion therapy in patients with anterior-wall acute myocardial infarction. J Am Soc Echocardiogr 21: 262–267.
7. Hung CL, Verma A, Uno H, Shin SH, Bourgoun M, et al. (2010) Longitudinal and circumferential strain rate, left ventricular remodeling, and prognosis after myocardial infarction. J Am Coll Cardiol 56: 1812–1822.
8. Ingul CB, Torp H, Aase SA, Berg S, Stoylen A, et al. (2005) Automated analysis of strain rate and strain: feasibility and clinical implications. J Am Soc Echocardiogr 18: 411–418.
9. Chan J, Hanekom L, Wong C, Leano R, Cho GY, et al. (2006) Differentiation of subendocardial and transmural infarction using two-dimensional strain rate imaging to assess short-axis and long-axis myocardial function. J Am Coll Cardiol 48: 2026–2033.
10. Wu KC, Kim RJ, Bluemke DA, Rochitte CE, Zerhouni EA, et al. (1998) Quantification and time course of microvascular obstruction by contrast-enhanced echocardiography and magnetic resonance imaging following acute myocardial infarction and reperfusion. J Am Coll Cardiol 32: 1756–1764.
11. Gerber BL, Lima JA, Garot J, Bluemke DA (2000) Magnetic resonance imaging of myocardial infarct. Top Magn Reson Imaging 11: 372–382.
12. Wu KC, Rochitte CE, Lima JA (1999) Magnetic resonance imaging in acute myocardial infarction. Curr Opin Cardiol 14: 480–484.
13. Wu KC, Zerhouni EA, Judd RM, Lugo-Olivieri CH, Barouch LA, et al. (1998) Prognostic significance of microvascular obstruction by magnetic resonance imaging in patients with acute myocardial infarction. Circulation 97: 765–772.
14. Gerber BL, Rochitte CE, Melin JA, McVeigh ER, Bluemke DA, et al. (2000) Microvascular obstruction and left ventricular remodeling early after acute myocardial infarction. Circulation 101: 2734–2741.
15. Hanekom L, Jenkins C, Jeffries L, Case C, Mundy J, et al. (2005) Incremental value of strain rate analysis as an adjunct to wall-motion scoring for assessment of myocardial viability by dobutamine echocardiography: a follow-up study after revascularization. Circulation 112: 3892–3900.
16. Leitman M, Lysyansky P, Sidenko S, Shir V, Peleg E, et al. (2004) Two-dimensional strain-a novel software for real-time quantitative echocardiographic assessment of myocardial function. J Am Soc Echocardiogr 17: 1021–1029.

17. Cerqueira MD, Weissman NJ, Dilsizian V, Jacobs AK, Kaul S, et al. (2002) Standardized myocardial segmentation and nomenclature for tomographic imaging of the heart: a statement for healthcare professionals from the Cardiac Imaging Committee of the Council on Clinical Cardiology of the American Heart Association. Circulation 105: 539–542.
18. Ortiz-Perez JT, Rodriguez J, Meyers SN, Lee DC, Davidson C, et al. (2008) Correspondence between the 17-segment model and coronary arterial anatomy using contrast-enhanced cardiac magnetic resonance imaging. JACC Cardiovasc Imaging 1: 282–293.
19. Bland JM, Altman DG (1986) Statistical methods for assessing agreement between two methods of clinical measurement. Lancet 1: 307–310.
20. Landis JR, Koch GG (1977) The measurement of observer agreement for categorical data. Biometrics 33: 159–174.
21. Kan G, Visser CA, Koolen JJ, Dunning AJ (1986) Short and long term predictive value of admission wall motion score in acute myocardial infarction. A cross sectional echocardiographic study of 345 patients. Br Heart J 56: 422–427.
22. Pfeffer MA, Braunwald E (1990) Ventricular remodeling after myocardial infarction. Experimental observations and clinical implications. Circulation 81: 1161–1172.
23. Kim RJ, Wu E, Rafael A, Chen EL, Parker MA, et al. (2000) The use of contrast-enhanced magnetic resonance imaging to identify reversible myocardial dysfunction. N Engl J Med 343: 1445–1453.
24. Gerber BL, Garot J, Bluemke DA, Wu KC, Lima JA (2002) Accuracy of contrast-enhanced magnetic resonance imaging in predicting improvement of regional myocardial function in patients after acute myocardial infarction. Circulation 106: 1083–1089.
25. Bolognese L, Neskovic AN, Parodi G, Cerisano G, Buonamici P, et al. (2002) Left ventricular remodeling after primary coronary angioplasty: patterns of left ventricular dilation and long-term prognostic implications. Circulation 106: 2351–2357.
26. Burns RJ, Gibbons RJ, Yi Q, Roberts RS, Miller TD, et al. (2002) The relationships of left ventricular ejection fraction, end-systolic volume index and infarct size to six-month mortality after hospital discharge following myocardial infarction treated by thrombolysis. J Am Coll Cardiol 39: 30–36.
27. Savoye C, Equine O, Tricot O, Nugue O, Segrestin B, et al. (2006) Left ventricular remodeling after anterior wall acute myocardial infarction in modern clinical practice (from the REmodelage VEntriculaire [REVE] study group). Am J Cardiol 98: 1144–1149.
28. Sutton JM, Ellis SG, Roubin GS, Pinkerton CA, King SB 3rd, et al. (1994) Major clinical events after coronary stenting. The multicenter registry of acute and elective Gianturco-Roubin stent placement. The Gianturco-Roubin Intracoronary Stent Investigator Group. Circulation 89: 1126–1137.
29. Lang RM, Bierig M, Devereux RB, Flachskampf FA, Foster E, et al. (2005) Recommendations for chamber quantification: a report from the American Society of Echocardiography's Guidelines and Standards Committee and the Chamber Quantification Writing Group, developed in conjunction with the European Association of Echocardiography, a branch of the European Society of Cardiology. J Am Soc Echocardiogr 18: 1440–1463.
30. Torrent-Guasp F, Kocica MJ, Corno AF, Komeda M, Carreras-Costa F, et al. (2005) Towards new understanding of the heart structure and function. Eur J Cardiothorac Surg 27: 191–201.
31. Amundsen BH, Helle-Valle T, Edvardsen T, Torp H, Crosby J, et al. (2006) Noninvasive myocardial strain measurement by speckle tracking echocardiography: validation against sonomicrometry and tagged magnetic resonance imaging. J Am Coll Cardiol 47: 789–793.
32. Reant P, Labrousse L, Lafitte S, Bordachar P, Pillois X, et al. (2008) Experimental validation of circumferential, longitudinal, and radial 2-dimensional strain during dobutamine stress echocardiography in ischemic conditions. J Am Coll Cardiol 51: 149–157.
33. Zhang Y, Chan AK, Yu CM, Yip GW, Fung JW, et al. (2005) Strain rate imaging differentiates transmural from non-transmural myocardial infarction: a validation study using delayed-enhancement magnetic resonance imaging. J Am Coll Cardiol 46: 864–871.
34. Antoni ML, Mollema SA, Delgado V, Atary JZ, Borleffs CJ, et al. (2010) Prognostic importance of strain and strain rate after acute myocardial infarction. Eur Heart J 31: 1640–1647.
35. Mollema SA, Delgado V, Bertini M, Antoni ML, Boersma E, et al. (2010) Viability assessment with global left ventricular longitudinal strain predicts recovery of left ventricular function after acute myocardial infarction. Circ Cardiovasc Imaging 3: 15–23.
36. Grabka M, Wita K, Tabor Z, Paraniak-Gieszczyk B, Chmurawa J, et al. (2013) Prediction of infarct size by speckle tracking echocardiography in patients with anterior myocardial infarction. Coron Artery Dis 24: 127–134.
37. Cimino S, Canali E, Petronilli V, Cicogna F, De Luca L, et al. (2013) Global and regional longitudinal strain assessed by two-dimensional speckle tracking echocardiography identifies early myocardial dysfunction and transmural extent of myocardial scar in patients with acute ST elevation myocardial infarction and relatively preserved LV function. Eur Heart J Cardiovasc Imaging 14: 805–811.
38. Munk K, Andersen NH, Schmidt MR, Nielsen SS, Terkelsen CJ, et al. (2010) Remote Ischemic Conditioning in Patients With Myocardial Infarction Treated With Primary Angioplasty: Impact on Left Ventricular Function Assessed by Comprehensive Echocardiography and Gated Single-Photon Emission CT. Circ Cardiovasc Imaging 3: 656–662.
39. Sjoli B, Orn S, Grenne B, Ihlen H, Edvardsen T, et al. (2009) Diagnostic capability and reproducibility of strain by Doppler and by speckle tracking in patients with acute myocardial infarction. JACC Cardiovasc Imaging 2: 24–33.
40. Bergerot C, Mewton N, Lacote Roiron C, Ernande L, Thibault H, et al. (2010) Influence of myocardial infarction size and micro-vascular obstruction on regional myocardial deformation. Eur Heart J 31: 1060.
41. Reant P, Barbot L, Touche C, Dijos M, Arsac F, et al. (2012) Evaluation of global left ventricular systolic function using three-dimensional echocardiography speckle-tracking strain parameters. J Am Soc Echocardiogr 25: 68–79.

Clinical Implications of Sleep Disordered Breathing in Acute Myocardial Infarction

Doron Aronson[1]*, Morad Nakhleh[1], Tawfiq Zeidan-Shwiri[1], Michael Mutlak[1], Peretz Lavie[2], Lena Lavie[2]

1 Department of Cardiology, Rambam Medical Center, Haifa, Israel, **2** Lloyd Rigler Sleep Apnea Research Laboratory, The Ruth and Bruce Rappaport Faculty of Medicine, Technion, Israel Institute of Technology, Haifa, Israel

Abstract

Background: Sleep disordered breathing (SDB), characterized by nightly intermittent hypoxia, is associated with multiple pathophysiologic alterations that may adversely affect patients with acute myocardial infarction (AMI). This prospective study investigated whether the metabolic perturbations associated with SDB are present when these patients develop AMI and if they affect clinical outcomes.

Methods: We prospectively enrolled 180 AMI patients. SDB was defined as oxygen desaturation index (ODI) >5 events/hour based on a Watch Pat-100 sleep study. Blood samples were obtained for high-sensitivity C-reactive protein (hs-CRP) and markers of oxidative stress (lipid peroxides [PD] and serum paraoxonase-1 [PON-1] (arylesterase activity). Echocardiography was performed to evaluate cardiac dimensions and pulmonary artery systolic pressure.

Results: SDB was present in 116 (64%) patients. Hs-CRP levels, PD and PON-1 were similar in patients with and without SDB. Echocardiography revealed higher left atrial dimension (4.1±0.5 vs 3.8±0.5 cm; $P = 0.003$) and a significant positive correlation between ODI and pulmonary artery systolic pressure ($r = 0.41$, $P < 0.0001$). After a median follow up of 68 months, no significant differences were observed between the study groups with regard to clinical outcomes, including death, heart failure, myocardial infarction and unstable angina.

Conclusion: There is a high prevalence of previously undiagnosed SDB among patients with AMI. SDB in the setting of AMI is associated with higher pulmonary artery systolic pressure. SDB was not associated with adverse clinical outcomes.

Editor: Mark A. Sussman, San Diego State University, United States of America

Funding: The study was funded by internal departmental sources and by the LEDLER Foundation. The funders had no role in study design, data collection and analysis, decision to publish, or preparation of the manuscript.

Competing Interests: The authors have declared that no competing interests exist.

* E-mail: daronson@tx.technion.ac.il

Introduction

Sleep disordered breathing (SDB), characterized by nightly intermittent hypoxia and sleeps fragmentation, is a highly prevalent disease in the adult population [1]. There is increasing evidence that SDB is a risk factor for the development of coronary disease [2] and may trigger cardiovascular events [3].

SDB is associated with multiple alterations that may have an adverse impact in the setting of acute myocardial infarction (AMI). These include exacerbation of myocardial ischemia [4], sympathetic activation [5], systemic inflammation [6], endothelial dysfunction [7], oxidative stress [8] and increased platelet activation [9]. Thus, concomitant SDB may aggravate the clinical outcome of patients with AMI.

However, SDB is frequently not considered and therefore underdiagnosed in patients with AMI. Few data are available on the prevalence and clinical consequences of SDB in patients with AMI. Furthermore, there is no data regarding the impact of SDB on various metabolic abnormalities in patients with AMI. We hypothesized that the metabolic perturbations that are known to occur in patients with SDB may be also present in patients with AMI. We further sought to assess the impact of metabolic change as well as structural and functional alterations in left ventricular function on the clinical outcome of patients with AMI.

Methods

Patients

Patients presenting to the intensive coronary care unit with AMI and surviving the first 5 days of the event were prospectively enrolled into the study. We excluded patients with previous heart failure and patients presenting with cardiogenic shock. The ethics committee of Rambam Health Care Campus reviewed and approved the study and each patient signed an informed consent.

Endpoints definitions

The primary endpoints of the study were cardiovascular mortality, re-admission for the treatment of new heart failure, recurrent myocardial infarction and readmission for unstable angina. Myocardial infarction was diagnosed according to the Universal Definition of Myocardial Infarction [10]. The diagnosis of heart failure was confirmed using hospital records and discharge summaries. Following hospital discharge, clinical endpoint information was acquired by reviewing the national death registry and by contacting each patient individually and independently reviewing the hospital course for major clinical events if the patient had been re-hospitalized. Each endpoint was evaluated separately and as a combined endpoint.

Diagnosis of SDB

Sleep studies were performed several days after admission and preferably during the night of the last hospital day, using the Watch-PAT 100 ambulatory device. The watch-PAT 100 consists of a battery-powered, wrist-mounted, recording device and software for viewing and analysis of the recorded data. The wrist unit contains an actigraph to differentiate wake time from sleep time and 2 finger-mounted sensors. 1) a PAT probe (Itamar Medical Ltd., Caesarea, Israel) and 2) a pulse oximeter sensor (Nonin 8000 J, Plymouth, Minn). The watch-PAT 100 has been extensively validated against polysomnographic recordings for SDB diagnosis [11].

The apnea-hypopnea index (AHI) was defined as the number of episodes of apnea plus hypopnea per hour of sleep; ODI was defined as the number of decreases in oxyhemoglobin saturation by at least 3% divided by hours of sleep. SDB was defined as present when the ODI was >5 events/h [12].

Blood sampling and laboratory procedures

Venous blood samples for high sensitivity CRP (hs-CRP) and markers of oxidative stress were obtained in the morning following the sleep study.

Blood Chemistry

The lipid profile (total cholesterol, LDL and HDL cholesterol, and triglycerides), glucose, and creatinine in serum were determined by routine laboratory techniques.

Lipid Peroxides

The lipid peroxides (PD) assay was based on the method by El-Saadani et al [13]. One milliliter of color reagent (CHOD-iodide-Merck cat. no 14106) was added to 100 μL diluted plasma samples, vortexed, and let stand for 30 minutes in the dark. Absorbance was read at 365 nm against the color reagent as the blank. Data are expressed as nmol PD/mL plasma.

Paraoxonase 1-arylesterase Activity

Serum paraoxonase-1 (PON-1) arylesterase activity was measured spectrophotometrically at 270 nm with phenyl acetate as the substrate. The assay mixture consisted of 1 mmol/L of phenyl acetate and 0.9 mmol/L CaCl2 in 20 mmol/L Tris HCl, pH of 8.0, at 25°C. Nonenzymatic hydrolysis of phenyl acetate was subtracted from the total rate of hydrolysis. The data are presented as Units per minute per milliliter of serum. One unit of arylestrase activity is equal to 1 μmol of phenyl acetate hydrolyzed per minute per milliliter of serum [14].

Echocardiographic studies

Echocardiography was performed during hospital stay after a median of 2 days from admission [interquartile range 1 to 3 days]. Left ventricular and left atrial dimensions were obtained using M-mode echocardiography, guided by two-dimensional imaging. Left ventricular internal dimension and interventricular septal and posterior wall thicknesses were measured at end diastole and end systole according to the American Society of Echocardiography recommendations.

Left ventricular ejection fraction (LVEF) was assessed by a combination of the Teichholz formula and visual estimation from multiple echocardiographic windows, and classified as normal (≥ 55%), mildly reduced (45–54%), moderately reduced (30–44%) or severely reduced (<30%).

The pulmonary artery systolic pressure (PASP) was calculated as the sum of the peak systolic pressure gradient across the tricuspid valve (using the modified Bernoulli equation), and the right atrial (RA) pressure. RA pressure was estimated according to the size and respiratory variation of the inferior vena caval diameter in the subcostal view [15].

Statistical analysis

Data are expressed as mean ± SD or median and interquartile range. The baseline characteristics and laboratory parameters of the study groups were compared using unpaired *t* test for continuous variables and by the χ^2 statistic for categorical variables. When continuous data was not normally distributed or had unequal variance, groups were compared with the nonparametric Mann-Whitney U test. Spearman rank-order correlations were calculated between the various biomarkers and echocardiographic data and the sleep studies data. Multivariable linear regression analysis was used to determine the relationship between ODI and biomarkers or echocardiographic parameters, adjusting for other relevant variables.

Event–free survival was estimated by the Kaplan–Meier method for each endpoint. Stepwise Cox proportional hazards models with backward selection were used to calculate hazard ratios (HRs) and 95% CI for SDB. We sought a final parsimonious model that included only those baseline variables that differed between patients with and without SDB.

Patients receiving CPAP therapy were censored at the time of therapy initiation. Differences were considered statistically significant at the 2-sided $P<0.05$ level. Statistical analyses were performed using the STATA Version 12.0 (College Station, TX).

Results

Between February 2005 and June 2009, 220 patients with AMI were enrolled. After exclusions for technical failures (n = 40), complete sleep analyses were obtained in 150 men and 30 women. The median duration from hospital admission to sleep study was 5 days. The median ODI and AHI of the study population were 8 (interquartile range 3 to 18 events/h) and 17 events/h (interquartile range 5 to 30 events/h), respectively. One hundred sixteen patients (64%) were diagnosed as having SDB with an ODI>5/hour. All patients in which SDB was detected were notified of the sleep study results and referred to sleep medicine specialists for consultations.

The clinical characteristics of patients with and without SDB are summarized in Table 1. Patients with SDB were more likely to be older and females, and had higher prevalence of hypertension and higher BMI.

Effect of SDB on markers of inflammation and oxidative stress

Plasma hs-CRP levels were nonsignificantly higher in patients with SDB. Both PON1 and PD were similar among patients with and without SDB (Table 2).

Effect of SDB on echocardiographic parameters

Left ventricular systolic and diastolic dimensions, LVEF and left ventricular wall motion score index were similar among patients with and without SDB, while left atrial dimension was larger in patients with SDB (Table 3). There was a moderate positive correlation between LA size and ODI (r = 0.39, $P<0.001$).

Table 1. Baseline Clinical Characteristics according to ODI.

	ODI≤5	ODI>5	
Characteristics	(n = 64)	(n = 116)	P value
Age (years)	56±11	59±9	0.03
Female gender	5 (8%)	25 (22%)	0.02
Previous infarction	10 (16%)	25 (22%)	0.34
Body mass index (Kg/m^2)	26±3	30±6	< 0.0001
Lipid profile			
Total cholesterol (mg/dl)	181±49	180±43	0.90
LDL cholesterol (mg/dl)	109±40	111±38	0.48
Triglycerides (mg/dl)	171±106	157±96	0.13
HDL cholesterol (mg/dl)	38±9	44±25	0.77
Hypertension	24 (38%)	62 (53%)	0.04
Current Smoking	22 (34%)	29 (25%)	0.18
Diabetes	13 (20%)	35 (30%)	0.15
Creatinine (mg/dl)	1.0±0.3	1.0±0.3	0.51
Killip Class II-IV	6 (10%)	16 (14%)	0.38
Anterior infarction	28 (44%)	44 (38%)	0.45
ST-elevation infarction	42 (66%)	66 (57%)	0.25
Medical therapy			
Aspirin	62 (97%)	115 (99%)	0.26
Clopidogrel	57 (89%)	106 (91%)	0.61
Beta blockers	55 (86%)	103 (89%)	0.58
ACE inhibitors/ARBs	82 (81%)	63 (80%)	0.81
Statins	61 (95%)	109 (94%)	0.71
Primary angioplasty	28 (44%)	45 (39%)	0.52
Coronary revascularization	47 (84%)	86 (85%)	0.84
Sleep parameters			
Apnea-hypopnea index (events/h)	8±5	32±21	< 0.0001
ODI (events/h)	2±2	21±18	< 0.0001
Minimal O^2 Saturation (%)	89±4	83±7	< 0.0001

Data are mean ± SD or number (%). Continuous variables were compared using unpaired *t* test. Categorical variables were compared by the χ^2 statistic. ACE = Angiotensin converting enzyme; ARBs = Angiotensin II receptor blockers.

Table 3. Echocardiographic characteristics of patients with and without SDB.

	ODI≤5	ODI>5	
Characteristics	(n = 64)	(n = 116)	P value
Left ventricular end systolic dimension (cm)	3.6± 0.7	3.4±0.8	0.76
Left ventricular end diastolic dimension (cm)	5.1±0.5	5.2±0.6	0.22
Interventricular septal thickness (cm)	1.0±0.2	1.0±0.2	0.76
Posterior wall thickness (cm)	0.8±0.1	0.9±0.1	0.32
Left ventricular ejection fraction (%)	48±12	47±13	0.43
Left ventricular wall motion score index	1.5±0.5	1.6±0.4	0.30
Left atrial dimension (cm)	3.8±0.5	4.1±0.5	0.003
Pulmonary artery systolic pressure (mm Hg)	29±7	33±9	0.006

PASP was evaluable in 120 patients (71 [70%] without and 49 [62%] with SDB, respectively, $P = 0.24$). PASP was higher in patients with SDB (Table 3). There was a moderate positive correlation between ODI and PASP ($r = 0.41$, $P < 0.0001$; Figure 1). In a multivariable linear regression model, adjusting for age, gender, BMI and left ventricular systolic function, the positive relationship between PASP and ODI remained highly significant ($P = 0.001$).

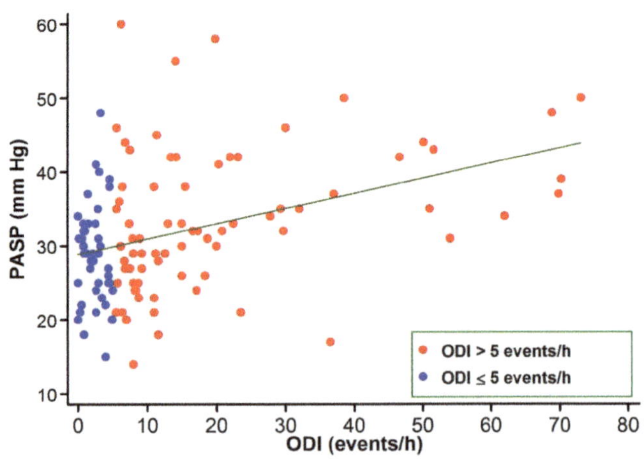

Figure 1.Correlation between ODI and pulmonary artery systolic pressure.

Table 2. Markers of inflammation and oxidative stress in patients with and without SDB.

	ODI≤5	ODI>5	
Characteristics	(n = 64)	(n = 116)	P value
C-reactive protein (mg/L)	9.4 [5.6–29.7]	15.3 [6.2–32.6]	0.33
Lipid peroxides (nmol/mL)	925 [802–1063]	897 [795–1055]	0.49
Paraoxonase 1-arylesterase Activity (U·min·^{1}ml^{-1})	76 [62–81]	71 [63–82]	0.91

Effect of SDB on clinical outcomes

The median follow-up after hospital discharge was 68 months. The rates of hard cardiovascular endpoints including death, readmission for CHF and recurrent infarctions were generally low. For the clinical outcomes analysis, 4 patients were censored at the time of CPAP therapy initiation. Figure 2 displays the Kaplan-Meier curves for the endpoint of mortality, readmission for heart failure, recurrent infarction and the combined endpoint of mortality heart failure and recurrent infarctions. Figure 3 shows the area under the ROC curves for the respective endpoints.

None of these endpoints were significantly different between patients with and without SDB with the exception of readmission for heart failure. However, after adjustments for other covariates in a Cox proportional hazards model, SDB was not an independent predictor of any of the endpoints (Table 4). Similar results were obtained in a sensitivity analysis using AHI >5 events/h for the diagnosis of SDB, and with the use of ROC-derived optimal ODI cutoffs.

Discussion

In this prospective study we found a high prevalence of previously undiagnosed SDB in patients admitted to the hospital for AMI. There were no structural and functional cardiac alterations among patients with SDB with the exception of increased left atrial dimension. However, pulmonary artery systolic pressures were elevated among patients with SDB and correlated with its severity. Contrary to our hypothesis SDB was not associated with any discernible impact on clinical outcomes with the possible exception of heart failure.

Prevalence of SDB in AMI patients

In the present study, 64% of patients admitted for AMI were diagnosed with SDB. Few data are available with regard to the prevalence of SDB among patients with acute coronary syndromes. However, although the method of diagnosis and definitions of SDB vary between studies, all have consistently demonstrated high prevalence of SDB ranging from 22% to 69% [16–21]. Similarly, in patients with stable coronary artery disease, the prevalence of SDB ranges from 30 to 54% [22,23].

The pathophysiological effects of SDB on the cardiovascular system involve complex mechanical, hemodynamic, neurohumoral, and inflammatory mechanisms [1,6]. The high prevalence of concomitant SDB in patients with acute coronary syndromes underscores the importance of better understanding of the consequences and clinical implications of SDB in these patients.

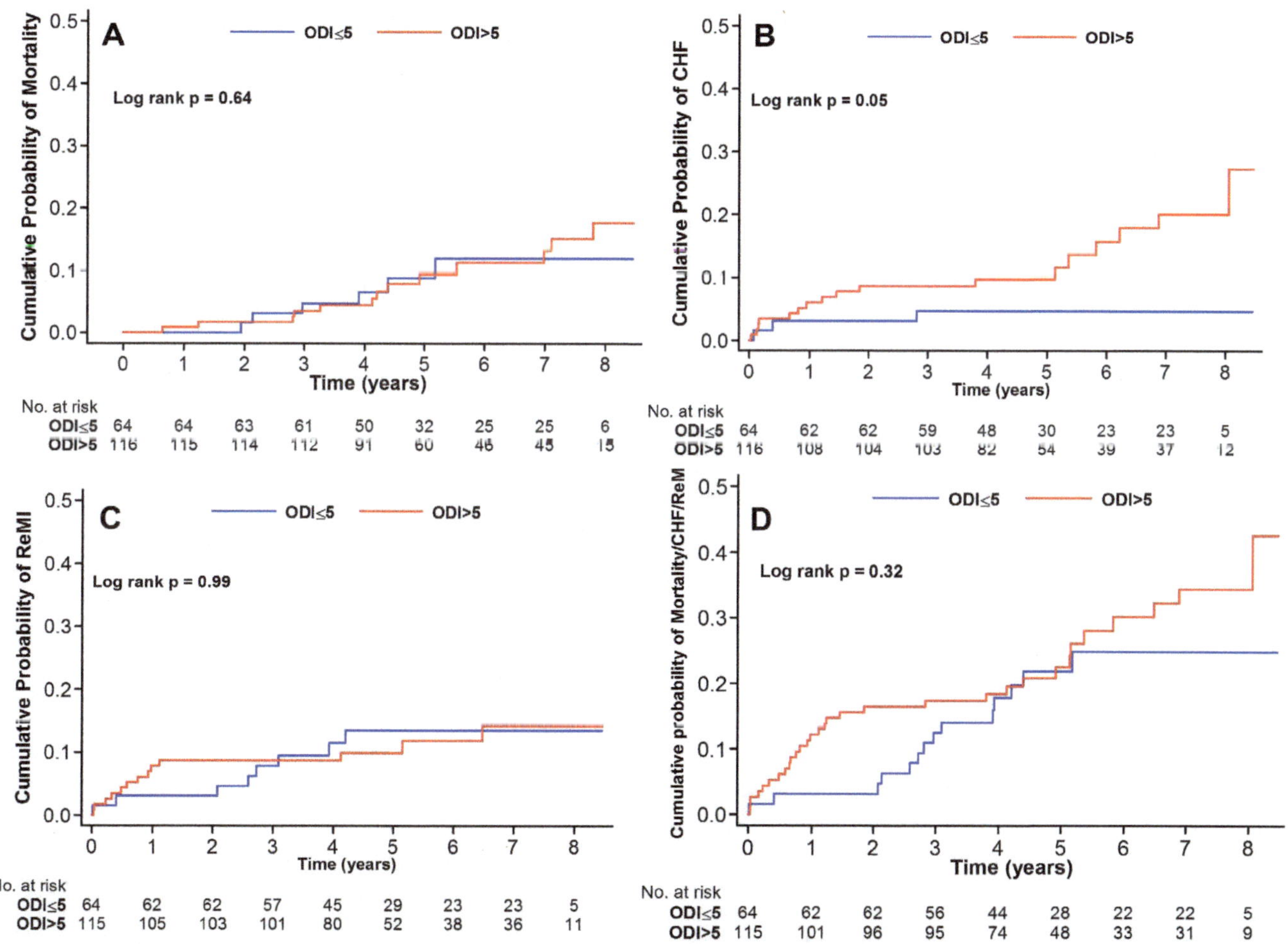

Figure 2. Kaplan-Meier curves for the clinical endpoints including mortality (A), readmission for heart failure (B), recurrent infarction (C) and the combined endpoint of mortality, readmission for heart failure and recurrent infarctions (D).

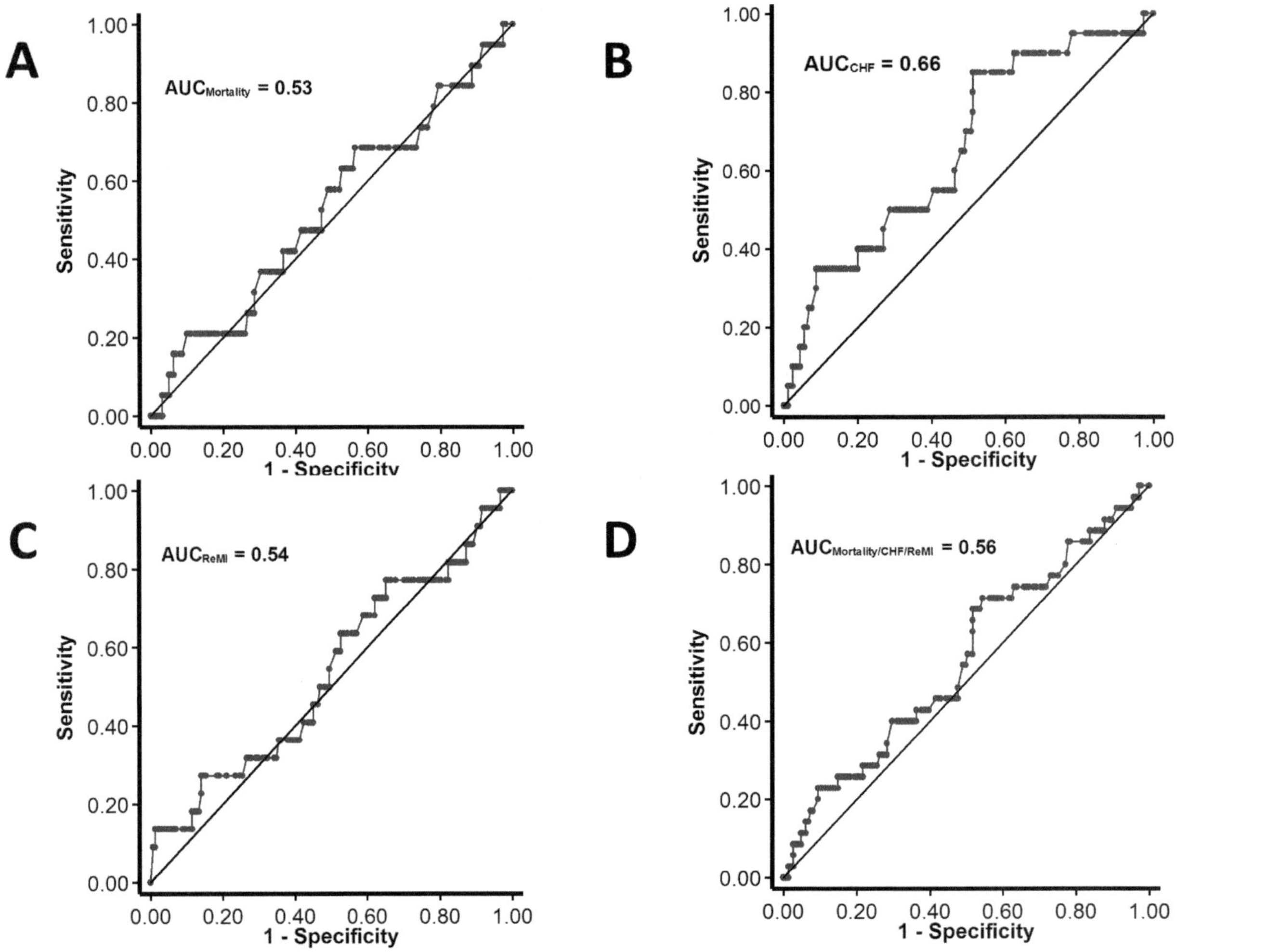

Figure 3. Receiver-operating characteristic curves for the performance of ODI in the prediction of mortality (A), congestive heart failure (B), recurrent infarction (C) and the combined endpoint of mortality, readmission for heart failure and recurrent infarctions (D).

Inflammation and oxidative stress

Previous studies have reported that patients with SDB have evidence of systemic inflammation—including elevated levels of CRP and pro-inflammatory cytokines such as tumor necrosis-α and interleukin-6 [24]. However, it remains controversial whether these findings depend more on obesity or sleep apnea. Oxidative stress has been hypothesized to be one of the plausible pathogenic mechanisms underlying the associations between SDB and coronary heart disease. There has been growing evidence that intermittent hypoxia (IH) and reoxygenation during repetitive SDB may elicit increased vascular oxidative stress [8,25]. However, few data are available regarding markers of inflammation or oxidative stress in patients with SDB in the setting of AMI [12].

Table 4. Unadjusted and Adjusted Cox's proportional Hazards Model for Clinical Endpoints in Patients with SDB.

	Unadjusted		**Adjusted**	
Endpoint	**HR (95% CI)**	***P* value**	**HR (95% CI)**	***P* value**
Mortality	1.19 (0.45–3.12)	0.73	0.88 (0.33–2.34)	0.79
Admission for heart failure	3.19 (0.93–10.88)	0.06	2.50 (0.71–8.77)	0.27
Recurrent infarction	0.93 (0.39–2.25)	0.88	0.94 (0.39–2.27)	0.89
Unstable Angina	1.40 (0.71–2.74)	0.33	1.38 (0.66–2.87)	0.39
Mortality/heart failure/recurrent infarction	1.34 (0.71–2.51)	0.37	1.05 (0.55–2.00)	0.15

Models were adjusted for age, gender, BMI and PASP.

In contrast to previous studies in stable subjects with SDB, hs-CRP, PD and the activity of the endogenous antioxidant enzyme PON1 were not affected by the presence of SDB. A possible explanation for these findings is that serum antioxidants are not elevated in patients with myocardial infarction but rather with cardiovascular risk factors, such as cigarette smoking [26] and diabetes [27]. In addition, HMG-CoA reductase inhibitors, which can reduce reactive oxygen species [28] were used in nearly all patients in the present study, potentially masking the differences between the groups.

Echocardiographic findings in SDB

In the general population, airway occlusion during sleep is associated with a reduced LVEF and increased LV end-systolic volume [29]. Recurrent acute increases in left ventricular volume might lead to eccentric remodeling and contribute to adverse left ventricular remodeling when superimposed on the acute ischemic injury in AMI patients. It is possible that the profound changes in loading conditions during apnea after an acute myocardial injury may impair the recovery of LV systolic function in patients after AMI [20]. However, in the present study, SDB was not associated with larger left ventricular internal dimensions or with reduced left ventricular systolic function. It is possible that the acute infarction was the dominant factor in determining left ventricular dimensions and function. By contrast, left atrial dimension was larger among patients with SDB. This finding may represent greater impairment of diastolic function in SDB patients [30], leading to left atrial enlargement.

Mild pulmonary hypertension is found in a sizable minority of patients with SDB, even in the absence of clinically recognizable lung disease or left-sided heart disease [31]. In the present study, pulmonary hypertension was higher in patients with SDB, and correlated positively with ODI. Pulmonary hypertension and SDB share common risk factors—namely, obesity and aging, which may confound risk factor associations [32]. Notwithstanding, the strong positive association between ODI and PASP remained significant after adjusting for age, sex, BMI and left ventricular systolic function. Importantly, elevated PASP after AMI frequently represents postcapillary pulmonary hypertension due to elevated capillary wedge pressures. As such, increased PASP is a marker of latent subclinical CHF and predicts the development of overt clinical CHF [15].

SDB and clinical outcome

In the general population, SDB is associated with increased risk for major cardiovascular events including AMI, heart failure, stroke and life-threatening arrhythmias [1,33,34]. Therefore, it may be postulated that untreated concomitant SDB might be a risk factor for adverse outcome after AMI. Potential mechanisms underlying such an association include recurrent episodes of hypoxemia and arousal from sleep after obstructive respiratory events, both of which cause an increase in sympathetic activity and blood pressure [5] that result in increased left ventricular afterload and the propensity for arrhythmias [33]. Furthermore, the forceful inspiratory efforts generated in the face of an obstructed airway result in large negative swings in intrathoracic pressure, which consequently increases transmyocardial pressure [35]. Despite of these considerations, that provided part of the rational for the present study, we observed no difference between patients with and without SDB with regard to hard clinical endpoints, with the potential exception of incident heart failure. These results are in agreement with previous studies on patients with SDB in the setting of acute coronary syndromes [16–18].

The sample size of the present study might have been insufficient to demonstrate a significant association between SDB and hard cardiovascular endpoints. In addition, survival bias toward a null result may be present as only patients who survived the first several days after the infarction were recruited. Notwithstanding, given the results of the present and previous studies [16–18], the clinical significance of SDB in the post-infarction setting remains to be established.

Although several mechanisms may promote CHF in SDB, there is also evidence that SDB might be associated with activation of cardiovascular adaptive mechanisms [12,36,37]. In this context, our group has recently demonstrated the existence of IH-associated protective mechanisms that are activated in patients with AMI. Specifically, endothelial progenitor cell numbers and proliferative and angiogenic properties are heightened in patients with AMI and coexistent SDB compared with patients with AMI without SDB [12]. Similarly, the proliferative and angiogenic properties of EPCs from healthy individuals were increased after exposure to IH *in vitro*, indicating that IH associated with SDB promotes EPC numbers and functions [12].

Conclusions

We found a high prevalence of previously undiagnosed SDB among patients admitted to the hospital with AMI. SDB in the setting of AMI is associated with higher pulmonary artery systolic pressure. SDB was not associated with adverse clinical outcomes.

Acknowledgments

We thank Ms. Eva Leder for her helpful technical support

Author Contributions

Conceived and designed the experiments: DA PL LL. Performed the experiments: MN MM TZ. Analyzed the data: DA. Wrote the paper: DA PL LL.

References

1. Somers VK, White DP, Amin R, Abraham WT, Costa F, et al. (2008) Sleep apnea and cardiovascular disease: an American Heart Association/American College of Cardiology Foundation Scientific Statement from the American Heart Association Council for High Blood Pressure Research Professional Education Committee, Council on Clinical Cardiology, Stroke Council, and Council on Cardiovascular Nursing. J Am Coll Cardiol 52: 686–717.
2. Shahar E, Whitney CW, Redline S, Lee ET, Newman AB, et al. (2001) Sleep-disordered breathing and cardiovascular disease: cross-sectional results of the Sleep Heart Health Study. Am J Respir Crit Care Med 163: 19–25.
3. Kuniyoshi FH, Garcia-Touchard A, Gami AS, Romero-Corral A, van der Walt C, et al. (2008) Day-night variation of acute myocardial infarction in obstructive sleep apnea. J Am Coll Cardiol 52: 343–346.
4. Franklin KA, Nilsson JB, Sahlin C, Naslund U (1995) Sleep apnoea and nocturnal angina. Lancet 345: 1085–1087.
5. Somers VK, Dyken ME, Clary MP, Abboud FM (1995) Sympathetic neural mechanisms in obstructive sleep apnea. J Clin Invest 96: 1897–1904.
6. McNicholas WT (2009) Obstructive sleep apnea and inflammation. Prog Cardiovasc Dis 51: 392–399.
7. Hamilton GS, Solin P, Walker A (2008) Coronary blood flow becomes uncoupled from myocardial work during obstructive sleep apnea in the presence of endothelial dysfunction. Sleep 31: 809–816.
8. Lavie L (2009) Oxidative stress--a unifying paradigm in obstructive sleep apnea and comorbidities. Prog Cardiovasc Dis 51: 303–312.
9. Hui DS, Ko FW, Fok JP, Chan MC, Li TS, et al. (2004) The effects of nasal continuous positive airway pressure on platelet activation in obstructive sleep apnea syndrome. Chest 125: 1768–1775.
10. Thygesen K, Alpert JS, White HD, Jaffe AS, Apple FS, et al. (2007) Universal definition of myocardial infarction. Circulation 116: 2634–2653.

11. Pittman SD, Ayas NT, MacDonald MM, Malhotra A, Fogel RB, et al. (2004) Using a wrist-worn device based on peripheral arterial tonometry to diagnose obstructive sleep apnea: in-laboratory and ambulatory validation. Sleep 27: 923–933.
12. Berger S, Aronson D, Lavie P, Lavie L (2013) Endothelial progenitor cells in acute myocardial infarction and sleep-disordered breathing. Am J Respir Crit Care Med 187: 90–98.
13. el-Saadani M, Esterbauer H, el-Sayed M, Goher M, Nassar AY, et al. (1989) A spectrophotometric assay for lipid peroxides in serum lipoproteins using a commercially available reagent. J Lipid Res 30: 627–630.
14. Lavie L, Vishnevsky A, Lavie P (2004) Evidence for lipid peroxidation in obstructive sleep apnea. Sleep 27: 123–128.
15. Mutlak D, Lessick J, Carasso S, Kapeliovich M, Dragu R, et al. (2012) Utility of pulmonary hypertension for the prediction of heart failure following acute myocardial infarction. Am J Cardiol 109: 1254–1259.
16. Marin JM, Carrizo SJ, Kogan I (1998) Obstructive sleep apnea and acute myocardial infarction: clinical implications of the association. Sleep 21: 809–815.
17. Lee CH, Khoo SM, Tai BC, Chong EY, Lau C, et al. (2009) Obstructive sleep apnea in patients admitted for acute myocardial infarction. Prevalence, predictors, and effect on microvascular perfusion. Chest 135: 1488–1495.
18. Yumino D, Tsurumi Y, Takagi A, Suzuki K, Kasanuki H (2007) Impact of obstructive sleep apnea on clinical and angiographic outcomes following percutaneous coronary intervention in patients with acute coronary syndrome. Am J Cardiol 99: 26–30.
19. Mehra R, Principe-Rodriguez K, Kirchner HL, Strohl KP (2006) Sleep apnea in acute coronary syndrome: high prevalence but low impact on 6-month outcome. Sleep Med 7: 521–528.
20. Nakashima H, Katayama T, Takagi C, Amenomori K, Ishizaki M, et al. (2006) Obstructive sleep apnoea inhibits the recovery of left ventricular function in patients with acute myocardial infarction. Eur Heart J 27: 2317–2322.
21. Konecny T, Kuniyoshi FH, Orban M, Pressman GS, Kara T, et al. (2010) Under-diagnosis of sleep apnea in patients after acute myocardial infarction. J Am Coll Cardiol 56: 742–743.
22. Mooe T, Rabben T, Wiklund U, Franklin KA, Eriksson P (1996) Sleep-disordered breathing in women: occurrence and association with coronary artery disease. Am J Med 101: 251–256.
23. Mooe T, Rabben T, Wiklund U, Franklin KA, Eriksson P (1996) Sleep-disordered breathing in men with coronary artery disease. Chest 109: 659–663.
24. Yokoe T, Minoguchi K, Matsuo H, Oda N, Minoguchi H, et al. (2003) Elevated levels of C-reactive protein and interleukin-6 in patients with obstructive sleep apnea syndrome are decreased by nasal continuous positive airway pressure. Circulation 107: 1129–1134.
25. Dyugovskaya L, Lavie P, Lavie L (2002) Increased adhesion molecules expression and production of reactive oxygen species in leukocytes of sleep apnea patients. Am J Respir Crit Care Med 165: 934–939.
26. Burke A, Fitzgerald GA (2003) Oxidative stress and smoking-induced vascular injury. Prog Cardiovasc Dis 46: 79–90.
27. Aronson D (2008) Hyperglycemia and the pathobiology of diabetic complications. Adv Cardiol 45: 1–16.
28. Haendeler J, Hoffmann J, Zeiher AM, Dimmeler S (2004) Antioxidant effects of statins via S-nitrosylation and activation of thioredoxin in endothelial cells: a novel vasculoprotective function of statins. Circulation 110: 856–861.
29. Chami HA, Devereux RB, Gottdiener JS, Mehra R, Roman MJ, et al. (2008) Left ventricular morphology and systolic function in sleep-disordered breathing: the Sleep Heart Health Study. Circulation 117: 2599–2607.
30. Kim SH, Cho GY, Shin C, Lim HE, Kim YH, et al. (2008) Impact of obstructive sleep apnea on left ventricular diastolic function. Am J Cardiol 101: 1663–1668.
31. Sajkov D, McEvoy RD (2009) Obstructive sleep apnea and pulmonary hypertension. Prog Cardiovasc Dis 51: 363–370.
32. Golbin JM, Somers VK, Caples SM (2008) Obstructive sleep apnea, cardiovascular disease, and pulmonary hypertension. Proc Am Thorac Soc 5: 200–206.
33. Zeidan-Shwiri T, Aronson D, Atalla K, Blich M, Suleiman M, et al. (2011) Circadian pattern of life-threatening ventricular arrhythmia in patients with sleep-disordered breathing and implantable cardioverter-defibrillators. Heart Rhythm 8: 657–662.
34. Gottlieb DJ, Yenokyan G, Newman AB, O'Connor GT, Punjabi NM, et al. (2010) Prospective Study of Obstructive Sleep Apnea and Incident Coronary Heart Disease and Heart Failure: The Sleep Heart Health Study. Circulation 122: 352–360.
35. Tkacova R, Rankin F, Fitzgerald FS, Floras JS, Bradley TD (1998) Effects of continuous positive airway pressure on obstructive sleep apnea and left ventricular afterload in patients with heart failure. Circulation 98: 2269–2275.
36. Steiner S, Schueller PO, Schulze V, Strauer BE (2010) Occurrence of coronary collateral vessels in patients with sleep apnea and total coronary occlusion. Chest 137: 516–520.
37. Lavie L, Lavie P (2010) Coronary collateral circulation in sleep apnea: a cardioprotective mechanism? Chest 137: 511–512.

18

Coronary Flow Reserve in Pregnant Rats with Increased Left Ventricular Afterload

Nils Thomas Songstad[1,2]*, Maria C. Serrano[3], Vasilis Sitras[1,4], Davis Johansen[5], Kirsti Ytrehus[5], Ganesh Acharya[1,4]

1 Women's Health and Perinatology Research Group, Institute of Clinical Medicine, Faculty of Health Sciences, UiT – The Arctic University of Norway, Tromsø, Norway, **2** Department of Pediatrics, University Hospital of Northern Norway, Tromsø, Norway, **3** Division of Pediatric Cardiology, Department of Pediatrics, University of Miami, Jackson Memorial Hospital, Miami, Florida, United States of America, **4** Department of Obstetrics and Gynecology, University Hospital of Northern Norway, Tromsø, Norway, **5** Cardiovascular Research Group, Department of Medical Biology, Faculty of Health Science, UiT – The Arctic University of Norway, Tromsø, Norway

Abstract

Background: Coronary flow reserve (CFR) is used as a measure of coronary endothelial function. We investigated the effect of increased afterload on CFR of pregnant and non-pregnant rats.

Methods: Afterload increase in Wister rats (both pregnant and non-pregnant) was achieved by the infusion of angiotensin II (Ang II) for ~10 days or by subjecting them to transverse aortic constriction (TAC) for ~14 days. Control groups were infused with 0.9% NaCl or had sham surgery, respectively. In pregnant rats, the experiments were performed close to term gestation. Doppler velocity waveforms of the left main coronary artery were recorded using a high resolution ultrasound imaging system (Vevo 770, VisualSonics, Canada) at baseline while the animals were anesthetized with 1.5% inhaled isoflurane, and during maximal coronary dilatation obtained by the inhalation of 3.5% of isoflurane. CFR was calculated as the ratio between the peak coronary flow velocities (CFR_{peak}) and the velocity-time integrals (CFR_{VTI}) recorded at hyperemia and at baseline.

Results: CFR could be calculated in 60 of 75 (80%) animals. There were no differences in CFR between intervention and control groups irrespective of whether afterload was increased by Ang II or TAC. In the TAC-study CFR_{peak} (1.54 ± 0.07 vs 1.85 ± 0.17; $p=0.03$) was decreased in pregnant compared to non-pregnant shams. When sham animals from both studies were pooled together both CFR_{peak} (1.42 ± 0.07 vs 1.86 ± 0.16; $p=0.005$) as well as CFR_{VTI} (1.45 ± 0.07 vs 1.78 ± 0.12; $p=0.03$) were significantly lower in pregnant rats compared to non-pregnant.

Conclusions: CFR can be measured non-invasively in rats using Doppler echocardiography and high concentrations of inhaled isoflurane as a coronary vasodilator. In pregnant rats, CFR is reduced close to term. CFR is not affected by increased left ventricular afterload caused by chronic Ang II infusion or TAC.

Editor: Rajesh Gopalrao Katare, University of Otago, New Zealand

Funding: This work was supported by research grants from the Northern Norway Regional Health Authority, grant numbers 1411, 1668 and 2038 (http://www.helse-nord.no/about-helse-nord/category5770.html). The funders had no role in study design, data collection and analysis, decision to publish, or preparation of the manuscript.

Competing Interests: The authors have declared that no competing interests exist.

* Email: Nils.songstad@unn.no

Introduction

Coronary flow reserve (CFR), i.e. the ratio of maximum to baseline coronary blood flow [1], is used as a measure of coronary endothelial function. Human studies have shown a link between impaired coronary microvascular function and adverse cardiovascular events [2,3]. In order to measure CFR, application of an agent with potent endothelium independent vasodilating properties is needed. Adenosine administered intravenously is usually preferred due to its rapid action and short half time [1,4], and has been used in both human [5,6] and animal studies [7,8]. Inhaled isoflurane, which is used as an anaesthetic in small animal research, is a potent coronary vasodilator. Hartley et al. have shown that the increase in coronary blood flow after administering high concentrations of inhaled isoflurane can be used to estimate CFR in mice [9,10].

Normal pregnancy is characterised by increased cardiac preload and decreased afterload [11,12]. However, in hypertensive disorders of pregnancy, and in some women with congenital heart defects, the heart may be exposed to pathologically increased afterload [13]. Increased afterload reduces CFR in humans with aortic stenosis [14], and in dogs [15] and mice [10] with cardiac hypertrophy following aortic banding. Endothelium-dependent vasodilatation can be examined non-invasively in humans measuring flow mediated dilatation (FMD) of the brachial artery [16,17], and several studies have evaluated FMD in pregnancy [18–24]. However, it is debated whether endothelial function in the peripheral vessels correlates with endothelial function in the coronary vascular bed [1,17,25,26]. Furthermore, we are not

A B C

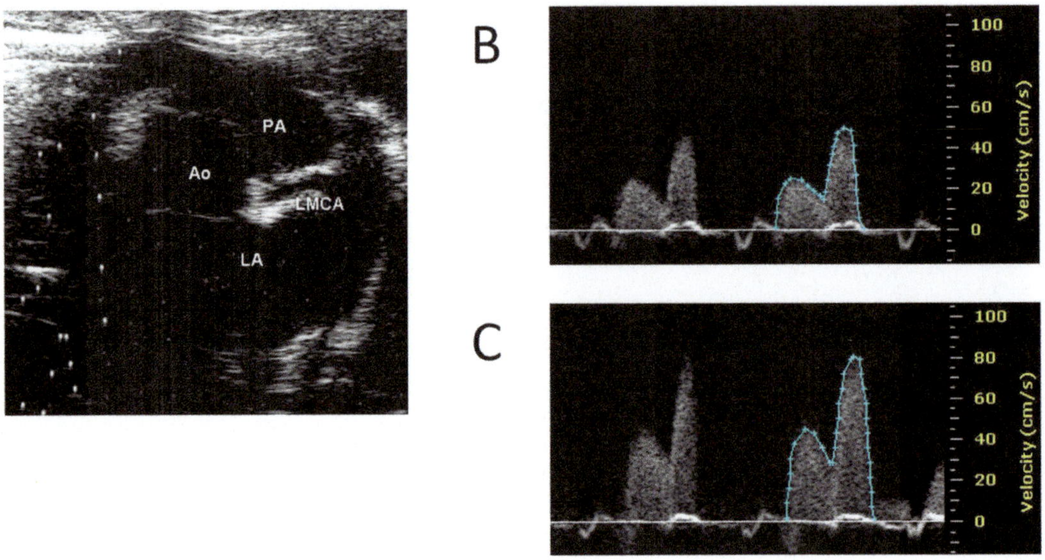

Figure 1. Measurement of coronary flow using Doppler echocardiography in rats. Parasternal short axis view of the heart (A) showing the Aorta (Ao), pulmonal artery (PA), left atrium (LA) and left main coronary artery (LMCA). Doppler velocity waveforms from the LMCA were traced and peak velocity and velocity time integrals were calculated during inhalation of 1.5% (B) and 3.5% (C) of isoflurane with oxygen.

aware of any published studies evaluating endothelial function in the coronary circulation during pregnancy, and to our knowledge the effect of increased afterload on CFR during pregnancy has not been reported.

The aims of this study were to (1) evaluate a non-invasive method of assessing CFR in rats using different concentrations of inhaled isoflurane for coronary vasodilation, (2) to investigate the differences in CFR between pregnant and non-pregnant rats and (3) to study how CFR is affected by increased afterload in pregnant and non-pregnant rats.

Materials and Methods

Ethics Statement

Animal experiments conformed to the Directive 2010/63/EU of the European Parliament on the protection of animals used for scientific purposes [27] and all procedures were approved by the Norwegian Committee on Ethics in Animal Experimentation (project ID 907 and 2177).

CFR was measured in young, female Wistar rats (Charles River, Sulzfeld, Germany) included in two experimental studies of increased cardiac afterload in pregnancy [28,29]. In the first study (Ang II-study) mini osmotic pumps (Alzet Model 2002, Cupertino, CA, USA) releasing 150 ng/kg/min of angiotensin (Ang) II (Calbiochem, Darmstadt, Germany) or 0.9% sodium chloride was implanted subcutaneously in the neck of pregnant and non-pregnant rats for ~10 days [28]. In the second study (TAC-study) transverse aorta constriction (TAC) or sham surgery was performed ~14 days before the experiments in pregnant (on gestational day 5–8) and non-pregnant rats [29]. Both interventions led to increased afterload and cardiac hypertrophy with increased mean pressure in ascending aorta (AngII-study: 110±5 mmHg vs 84±5 mmHg, $p = 0.001$. TAC-study: 127±3 mmHg vs 96±5 mmHg, $p < 0.001$) and heart weight (AngII-study: 896±30 mg vs 768±15 mg, $p = 0.001$. TAC-study: 845±29 mg vs 671±14 mg, $p < 0.001$) as well as increased expression of B-type natriuretic peptide [28,29]. In both studies the pregnant rats were examined close to term gestation (term = ~21 days). Ten male rats were used to practice and evaluate the experimental procedure, dose of inhaled isoflurane and timing of CFR measurement using Doppler echocardiography. In four non-pregnant rats we compared the effect of 140 µg/kg/min continuous adenosine [8] infusion through the external jugular vein to 3.5% isoflurane inhalation.

Echocardiography was performed using a high resolution ultrasound imaging system equipped with a RMV-710B transducer with a frequency of 25 MHz and a fixed focal length of 15 mm mounted on an integrated rail system (Vevo 770, Visualsonics, Toronto, Canada) as described earlier [28,29]. Anesthesia was induced with isoflurane 4% in 100% oxygen in an induction chamber. The rats were placed supine on a warm electric pad and inhaled isoflurane 1.5% in 100% oxygen was provided via a mask covering the rat's snout (Vevo Compact Anesthesia System, VisualSonics, Toronto, Canada) in spontaneously breathing rats (Ang II-study) or via an endotracheal tube in ventilated rats (TAC-study). The Doppler signals from the left main coronary artery (LMCA) was obtained from the parasternal short-axis view (Fig. 1A) by visualizing the aortic root and then moving the Doppler gate slightly anterior and to the left of the aorta. Doppler velocity waveforms with the highest peak flow velocity were recorded (Fig. 1B). Doppler signals could be detected even when the LMAC was not clearly visualized in B-mode echocardiography. After performing baseline measurements, the isoflurane concentration was increased to 3.5% and another recording of the LMCA Doppler signals was obtained after 2 minutes with the ultrasound probe fixed in the same position (Fig. 1C).

Echocardiography was performed without the knowledge of intervention, but the operator could not be blinded for pregnancy status. All ultrasound measurements were performed off-line without the knowledge of the animals' pregnancy status and intervention. Three consecutive cycles with good quality signals were measured and the average value was used for the statistics. Velocity-time integral (VTI) was outlined manually using the software provided with the ultrasound equipment (VisualSonics Vevo 770 v.3.0.0, Fig. 1BC), and peak velocity and VTI were calculated by the software. Angle correction was not used. CFR was calculated as the ratio between coronary flow velocities recorded at hyperemia (3.5% isoflurane) and at baseline (1.5% isoflurane). CFR_{peak} was calculated as peak velocity at hyperemia/ peak velocity at baseline and CFR_{VTI} was calculated as VTI at hyperemia/VTI at baseline. Only echocardiographic examinations performed by a single operator were included in each study (Ang II-study: M.C.S., TAC-study: N.T.S.). After ultrasound, blood pressure (BP) was measured invasively via a 2F microtip pressure-volume catheter (SPR-838; Millar Instruments Inc, Houston, TX, USA) in the ascending aorta [28,29].

Statistics

Data are reported as mean±standard error of the mean (SEM). One way analysis of variance (ANOVA) was used to compare groups and the Holm–Sidak method was used as post-hoc test. Independent-Samples T-test was used to compare two groups. Correlation between parametric variables was checked using Pearson Correlation coefficient. A p-value of <0.05 was considered statistically significant. PASW Statistics 18.0.3 (SPSS Inc., Chigaco, IL, USA) software was used for statistical analyses.

Results

In the Ang II-study we were able to obtain reliable Doppler flow velocity waveforms from the LMCA in 28 (85%) of 33 animals that had an echocardiography by the most experienced operator (M.C.S.); 13 pregnant sham, 11 pregnant Ang II, 2 non-pregnant sham, and 2 non-pregnant Ang II. Due to low numbers of non-pregnant animals, only data from pregnant animals are presented in Fig. 2. In the TAC-study echocardiography was performed by one operator (N.T.S.) in all animals. LMCA flow velocity was recorded in 36 of the 42 animals included. Four animals were excluded due to poor signal quality or inability to repeat measurements after increase of isoflurane concentration. Thus CFR measurements from 32 (76%) animals were eligible for analysis; 10 pregnant sham, 7 pregnant TAC, 7 non-pregnant sham, and 8 non-pregnant TAC.

Ten male rats were used to evaluate the effect of inhaled isoflurane on coronary flow. Coronary flow velocities increased and stabilized one to two minutes after the concentration of inhaled isoflurane was increased from 1.5% to 3.5%, and returned to baseline values three to five minutes after the isoflurane concentration was reduced to 1.5%. Increase in inhaled isoflurane concentration above 3.5% in four rats did not lead to further increase in coronary flow velocities, and there was no difference in calculated CFR_{peak} or CFR_{VTI} at 3.5% compared to 4.5% (two rats) or 5.0%(two rats) concentration of inhaled isoflurane (CFR_{peak}:1.78±0.13 vs 1.63±0.11, $p=0.4$. CFR_{VTI}: 1.96±0.29 vs 2.05±0.27, $p=0.3$). In most animals measurement of coronary flow was not feasible when the inhaled isoflurane concentration was below 1.5% as the animals would start moving and the coronary flow signals were lost. In two rats blood flow velocities were similar at 1.0% and 1.5% isoflurane.

Adenosine infusion led to a significant increase in coronary flow velocity only in one of four rats. In this rat the calculated CFR_{peak} was similar following adenosine infusion and isoflurane inhalation (1.82 and 1.89 respectively). In three rats not responding to adenosine the calculated CFR_{peak} following isoflurane inhalation was 1.11, 1.67 and 1.72.

Calculated CFR_{peak} and CFR_{VTI} values are presented in Fig. 2. There were no differences in CFR_{peak} or CFR_{VTI} between pregnant sham and pregnant AngII-infused rats. In the TAC-study CFR_{peak} (1.54±0.07 vs 1.85±0.17, $p=0.03$) but not CFR_{VTI} (1.57±0.08 vs 1.72±0.06, $p=0.3$) was decreased in pregnant compared to non-pregnant sham. TAC did not significantly affect CFR_{peak} or CFR_{VTI} in pregnant or non-pregnant animals. When pregnant ($n=23$) and non-pregnant ($n=9$) sham animals from both studies were pooled together and compared, both CFR_{peak} (1.42±0.07 vs 1.86±0.16, $p=0.005$, Fig. 3) and CFR_{VTI} (1.45±0.07 vs 1.78±0.12; $p=0.03$) were significantly decreased in pregnant animals. There was no correlation between CFR_{peak} and systolic or diastolic BP, heart weight or left ventricular contractility measured as left ventricular fractional shortening by m-mode echocardiography.

Discussion

We measured CFR non-invasively in pregnant and non-pregnant rats using high concentrations of inhaled isoflurane as a vasodilating agent. We were able to calculate CFR using Doppler flow velocity waveforms of LMCA in most animals. CFR was reduced in pregnant rats compared to non-pregnant. Furthermore, we investigated whether increased afterload has an effect on CFR in pregnant and non-pregnant rats and found that neither chronic Ang II infusion nor aorta constriction affected CFR.

In the TAC-study CFR_{peak} was reduced in pregnant compared to non-pregnant sham operated rats. The same trend was observed in sham treated rats in the AngII-study (Fig. 2A), however only two non-pregnant rats were examined and difference was not statistically significant. Combining data on sham animals from two studies, we found that both CFR_{peak} and CFR_{VTI} were significantly lower in pregnant compared to non-pregnant rats. There are no published studies on CFR in pregnancy. FMD reflects the endothelial function in the peripheral resistance vessels but may not correlate with that of the coronary vascular bed [17,25,26,30]. Studies in pregnant women have shown that FMD decreases towards term [19,20,23] which is in line with our findings.

To our knowledge, the effects of pregnancy on CFR have not been studied before, and it is not known if reduced CFR increases the risk of adverse cardiovascular events in pregnancy. A recent study showed that the utero-placental blood flow is impaired in pregnant women with congenital heart diseases [31].The course and outcome of pregnancy may be affected by maternal heart disease [32]. Death from heart disease is the leading cause of indirect maternal death in the UK [33]. Hirata et al. have shown an increase in CFR associated with increasing levels of 17β-estrogen in the follicular phase of the menstrual cycle in young, healthy women and after administration of conjugated estrogen in postmenopausal women [34]. Profound hormonal changes that occur during pregnancy could be responsible for reduced CFR that we observed in rats close to term. There is a need for non-invasive tests to asses risk and predict outcome in pregnant women at risk. Thus, studies of CFR in healthy human pregnancies and in pregnant women with hypertension or heart diseases using non-invasive methods and safe vasodilating agents (e.g. dipyridamole, a FDA category B drug) are warranted.

In contrast to previous findings in dogs [15] and mice [10] with increased afterload, in our study CFR was not reduced by Ang II infusion or TAC in rats. In addition to species differences, there could be several other reasons for this discrepancy. Hittinger et al. found that CFR was preserved in dogs with compensated heart hypertrophy, but was exhausted when the dogs developed decompensated pressure overload left ventricular hypertrophy [15]. In our studies the animals did not have decompensated heart failure when CFR was measured [28,29]. The coronary circula-

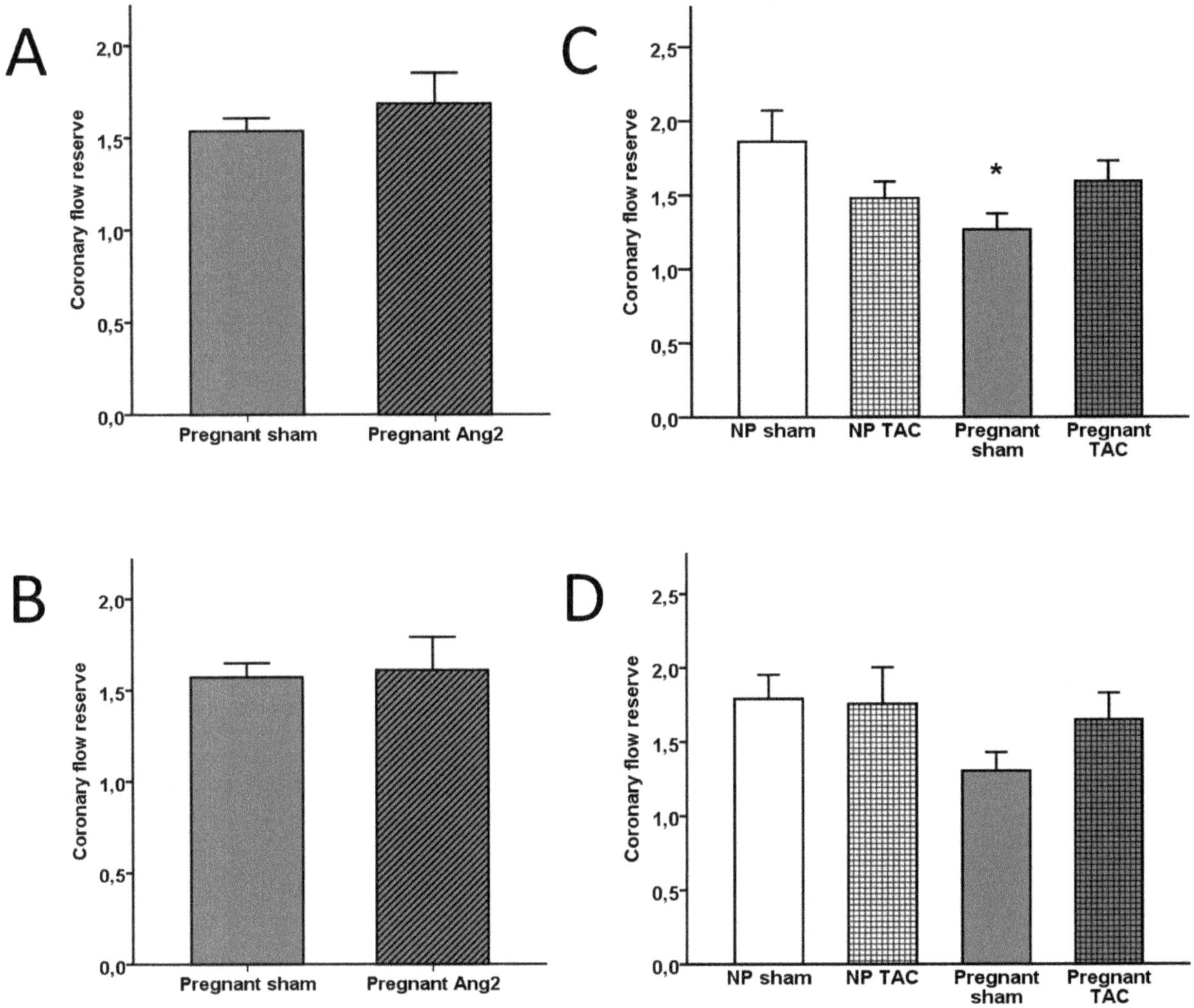

Figure 2. Coronary flow reserve in pregnant and non-pregnant rats. Mean ±SEM for coronary flow reserve calculated from peak velocities (A, C) and velocity time integrals (B, D). Comparisons between groups were made using independent samples T-test (A, B) and one-way ANOVA and Holm-Sidak post hoc test (C, D). SEM, standard error of the mean, NP, non-pregnant, Ang2, Angiotensin II, TAC, transverse aorta constriction, $p<0.05$ compared to non-pregnant sham (*).

tion is subjected to autoregulation and coronary blood flow is constant over a wide range of pressures, referred to as the 'zero pressure flow phenomenon' [1,35]. When the vascular bed of the heart is maximally vasodilated (e.g. by adenosine or isoflurane) the coronary autoregulation is revoked and coronary blood flow exhibits a linear relationship with the myocardial perfusion pressure [1,36]. Therefore, a change in blood pressure will affect CFR. As coronary flow is predominantly diastolic in the rat LMCA (Fig. 1BC), an increase in diastolic BP may increase calculated CFR. In our study, systolic rather than diastolic BP was increased following TAC and the pregnant sham animals had a significantly lower diastolic BP than all other groups [29]. Therefore, the reduced CFR in late pregnancy may be a result of reduced diastolic BP rather than impaired coronary endothelial function. Examining CFR and BP at mid-term could have added valuable information, but we refrained from anaesthetising the animals twice during pregnancy to avoid adverse effects on mother and fetuses.

In contrary to TAC, chronic Ang II infusion led to significantly increased diastolic as well as systolic pressure [28]. Furthermore, Ang II infusion led to significant fibrosis of the heart tissue, whereas TAC did not [28,29]. Thus the Ang II infused rats probably were closer to heart failure. According to the 'zero pressure flow phenomenon' an increased diastolic BP in Ang II infused rats will increase calculated CFR and may mask an actual impairment of the coronary vessels ability to dilate [1,35]. Hoffmann et al. defined CFR as the maximal increase in coronary blood flow above its basal level for a given perfusion pressure when coronary circulation is maximally dilated [37], and ideally speaking, perfusion pressure needs to be taken into account while comparing coronary flows in different animals. Thus, even though the CFR was not significantly affected by Ang II infusion, we cannot conclude that coronary microvascular dilatation is not impaired by Ang II.

The gold standard method for measuring CFR is by using adenosine infusion. We used inhaled isoflurane which is commonly used as a safe anesthetic in rats. This method is non-invasive and does not require insertion of an intravenous cannula and is more practical. We found that this method of measuring CFR in rats using different concentrations of inhaled isoflurane and echocar-

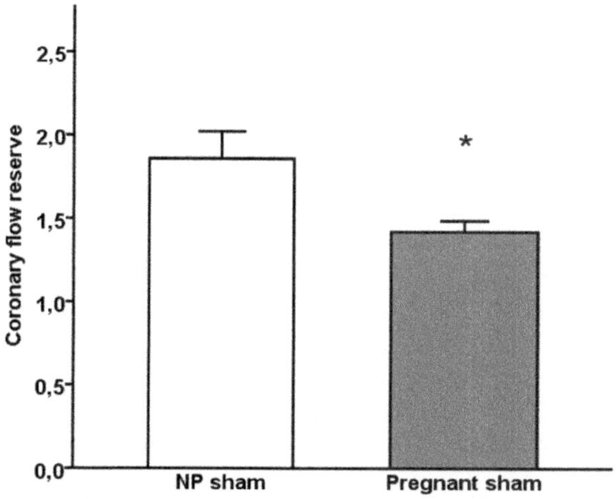

Figure 3. Coronary flow reserve in sham rats. Mean ±SEM for coronary flow reserve calculated from peak velocities in non-pregnant (NP) and pregnant sham animals from both studies. Independent-Samples T-test was used to compare groups. SEM, standard error of the mean, NP, non-pregnant, $p<0.05$ compared to non-pregnant sham (*).

diography is feasible in a laboratory setting. The operator of the Ang II-study was more experienced in small-animal echocardiography than the operator of the TAC-study and had a higher success rate in obtaining reliable CFR measurements. However, the difference between operators was not significant ($p = 0.4$). The most frequent cause of not obtaining CFR measurements was inability to detect LMCA flow velocity signals consistently. Using an ultrasound system equipped with color Doppler could facilitate the identification of coronary artery, and increase the success rate.

3.5% of isoflurane was chosen as high-concentration as this was set as the maximum maintenance dose used in rats in our laboratory. High concentrations of inhaled isoflurane may lead to reduced cardiac output, reduced BP, circulatory collapse and cardiac arrest. In four male rats an increase in isoflurane concentration above 3.5% did not lead to further increase in coronary flow velocity indicating that the coronary vessels were maximally dilated at 3.5%.

Due to the small caliber of coronary artery and limited image resolution, its diameter is difficult to measure and coronary volume blood flow cannot be calculated non-invasively. However, coronary flow reserve estimated using Doppler flow velocity waveforms correlates well with invasively measured CFR [38]. Previous studies mostly report CFR_{peak} rather than CFR_{VTI}. We have presented both the CFR_{peak} and CFR_{VTI} in our results.

An increase in peak velocity during the diastole is expected following coronary vasodilatation. However, an increase in systolic component was also observed during hyperemia (Fig. 1BC). Therefore measuring VTI of the flow velocity waveform during the whole cardiac cycle might be a better estimate of coronary flow than just the peak velocity.

Conclusions

It is feasible to measure CFR in rats non-invasively using Doppler echocardiography and high concentration of inhaled isoflurane as the vasodilating agent. CFR was not affected by increased left ventricular cardiac afterload caused by chronic Ang II infusion or TAC both in pregnant and non-pregnant rats. CFR is reduced in late pregnancy (close to term) in rats. Whether this reduction is a result of impaired coronary endothelial function or is merely a reflection of reduced diastolic BP in late pregnancy remains to be elucidated.

Author Contributions

Conceived and designed the experiments: NTS VS DJ KY GA. Performed the experiments: NTS MCS VS DJ. Analyzed the data: NTS MCS GA. Contributed reagents/materials/analysis tools: KY GA. Wrote the paper: NTS GA.

References

1. Hirata K, Amudha K, Elina R, Hozumi T, Yoshikawa J, et al. (2004) Measurement of coronary vasomotor function: getting to the heart of the matter in cardiovascular research. Clin Sci 107: 449–460.
2. Al Suwaidi J, Hamasaki S, Higano ST, Nishimura RA, Holmes DR Jr, et al. (2000) Long-term follow-up of patients with mild coronary artery disease and endothelial dysfunction. Circulation 101: 948–954.
3. Schächinger V, Britten MB, Zeiher AM (2000) Prognostic impact of coronary vasodilator dysfunction on adverse long-term outcome of coronary heart disease. Circulation 101: 1899–1906.
4. Gan LM, Wikstrom J, Fritsche-Danielson R (2013) Coronary Flow Reserve from Mouse to Man-from Mechanistic Understanding to Future Interventions. J Cardiovasc Transl Res 6: 715–728.
5. Hozumi T, Yoshida K, Ogata Y, Akasaka T, Asami Y, et al. (1998) Noninvasive Assessment of Significant Left Anterior Descending Coronary Artery Stenosis by Coronary Flow Velocity Reserve With Transthoracic Color Doppler Echocardiography. Circulation 97: 1557–1562.
6. Lethen H, Tries HP, Brechtken J, Kersting S, Lambertz H (2003) Comparison of transthoracic Doppler echocardiography to intracoronary Doppler guidewire measurements for assessment of coronary flow reserve in the left anterior descending artery for detection of restenosis after coronary angioplasty. Am J Cardiol 91: 412–417.
7. Wold LE, Ying Z, Hutchinson KR, Velten M, Gorr MW, et al. (2012) Cardiovascular Remodeling in Response to Long-Term Exposure to Fine Particulate Matter Air Pollution/Clinical Perspective. Circulation: Heart Failure 5: 452–461.
8. Hagg U, Gronros J, Wikstrom J, Jonsdottir IH, Bergstrom G, et al. (2005) Voluntary physical exercise and coronary flow velocity reserve: a transthoracic colour Doppler echocardiography study in spontaneously hypertensive rats. Clin Sci (Lond) 109: 325–334.
9. Hartley CJ, Reddy AK, Madala S, Michael LH, Entman ML, et al. (2007) Effects of Isoflurane on Coronary Blood Flow Velocity in Young, Old and ApoE−/− Mice Measured by Doppler Ultrasound. Ultrasound in Medicine & Biology 33: 512–521.
10. Hartley CJ, Reddy AK, Madala S, Michael LH, Entman ML, et al. (2008) Doppler Estimation of Reduced Coronary Flow Reserve in Mice with Pressure Overload Cardiac Hypertrophy. Ultrasound in Medicine & Biology 34: 892–901.
11. Valensise H, Novelli GP, Vasapollo B, Borzi M, Arduini D, et al. (2000) Maternal cardiac systolic and diastolic function: relationship with uteroplacental resistances. A Doppler and echocardiographic longitudinal study. Ultrasound in Obstetrics and Gynecology 15: 487–497.
12. Blanco PG, Tórtora M, Rodríguez R, Arias DO, Gobello C (2011) Ultrasonographic assessment of maternal cardiac function and peripheral circulation during normal gestation in dogs. The Veterinary Journal 190: 154–159.
13. Lang RM, Pridjian G, Feldman T, Neumann A, Lindheimer M, et al. (1991) Left ventricular mechanics in preeclampsia. Am Heart J 121: 1768–1775.
14. Marcus ML, Doty DB, Hiratzka LF, Wright CB, Eastham CL (1982) Decreased Coronary Reserve. New England Journal of Medicine 307: 1362–1366.
15. Hittinger L, Shannon RP, Bishop SP, Gelpi RJ, Vatner SF (1989) Subendomyocardial exhaustion of blood flow reserve and increased fibrosis in conscious dogs with heart failure. Circ Res 65: 971–980.
16. Celermajer DS, Sorensen KE, Gooch VM, Miller, Sullivan ID, et al. (1992) Non-invasive detection of endothelial dysfunction in children and adults at risk of atherosclerosis. The Lancet 340: 1111–1115.
17. Acharya G, Kiserud T, Lunde P (2009) Ultrasound assessment of maternal endothelial function: a tool for epidemiology. Norsk epidemiologi 19.
18. Dørup I, Skajaa K, Sørensen KE (1999) Normal pregnancy is associated with enhanced endothelium-dependent flow-mediated vasodilation. American Journal of Physiology-Heart and Circulatory Physiology 276: H821-H825.
19. Savvidou M, Kametas N, Donald A, Nicolaides K (2000) Non-invasive assessment of endothelial function in normal pregnancy. Ultrasound in obstetrics & gynecology 15: 502–507.

20. Kinzler WL, Smulian JC, Ananth CV, Vintzileos AM (2004) Noninvasive ultrasound assessment of maternal vascular reactivity during pregnancy: a longitudinal study. Obstetrics & Gynecology 104: 362.
21. Sierra-Laguado J, Garcia R, Lopez-Jaramillo P (2006) Flow-mediated dilatation of the brachial artery in pregnancy. International journal of gynecology & obstetrics 93: 60–61.
22. Saarelainen H, Laitinen T, Raitakari OT, Juonala M, Heiskanen N, et al. (2006) Pregnancy-related hyperlipidemia and endothelial function in healthy women. Circulation journal: official journal of the Japanese Circulation Society 70: 768.
23. Quinton AE, Cook C-M, Peek MJ (2007) A Longitudinal Study Using Ultrasound to Assess Flow-Mediated Dilatation in Normal Human Pregnancy. Hypertension in Pregnancy 26: 273–281.
24. Seeliger C, Brueckmann A, Schleussner E (2012) [Maternal endothelial function in the course of pregnancy and postpartum - ultrasound-based longitudinal assessment using flow-mediated dilatation (FMD)]. Ultraschall Med 33: E126–131.
25. Bøttcher M, Madsen MM, Refsgaard J, Buus NH, Dørup I, et al. (2001) Peripheral flow response to transient arterial forearm occlusion does not reflect myocardial perfusion reserve. Circulation 103: 1109–1114.
26. Khan F, Patterson D, Belch J, Hirata K, Lang C (2008) Relationship between peripheral and coronary function using laser Doppler imaging and transthoracic echocardiography. Clinical Science 115: 295–300.
27. European Parliament, Council of the European Union (2010) Directive 2010/63/EU of the European Parliament and of the Council of 22 September 2010 on the protection of animals used for scientific purposes. Official J Eur Union.
28. Aljabri MB, Songstad NT, Lund T, Serrano MC, Andreasen TV, et al. (2011) Pregnancy protects against antiangiogenic and fibrogenic effects of angiotensin II in rat hearts. Acta Physiol (Oxf) 201: 445–456.
29. Songstad NT, Johansen D, How O-J, Kaaresen PI, Ytrehus K, et al. (2014) Effect of Transverse Aortic Constriction on Cardiac Structure, Function and Gene Expression in Pregnant Rats. PLoS ONE 9: e89559.
30. Hirata K, Kadirvelu A, Kinjo M, Sciacca R, Sugioka K, et al. (2007) Altered coronary vasomotor function in young patients with systemic lupus erythematosus. Arthritis & Rheumatism 56: 1904–1909.
31. Pieper PG, Balci A, Aarnoudse JG, Kampman MAM, Sollie KM, et al. (2013) Uteroplacental Blood Flow, Cardiac Function, and Pregnancy Outcome in Women With Congenital Heart Disease. Circulation 128: 2478–2487.
32. Roos-Hesselink JW, Ruys TPE, Stein JI, Thilén U, Webb GD, et al. (2013) Outcome of pregnancy in patients with structural or ischaemic heart disease: results of a registry of the European Society of Cardiology. European Heart Journal 34: 657–665.
33. Enquiries CfMaC (2011) Saving Mothers' Lives: Reviewing maternal deaths to make motherhood safer: 2006–2008. BJOG: An International Journal of Obstetrics & Gynaecology 118: 1–203.
34. Hirata K, Shimada K, Watanabe H, Muro T, Yoshiyama M, et al. (2001) Modulation of coronary flow velocity reserve by gender, menstrual cycle and hormone replacement therapy. Journal of the American College of Cardiology 38: 1879–1884.
35. Hoffman JI, Spaan JA (1990) Pressure-flow relations in coronary circulation. Physiol Rev 70: 331–390.
36. Baumgart D, Haude M, Liu F, Ge J, Goerge G, et al. (1998) Current concepts of coronary flow reserve for clinical decision making during cardiac catheterization. Am Heart J 136: 136–149.
37. Hoffman JI (1984) Maximal coronary flow and the concept of coronary vascular reserve. Circulation 70: 153–159.
38. Wilson RF, Laughlin DE, Ackell PH, Chilian WM, Holida MD, et al. (1985) Transluminal, subselective measurement of coronary artery blood flow velocity and vasodilator reserve in man. Circulation 72: 82–92.

The Effect of Rosuvastatin on Inflammation, Matrix Turnover and Left Ventricular Remodeling in Dilated Cardiomyopathy

Kaspar Broch[1,7*◑], Erik T. Askevold[1,2◑], Erik Gjertsen[6], Thor Ueland[2,7], Arne Yndestad[2], Kristin Godang[3], Wenche Stueflotten[1], Johanna Andreassen[1], Rolf Svendsmark[4], Hans-Jørgen Smith[4,7], Svend Aakhus[1], Pål Aukrust[2,5,7], Lars Gullestad[1,7,8]

1 Department of Cardiology, Oslo University Hospital Rikshospitalet, Oslo, Norway, **2** Research Institute of Internal Medicine, Oslo University Hospital Rikshospitalet, Oslo, Norway, **3** Department of Endocrinology, Oslo University Hospital Rikshospitalet, Oslo, Norway, **4** Department of Radiology, Oslo University Hospital Rikshospitalet, Oslo, Norway, **5** Section of Clinical Immunology and Infectious Diseases, Oslo University Hospital Rikshospitalet, Oslo, Norway, **6** Department of Internal Medicine, Drammen Hospital, Vestre Viken Hospital Trust; Drammen, Norway, **7** Faculty of Medicine, University of Oslo, Oslo, Norway, **8** K. G. Jebsen Cardiac Research Centre and Center for Heart Failure Research, Faculty of Medicine, University of Oslo, Oslo, Norway

Abstract

Background: Dilated cardiomyopathy is characterized by left ventricular dilatation and dysfunction. Inflammation and adverse remodeling of the extracellular matrix may be involved in the pathogenesis. Statins reduce levels of low density lipoprotein cholesterol, but may also attenuate inflammation and affect matrix remodeling. We hypothesized that treatment with rosuvastatin would reduce or even reverse left ventricular remodeling in dilated cardiomyopathy.

Materials and Methods: In this multicenter, randomized, double blind, placebo-controlled study, 71 patients were randomized to 10 mg of rosuvastatin or matching placebo. Physical examination, blood sampling, echocardiography and cardiac magnetic resonance imaging were performed at baseline and at six months' follow-up. The pre-specified primary end point was the change in left ventricular ejection fraction from baseline to six months.

Results: Over all, left ventricular ejection fraction improved 5 percentage points over the duration of the study, but there was no difference in the change in left ventricular ejection fraction between patients allocated to rosuvastatin and those allocated to placebo. Whereas serum low density lipoprotein cholesterol concentration fell significantly in the treatment arm, rosuvastatin did not affect plasma or serum levels of a wide range of inflammatory variables, including C-reactive protein. The effect on markers of extracellular matrix remodeling was modest.

Conclusion: Treatment with rosuvastatin does not improve left ventricular ejection fraction in patients with dilated cardiomyopathy.

Trial Registration: ClinicalTrials.gov NCT00505154

Editor: Sudhiranjan Gupta, Texas A & M, Division of Cardiology, United States of America

Funding: The trial was supported by an unrestricted grant from AstraZeneca®. The trial was also sponsored by an anonymous donor. The funders had no role in study design, data collection and analysis, decision to publish, or preparation of the manuscript.

Competing Interests: This work was supported by AstraZeneca®, providing an unrestricted grant and the active drug and placebo tablets used in this study. Dr Gjertsen has received lecture fees from AstraZeneca®. In addition, the authors would like to state that 1) No research cost or salaries relevant to this work were funded, in whole or in part, by a tobacco company; 2) The anonymous donor has no competing interest in relation to this work; 3) The identity of the anonymous donor, as disclosed in an e-mail to the editorial office, is not relevant to the editors or the reviewers' assessment of the current work; 4) The authors are not aware of any competing interests.

* E-mail: kaspar.broch@ous-hf.no

◑ These authors contributed equally to this work.

Introduction

Statins are inhibitors of 3-hydroxy 3-methylglutaryl coenzyme A reductase, the rate-limiting enzyme in cholesterol synthesis. Statins significantly reduce the risk of coronary events in patients with, or at risk of developing, coronary artery disease [1] [2]. While these effects are clearly related to lipid lowering, statins also possess anti-inflammatory and matrix stabilizing properties of potential relevance to their cardioprotective effects [3]. The relative risk reduction observed in statin trials is independent of baseline cholesterol levels [1] and is associated with a treatment-induced reduction of C-reactive protein (CRP) serum concentration [4].

The role of statins in heart failure (HF) has been under debate. Two major, randomized controlled trials in patients with HF, the CORONA [5] and GISSI-HF [6] trials, did not show any effect on survival with treatment with rosuvastatin, a statin that effectively reduces the number of coronary events in a low risk population [2]. However, in several small, randomized trials, treatment with a statin has been associated with improved left ventricular (LV) function and a reduction in markers of inflammation in patients with dilated cardiomyopathy (DCM) [7] [8] [9] [10]. A meta-analysis, including the CORONA and GISSI trials, recently concluded that there is evidence to suggest that in patients with HF, statins may improve LV ejection fraction (LVEF) and reduce the number of hospitalizations for worsening HF [11]. It is unclear, however, if these effects are related to changes in immunological parameters or remodeling of the extracellular matrix.

Approximately 10% of HF cases are due to DCM [12]. Dilated cardiomyopathy is a clinical entity based on morphological criteria and exclusion of specific causes of LV dysfunction such as coronary artery disease, valvular disease or hypertension [13]. This phenotype is probably the result of a multifactorial process where external or internal stressors induce structural changes in the myocardium of individuals at risk. Dilated cardiomyopathy may thus serve as a model for studying pathogenic mechanisms in the failing myocardium *per se*, without one having to account for the confounding effect of coronary atherosclerosis. In the present study, we evaluated the effect of rosuvastatin in patients with idiopathic DCM, hypothesizing that rosuvastatin would reduce or even reverse LV remodeling in this patient population through effects on inflammation and matrix remodeling.

Materials and Methods

Study Procedures

This is a multicenter, randomized, double blind, placebo-controlled trial designed to assess the effect of rosuvastatin on LV function in patients with DCM (ClinicalTrials.gov, registration number NCT00505154; http://clinicaltrials.gov/ct2/show/NCT00505154). It was conducted at three sites in Norway. The investigation conforms with the principles outlined in the Declaration of Helsinki and was approved by the Regional Committee for Medical and Health Research Ethics South East and the Norwegian Medicines Agency. All patients provided written, informed consent. The study was performed in accordance with the Consolidated Standards of Reporting Trials (CONSORT) statement [14]. The protocol for this trial and supporting CONSORT checklist are available as supporting information; see Protocol S1 and Checklist S1.

At baseline, all participants underwent physical examination, blood tests, echocardiography and, unless contraindicated, cardiac magnetic resonance imaging (MRI). Patients were then randomized to 10 mg of rosuvastatin or matching placebo, once daily, in a 1:1 fashion. After four weeks and three months, the patients were reassessed for safety. Physical examination, blood tests, echocardiography and cardiac MRI were repeated after six months of intervention.

Patient population

Patients between 18 and 80 years old with symptoms and/or signs of HF for at least three months and with LVEF $\leq$ 40% were eligible, provided that treatment with a cholesterol-lowering drug was not otherwise indicated. Criteria for exclusion included decompensated HF requiring mechanical or inotropic support; HF of ischemic etiology; hemodynamically significant valvular disease not considered to be secondary to ventricular dilatation; recent or planned surgical procedures or operations; significant concomitant disease such as infection, severe pulmonary disease or connective tissue disease; acute or chronic liver disease; current statin treatment; or contraindications to statin therapy defined as hypersensitivity to any statin, alanine transaminase $\geq$ 2 times the upper limit of normal, serum creatinine $\geq$ 2 mg/dL, an unexplained creatine kinase $\geq$ 3 times the upper limit of normal, current or planned pregnancy, or breast feeding.

Drug handling, randomization and blinding

Rosuvastatin and matching placebo tablets were provided by the manufacturer (AstraZeneca) and appropriately stored. A randomization list was produced by an external department by computer block randomization and placed in a concealed envelope. Study drugs were provided in numbered, otherwise indistinguishable containers and dispensed in a double blind fashion by a dedicated study nurse. Study drug adherence was evaluated at one, three and six months' follow-up based on pill counts of returned, unused study medication. Compliance was considered good if more than 80% of the appropriate number of tablets had been taken.

Study outcomes

The primary objective of this study was to evaluate the effect of rosuvastatin on LV remodeling in patients with HF due to idiopathic DCM. The pre-specified primary end point was the change in LVEF from baseline to follow-up as analyzed by MRI. Due to the fact that many otherwise eligible patients had contraindications to cardiac MRI, we chose to report the change in LVEF as determined by MRI or, if the latter result was not available at both baseline and follow-up, by echocardiography. Secondary endpoints were effects on neurohormonal variables, immunological variables and markers of extracellular matrix remodeling; LV end-diastolic and end-systolic volumes as measured by MRI and echocardiography; New York Heart Association (NYHA) functional class; and quality of life. Withdrawals and side effects were recorded.

Imaging

MRI and echocardiography were performed at baseline, before study drug administration, and after six months, prior to study drug discontinuation. All image analyses were performed at Oslo University Hospital, Rikshospitalet, which served as the core laboratory. Image analyses were performed by operators blinded to patient treatment allocation.

Magnetic resonance imaging

Siemens 1.5 tesla scanners were used for MRI (Siemens Avanto and Siemens Sonata; Siemens Medical Systems, Erlangen, Germany). LV long axis and short axis views were acquired using a breath-hold, prospectively ECG-triggered, segmented, balanced, steady-state free precession gradient-echo cine sequence with minimum echo and repetition times, 6 mm slice thickness, 4 mm short-axis interslice gap, spatial resolution 1.9 mm×1.3 mm, and temporal resolution 30–35ms. LV endocardial borders were traced manually using a PACS work station (Sectra Medical Systems AB, Linköping, Sweden), and LV volumes and ejection fractions were calculated by short axis slice summation.

Echocardiography

Echocardiography was performed with Vivid 7 or E9 ultrasound scanners (GE Vingmed Ultrasound, Horten, Norway), using phased array transducers. Cine loops were digitally stored and later analyzed off line using Echo-Pac (GE Vingmed). 2D parameters and conventional Doppler parameters were measured according to current recommendations [15] [16]. Valvular regurgitations were graded as mild, moderate or severe by visual assessment [17]. LVEF was measured by Simpson's biplane method [15].

Blood sampling

Peripheral blood was collected in pyrogen-free tubes without any additives (serum) or with EDTA as anticoagulant (plasma). The tubes were allowed to coagulate at room temperature (serum) or put on melting ice (plasma) and centrifuged after coagulation (1000*g* at 10 minutes) or within 10 minutes (2000 *g* at 20 minutes) to obtain serum and platelet-poor plasma, respectively. Serum and plasma samples were stored at −80°C in multiple aliquots and thawed once only.

Biochemical analyses

N-terminal pro-B-type natriuretic peptide (NT-proBNP) was analyzed by routine methods on a MODULAR analytical platform by an electrochemiluminescence immunoassay (Roche proBNP II, Roche Diagnostic, Basel, Switzerland). Levels of CRP were determined on a MODULAR Analytical platform, P800 module (Roche Diagnostics) using a particle-enhanced immunoturbidimetric assay (Tina-Quant CRP Gen.3). Soluble tumor necrosis factor receptor type 1 (sTNF-R1), osteoprotegerin (OPG), soluble glycoprotein 130 (sgp130), matrix metalloproteinase-9 (MMP-9) and monocyte chemotactic protein-1 (MCP-1)/CCL2 were analyzed by enzyme immunoassays obtained from R&D Systems (Minneapolis, MN).

Procollagen type I and III N-terminal pro-peptides (PINP and PIIINP, respectively) were analyzed by radioimmunoassays (UniQ PINP RIA and UniQ PIIINP RIA, Orion Diagnostica, Espoo, Finland). Von Willebrand factor (vWF) was determined by an enzyme immunoassay as previously reported [18]. Inter-and intra-assay coefficients of variation were < 10% for all biochemical analyses.

Quality of life assessment

Quality of life was assessed at baseline and after six months using self-report inventories. Heart failure related symptoms were measured with the Minnesota Living with Heart Failure Questionnaire (MLHFQ) and the EuroQol visual analogue scale. Symptoms of depression were assessed using the Beck Depression Inventory.

Statistics

Assuming a standard deviation of 7.5% in LVEF measurement, we calculated that with an α of 5% and power of 80% we would need 32 patients in each group in order to observe a 5 per cent points difference in the change in LVEF between the rosuvastatin and placebo arms at follow-up. To allow for drop out, we aimed to enroll 75 patients.

To assess total population differences between baseline and follow-up, we used paired parametric (t-tests) or non-parametric (Wilcoxon signed rank) tests depending on distribution. Differences in numerical outcome variables between patients treated with rosuvastatin and patients treated with placebo were analyzed using analysis of covariance (ANCOVA), adjusting for baseline values [19]. Highly skewed parameters were log transformed prior to analysis. The number of adverse events was compared across treatment groups by Poisson regression. The between-group difference in the change in NYHA class from baseline to follow-up was analyzed by general estimating equations. All end point analyses were performed according to the intention-to-treat principle. Numerical values are presented as mean values ± SD or median (interquartile range) as appropriate. All statistical analyses were performed with the Statistical Package for Social Sciences version 18 software (SPSS Inc. Chicago, IL). Two-sided probability values were considered significant at $p < 0.05$.

Results

Patients

From the 20th of September 2007 to the 15th of February 2012, a total of 72 patients were included in Oslo (n = 57), Drammen (n = 12) and Trondheim (n = 3). A DCM phenotype had been confirmed by echocardiography prior to inclusion. Ischemic etiology had been excluded by a combination of patient history, coronary angiography (n = 71) and/or myocardial scintigraphy. Primary valvular disease was excluded by a combination of patient history and echocardiography. For administrative reasons, one patient was never randomized and was excluded from further participation in the study. Seventy-one patients were thus randomized, of whom 36 were allocated to treatment with rosuvastatin and 35 to placebo. Baseline characteristics stratified by treatment allocation are presented in Table 1. Sixty seven patients were naïve to statins, whereas five patients had stopped taking statins 5 – 61 months prior to inclusion. Throughout the study period, heart failure treatment was adjusted in an individualized fashion according to current guidelines [20]. One patient discontinued study drug treatment after 5 days and was later lost to follow up. One patient withdrew consent without stating any particular reason. Both of these patients were in the rosuvastatin arm. A total of 69 patients were thus re-evaluated after 182±20 days. In one patient, imaging data were incomplete, and this patient was excluded from analysis of the primary endpoint (Figure 1).

Left ventricular remodeling and function

Magnetic resonance imaging was performed in 53 patients at baseline. Thirteen patients had an implantable device prohibiting cardiac MRI, in one patient MRI was contraindicated due to anxiety, and in three patients, MRI was not performed for administrative reasons. Fifty of the patients in whom MRI was performed at baseline, also had an MRI at six months' follow-up. Echocardiographic images were available for all participants who were not lost to follow up, but in four patients, echocardiographic image quality did not allow for quantification of LVEF. In 68 patients, 34 in the rosuvastatin group and 34 in the placebo group, LVEF was available by MRI and/or echocardiography at baseline as well as follow-up.

Over all, LVEF improved 4.6 percentage points over the duration of the study (95% confidence interval 2.2–7.0; $p < 0.001$), but there was no difference in the adjusted LVEF between the two treatment groups after six months (Figure 2 and Table 2). The two treatment groups were well balanced for baseline characteristics. However, there was a four times higher proportion of previously hypertensive patients in the rosuvastatin arm, and a four times higher proportion of patients with atrial fibrillation in the placebo arm. Adjusting for these differences did not affect the main result. A similar pattern as for LVEF was seen for LV end diastolic and end systolic size; despite a reduction in volumes across both treatment arms, there was no between-group difference in the outcome (Table 2). Results obtained by cardiac MRI and echocardiography were highly congruous (Figure 3).

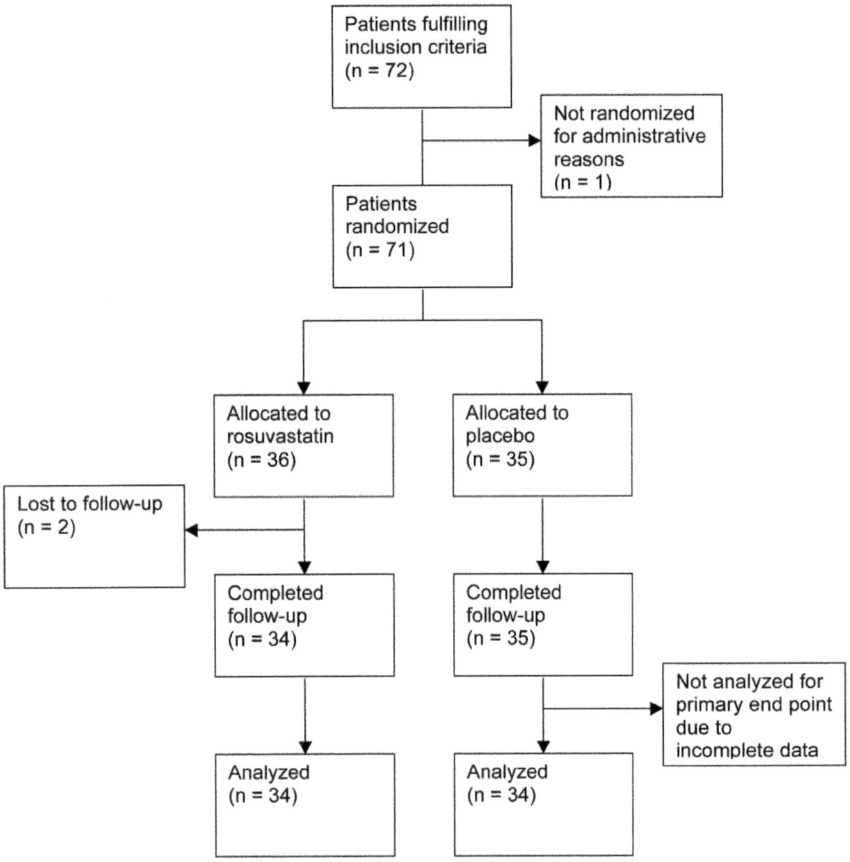

Figure 1. Trial flow chart.

Lipids and markers of inflammation, endothelial reactivity and extracellular matrix turnover

Laboratory results are presented in Table 3. Consistent with a high level of adherence to the study drug regimen, a substantial reduction in total and LDL cholesterol was observed in patients treated with rosuvastatin, resulting in a highly significant between-group difference (Figure 2 and table 3). In contrast, markers of inflammation, i.e. CRP, sTNF-R1, MCP1, sgp130 and OPG [21] and endothelial reactivity (vWF) [22] remained essentially unchanged throughout the study, and no difference was observed between treatment groups (Table 3 and Figure 4).

Among the candidate markers of extracellular matrix remodeling: MMP-9, PINP and PIIINP [23] [24] [25]; PINP and MMP-9 increased significantly throughout the study period for the population as a whole ($p = 0.03$ and 0.03, respectively).

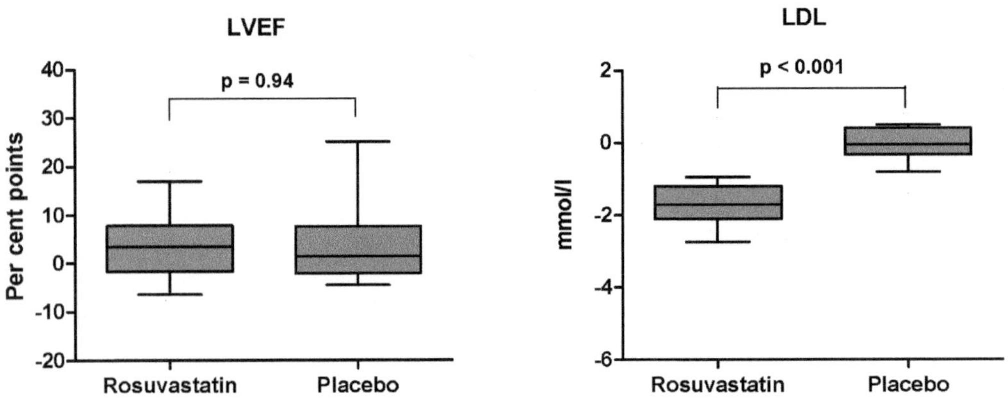

Figure 2. Changes in left ventricular ejection fraction and LDL cholesterol. The left panel illustrates the change in left ventricular ejection fraction (LVEF) stratified by treatment allocation. There was no difference in the change in LVEF between the two groups as analyzed by an independent group t-test ($p = 0.94$). The right panel illustrates the change in LDL cholesterol stratified by treatment allocation. The fall in LDL cholesterol occurred in patients allocated to rosuvastatin (p for difference < 0.001). Boxes: 25–75 percentiles; whiskers: 10–90 percentiles.

Table 1. Baseline data stratified according to treatment allocation.

Variable	All patients	Rosuvastatin (N = 36)	Placebo (N = 35)
Clinical characteristics			
Age - years	58±11	58±11	58±11
Men – no (%)	55 (78)	27 (75)	28 (80)
Body mass index	28±5	28±5	28±5
Systolic blood pressure - mm Hg	125±20	128±23	123±17
Diastolic blood pressure - mm Hg	77±10	77±11	76±9
Heart rate – beats/minute	67±12	66±11	69±13
Atrial fibrillation – no (%)	15 (21)	3 (8)	12 (34)
NYHA class I – no (%)	8 (11)	4 (11)	4 (11)
NYHA class II – no (%)	43 (62)	21 (58)	22 (63)
NYHA class III – no (%)	20 (28)	11 (31)	9 (26)
Medical history			
Smokers – no (%)	13 (18)	6 (17)	7 (20)
History of hypertension – no (%)	21 (30)	17 (47)	4 (11)
Diabetes mellitus – no (%)	10 (14)	7 (19)	3 (7)
Prior stroke/TIA – no (%)	2 (3)	1 (3)	1 (3)
Baseline medication			
ACEI and/or ARB no (%)	71 (100)	36 (100)	35 (100)
Beta blocker – no (%)	70 (99)	35 (97)	35 (100)
Aldosterone antagonist – no (%)	30 (42)	18 (50)	12 (34)
Diuretic – no (%)	49 (69)	26 (72)	23 (66)
Digoxin or digitoxin – no (%)	13 (18)	5 (14)	8 (23)
Laboratory values			
Creatinine (mmol/l) [mg/dl]	85±19 [0.96±0.21]	86±18 [0.97±0.21]	84±20.[0.95±0.22]
Total serum cholesterol – mmol/l	5.8±1.2	5.9±1.6	5.6±0.8
C-reactive protein – mg/l	2.2 (1.0–5.3)	1.7 (1.0–1.4)	2.7 (1.3–6.2)
N-terminal pro-B-type natriuretic peptide – pg/dl	592 (236–1607)	600 (186–1630)	588 (243–1643)

NYHA: New York Heart Association; TIA: transient ischemic attack; ACEI: angiotensin converting enzyme inhibitor; ARB: angiotensin receptor blocker.

Procollagen type I N-terminal pro-peptide increased more in patients treated with rosuvastatin as compared with patients treated with placebo (Table 3 and Figure 4), while for MMP-9 there was a trend toward a more pronounced increase in the placebo group (p = 0.08) (Table 3).

New York Heart Association class and quality of life

At baseline, 8/43/20 patients were in NYHA class I/II/III, respectively. In the 69 patients who completed the study, the corresponding figures were 12/48/9 at follow-up, indicating a significant improvement (p = 0.003). However, no difference was observed between patients treated with rosuvastatin and those treated with placebo (p = 0.90). Likewise, quality of life improved significantly in the population as a whole, but adjusted for baseline values, there was no between-group difference at follow-up (Table 2).

Compliance, safety, and side effects

In the rosuvastatin arm, two patients, one of whom was later lost to follow-up, prematurely discontinued study drug due to mild side-effects. One patient in the placebo arm stopped taking the study drug after a few days due to stomach pain and diarrhea. Throughout the study period, a total of fifty adverse clinical events were recorded in 33 patients. Twenty-six events were recorded in 16 patients who were allocated to rosuvastatin, and 24 events were recorded in 17 patients allocated to placebo (p = 0.80). Four serious adverse events were recorded in four patients allocated to rosuvastatin (surgery for colon cancer; development of atrial fibrillation; hospitalization for worsening HF; and an accidental fracture), and seven serious adverse events occurred in five patients allocated to placebo (development of dementia; and hospitalizations for hypotension, pneumonia, newly developed symptomatic coronary artery disease, and severe nose bleed). There were no episodes of rhabdomyolysis or on-treatment elevation in alanine transaminase. No patient died during follow-up.

Discussion

Assuming that statins modulate inflammation and the extracellular matrix, we hypothesized that treatment with rosuvastatin would mitigate LV remodeling in patients with DCM. However, we did not find that six months of treatment with this potent statin influenced any measure of LV function or size in our patients. Moreover, while treatment with rosuvastatin was associated with a pronounced reduction in serum cholesterol, it did not affect plasma/serum levels of a wide range of inflammatory variables. The effect on markers of extracellular matrix turnover was modest.

Table 2. Results from cardiac imaging exams, New York Heart Association (NYHA) classification and quality of life measurements.

Variable	Placebo			Rosuvastatin			p-value for between-group difference
	Baseline	Follow-up	Change (95% CI)	Baseline	Follow-up	Change (95% CI)	
Imaging							
LVEF (%)*	36±13	40±14	4.7 (0.9 – 8.5)†	36±13	41±15	4.5 (1.5 – 7.5)†	0.98
EDV by MRI (ml)	249 (185 – 325)	202 (160 – 303)	−36 (−61 – −10)†	242 (191 – 326)	193 (169 – 326)	−26 (−48 – −3)†	0.56
ESV by MRI (ml)	159 (93 – 242)	118 (79–216)	−35 (−60 – −9)†	154 (92 – 236)	102 (67 – 176)	−28 (−49 – −7)†	0.76
LVEF by MRI (%)	36±14	41±15	5.4 (0.9 – 9.9)†	38±14	44±15	5.8 (2.0 – 9.5)†	0.75
EDV by E/D (ml)	188 (141 – 228)	151 (134 – 210)	−19 (−32 – −7)†	202 (145 – 278)	186 (138 – 270)	−2 (−17 – 13)	0.07
ESV by E/D (ml)	129 (87 – 165)	95 (79 – 148)	−19 (−32 – −6)†	135 (99 – 203)	126 (78 – 204)	−6 (−20 – 7)	0.16
LVEF by E/D (%)	32±10	36±10	3.9 (1.0 – 6.6)†	31±8	34±11	3.7 (0.9 – 6.6)†	0.81
NYHA class							
NYHA class (I/II/III)	4/22/9	7/22/6		4/21/11	5/26/3		0.90
Quality of life							
MLHFQ	23 (4 – 35)	14 (3 – 23)	−3 (−9 – 2)	30 (16 – 56)	20 (9 – 44)	−7 (−12 – −1)†	0.39
Beck depression inventory	4 (2 – 7)	3 (1 – 5)	−1 (−2 – 0)	6 (2 – 9)	3 (1 – 9)	−1 (−3 – 0)	0.91
EuroQoL VAS (%)	66±17	68±15	2 (−4 – 7)	64±18	66±18	1 (−7 – 8)	0.68

*This row represents left ventricular ejection fraction (LVEF) by magnetic resonance imaging (MRI) or, if the latter result was not available at both baseline and follow-up, LVEF by echocardiography (E/D, N = 18). † $p < 0.05$ for difference between baseline and follow-up. CI: confidence interval; EDV: end diastolic left ventricular internal volume; ESV: end systolic left ventricular internal volume; NT-proBNP: N-terminal pro-B-type natriuretic peptide; LDL: low density lipoprotein; MLHFQ: Minnesota Living with Heart Failure Questionnaire; VAS: visual analogue scale.

There is a large body of evidence indicating that inflammation is involved in the pathogenesis of HF [26]. The anti-inflammatory effect of statins has also been extensively studied [27]. Almost uniformly, an on-treatment fall in CRP has been observed in major statin trials, most of which have been performed in patients with, or at increased risk of, atherosclerotic disease [2] [28] [29]. We have previously demonstrated that the anti-inflammatory effects of these drugs extend beyond a reduction in CRP [30] [31]. However, in the present study, rosuvastatin had no effect on markers of inflammation, including CRP.

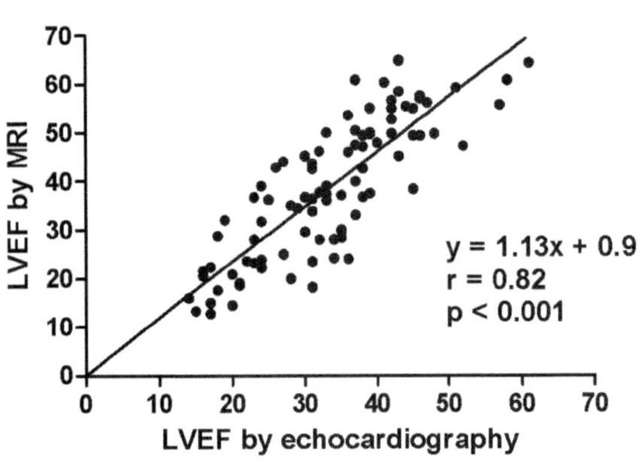

Figure 3. Correlation between left ventricular ejection fraction as measured by echocardiography and as measured by magnetic resonance imaging. Data from baseline and follow-up are pooled. The Pearson correlation coefficient between results obtained by magnetic resonance imaging (MRI) and results obtained by echocardiography was 0.82 ($p < 0.001$).

The precise mechanisms underlying the proposed anti-inflammatory effect of statins have not been fully elucidated. The so called pleiotropic effects of statins could at least partly involve reduced inflammation secondary to a reduction in LDL levels [32]. In our patients, however, we observed a substantial on-treatment decrease in LDL, without this translating to an effect on inflammatory markers. It is possible that the anti-inflammatory effects of statins observed in atherosclerotic disease can be directly attributed to an amelioration of the atherosclerotic burden. However, in a large population of elderly patients with HF of ischemic etiology, rosuvastatin reduced levels of CRP [33], but its effect on other inflammatory markers has been disappointing [34] [35] [36]. Although the exact mechanism is not clear, it is therefore possible that the ability of statins to modulate inflammation in HF is questionable.

In the UNIVERSE trial [37], assessing the effect of rosuvastatin in DCM, an increase in PIIINP was observed in the rosuvastatin group. The authors speculated that an on-treatment increase in extracellular fibrosis might offset other, potentially beneficial effects of rosuvastatin, explaining the neutral result on LVEF in this study [38]. In the present trial, rosuvastatin was associated with an increase in PINP and an attenuated increase in MMP-9, potentially reflecting increased collagen synthesis and inhibited matrix degradation, respectively. While these processes could influence myocardial remodeling, the between-group differences were modest and, in the case of MMP-9, not significant. Most importantly, they were not accompanied by a treatment induced effect on LV function.

In the population as a whole, we observed a substantial increase in LVEF from baseline to follow-up. Implicitly, our study demonstrates the inherent potential for improvement in patients with DCM, and that adverse remodeling is not an irreversible process. The high degree of spontaneous recovery may have

Table 3. Results of blood tests.

Variable	Placebo			Rosuvastatin			p-value for between-group difference
	Baseline	Follow-up	Change (95% CI)	Baseline	Follow-up	Change (95% CI)	
Lipids							
Cholesterol (mmol/l)	5.6±0.8	5.6±0.8	−0.1 (−0.3 - 0.2)	5.9±1.6	4.3±1.0	−1.7 (−2.1 – −1.3)*	<0.001
LDL cholesterol (mmol/l)	3.7±0.8	3.6±0.9	−0.1 (−0.2 – 0.1)	3.8±1.2	2.1±0.8	−1.7 (−2.0 – −1.4)*	<0.001
HDL cholesterol (mmol/l)	1.2±0.3	1.2±0.4	0 (−0.1 – 0.1)	1.3±0.4	1.4±0.5	0.1 (0 – 0.2)	0.19
Natriuretic peptides							
NT-ProBNP (pg/dl)	617 (245 – 1581)	499 (167 – 1226)	−79 (−347 – 307)	567 (186 – 1615)	431 (169 – 983)	−19 (−418 – 475)	0.73
Kidney function							
Creatinine (μmol/l) [mg/dl]	84±20	82±14	−2 (−6 – 3)	86±18	86±18	1 (−2 – 3)	0.23
Markers of inflammation							
C−reactive protein (mg/l)	2.7 (1.3 – 6.2)	3.2 (1.2 – 10.1)	1.1 (−1.3 – 3.5)	1.7 (1.0 – 4.0)	2.1 (1.0 – 4.9)	1.2 (−1.1 – 3.4)	0.14
sTNF-R1 (pg/ml)	1039±271	1038 ± 304	−1 (−71 – 68)	1134±327	1082 ± 235	−53 (−141 – 36)	0.72
MCP-1 (pg/ml)	115 (72 - 160)	117 (76 - 142)	−5 (−21 – 10)	103 (87 - 146)	94 (70−127)	−6 (−21 - 8)	0.77
gp130 (ng/ml)	92±23	96 ± 23	4 (−5 – 14)	91±18	97±22	6 (−3 - 15)	0.83
Osteoprotegerin (pg/ml)	666±243	610 ± 193	−56 (−127 - 16)	600±203	643±248	42 (−34 - 118)	0.13
Endothelial reactivity							
vWF (ng/ml)	21±14	22 ± 13	1 (−3 – 5)	23±16	23 ± 12	0 (−4 - 4)	0.99
Matrix turnover							
MMP-9 (ng/ml)	247 (50 - 386)	354 (162 - 467)	68 (11 - 124)*	220 (64 - 302)	243 (106 - 367)	13 (−33 - 59)	0.08
PINP (μg/l)	40 (29 - 47)	40 (27 - 50)	0 (−5 – 4)	38 (32 - 46)	45 (37 - 68)	8 (2 - 13)*	0.02
PIIINP (μg/l)	3.7 (3.3 - 4.4)	3.8 (3.4 - 5.0)	0.0 (−0.6 - 0.5)	3.8 (2.9 - 4.5)	3.8 (3.4−5.0)	−0.2 (−0.4 - 0.8)	0.27

* $p < 0.05$ for difference between baseline and follow-up. CI: confidence interval; LDL: low density lipoprotein; HDL: high density lipoprotein; NT-proBNP: N-terminal pro-B-type natriuretic peptide; sTNF-R1: soluble tumour necrosis factor receptor 1; MCP-1: monocyte chemotactic protein-1; gp130: Soluble glycoprotein 130; MMP-9: matrix metalloproteinase-9; PINP: procollagen type I N-terminal pro-peptide; PIIINP: procollagen type III N-terminal pro-peptide.

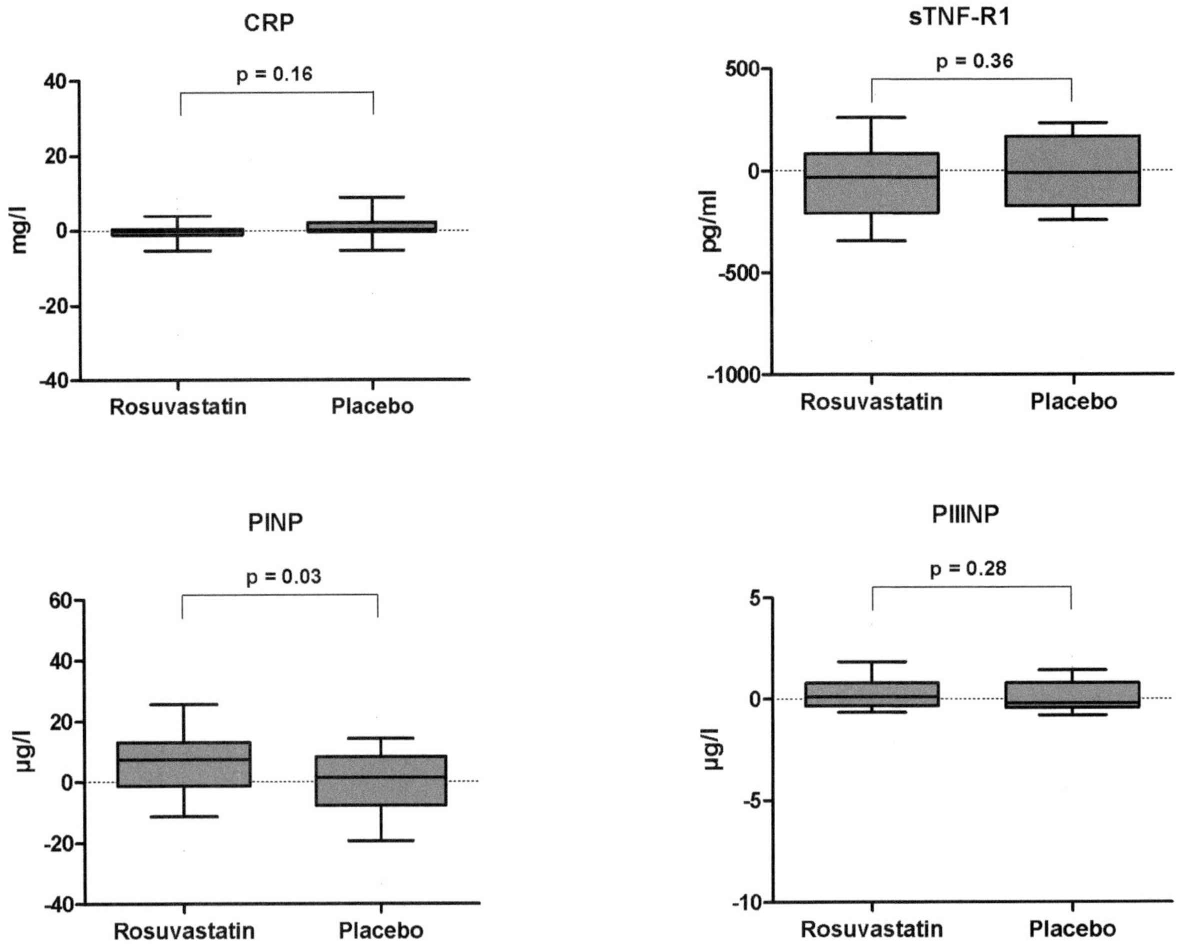

Figure 4. Changes in markers of inflammation and extracellular matrix turnover. Changes in C-reactive protein (CRP), soluble tumor necrosis factor receptor type 1 (sTNF-R1), and procollagen type I and III N-terminal pro-peptides (PINP and PIIINP) stratified by treatment allocation. p-values for between-group differences in changes were computed by independent group t-tests. While PINP increased more in patients treated with rosuvastatin as compared to patients treated with placebo ($p = 0.03$), treatment did not affect any of the other markers of inflammation or matrix remodeling. Boxes: 25–75 percentiles; whiskers: 5–95 percentiles.

influenced our results. If new treatments for DCM are to prove better than placebo, they will have to not only attenuate adverse remodeling, but also contribute to a marked improvement in LV function.

Limitations

The present study was powered to detect a five per cent point difference in LVEF between the two treatment arms. It could be argued that this endpoint was overly ambitious, necessitating a neutral outcome of the trial. On the other hand, we did not observe differences across treatment arms on any measure of LV size or function, including NT-pro-BNP, indicating that rosuvastatin did in fact not impact LV remodeling. Nonetheless, our study was underpowered to detect small, but potentially relevant changes in LV function. Due to the limited number of patients and short observation period, we cannot conclude that statin treatment does not reduce morbidity or mortality in patients with DCM.

"Idiopathic" DCM is a category that includes different disease entities with a common structural phenotype. While subgroups of these patients might benefit from statin treatment, others may not. This fact may limit the generalizability of our findings.

Finally, unlike most statins, rosuvastatin is a hydrophilic compound. Accordingly, it has been suggested that it does not have the same pleiotropic profile as the lipid soluble statins [11], and we cannot exclude that other statins might have performed differently in our patient population. In patients at risk of coronary disease, however, rosuvastatin is highly effective not only when it comes to reducing LDL cholesterol; it also effectively reduces CRP, as well as the number of cardiovascular events and death [2].

Conclusion

This small, randomized study did not provide evidence that treatment with a potent statin improves LV function in patients with DCM. While safe, rosuvastatin should not be prescribed routinely in patients with HF. Whether treatment with a statin might benefit subgroups of patients with DCM, remains to be elucidated.

Supporting Information

Checklist S1 Consolidated Standards of Reporting Trials (CONSORT) checklist to show that the trial conforms to the CONSORT requirements.

Protocol S1 The full version of the trial protocol.

Acknowledgments

We would like to thank Dr Rune Mo at the Department of Cardiology, St Olav's Hospital, Trondheim University Hospital, and Else-Marie Christiansen at the Department of Internal Medicine, Drammen Hospital, Vestre Viken Hospital Trust for their contribution to this work.

Author Contributions

Conceived and designed the experiments: ETA TU AY H-JS SA PA LG. Performed the experiments: KB ETA EG WS JA LG. Analyzed the data: KB TU AY KG JA RS. Contributed reagents/materials/analysis tools: TU AY KG. Wrote the paper: KB PA LG.

References

1. Randomised trial of cholesterol lowering in 4444 patients with coronary heart disease: the Scandinavian Simvastatin Survival Study (4S) (1994) Lancet 344: 1383–1389.
2. Ridker PM, Danielson E, Fonseca FA, Genest J, Gotto AM Jr, et al. (2008) Rosuvastatin to prevent vascular events in men and women with elevated C-reactive protein. N Engl J Med 359: 2195–2207.
3. Mihos CG, Salas MJ, Santana O (2010) The pleiotropic effects of the hydroxy-methyl-glutaryl-CoA reductase inhibitors in cardiovascular disease: a comprehensive review. Cardiol Rev 18: 298–304.
4. Ridker PM, Rifai N, Clearfield M, Downs JR, Weis SE, et al. (2001) Measurement of C-reactive protein for the targeting of statin therapy in the primary prevention of acute coronary events. N Engl J Med 344: 1959–1965.
5. Kjekshus J, Apetrei E, Barrios V, Bohm M, Cleland JG, et al. (2007) Rosuvastatin in older patients with systolic heart failure. N Engl J Med 357: 2248–2261.
6. Tavazzi L, Maggioni AP, Marchioli R, Barlera S, Franzosi MG, et al. (2008) Effect of rosuvastatin in patients with chronic heart failure (the GISSI-HF trial): a randomised, double-blind, placebo-controlled trial. Lancet 372: 1231–1239.
7. Node K, Fujita M, Kitakaze M, Hori M, Liao JK (2003) Short-term statin therapy improves cardiac function and symptoms in patients with idiopathic dilated cardiomyopathy. Circulation 108: 839–843.
8. Sola S, Mir MQ, Lerakis S, Tandon N, Khan BV (2006) Atorvastatin improves left ventricular systolic function and serum markers of inflammation in nonischemic heart failure. J Am Coll Cardiol 47: 332–337.
9. Wojnicz R, Wilczek K, Nowalany-Kozielska E, Szygula-Jurkiewicz B, Nowak J, et al. (2006) Usefulness of atorvastatin in patients with heart failure due to inflammatory dilated cardiomyopathy and elevated cholesterol levels. Am J Cardiol 97: 899–904.
10. Bielecka-Dabrowa A, Goch JH, Mikhailidis DP, Rysz J, Maciejewski M, et al. (2009) The influence of atorvastatin on parameters of inflammation and function of the left ventricle in patients with dilated cardiomyopathy. Med Sci Monit 15: MS12–MS23.
11. Lipinski MJ, Cauthen CA, Biondi-Zoccai GG, Abbate A, Vrtovec B, et al. (2009) Meta-analysis of randomized controlled trials of statins versus placebo in patients with heart failure. Am J Cardiol 104: 1708–1716.
12. Cleland JG, Swedberg K, Follath F, Komajda M, Cohen-Solal A, et al. (2003) The EuroHeart Failure survey programme— a survey on the quality of care among patients with heart failure in Europe. Part 1: patient characteristics and diagnosis. Eur Heart J 24: 442–463.
13. Elliott P, Andersson B, Arbustini E, Bilinska Z, Cecchi F, et al. (2008) Classification of the cardiomyopathies: a position statement from the European Society Of Cardiology Working Group on Myocardial and Pericardial Diseases. Eur Heart J 29: 270–276.
14. Schulz KF, Altman DG, Moher D (2010) CONSORT 2010 Statement: updated guidelines for reporting parallel group randomised trials. BMC Med 8: 18.
15. Lang RM, Bierig M, Devereux RB, Flachskampf FA, Foster E, et al. (2006) Recommendations for chamber quantification. Eur J Echocardiogr 7: 79–108.
16. Galderisi M, Henein MY, D'hooge J, Sicari R, Badano LP, et al. (2011) Recommendations of the European Association of Echocardiography: how to use echo-Doppler in clinical trials: different modalities for different purposes. Eur J Echocardiogr 12: 339–353.
17. Rivera JM, Vandervoort PM, Morris E, Weyman AE, Thomas JD (1994) Visual assessment of valvular regurgitation: comparison with quantitative Doppler measurements. J Am Soc Echocardiogr 7: 480–487.
18. Bollerslev J, Ueland T, Jorgensen AP, Fougner KJ, Wergeland R, et al. (2006) Positive effects of a physiological dose of GH on markers of atherogenesis: a placebo-controlled study in patients with adult-onset GH deficiency. Eur J Endocrinol 154: 537–543.
19. Vickers AJ, Altman DG (2001) Statistics notes: Analysing controlled trials with baseline and follow up measurements. BMJ 323: 1123–1124.
20. Dickstein K, Cohen-Solal A, Filippatos G, McMurray JJ, Ponikowski P, et al. (2008) ESC Guidelines for the diagnosis and treatment of acute and chronic heart failure 2008 The Task Force for the Diagnosis and Treatment of Acute and Chronic Heart Failure 2008 of the European Society of Cardiology. Developed in collaboration with the Heart Failure Association of the ESC (HFA) and endorsed by the European Society of Intensive Care Medicine (ESICM). Eur J Heart Fail.
21. Gullestad L, Ueland T, Vinge LE, Finsen A, Yndestad A, et al. (2012) Inflammatory cytokines in heart failure: mediators and markers. Cardiology 122: 23–35.
22. Constans J, Conri C (2006) Circulating markers of endothelial function in cardiovascular disease. Clin Chim Acta 368: 33–47.
23. D'Armiento J (2002) Matrix metalloproteinase disruption of the extracellular matrix and cardiac dysfunction. Trends Cardiovasc Med 12: 97–101.
24. Cicoira M, Rossi A, Bonapace S, Zanolla L, Golia G, et al. (2004) Independent and additional prognostic value of aminoterminal propeptide of type III procollagen circulating levels in patients with chronic heart failure. J Card Fail 10: 403–411.
25. Zile MR, Desantis SM, Baicu CF, Stroud RE, Thompson SB, et al. (2011) Plasma biomarkers that reflect determinants of matrix composition identify the presence of left ventricular hypertrophy and diastolic heart failure. Circ Heart Fail 4: 246–256.
26. Yndestad A, Damas JK, Oie E, Ueland T, Gullestad L, et al. (2006) Systemic inflammation in heart failure--the whys and wherefores. Heart Fail Rev 11: 83–92.
27. Bu DX, Griffin G, Lichtman AH (2011) Mechanisms for the anti-inflammatory effects of statins. Curr Opin Lipidol 22: 165–170.
28. Crea F, Monaco C, Lanza GA, Maggi E, Ginnetti F, et al. (2002) Inflammatory predictors of mortality in the Scandinavian Simvastatin Survival Study. Clin Cardiol 25: 461–466.
29. Chan KY, Boucher ES, Gandhi PJ, Silva MA (2004) HMG-CoA reductase inhibitors for lowering elevated levels of C-reactive protein. Am J Health Syst Pharm 61: 1676–1681.
30. Waehre T, Damas JK, Gullestad L, Holm AM, Pedersen TR, et al. (2003) Hydroxymethylglutaryl coenzyme a reductase inhibitors down-regulate chemokines and chemokine receptors in patients with coronary artery disease. J Am Coll Cardiol 41: 1460–1467.
31. Waehre T, Yndestad A, Smith C, Haug T, Tunheim SH, et al. (2004) Increased expression of interleukin-1 in coronary artery disease with downregulatory effects of HMG-CoA reductase inhibitors. Circulation 109: 1966–1972.
32. Robinson JG, Smith B, Maheshwari N, Schrott H (2005) Pleiotropic effects of statins: benefit beyond cholesterol reduction? A meta-regression analysis. J Am Coll Cardiol 46: 1855–1862.
33. McMurray JJ, Kjekshus J, Gullestad L, Dunselman P, Hjalmarson A, et al. (2009) Effects of statin therapy according to plasma high-sensitivity C-reactive protein concentration in the Controlled Rosuvastatin Multinational Trial in Heart Failure (CORONA): a retrospective analysis. Circulation 120: 2188–2196.
34. Ueland T, Dahl CP, Kjekshus J, Hulthe J, Bohm M, et al. (2011) Osteoprotegerin predicts progression of chronic heart failure: results from CORONA. Circ Heart Fail 4: 145–152.
35. Broch K, Ueland T, Nymo SH, Kjekshus J, Hulthe J, et al. (2012) Soluble ST2 is associated with adverse outcome in patients with heart failure of ischaemic aetiology. Eur J Heart Fail 14: 268–277.
36. Askevold ET, Nymo S, Ueland T, Gravning J, Wergeland R, et al. (2013) Soluble glycoprotein 130 predicts fatal outcomes in chronic heart failure: analysis from the Controlled Rosuvastatin Multinational Trial in Heart Failure (CORONA). Circ Heart Fail 6: 91–98.
37. Krum H, Ashton E, Reid C, Kalff V, Rogers J, et al. (2007) Double-blind, randomized, placebo-controlled study of high-dose HMG CoA reductase inhibitor therapy on ventricular remodeling, pro-inflammatory cytokines and neurohormonal parameters in patients with chronic systolic heart failure. J Card Fail 13: 1–7.
38. Ashton E, Windebank E, Skiba M, Reid C, Schneider H, et al. (2011) Why did high-dose rosuvastatin not improve cardiac remodeling in chronic heart failure? Mechanistic insights from the UNIVERSE study. Int J Cardiol 146: 404–407.

20

Silencing of miR-34a Attenuates Cardiac Dysfunction in a Setting of Moderate, but Not Severe, Hypertrophic Cardiomyopathy

Bianca C. Bernardo[1]*, Xiao-Ming Gao[1], Yow Keat Tham[1], Helen Kiriazis[1], Catherine E. Winbanks[1], Jenny Y. Y. Ooi[1], Esther J. H. Boey[1], Susanna Obad[2], Sakari Kauppinen[3], Paul Gregorevic[1], Xiao-Jun Du[1], Ruby C. Y. Lin[4], Julie R. McMullen[1,5,6]*

1 Baker IDI Heart and Diabetes Institute, Melbourne, Victoria, Australia, **2** Santaris Pharma, Horsholm, Denmark, **3** Department of Haematology, Aalborg University Hospital, Copenhagen, Denmark, **4** Ramaciotti Centre for Genomics, School of Biotechnology & Biomolecular Sciences, University of New South Wales, Sydney, New South Wales, Australia, **5** Departments of Medicine Monash University, Clayton, Victoria, Australia, **6** Departments of Physiology, Monash University, Clayton, Victoria, Australia

Abstract

Therapeutic inhibition of the miR-34 family (miR-34a,-b,-c), or miR-34a alone, have emerged as promising strategies for the treatment of cardiac pathology. However, before advancing these approaches further for potential entry into the clinic, a more comprehensive assessment of the therapeutic potential of inhibiting miR-34a is required for two key reasons. First, miR-34a has ~40% fewer predicted targets than the miR-34 family. Hence, in cardiac stress settings in which inhibition of miR-34a provides adequate protection, this approach is likely to result in less potential off-target effects. Secondly, silencing of miR-34a alone may be insufficient in settings of established cardiac pathology. We recently demonstrated that inhibition of the miR-34 family, but not miR-34a alone, provided benefit in a chronic model of myocardial infarction. Inhibition of miR-34 also attenuated cardiac remodeling and improved heart function following pressure overload, however, silencing of miR-34a alone was not examined. The aim of this study was to assess whether inhibition of miR-34a could attenuate cardiac remodeling in a mouse model with pre-existing pathological hypertrophy. Mice were subjected to pressure overload via constriction of the transverse aorta for four weeks and echocardiography was performed to confirm left ventricular hypertrophy and systolic dysfunction. After four weeks of pressure overload (before treatment), two distinct groups of animals became apparent: (1) mice with moderate pathology (fractional shortening decreased ~20%) and (2) mice with severe pathology (fractional shortening decreased ~37%). Mice were administered locked nucleic acid (LNA)-antimiR-34a or LNA-control with an eight week follow-up. Inhibition of miR-34a in mice with moderate cardiac pathology attenuated atrial enlargement and maintained cardiac function, but had no significant effect on fetal gene expression or cardiac fibrosis. Inhibition of miR-34a in mice with severe pathology provided no therapeutic benefit. Thus, therapies that inhibit miR-34a alone may have limited potential in settings of established cardiac pathology.

Editor: Junichi Sadoshima, Rutgers New Jersey Medical School, United States of America

Funding: This study was funded by National Health and Medical Research Council Project Grant 586603 (to J.R.M and R.C.Y.L), and also supported in part by the Victorian Government's Operational Infrastructure Support Program. X.J.D. and J.R.M are National Health and Medical Research Council Senior Research Fellows (APP1043026 and 586604). J.R.M, R.C.Y.L., and P.G. are supported by an Australian Research Council Future Fellowship (FT0001657), a University of New South Wales Vice Chancellor Research Fellowship, and a Pfizer Australia Senior Research Fellowship, respectively. The funders had no role in study design, data collection and analysis, decision to publish, or preparation of the manuscript.

Competing Interests: S.O. is an employee of Santaris Pharma A/S, a clinical stage biopharmaceutical company that develops RNA-based therapeutics. S.K. is a former employee of Santaris Pharma A/S and is now Professor at the Department of Haematology, Aalborg University Hospital. Depending on the field of use, LNA oligonucleotides can be obtained from Santaris Pharma A/S or Exiqon.

* E-mail: bianca.bernardo@bakeridi.edu.au (BCB); julie.mcmullen@bakeridi.edu.au (JRM)

Introduction

Cardiovascular disease remains the leading cause of morbidity and mortality worldwide and whilst current drugs (e.g. angiotensin-converting enzyme inhibitors, beta blockers) improve symptoms and reduce hospital admissions, the prevalence of cardiovascular disease is still increasing, highlighting the need for the identification of novel and efficacious therapies that can prevent cardiovascular disease. microRNAs (miRNAs) are an abundant class of small, non-coding RNAs that target partially complementary sequences in the 3' untranslated region of target mRNA, leading to mRNA cleavage and/or translational repression [1]. Whilst miRNAs regulate a wide range of biological processes, recent studies have unveiled critical roles of miRNAs in cardiovascular disease (reviewed in [2–6]). These studies highlight their potential as novel therapeutic targets. miRNA inhibitors or antimiRs have been shown to be efficient in silencing miRNAs in mice [7], and non-human primates [8], and the first miRNA-targeted drug, miravirsen, has advanced into clinical phase 2 trials for the treatment of hepatitis C virus infection [9]. Although miRNA based therapies for cardiovascular disease have not yet reached clinical trials, a number of successful preclinical studies in animal models of heart failure, cardiac hypertrophy and remodeling highlight the translational potential of targeting miRNAs in human heart failure [10–15]. Most preclinical studies have focused on inhibiting individual miRNAs in the heart [11,13,15]. However, more recent studies have demonstrated the therapeutic potential of targeting disease-implicated miRNA-families [10,14,16,17]. Though a potential disadvantage of inhibiting an entire miRNA family is the increased risk of generating off-target effects. Thus it is important to assess whether the effects of silencing miRNA families can yield more therapeutic benefit in settings of cardiac stress than the targeting of individual miRNAs.

We and others have previously shown that expression of miR-34a is elevated in settings of cardiac stress [10,18] and ageing [11], and that miR-34 family members, 34b and 34c, are also elevated in the mouse heart following a cardiac insult [10,18]. Furthermore, expression of miR-34 family members was found to be elevated in cardiac tissue from patients with heart disease [19,20]. We recently found that inhibition of the miR-34 family, but not miR-34a alone, displayed a therapeutic benefit in a chronic model of myocardial infarction (MI, with pre-existing cardiac dysfunction and significant left ventricular (LV) remodeling; antimiR delivered 2 days after MI) [10]. Inhibition of the miR-34 family also improved cardiac function and attenuated LV remodeling in a mouse model with pre-existing pathological cardiac remodeling and dysfunction due to pressure overload by transverse aortic constriction (TAC) [10], however the therapeutic impact of inhibiting miR-34a alone was not assessed in that study. More recently, it was shown that inhibition of miR-34a prevented cardiac contractile dysfunction, and reduced apoptosis and fibrosis following acute MI, but the first dose of the miRNA-based therapy was administered 3 hours after acute MI, before any chronic LV remodeling had occurred [11]. Collectively, these findings suggest that inhibition of miR-34a might be beneficial in acute settings of cardiac stress or conditions with moderate pathology, but not chronic or severe settings. Given the current enthusiasm and anticipation regarding therapeutic development of miR-34a and miR-34 family-targeted antimiRs [11,21–23], and the differences in cardiac protection in acute versus chronic settings [10,11], it is important to assess the therapeutic potential of inhibiting miR-34a in more sustained pathological settings. This is also important because a challenge facing miRNA-based therapies is the vast number of predicted targets which could result in off-target effects. Since the miR-34 family has approximately 31–55% more targets in humans (which is dependent on the particular target prediction algorithm used) than miR-34a alone, interventions that modulate the entire miRNA family have greater theoretical potential to generate off-target effects. Thus, if manipulation of a single miRNA can provide adequate cardiac protection, this approach may be an advisable alternative means of obtaining a therapeutic effect with lower risk of off-target complications.

In the current study, we assessed the therapeutic potential of inhibiting miR-34a in a mouse model with pre-existing pathological hypertrophy and systolic dysfunction due to pressure overload induced by TAC. We report here, that administration of a locked nucleic acid (LNA)-antimiR-34a in a model of pressure overload-induced hypertrophic cardiomyopathy with moderate systolic dysfunction was able to prevent further deterioration in cardiac function over an eight week period. In contrast, this approach was unable to attenuate pathological remodeling in a model of pressure overload with severe systolic dysfunction, whereby systolic function continued to decline eight weeks after treatment.

Methods

Experimental animals

All experiments using animals were conducted in accordance with the Australian code of practice for the care and use of animals for scientific purposes (National Health & Medical Research Council of Australia, 8th Edition, 2013). Animal care and experimental procedures were approved by the Alfred Medical Research and Education Precinct's Animal Ethics Committee. All surgery was performed under anesthesia (ketamine:xylazine:atropine) with post-operative analgesia (carprofen), and all efforts were made to minimize animals' discomfort.

Pressure overload

Adult (12 week old) male C57BL/6 mice were subjected to a pressure overload surgery induced TAC as previously described [24]. In brief, mice were anaesthetized with ketamine:xylazine:atropine (100:20:1.2 mg/kg, i.p.), administered an analgesic (carprofen, 5 mg/kg, s.c.) and intubated for ventilation. A sternectomy was performed to access the aorta and a non-absorbable 5–0 braided silk suture was tied around the aorta between the right innominate and left carotid arteries, causing a constriction of approximately 65% using a 0.45 mm probe as a guide. Mice were monitored and studied for 12 weeks. Controls were unoperated aged matched male mice.

LV structure and function

Transthoracic echocardiography (M-mode two-dimensional echocardiography) was performed on anaesthetized mice (1.8% isoflurane, inhalation) using a Philips iE33 ultrasound machine with a 15 mHz liner array transducer, prior to surgery (baseline), four weeks post TAC, and endpoint echocardiography was performed eight weeks post treatment (i.e. 12 weeks post TAC). LV chamber dimensions (LV end-diastolic dimension, LVEDD; LV end-systolic dimension, LVESD), LV wall thicknesses (LV posterior wall, LVPW; interventricular septum, IVS), heart rate (HR), fractional shortening (FS, calculated as [(LVEDD – LVDSD)/LVEDD] × 100%) and ejection fraction (EF, calculated as [($LVEDD^3$ – $LVDSD^3$)/$LVEDD^3$] × 100%) were analyzed offline using dedicated software (ProSolv Cardiovascular Analyzer version 3.5; ProSolv, Indianapolis, IN) obtained from M-mode traces.

Classification of cardiac phenotype

The TAC model is associated with pathological hypertrophy and systolic dysfunction within four weeks of surgery [25,26]. Cardiac function was assessed before surgery and at four weeks post-surgery. At four weeks post surgery, the analysis of echocardiography parameters (i.e. FS, EF) was used to define mice as exhibiting either a moderate ($n = 9$) or severe phenotype ($n = 6$).

LNA-oligonucleotide synthesis

The antimiR-34a was synthesized as a LNA:DNA mixmer with a complete phosphorothioate backbone (Santaris Pharma A/S, Denmark). The sequence of the 15-mer antimiR-34a was: 5′ – AgCtaAGacACTgCC – 3′ (LNA uppercase, DNA lowercase), and was specifically designed to target miR-34a, as previously reported [10]. The 15-mer LNA-control was synthesized (Santaris Pharma A/S, Denmark) with the following sequence: 5′ – TcAtcCTatAtGaCA – 3' (LNA uppercase, DNA lowercase). The LNA-control sequence was randomly chosen using a well-validated and established antimiR design. It was checked against a number of databases and shown not to have any perfect match binding sites in the transcriptome. Validation with *in vitro* and *in vivo* assays demonstrated that the control did not differ from un-transfected/mock or saline samples [27].

In vivo delivery of LNA-antimiR oligonucleotides

Four weeks post TAC (after echocardiography), TAC mice were randomized into control or treated groups. Mice were subcutaneously administered either a LNA-control or LNA-antimiR-34a (25 mg/kg/day) over three consecutive days and left for a period of eight weeks (Figure S1). Studies conducted in our laboratory have demonstrated that LNA-control itself has no effect on body weight, tibia length, and other organ weights (including heart, atria, lung, kidney and liver) compared with the same dosing regime of saline [comparison of LNA-control (3 daily doses: 25 mg/kg/day) or saline and 8 week follow-up in adult C57BL/6 mice; Bernardo BC., unpublished data].

Control mice were unoperated, untreated aged matched male mice. Our previous study demonstrated that administration of LNA-antimiR-34a had no effect in sham mice when compared to LNA-control mice, and that this dosing regimen is sufficient to silence miRNAs in the heart for at least two months [10]. In male C57BL/6 mice, administration of LNA-antimiR-34a had no effect on body weight (BW), tibial length (TL), heart weight (HW), atrial weight (AW) and lung weight (LW) after two months (Table S1). Therefore we used unoperated/untreated mice as controls.

RNA and protein isolation

Total RNA was isolated from frozen mouse ventricles using TRI Reagent (Sigma-Aldrich, St Louis, MO) and quantitated on a Nanodrop Spectrometer (Thermo Scientific, Waltham, MA). For protein lysates, frozen mouse ventricles were homogenized in a lysis buffer (10% glycerol, 137 mM NaCl, 20 mM Tris-HCl (pH 7.4), 20 mM NaF, 10 mM EDTA, 1 mM EGTA, 1 mM sodium pyrophosphate, 1 mM vanadate, 1 mM PMSF, 4 µg/mL pepstatin, 4 µg/mL aprotinin, 4 µg/mL leupeptin) and total protein concentration was determined using a Pierce micro protein assay kit (Thermo Scientific).

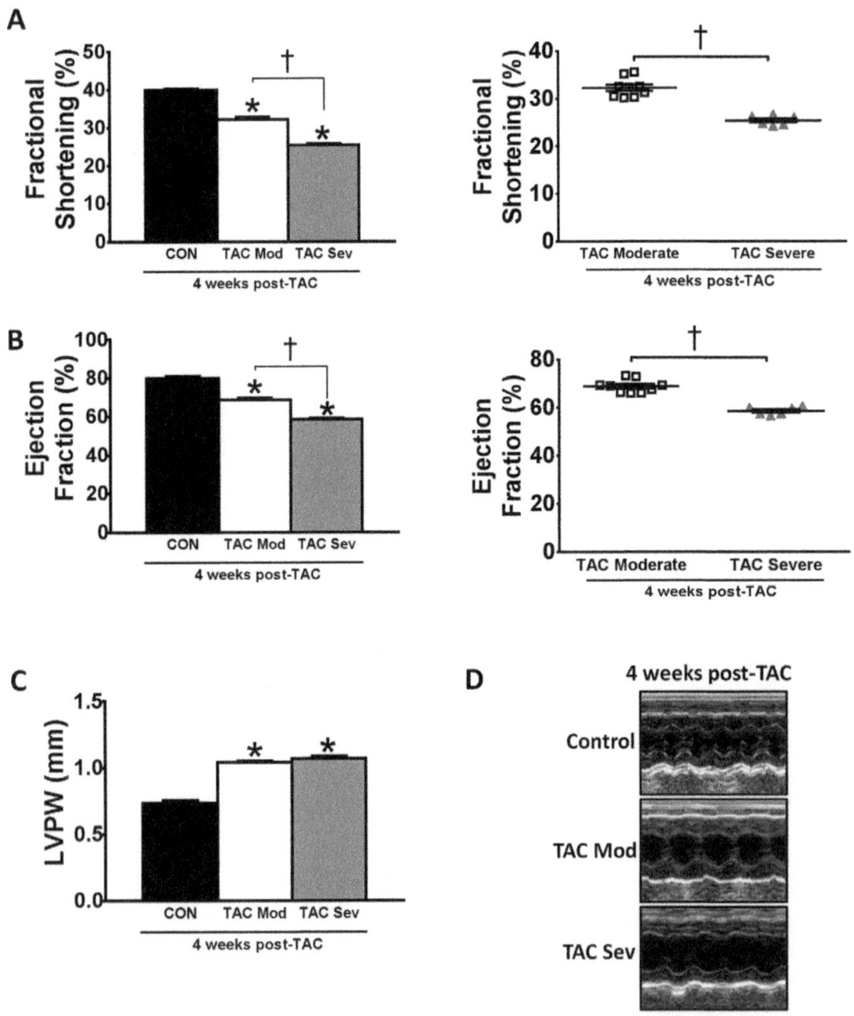

Figure 1. Mice with moderate or severe cardiac dysfunction following four weeks of pressure overload. Quantification of (A) fractional shortening, (B) ejection fraction and (C) left ventricular posterior wall thickness (LVPW) at four weeks post-TAC in control (CON), TAC moderate (TAC mod) and TAC severe (TAC sev) mice. Scatter plots demonstrate no overlap of fractional shortening and ejection fraction between TAC moderate and TAC severe groups. (D) Representative M-mode echocardiograms. N = 4–9 per group. *P<0.05 vs. control at four weeks post-TAC. †P<0.05. 1 way ANVOA followed by Fisher's Post Hoc Test.

Table 1. Echocardiography data of control and TAC mice at baseline and four weeks post-TAC.

	Baseline			Four weeks post-TAC		
	Control	TAC moderate	TAC severe	Control	TAC moderate	TAC severe
Number of animals	4	9	6	4	9	6
BW (g)	28.6±0.4	28.1±0.8	27.4±1.1	30.3±0.7	29.2±0.5	29.0±0.6
Heart rate, bpm	608±9	567±13	555±28	643±21	597±15	580±17
LVPW, mm	0.67±0.01	0. 69±0.01	0.73±0.03	0.73±0.02	1.04±0.01*	1.06±0.02*
IVS, mm	0.75±0.01	0.74±0.01	0.73±0.01	0.78±0.01	1.15±0.02*	1.19±0.02*†
LVEDD, mm	3.81±0.12	4.01±0.08	4.01±0.11	3.89±0.21	4.03±0.10	4.34±0.13
LVESD, mm	2.23±0.08	2.40±0.07	2.41±0.08	2.33±0.11	2.73±0.08*	3.24±0.11*†
FS, %	41±1	40±1	40±1	40±0	32±1*	25±0*†
EF, %	80±1	79±1	78±1	78±0	69±1*	59±1*†

BW, body weight; LV, left ventricular; LVPW, LV posterior wall thickness; IVS, interventricular septum thickness; LVEDD, LV end-diastolic dimension; LVESD, LV end-systolic dimension; FS, fractional shortening; EF, ejection fraction. Data are shown as mean ± SEM. One way ANOVA followed by Fisher's Post hoc Test. *P<0.05 vs. baseline of same group and control at same time point, †P<0.05 vs. TAC moderate at same time point.

Quantitative PCR (qPCR)

For mRNA expression analysis, 2 µg of total RNA was reverse transcribed using the High Capacity RNA-to-cDNA kit (Life Technologies, Carlsbad, CA) according to manufacturer's recommendations. qPCR was performed using TaqMan probes (Life Technologies) and amplified on an Applied Biosystems 7500 real-time PCR instrument according to manufacturer's instructions. Hypoxanthine phosphoribosyltransferase 1 *(Hprt1)* was used to standardize for cDNA concentration and data was analyzed using the $2^{-\Delta\Delta Ct}$ method of quantification [28]. For miRNA expression analysis, 50 ng of total RNA was reversed transcribed for each miRNA of interest using TaqMan® MicroRNA Reverse Transcription Kit (Life Technologies) according to manufacturer's recommendations. qPCR was performed using TaqMan® MicroRNA Assays (Life Technologies) according to manufacturer's instructions. Expression was normalized against snoU6 and data analyzed using the $2^{-\Delta\Delta Ct}$ algorithm [28].

Northern blotting

10 µg of total RNA was separated on a formaldehyde denaturing agarose gel and transferred to a Hybond-N membrane (GE Healthcare, Pittsburgh, PA) in 20X SSC by upward capillary transfer, and probed for atrial natriuretic peptide *(Anp)*, B type natriuretic peptide *(Bnp)*, β myosin heavy chain *(β-MHC)*, sarcoplasmic/endoplasmic reticulum Ca^{2+}-ATPase 2a *(Serca2a)*, and glyceraldehyde-3-phosphate dehydrogenase *(Gapdh)* as previously described [29]. Membranes were stripped and re-probed for subsequent analyses. Signals were quantitated using ImageJ 1.44p pixel analysis (NIH Image Software) and data normalized to a control value of 1.

Western blotting

20 µg of protein lysates were separated by SDS-PAGE using pre-cast 4–12% Bis-Tris gels (Life Technologies), blotted onto nitrocellulose membrane (BioRad, Hercules, CA), incubated with antibody overnight (VEGF-A, Santa Cruz, Santa Cruz, CA, sc-152, 1:500; vinculin, Sigma Aldrich, clone hVIN-1, V9131, 1:2000; GAPDH, Santa Cruz, sc-32233, 1:5000) and detected by chemiluminescence. Membranes were stripped and re-probed for subsequent analyses. Signals were quantitated using ImageJ 1.44p pixel analysis (NIH Image Software) and data normalized to a control value of 1 [30].

Fibrosis

Ventricle samples were fixed in 4% paraformaldehyde and paraffin embedded for histological analysis at 6 µm cross-sections. Cardiac collagen deposition/interstitial fibrosis was assessed by Masson's trichrome stain (Alfred Pathology, Melbourne, Australia). Images of the LV were obtained using an Olympus light microscope at 40x magnification. Collagen stained blue, which was measured and analyzed using Olympus Image-Pro Plus version 6.0. The percentage fibrosis was calculated by dividing the total area of collagen by the total area of the LV and multiplying by 100%. Data were normalized to a control value of 1 and presented as a fold change.

Cardiomyocyte area

Ventricle samples were fixed in 4% paraformaldehyde and paraffin embedded for cardiomyocyte area analysis at 4 µm cross-sections. Cell membranes were stained with Fluorescein Wheat Germ Agglutinin (WGA; Vector Laboratories Inc; Burlingame, CA, USA). Cardiomyocyte size was analysed using ImageJ software (Bethesda, MD, USA) by averaging the measurements (arbitrary units) of at least 60 individual cardiomyocytes per heart, as previously described [10].

Statistical analyses

Statistical analyses was performed using StatView (Version 5.0.1, SAS Institute Inc.). Results are presented as mean ± SEM. Differences between groups were identified using one-way analysis of variance (ANOVA) followed by *Fisher's* post-hoc tests, unless otherwise indicated. Unpaired t-tests were used when comparing two groups for a single measure. A value of P<0.05 was considered significant. All relative units are expressed as a fold change with the relevant control group normalized to 1.

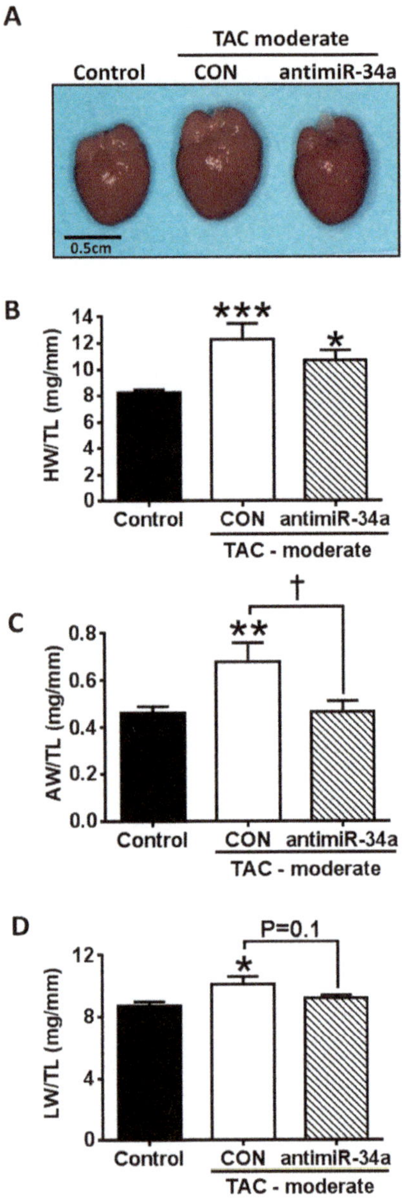

Figure 2. LNA-antimiR-34a is associated with modest improvements in cardiac remodeling in a moderate model of pressure overload. (A) Representative heart images of control, TAC moderate LNA control (CON) and TAC moderate LNA-antimiR-34a (anti-34a) at dissection. Scale bar = 0.5 cm. (B-D) Graphs of HW/TL, AW/TL and LW/TL. N=4–8 per group. ***P<0.001 vs. control, **P<0.01 vs. control, *P<0.05 vs. control, †P<0.05. 1 way ANVOA followed by Fisher's Post Hoc Test.

Results

Distinct remodeling and function in a moderate and severe model of pressure overload induced hypertrophy

To determine whether inhibition of miR-34a could improve systolic function in a mouse model with pre-existing pathological hypertrophy and systolic dysfunction, we subjected mice to TAC for four weeks. After four weeks of pressure overload, LV remodeling was confirmed by echocardiography. On the basis of the echocardiography results measured four weeks after TAC (and before administration of LNA-control or LNA-antimiR-34a), two distinct groups of mice became apparent: 1) mice with a moderate hypertrophic cardiomyopathy phenotype, i.e. increased wall thickness, and moderate cardiac dysfunction (fractional shortening >30% but significantly less than control unoperated mice, Figure 1, Table 1); and 2) mice with a more severe cardiac hypertrophic cardiomyopathy; i.e. increased wall thickness and more significant cardiac dysfunction (fractional shortening <30%, Figure 1, Table 1). Thus, mice were classified as having a moderate or severe cardiomyopathy phenotype based on echocardiography parameters prior to treatment (subsequently referred to as TAC moderate and TAC severe, respectively). The reason the TAC surgery resulted in mice with either a moderate or severe pathology is not apparently obvious but is consistent with our previous report [31].

TAC moderate mice displayed a 20% and 13% decrease in fractional shortening and ejection fraction respectively, compared to the performances of hearts evaluated pre-surgery (Figure 1A & B, Table 1). In contrast, the hearts of TAC severe mice displayed a greater decrease in fractional shortening (37%) and ejection fraction (25%) (Figure 1A & B, Table 1). There was no overlap in fractional shortening or ejection fraction from individual mice in the two groups (Figure 1A & B). Mice with moderate and severe cardiomyopathy were further subdivided and randomized into LNA-control or LNA-antimiR-34a treatment groups. Moderate and severe aortic-banded mice received three consecutive daily injections (subcutaneously) of LNA-oligonucleotides and were then left for eight weeks (Figure S1).

Inhibition of miR-34a had modest protective actions in a moderate but not severe model of pressure overload

We previously showed that three consecutive daily subcutaneous injections of an LNA-antimiR in mice is sufficient to silence miRNA expression in the heart for at least two months [10]. At eight weeks post-treatment, we confirmed that miR-34a was effectively silenced in heart tissue of TAC moderate and TAC severe LNA-antimiR-34a mice compared to LNA-control mice (Figure S2).

Compared to control mice, HW/TL increased more significantly in LNA-control TAC moderate mice (~50%) than LNA-antimiR-34a TAC moderate mice (~30%; Figure 2B, Table 2). Furthermore, while TAC moderate LNA-control mice displayed significant atrial enlargement (47% increase in atrial weight/TL, AW/TL, Figure 2C, Table 2) and developed lung congestion (15% increase in lung weight/TL, LW/TL, Figure 2D, Table 2), there was no significant increase in AW/TL and LW/TL with LNA-antimiR-34a treatment in TAC moderate mice (Figure 2C & D, Table 2). Therefore, LNA-antimiR-34a treatment attenuated, in part, adverse cardiac remodeling in a setting of moderate pathology.

By contrast, LNA-antimiR-34a treatment provided no protection in those mice classified as having a severe hypertrophic cardiomyopathy phenotype four weeks post TAC. Severe TAC mice administered LNA-control or LNA-antimiR-34a displayed significant increases in HW/TL (110–130% increase vs. control, Figure 3A, Table 2), developed significant atrial enlargement (Figure 3A, Table 2) and lung congestion (increased LW/TL, Figure 3A, Table 2); each significantly greater than that observed in TAC moderate mice (Figure 3A). In the TAC severe model, treatment with LNA-antimiR-34a was unable to attenuate hypertrophy, atrial enlargement and lung congestion, demonstrating that LNA-antimiR-34a was not protective in a severe disease setting (Figure 3A, Table 2). The changes in heart size in both moderate and severe TAC groups were accompanied by similar changes in cardiomyocyte size (Figure 3A and B).

Table 2. Morphological data for control and TAC moderate and severe mice following four weeks of pressure overload and eight weeks after treatment with LNA-control or LNA-antimiR-34a.

	Control	TAC moderate		TAC severe	
		LNA control	LNA antimiR-34a	LNA control	LNA antimiR-34a
Number of animals	8	5	4	3	3
BW (g)	33.8±0.7	32.3±1.0	31.1±1.0	33.5±1.2	28.3±2.7*§
TL (mm)	16.2±0.1	16.2±0.0	16.1±0.1	16.5±0.1	16.1±0.2
HW (mg)	133.6±3.7	198.8±20.0‡	172.1±11.1*	285.8±5.6‡‖	307.0±14.1‡‖
AW (mg)	7.5±0.5	11.0±1.3#	7.5±0.7**	26.5±1.8†‖	47.3±13.6‡§‖
LW (mg)	141.9±4.1	163.2±8.4#	148.2±3.9	398.8±34.2‡‖	393.4±59.0‡‖
HW/TL (mg/mm)	8.25±0.22	12.28±1.23‡	10.70±0.73*	17.34±0.32‡‖	19.07±1.00‡‖
AW/TL (mg/mm)	0.46±0.03	0.68±0.08#	0.47±0.05**	1.61±0.11†‖	2.93±0.84‡§‖
LW/TL (mg/mm)	8.76±0.23	10.09±0.52#	9.20±0.22	24.17±1.90‡‖	24.50±4.00‡‖

BW: body weight, HW: heart weight, AW: atria weight, LW: lung weight, TL: tibia length, HW/TL: heart weight/ tibia length ratio, AW/TL: atria weight/ tibia length ratio, LW/TL: lung weight/ tibia length ratio. Data are shown as mean ± SEM. One-way ANOVA followed by Fisher's post-hoc test (comparing 5 groups): *P<0.05 vs. control, †P<0.05 vs. control, ‡P<0.001 vs. control, §P<0.05 vs. TAC LNA control of the same group, ‖P<0.05 vs. TAC-moderate of the same treatment group. One-way ANOVA followed by Fisher's post-hoc test (comparing TAC moderate groups to control, i.e. 3 groups only): #P<0.05 vs. control, **P<0.05 vs. TAC LNA control.

After four weeks of pressure overload, fractional shortening decreased by ~20% in TAC moderate mice and by ~37% in TAC severe mice (Figure 3C, Table 3). At eight weeks post-treatment (i.e. 12 weeks post-TAC), fractional shortening decreased further in the TAC moderate LNA-control mice compared with pretreatment values at four weeks post-TAC (Figure 3C, Table 3). However, treatment with LNA-antimiR-34a prevented further deterioration as reflected in the fractional shortening after 12 weeks of TAC compared to pretreatment values at four weeks post-TAC. Furthermore, fractional shortening tended to be higher (P = 0.06) in the moderate TAC antimiR-34a treated mice at 12 weeks post-TAC compared with LNA-control mice at the same time point (Figure 3C, Table 3). In contrast, fractional shortening in the severe model of pressure overload was further decreased at eight weeks post-treatment (i.e. 12 weeks post-TAC) in both TAC LNA-control and TAC LNA-antimiR-34a mice compared with pretreatment values at four weeks post-TAC (Figure 3C, Table 3). Interestingly, fractional shortening in TAC severe LNA-antimiR-34a treated mice was significantly decreased at 12 weeks post-TAC compared to TAC severe LNA-control mice at the same time point (Figure 3C, Table 3). Finally, fractional shortening was further compromised in TAC severe groups compared to TAC moderate groups at 12 weeks post-TAC (Figure 3C, Table 3). Thus, treatment with antimiR-34a prevented further deterioration in cardiac function in a moderate model of pressure overload, but was unable to improve or maintain cardiac function in a severe model of pressure overload.

Inhibition of miR-34a did not alter the expression of cardiac stress genes following pressure overload

Pathological hypertrophy is typically associated with the re-expression of the cardiac fetal gene program, accumulation of collagen in the extracellular matrix (interstitial fibrosis) and down-regulation of calcium handling proteins [32]. Cardiac dysfunction in TAC moderate and TAC severe LNA-control treated mice was accompanied by increased expression of fetal genes, including atrial natriuretic peptide (*Anp*), B type natriuretic peptide (*Bnp*) and β myosin heavy chain (*β-MHC*), which were exacerbated in the TAC severe model (Figure 4A). Although *Anp* and *Bnp* were not attenuated with LNA-antimiR-34a treatment in moderate and severe TAC groups, there was a trend for decreased *β-MHC* in TAC moderate mice treated with LNA-antimiR-34a, but not in TAC severe mice treated with LNA-antimiR-34a (Figure 4B).

There was no change in sarcoplasmic/endoplasmic reticulum Ca^{2+}-ATPase 2a (*Serca2a*) gene expression in TAC moderate LNA-control or LNA-antimiR-34a treated mice, most likely as severe cardiac dysfunction was not present (Figure 4A). In contrast, TAC severe LNA-control and LNA-antimiR-34a mice exhibited significantly decreased *Serca2a* expression, which was not different between treatment cohorts (Figure 4A). Decreased *Serca2a* expression is a hallmark of heart failure that results in abnormal calcium handling. The disturbances in calcium metabolism contribute significantly to the contractile dysfunction observed in heart failure [33,34], which may explain why mice exhibiting altered *Serca2a* expression have more severe cardiac dysfunction.

Pathological hypertrophy is associated with progressive accumulation of collagen in the interstitial space which adversely influences contractile performance. There was a significant increase in LV fibrosis in TAC moderate mice, independent of treatment, which was further increased in TAC severe mice (Figure 4C). Treatment with LNA-antimiR-34a did not attenuate fibrosis in either the TAC moderate or TAC severe groups (Figure 4C).

Impact of miR-34a inhibition on the expression of validated targets

Identified targets of miR-34a and the miR-34 family which have been associated with improved cardiac outcomes due to their roles related to cell survival, proliferation, cardiac repair and regeneration, maintenance of cardiac function, and angiogenesis include vinculin (*Vcl*), phosphatase 1 nuclear targeting subunit (also known as PNUTS), vascular endothelial growth factor–A and B (*Vegfa, Vegfb*), Cyclin D1, Sirt1, Notch1, protein O-fucosyltransferase 1 (*Pofut1*) and semaphorin 4b (*Sema4b*) [10,11]. In this study, there was a trent for increased *Sirt1* mRNA levels in TAC moderate LNA-antimiR-34a hearts when compared to control hearts (Figure 5B). However, protein levels of vinculin (VCL), and mRNA levels of PNUTS (*Ppp1r10*), *Notch1*, *Pofut1*, Cyclin DI (*Ccnd1*), *Vegfb* and *Sema4b*, did not change in either the TAC moderate or TAC severe models of pressure overload with LNA-antimiR-34a treatment (Figure 5A & B). Protein levels of VEGF-A, which

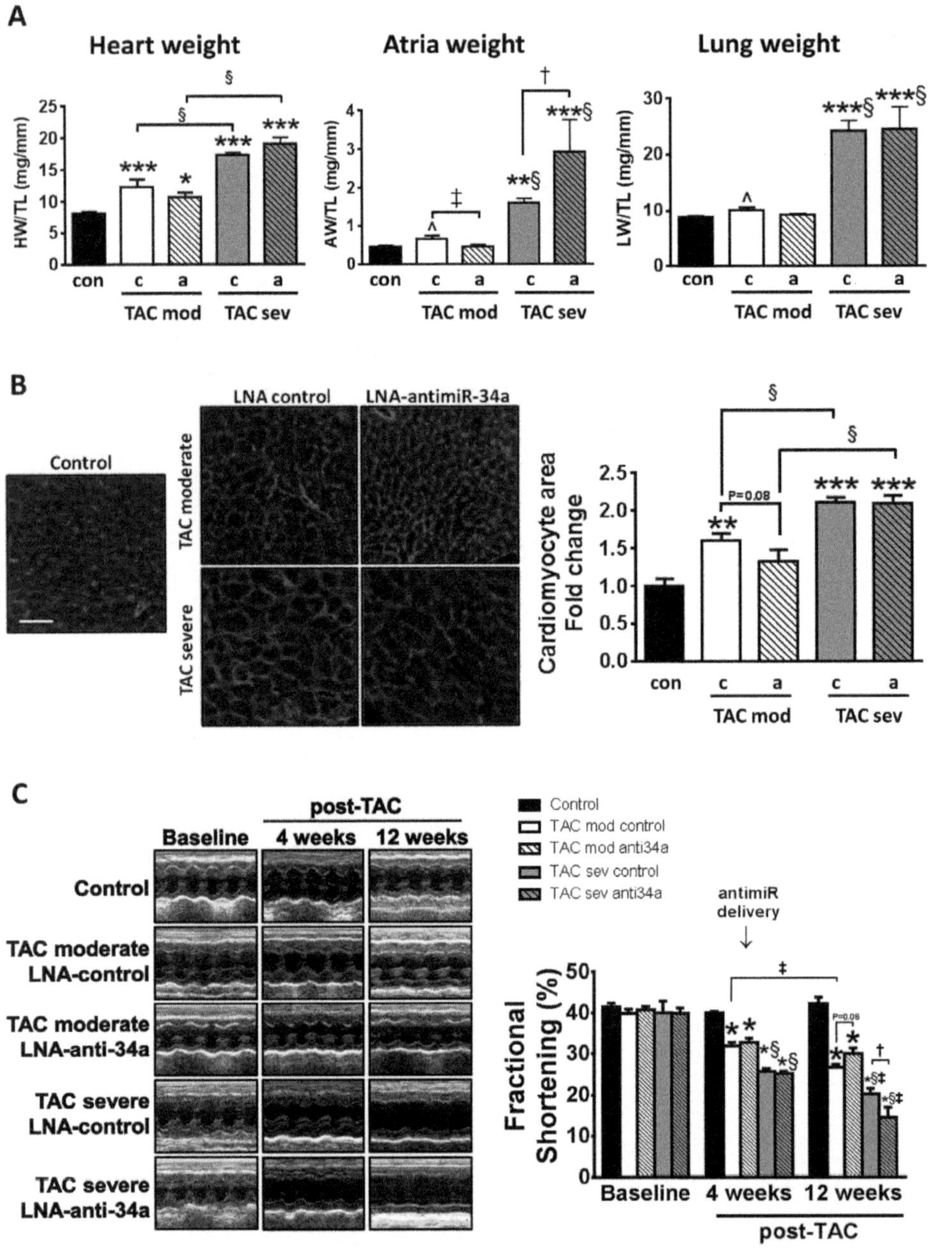

Figure 3. LNA-antimiR-34a maintains cardiac function in a moderate model of pressure overload, but not in a severe model. (A) Graphs of HW/TL, AW/TL and LW/TL in control, TAC moderate (TAC mod) and TAC severe (TAC sev) LNA-control (c) and LNA-antimiR-34a (a) groups. N = 3–8 per group. ***P<0.001 vs. control, **P<0.01 vs. control, *P<0.05 vs. control, †P<0.05, §P<0.05 vs. TAC-moderate of same treatment group. 1 way ANOVA followed by Fisher's Post Hoc Test (comparing all five groups). When performing 1 way ANOVA followed by Fisher's Post Hoc Test on control and TAC moderate groups only (i.e. comparing three groups), n = 4–8 per group, ^P<0.05 vs. control, ‡P<0.05. (B) Representative LV cross-sections stained with wheat germ agglutinin from control and TAC moderate and severe LNA-control and LNA-antimiR-34a mice, and quantification of cell area. Scale bar = 50 μM. Data are expressed as mean ± SEM. N = 3–5 per group. **P<0.01 vs. control, ***P<0.001 vs. control, §P<0.05. 1 way ANOVA followed by Fisher's Post Hoc Test (comparing all five groups). (C) Quantification of fractional shortening at baseline (pre-surgery), four weeks post TAC (before LNA oligonucleotide administration) and 12 weeks post (i.e. eight weeks post treatment) and representative M-mode echocardiograms. N = 4–5 per group. *P<0.05 vs. baseline of the same groups and control at the same time point, †P<0.05, ‡P<0.05 vs. same group at 4 weeks post TAC, §P<0.05 vs. TAC-moderate at same time point. 1 way ANOVA followed by Fisher's Post Hoc Test.

were associated with increased capillary density in our previous report (compared to TAC LNA-control mice) [10], did not increase with LNA-antimiR-34a treatment in TAC moderate or TAC severe mice. The lower levels of VEGF-A protein and *Sema4b* mRNA in hearts of TAC severe mice compared with control mice are consistent with the more severe cardiomyopathy phenotype in these animals (Figure 5A). In summary, treatment with LNA-atimiR-34a was unable to attenuate the expression of cardiac stress and fibrotic genes, improve/maintain *Serca2a* expression and significantly derepress validated targets in both

Table 3. Echocardiography data of control and TAC mice at baseline, four weeks post-TAC and eight weeks after treatment with either LNA-control or LNA-antimiR-34a.

	Baseline					Four weeks post-TAC					Eight weeks post treatment				
	Control	TAC Moderate		TAC severe		Control	TAC Moderate		TAC Severe		Control	TAC Moderate		TAC Severe	
		LNA control	LNA antimiR-34a	LNA control	LNA antimiR-34a		LNA control	LNA antimiR-34a	LNA control	LNA antimiR-34a		LNA control	LNA antimiR-34a	LNA control	LNA antimiR-34a
Number of animals	4	5	4	3	3	4	5	4	3	3	4	5	4	3	3
BW (g)	28.6±0.4	28.5±1.3	27.5±0.7	27.3±2.1	27.6±1.0	30.3±0.7	29.6±0.7	28.7±0.6	29.7±0.8	28.4±0.7	34.7±0.9	32.3±0.8	30.7±1.1	33.9±0.9	28.1±2.3†
Heart rate, bpm	608±9	564±22	570±15	500±29	611±11	643±21	584±19	613±25	572±31	587±20	598±20	569±18	597± 11	573±11	614±49
LVPW, mm	0.67±0.01	0.71±0.01	0.66±0.01	0.70±0.05	0.75±0.02	0.73±0.02	1.05±0.00*	1.03±0.02*	1.05±0.02*	1.08±0.04*	0.78±0.02*	1.17±0.03*‡	1.07±0.02*†	1.21±0.02*#§	1.22±0.01*‡§
IVS, mm	0.75±0.01	0.74±0.01	0.74±0.01	0.73±0.01	0.73±0.0[illegible]	0.78±0.01	1.17±0.02*	1.12±0.01*	1.22±0.03*	1.17±0.04*	0.81±0.02	1.18±0.04*	1.09±0.02*†	1.19±0.03*	1.25±0.02*‡§
LVEDD, mm	3.81±0.12	4.11±0.09	3.89±0.12	4.20±0.11	3.82±0.1[illegible]	3.89±0.21	4.16±0.[illegible]5	3.87±0.07	4.45±0.21	4.23±0.18	3.75±0.17	4.33±0.11	4.12±0.14	4.80±0.30*§	5.31±0.08*†‡§
LVESD, mm	2.23±0.08	2.47±0.10	2.39±0.13	2.50±0.10	2.30±0.1[illegible]	2.33±0.11	2.83±0.[illegible]2*	2.60±0.07‖	3.31±0.19*§	3.16±0.14*§	2.18±0.14	3.18±0.10*‡	2.89±0.15*# (P=0.08)	3.82±0.18*#§	4.54±0.11*†‡§
FS, %	41±1	40±1	41±1	40±3	40±1	40±0	32±1*	33±1*	26±1*§	25±1*§	42±2	27±1*‡	30±1* # (P=0.06)	20±1*#§	14±2*†‡§
EF, %	80±1	78±1	79±1	78±3	78±1	78±0	69±1*	68±1*	59±1*§	58±1*§	81±2	61±1*‡	65±2*†	49±2*#§	37±5*†‡§

BW, body weight; LV, left ventricular; LVPW, LV posterior wall thickness; IVS, interventricular septum thickness; LVEDD, LV end-diastolic dimension; LVESD, LV end-systolic dimension; FS, fractional shortening.
Data are shown as mean ± SEM. One way ANOVA followed by Fisher's Post hoc Test.
*P<0.05 vs. baseline of same group and control at same time point, †P<0.05 vs. TAC LNA control of same group at same time point, ‡P<0.05 vs. same group at 4 weeks post TAC,§P<0.05 vs. TAC moderate of same treatment group at same timepoint, ||P<0.1 vs. baseline of same group and control at same time point, #P<0.1 vs. TAC LNA control of same group at same time point.

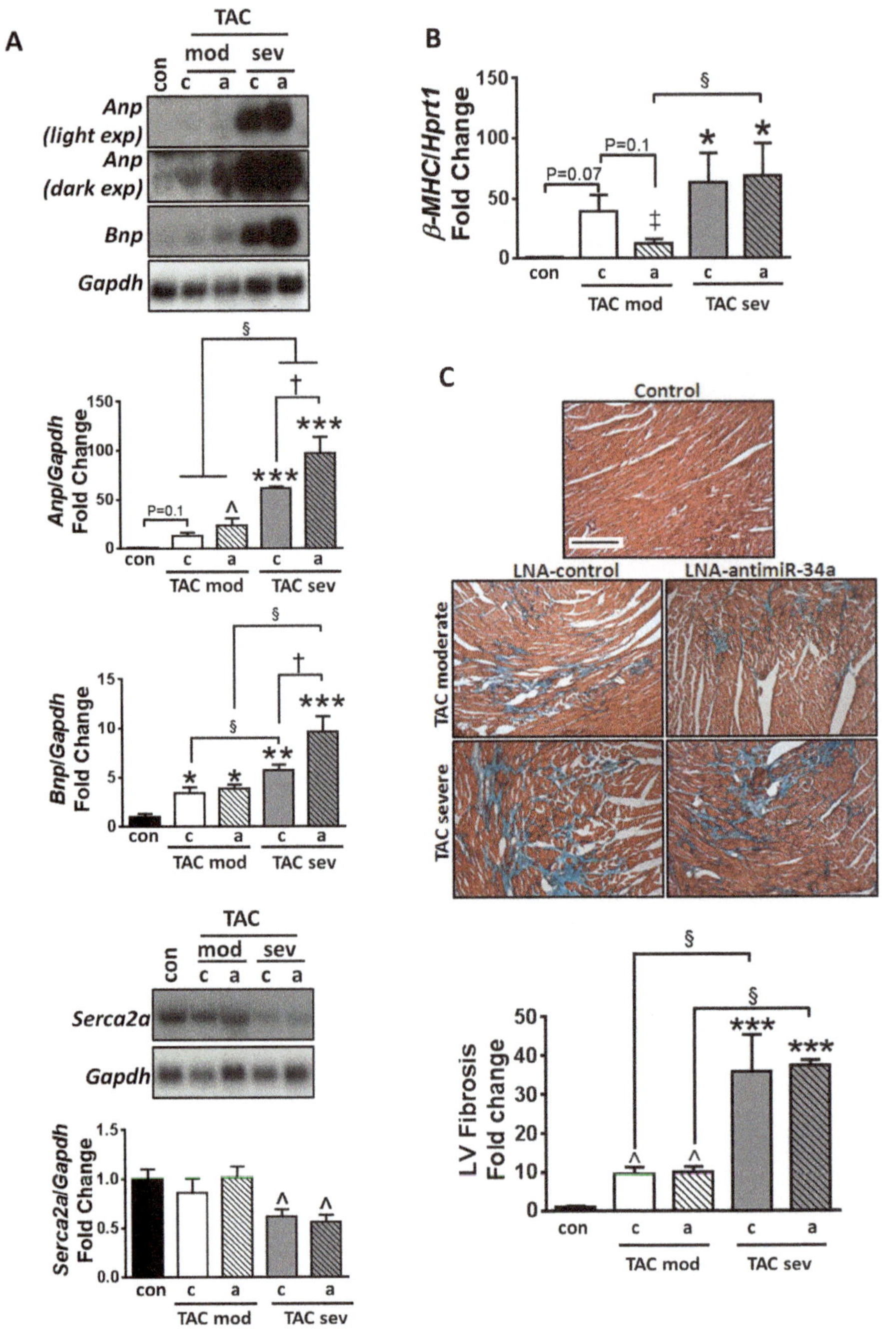

Figure 4. Cardiac stress gene expression and fibrosis in moderate and severe models of pressure overload. (A) Northern blots and quantification of *Anp*, *Bnp*, and *Serca2a* relative to *Gapdh*, in hearts of control (con), TAC moderate (mod), TAC severe (sev) mice dosed with either LNA-control (c) or LNA-antimiR-34a (a). For Northern blot of *Anp*, a light exposure (light exp) and dark exposure (dark exp) has been included. N = 3–5 per group. ***P<0.001 vs. control, **P<0.01 vs. control, *P<0.05 vs. control, §P<0.05, †P<0.05, 1 way ANOVA followed by Fisher's Post Hoc Test (comparing all five groups). When performing 1 way ANOVA followed by Fisher's Post Hoc Test on control and TAC severe groups only (comparing three groups), N = 3 per group, or control and TAC moderate groups only (comparing three groups), N = 3–5 per group, ^P<0.05 vs. control. (B) qPCR of *β-MHC* relative to *Hprt1* in control, TAC moderate and TAC severe mice dosed with LNA-control or LNA-antimiR-34a. N = 3–5 per group. *P<0.05 vs. control, §P<0.05, ‡P<0.05 vs. control, 1 way ANOVA followed by Fisher's Post Hoc Test (comparing all 5 groups). (C) LV cross-sections stained with Masson's trichrome and quantification of LV fibrosis in control, TAC moderate and TAC severe mice dosed with LNA-control or LNA-antimiR-34a. Scale = 200 μM. N = 4–5 per group. ***P<0.001 vs. control, §P<0.05 vs. TAC-moderate of the same treatment group, 1 way ANOVA followed by Fisher's Post Hoc Test (comparing all five groups). When comparing control and TAC moderate groups only (comparing three groups), N = 4–5 per group, ^P<0.05 vs. control, 1 way ANOVA followed by Fisher's Post Hoc Test.

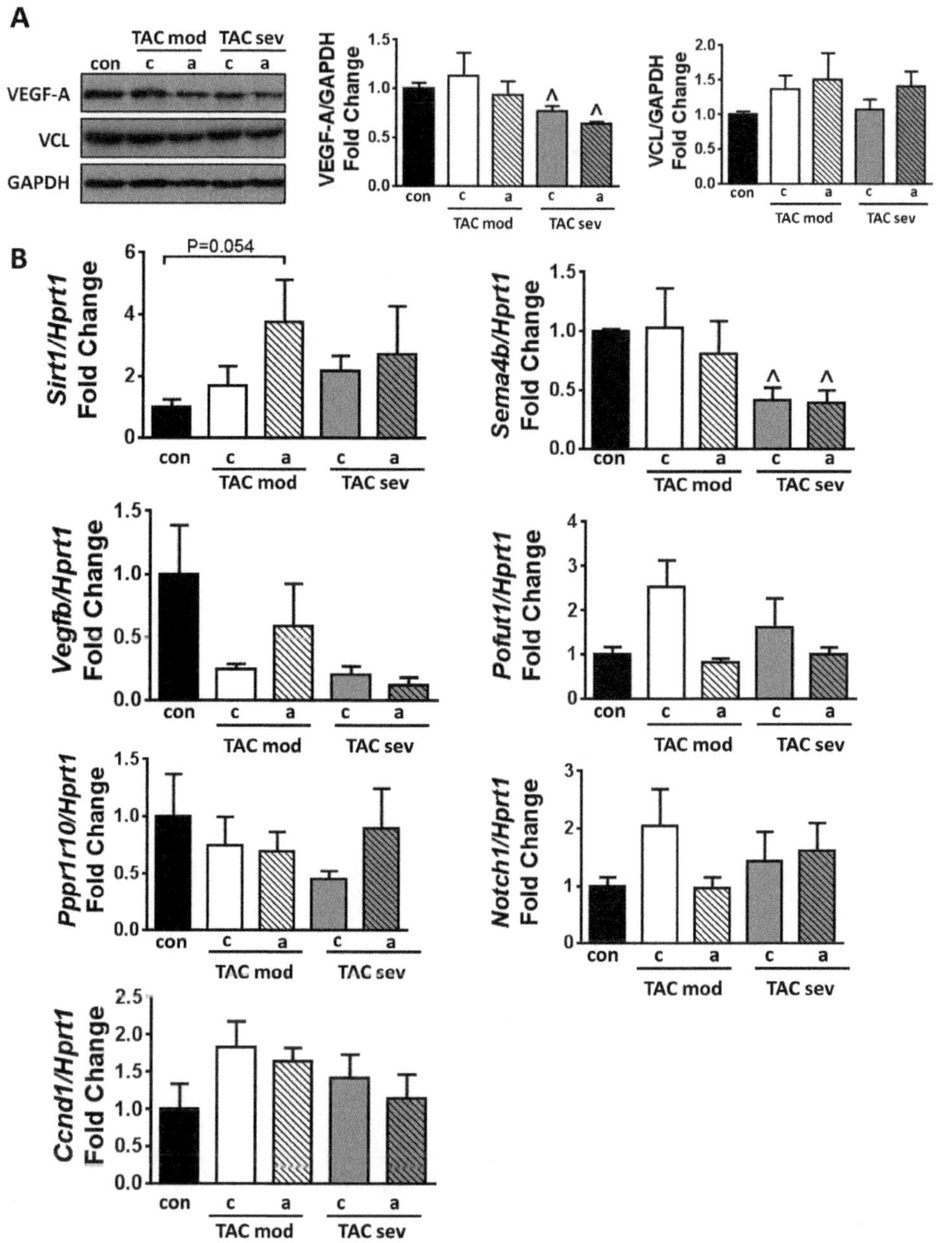

Figure 5. Analysis of miR-34a target gene or protein expression. (A) Representative Western blots and quantification of VEGF-A and VCL relative to GAPDH in hearts of control (con), TAC moderate (mod), TAC severe (sev) mice dosed with either LNA-control (c) or LNA-antimiR-34a (a). N = 3–5 per group. ^P<0.05 vs. control when using 1 way ANOVA followed by Fisher's Post Hoc test on severe group only. (B) qPCR analysis of *Sirt1, Sema4b, Vegfb, Pofut1,* PNUTS *(Pppr10), Notch 1* and Cyclin D1 *(Ccnd1)* relative to *Hprt1*. N = 3–5 per group. ^P<0.05 vs. control when using 1 way ANOVA followed by Fisher's Post Hoc test on control and TAC severe groups only (comparing three groups).

moderate and severe mouse models of pressure overload induced by TAC.

Expression of miR-34 family members, miR-34b and miR-34c, is elevated in moderate and severe models of pressure overload

We have previously shown that expression of other miR-34 family members, miR-34b and miR-34c, are elevated in settings of cardiac stress [10,18]. Since we identified only modest protection in the moderate model of TAC, and no protection in the severe model of TAC with LNA-antimiR-34a administration in the present study, we analyzed the expression of the other miR-34 family members (i.e. miR-34b and -34c) in control mice, TAC moderate LNA-control and TAC severe LNA-control mice. There was a significant increase in 34a, miR-34b and miR-34c in TAC moderate LNA-control mice compared to control mice (Figure 6). Interestingly, only miR-34b and miR-34c were significantly increased in TAC severe LNA-control mice (and at higher levels compared to TAC moderate), but not miR-34a. This may explain the partial protection observed in TAC moderate mice, but no protection in TAC severe mice, given that only miR-34a was inhibited in this study (Figure 6). We have previously shown that

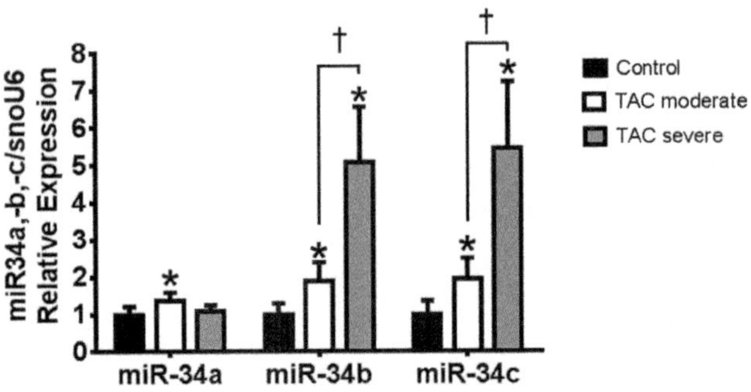

Figure 6. Expression of miR-34a, miR-34b and miR-34c in control and TAC mice. qPCR of miR-34a, miR-b and miR-34c in hearts of control, TAC moderate and TAC severe mice. N = 3–5 per group. *P<0.05 vs. control, †P<0.05. 1 way ANOVA followed by Fisher's Post Hoc test.

LNA-antimiR-34a does not significantly silence miR-34b and miR-34c in the heart [10].

Discussion

In a previous study, we reported that inhibition of the miR-34 family attenuated LV remodeling and atrial enlargement in mouse models with established cardiac dysfunction due to MI or pressure overload [10]. Interestingly, inhibition of miR-34a alone provided no significant benefit in the MI setting, but was not explored in the pressure overload model [10]. Given that inhibition of miR-34a is being considered as a possible therapy for cardiovascular disease [11,21,22], we set out to determine whether miR-34a inhibition could provide benefit in a mouse model of pressure overload-induced pathological hypertrophy. A potential advantage of inhibiting miR-34a alone, as opposed to the entire family, is related to fewer possible off-target effects.

The major finding of the present study is that inhibition of miR-34a provided some protection in the TAC moderate model, but not in the TAC severe model. LNA-antimiR-34a treated TAC moderate mice did not develop lung congestion, atrial enlargement was attenuated, and importantly, there was no further deterioration in cardiac function at 12 weeks post TAC compared to pretreatment values at four weeks post TAC. In contrast, systolic function continued to fall in TAC moderate LNA-control mice. HW/TL increased by approximately 49% in TAC moderate LNA-control mice, and only 30% in TAC moderate LNA-antimiR-34a mice. Despite attenuation of adverse cardiac remodeling, treatment with LNA-antimiR-34a was not associated with a more favorable cardiac molecular signature or less fibrosis. The only parameter which showed a tendency to be attenuated in antimiR-34a treated mice was β-MHC expression. Treatment with LNA-antimiR-34a was associated with a trend for increased *Sirt1* expression. *Sirt1* protects the heart against ageing and stress [35], thus increased *Sirt1* mRNA may contribute to the modest cardiac protection observed in TAC moderate mice. However, treatment with LNA-antimiR-34a was unable to increase the expression of other validated targets that have been associated with improved outcomes in settings of cardiac stress (VEGF-A, VEGF-B, VCL, PNUTS, Cyclin D1). This is in contrast to the more favorable effect of inhibiting the entire miR-34 family in the pressure overload mouse model in our previous report [10]. Inhibition of the entire miR-34 family improved cardiac function, and this was associated with reduced fibrosis, decreased *Anp* expression, increased angiogenesis, maintenance of *Serca2a* expression, and up-regulation of several direct targets, including VEGFs, Pofut1, Notch1 and Sema4b [10]. As miRNAs target several hundred mRNAs, it is possible that other targets could contribute to the modest cardiac benefit in the moderate model of pressure overload with LNA-antimiR-34a treatment. Finally, inhibition of miR-34a was not protective in a severe model of pressure overload since treatment with LNA-antimiR-34a did not attenuate LV remodeling, improve cardiac function or cardiac stress gene expression, and fibrosis. This finding is consistent with our previous report in which inhibition of miR-34a did not prevent LV remodeling or improve cardiac function following chronic MI [10]. Collectively, these studies suggest that inhibition of miR-34a provides some benefit in an acute setting of cardiac stress or conditions with moderate pathology, but not in chronic or severe settings.

A possible explanation for the reduced capacity of LNA-antimiR-34a to provide protection in chronic or severe settings of cardiac pathology may be due to increased expression of two other miR-34-family members, miR-34b and miR-34c (ranging from a ~1.7 to 4-fold increase in MI or TAC [10]). We have previously shown that LNA-antimiR-34a does not inhibit miR-34b and miR-34c [10], which were both elevated in the TAC severe model in this study. Interestingly, miR-34a was elevated in the hearts of the TAC moderate but not TAC severe model. Thus, this could explain why pharmacologic inhibition was not effective in the TAC severe model, and only partially protective in the TAC moderate model of pressure overload, which had increased levels of all miR-34 family members (i.e. miR-34a, miR-34b and miR-34c).

miRNA-based therapies are advancing at a rapid rate, with successful completion of phase 1 and phase 2 clinical trials of Santaris Pharma's LNA-modified antimiR, miravirsen, targeting miR-122 for the treatment of hepatitis C virus infection [9]. Thus, there is great enthusiasm for the development of miRNA-based therapies for cardiovascular disease. The different degrees of efficacy upon inhibition of miR-34a in different cardiac disease models highlights the importance of assessing therapeutic targeting of candidate miRNAs over a broad spectrum of cardiac conditions, as some miRNAs may be more effective than others under particular settings (e.g. acute vs. chronic). In recognition that cardiovascular disease and cardiac remodeling is associated with simultaneous dysregulation of several miRNAs (e.g. miR-1, miR-34a, miR-133, miR-199b, miR-320 [11,15,36–38]) or miRNA families (e.g. miR-34 family [10], miR-208 family [39]), tiny 8-mer seed-targeting LNA-antimiRs could provide an advantage by simultaneous inhibition of entire miRNA seed families [10,27]. The current study and our previous work [10] highlight a different therapeutic benefit of inhibiting a single miRNA (miR-34a) or a miRNA family (miR-34 family) in moderate and severe models of sustained cardiac stress. Greater therapeutic benefit of inhibiting the entire miR-34 family may be related to the regulation of more target genes. As shown by miRNA target prediction databases based on different algorithms (MiRanda, DIANA, PicTar), the miR-34 family is predicted to repress 24–40% (mouse) or 31–55% (human) more mRNAs than miR-34a alone (Figure S3). Thus, targeting miRNA families may be able to regulate multiple additional biological networks. However, this may have both favorable and unfavorable consequences, and the potential off-target effects must be carefully assessed when developing miRNA therapeutics [10].

Although there are several advantages of developing miRNA-based therapeutics, many miRNAs are ubiquitously expressed and miRNA-based therapeutics are taken up by various organs upon systemic delivery, making clinical intervention complex. Whilst inhibition of miR-34a and the miR-34 family is protective in the hearts of mice [10,11], the effect of prolonged/chronic inhibition of miR-34a and its family members may not be ideal because of its ability to drive tumorigenesis [40,41], although a recent study has shown that the miR-34 family is not required for tumor suppression in mice [42]. Conversely, miR-34a replacement therapy as a cancer therapeutic may have adverse affects on the heart or render the heart more susceptible to dysfunction in settings of stress. Following successful pre-clinical work that has demonstrated potent anti-tumor effects by introducing miR-34a mimics in different mouse models of cancer [43,44], Mirna Therapeutics have developed MRX34 to restore the expression of miR-34a in tumor cells and are currently conducting a Phase 1 study in patients with primary liver cancer or metastatic cancer with liver involvement [45,46]. In addition to the tumor suppressive role of miR-34a, miR-34 expression is important for long-term maintenance of the brain, healthy aging and modulation of protein homeostasis with age in *Drosophila* [47], and miR-34b and miR-34c are key regulators of skeletogenesis [48]. Therefore, while miR-34 has marked therapeutic potential in conditions of heart stress, it will be critical to assess the impact of miR-34 in brain, bone and other organs during its development as a therapeutic agent, or may require the development of cardiac-specific approaches[27, 32, 45,] [49].

In summary, administration of LNA-antimiR-34a in a moderate model of pressure overload was able to attenuate atrial enlargement, prevent lung congestion and maintain cardiac function, but was unable to attenuate pathological cardiac remodeling or prevent further cardiac dysfunction in a severe model of pressure overload. Thus, drugs that target the entire miR-34 family are likely to have greater therapeutic benefit in settings of sustained cardiac stress and severe pathology than inhibition of miR-34a alone.

Supporting Information

Figure S1 Experimental Timeline and dosing regimen of LNA-control/antimiR-34a for mice subjected to pressure overload (TAC).

Figure S2 Administration of LNA-antimiR-34a silences miR-34a in the heart. qPCR showing inhibition of miR-34a in hearts of TAC moderate and TAC severe mice dosed with LNA-antimiR-34a vs. LNA-control. N = 3-5 per group. *P<0.05 vs. LNA-control. Unpaired t-test.

Figure S3 Number of predicted targets of miR-34a versus the miR-34 family. Bar graphs showing the number of predicted targets of miR-34a versus the miR-34 family using three target prediction algorithms in mice and humans (MiRanda 4.0, PicTar, DIANA microT v5.0). All miR-34a targets are also predicted targets of miR-34 family.

Table S1 Morphological data for control adult male mice eight weeks after administration of a LNA-control or LNA-antimiR-34a.

Acknowledgments

We thank Nicole Jennings for assistance with echocardiography.

Author Contributions

Conceived and designed the experiments: BCB SO SK RCYL JRM. Performed the experiments: BCB XMG YKT HK CEW JYYO EJHB XJD JRM. Analyzed the data: BCB CEW JYYO YKT JRM. Contributed reagents/materials/analysis tools: SO SK PG. Wrote the paper: BCB JRM.

References

1. Bernardo BC, Charchar FJ, Lin RCY, McMullen JR (2012) A MicroRNA Guide for Clinicians and Basic Scientists: Background and Experimental Techniques. Heart, Lung and Circulation 21: 131–142.
2. Kumarswamy R, Thum T (2013) Non-coding RNAs in Cardiac Remodeling and Heart Failure. Circulation Research 113: 676–689.
3. Leite-Moreira AM, Lourenco AP, Falcao-Pires I, Leite-Moreira AF (2013) Pivotal role of microRNAs in cardiac physiology and heart failure. Drug Discov Today: doi:10.1016/j.drudis.2013.1007.1025 [Epub ahead of print].
4. Dangwal S, Thum T (2014) microRNA Therapeutics in Cardiovascular Disease Models. Annual Review of Pharmacology and Toxicology 54: doi:10.1146/annurev-pharmtox-011613-135957
5. Latronico MVG, Condorelli G (2009) MicroRNAs and cardiac pathology. Nature Reviews Cardiology 6: 418–429.
6. Latronico MV, Condorelli G (2011) microRNAs in hypertrophy and heart failure. Exp Biol Med (Maywood) 236: 125–131.
7. Elmen J, Lindow M, Silahtaroglu A, Bak M, Christensen M, et al. (2008) Antagonism of microRNA-122 in mice by systemically administered LNA-antimiR leads to up-regulation of a large set of predicted target mRNAs in the liver. Nucl Acids Res 36: 1153–1162.
8. Elmen J, Lindow M, Schutz S, Lawrence M, Petri A, et al. (2008) LNA-mediated microRNA silencing in non-human primates. Nature 452: 896–899.
9. Janssen HL, Reesink HW, Lawitz EJ, Zeuzem S, Rodriguez-Torres M, et al. (2013) Treatment of HCV infection by targeting microRNA. N Engl J Med 368: 1685–1694.
10. Bernardo BC, Gao XM, Winbanks CE, Boey EJ, Tham YK, et al. (2012) Therapeutic inhibition of the miR-34 family attenuates pathological cardiac remodeling and improves heart function. Proc Natl Acad Sci U S A 109: 17615–17620.
11. Boon RA, Iekushi K, Lechner S, Seeger T, Fischer A, et al. (2013) MicroRNA-34a regulates cardiac ageing and function. Nature 495: 107–110.
12. Hullinger TG, Montgomery RL, Seto AG, Dickinson BA, Semus HM, et al. (2012) Inhibition of miR-15 Protects Against Cardiac Ischemic Injury/Novelty and Significance. Circulation Research 110: 71–81.
13. Montgomery RL, Hullinger TG, Semus HM, Dickinson BA, Seto AG, et al. (2011) Therapeutic Inhibition of miR-208a Improves Cardiac Function and Survival During Heart Failure/Clinical Perspective. Circulation 124: 1537–1547.
14. Porrello ER, Mahmoud AI, Simpson E, Johnson BA, Grinsfelder D, et al. (2013) Regulation of neonatal and adult mammalian heart regeneration by the miR-15 family. Proc Natl Acad Sci U S A 110: 187–192.
15. da Costa Martins PA, Salic K, Gladka MM, Armand AS, Leptidis S, et al. (2010) MicroRNA-199b targets the nuclear kinase Dyrk1a in an auto-amplification loop promoting calcineurin/NFAT signalling. Nat Cell Biol 12: 1220–1227.
16. Murphy BL, Obad S, Bihannic L, Ayrault O, Zindy F, et al. (2013) Silencing of the miR-17~92 cluster family inhibits medulloblastoma progression. Cancer Research: doi:10.1158/0008-5472.CAN-1113-0927.
17. Pecot CV, Rupaimoole R, Yang D, Akbani R, Ivan C, et al. (2013) Tumour angiogenesis regulation by the miR-200 family. Nat Commun 4: doi:10.1038/ncomms3427.
18. Lin RCY, Weeks KL, Gao X-M, Williams RBH, Bernardo BC, et al. (2010) PI3K(p110α) protects against myocardial infarction-induced heart failure/ Identification of PI3K-regulated miRNAs and mRNAs. Arteriosclerosis, Thrombosis, and Vascular Biology 30: 724–732.
19. Greco S, Fasanaro P, Castelvecchio S, D'Alessandra Y, Arcelli D, et al. (2012) MicroRNA Dysregulation in Diabetic Ischemic Heart Failure Patients. Diabetes 61: 1633–1641.
20. Thum T, Galuppo P, Wolf C, Fiedler J, Kneitz S, et al. (2007) MicroRNAs in the Human Heart: A Clue to Fetal Gene Reprogramming in Heart Failure. Circulation 116: 258–267.
21. Loffredo FS, Pancoast JR, Lee RT (2013) Keep PNUTS in Your Heart. Circulation Research 113: 97–99.
22. Emanueli C, Thum T (2013) miRNAGE-34 induces cardiac damAGE. Cell Res 23: 866–867.
23. Lou K (2012) Distillery highlight: This week in therapeutics - Cardiovascular disease. SciBX 5: doi:10.1038/scibx.2012.1084.
24. Xu Q, Lekgabe ED, Gao X-M, Ming Z, Tregear GW, et al. (2008) Endogenous Relaxin Does Not Affect Chronic Pressure Overload-Induced Cardiac Hypertrophy and Fibrosis. Endocrinology 149: 476–482.
25. Gao X-M, Kiriazis H, Moore X-L, Feng X-H, Sheppard K, et al. (2005) Regression of pressure overload-induced left ventricular hypertrophy in mice. Am J Physiol Heart Circ Physiol 288: H2702-2707.

26. Weeks KL, Gao X, Du XJ, Boey EJ, Matsumoto A, et al. (2012) Phosphoinositide 3-kinase p110alpha is a master regulator of exercise-induced cardioprotection and PI3K gene therapy rescues cardiac dysfunction. Circ Heart Fail 5: 523–534.
27. Obad S, dos Santos CO, Petri A, Heidenblad M, Broom O, et al. (2011) Silencing of microRNA families by seed-targeting tiny LNAs. Nat Genet 43: 371–378.
28. Pfaffl MW (2001) A new mathematical model for relative quantification in real-time RT-PCR. Nucleic Acids Res 29: e45.
29. Shioi T, Kang PM, Douglas PS, Hampe J, Yballe CM, et al. (2000) The conserved phosphoinositide 3-kinase pathway determines heart size in mice. EMBO J 19: 2537–2548.
30. Winbanks CE, Beyer C, Hagg A, Qian H, Sepulveda PV, et al. (2013) miR-206 Represses Hypertrophy of Myogenic Cells but Not Muscle Fibers via Inhibition of HDAC4. PLoS One 8: e73589.
31. McMullen JR, Sherwood MC, Tarnavski O, Zhang L, Dorfman AL, et al. (2004) Inhibition of mTOR signaling with rapamycin regresses established cardiac hypertrophy induced by pressure overload. Circulation 109: 3050–3055.
32. Bernardo BC, Weeks KL, Pretorius L, McMullen JR (2010) Molecular distinction between physiological and pathological cardiac hypertrophy: experimental findings and therapeutic strategies. Pharmacology & Therapeutics 128: 191–227.
33. Inesi G, Prasad AM, Pilankatta R (2008) The Ca2+ ATPase of cardiac sarcoplasmic reticulum: Physiological role and relevance to diseases. Biochem Biophys Res Commun 369: 182–187.
34. Eisner D, Caldwell J, Trafford A (2013) Sarcoplasmic Reticulum Ca-ATPase and Heart Failure 20 Years Later. Circulation Research 113: 958–961.
35. Hsu CP, Odewale I, Alcendor RR, Sadoshima J (2008) Sirt1 protects the heart from aging and stress. Biol Chem 389: 221–231.
36. Care A, Catalucci D, Felicetti F, Bonci D, Addario A, et al. (2007) MicroRNA-133 controls cardiac hypertrophy. Nature Medicine 13: 613–618.
37. Ren XP, Wu J, Wang X, Sartor MA, Qian J, et al. (2009) MicroRNA-320 is involved in the regulation of cardiac ischemia/reperfusion injury by targeting heat-shock protein 20. Circulation 119: 2357–2366.
38. Yang B, Lin H, Xiao J, Lu Y, Luo X, et al. (2007) The muscle-specific microRNA miR-1 regulates cardiac arrhythmogenic potential by targeting GJA1 and KCNJ2. Nat Med 13: 486–491.
39. van Rooij E, Quiat D, Johnson BA, Sutherland LB, Qi X, et al. (2009) A family of microRNAs encoded by myosin genes governs myosin expression and muscle performance. Dev Cell 17: 662–673.
40. Silber J, Jacobsen A, Ozawa T, Harinath G, Pedraza A, et al. (2012) miR-34a Repression in Proneural Malignant Gliomas Upregulates Expression of Its Target PDGFRA and Promotes Tumorigenesis. PLoS One 7: e33844.
41. Wong MY, Yu Y, Walsh WR, Yang JL (2011) microRNA-34 family and treatment of cancers with mutant or wild-type p53 (Review). Int J Oncol 38: 1189–1195.
42. Concepcion CP, Han Y-C, Mu P, Bonetti C, Yao E, et al. (2012) Intact p53-Dependent Responses in miR-34 Deficient Mice. PLoS Genet 8: e1002797.
43. Liu C, Kelnar K, Liu B, Chen X, Calhoun-Davis T, et al. (2011) The microRNA miR-34a inhibits prostate cancer stem cells and metastasis by directly repressing CD44. Nat Med 17: 211–215.
44. Trang P, Wiggins JF, Daige CL, Cho C, Omotola M, et al. (2011) Systemic delivery of tumor suppressor microRNA mimics using a neutral lipid emulsion inhibits lung tumors in mice. Mol Ther 19: 1116–1122.
45. Hydbring P, Badalian-Very G (2013) Clinical Applications of microRNAs. F1000Research 2: 136 doi:110.12688/f11000research.12682-12136.v12682
46. Bader AG (2012) miR-34 - a microRNA replacement therapy is headed to the clinic. Front Genet 3: 120.
47. Liu N, Landreh M, Cao K, Abe M, Hendriks GJ, et al. (2012) The microRNA miR-34 modulates ageing and neurodegeneration in Drosophila. Nature 482: 519–523.
48. Wei J, Shi Y, Zheng L, Zhou B, Inose H, et al. (2012) miR-34s inhibit osteoblast proliferation and differentiation in the mouse by targeting SATB2. The Journal of Cell Biology 197: 509–521.
49. Ebert MS, Sharp PA (2010) MicroRNA sponges: Progress and possibilities. RNA 16: 2043–2050.

21

Extracellular Matrix Biomarker, Fibulin-1, Is Closely Related to NT-proBNP and Soluble Urokinase Plasminogen Activator Receptor in Patients with Aortic Valve Stenosis (The SEAS Study)

Ruan Kruger[1,2]*, Lars M. Rasmussen[3], William S. Argraves[4], Jesper Eugen-Olsen[5], Olav W. Nielsen[6], Adam Blyme[7], Ronnie Willenheimer[8], Kristian Wachtell[9], Michael H. Olsen[1,2]

1 Hypertension in Africa Research Team (HART), North-West University, Potchefstroom, South Africa, **2** The Cardiovascular and Metabolic Preventive Clinic, Department of Endocrinology, Centre for Individualized Medicine in Arterial Diseases (CIMA), Odense University Hospital, Odense, Denmark, **3** Department of Clinical Biochemistry and Pharmacology, Centre for Individualized Medicine in Arterial Diseases (CIMA), Odense University Hospital, Odense, Denmark, **4** Medical University of South Carolina, Department of Cell Biology, Charleston, South Carolina, United States of America, **5** Clinical Research Centre 136, Hvidovre Hospital, Copenhagen, Denmark, **6** Department of Cardiology, Bispebjerg Hospital, Copenhagen, Denmark, **7** Department of Cardiology, Glostrup Hospital, Copenhagen, Denmark, **8** Lund University and Heart Health Group, Malmö, Sweden, **9** Department of Medicine, Glostrup Hospital, Copenhagen, Denmark

Abstract

Background: Fibulin-1, a circulating extracellular matrix glycoprotein, has been associated with arterial disease and elevated N-terminal prohormone B-type natriuretic peptide (NT-proBNP) in diabetes. Soluble urokinase plasminogen activator receptor (suPAR), a marker of inflammation, has been associated with subclinical atherosclerosis. Therefore, we aimed to explore the interplay between these biomarkers and mild to moderate aortic valve stenosis (AS).

Methods: In 374 patients with mild to moderate AS, we investigated the relationship of fibulin-1 with NT-proBNP, levels of suPAR and the degree of AS at baseline and after one and four years of treatment with Simvastatin 40 mg and Ezetimibe 10 mg or placebo.

Results: During treatment, fibulin-1 became more closely associated with NT-proBNP ($\beta_{year0} = 0.10$, $p = 0.08$, $\beta_{year1} = 0.16$, $p = 0.005$, $\beta_{year4} = 0.22$, $p < 0.001$) and suPAR ($\beta_{year0} = 0.05$, $p = 0.34$, $\beta_{year1} = 0.16$, $p = 0.006$, $\beta_{year4} = 0.13$, $p = 0.03$) at the expense of the association to aortic valve area index (AVAI) ($\beta_{year0} = -0.14$, $p = 0.005$, $\beta_{year1} = -0.08$, $p = 0.11$, $\beta_{year4} = -0.06$, $p = 0.22$) independently of age, gender, creatinine, and serum aspartate aminotransferase ($Adj.R_{year0}^2 = 0.19$, $Adj.R_{year1}^2 = 0.22$, $Adj.R_{year4}^2 = 0.27$). Fibulin-1 was unrelated to aortic regurgitation, left ventricular mass, and ejection fraction. In patients with baseline AVAI$<$0.58 cm^2/m^2 (median value), fibulin-1 was more closely associated to NT-proBNP ($\beta_{year0} = 0.25$, $\beta_{year1} = 0.21$, $\beta_{year4} = 0.22$, all $p < 0.01$), and suPAR ($\beta_{year0} = 0.09$, $p = 0.26$, $\beta_{year1} = 0.23$, $\beta_{year4} = 0.21$, both $p <$ 0.01) independently of age, gender, AST and treatment allocation.

Conclusions: Increased levels of fibulin-1 were independently associated with higher levels of suPAR and NT-proBNP especially in patients with lower AVAI, suggesting that fibulin-1 may be an early marker of AS as well as cardiac fibrosis secondarily to elevated left ventricular hemodynamic load.

Editor: Giacomo Frati, Sapienza University of Rome, Italy

Funding: These authors have no support or funding to report.

Competing Interests: Roche Diagnostics have performed the NT-proBNP measurements for this study, without requiring any restrictions for the investigators. Roche Diagnostics was completely blinded for the clinical data and had no influence on the hypotheses, data collection and analyses, decision to publish, or preparation of the manuscript. There are no patents, products in development or marketed products to declare.

* Email: ruan.kruger@nwu.ac.za

Introduction

Aortic stenosis is a slow progressing condition developing with increasing age and abnormal calcium build up in the aortic valve [1,2]. Consequences of aortic stenosis normally include myocardial hypertrophy and fibrosis [3,4], finally cascading into heart failure, angina and sudden death [5]. Particularly soluble urokinase plasminogen activator receptor (suPAR)) has an overlapping interaction with atherosclerotic formation [6] and stiffness related to aortic stenosis [3,4,7]. Adverse hemodynamic alterations contribute to alter the integrity of structural components necessary to maintain healthy cardiovascular function, hence promoting extracellular matrix remodelling [8].

Fibulin-1, a calcium-binding extracellular matrix glycoprotein, recently received interest on its association with elastin fibres within cardiovascular tissue and fibrinogen cross-linking [9,10]. A study on rats found that levels of fibulin-1 are down-regulated in events related to cardiac ischemia [8]. However, no data is available on its potential involvement in fibrogenesis of heart failure progression. In addition, fibulin-1 is related to the amino-terminal prohormone B-type natriuretic peptide (NT-proBNP) in type 2 diabetes [11] and African patients subjected to early vascular ageing [12]. In cardiovascular disease states subjected to extracellular matrix turnover, fibulin-1 participates in an augmenting fashion and gradually contributes to the progression of tissue remodelling.

Due to the known associations of fibulin-1 with cardiac overload, as well as restrictive cardiomyopathy and decreased left ventricular (LV) systolic function in patients with symptomatic severe aortic stenosis [13], we hypothesize that fibulin-1 could be a potential biomarker of either early cardiac or valvular fibrosis. Currently, aortic stenosis is quantified by echocardiography demanding trained technicians or physicians. Therefore, biomarkers to screen for disease onset and progression of aortic stenosis would be very helpful especially in hospitals and clinics with limited health care facilities. Currently clinicians have a dilemma because many people slowly develop asymptomatic aortic valve sclerosis with increasing age, but may not necessarily progress to clinical pathology, whereas in some patients the process starts earlier and/or progress faster. Furthermore, the relationships between echocardiography findings and symptoms as well as the development of concomitant LV hypertrophy and improvement of symptoms vary between individuals. Therefore, new tools such as new biomarkers are needed to predict both anatomical and symptomatic progression as well as the cardiovascular risk in order to time operation better.

The aim of this study was to investigate whether fibulin-1 was associated with NT-proBNP, suPAR and echocardiography measures in patients with mild to moderate aortic valve stenosis before and during lipid-lowering treatment.

Methods

Study design and patient population

Ethics statement – All patients gave written informed consent and the ethical committees from all participating countries (Norway, Sweden, Denmark, Finland, Germany, the United Kingdom, and Ireland) approved the study.

The current study formed part of the Simvastatin and Ezetimibe in Aortic Stenosis (SEAS) trial which was originally designed to investigate the potential of lipid lowering drug treatment to minimise aortic valve replacements and to curb the risk of cardiovascular disease and death. The outline of the larger study and SEAS protocol was published in detail elsewhere [18]. Participants aged 45 years and older were included in this study, whereas patients with known rheumatic disease or congenital cardiomyopathy were excluded. Patients aged between 45–85 years, with asymptomatic aortic stenosis, as determined with Doppler ultrasound (aortic peak velocity ≥2.5 and ≤4.0 m/sec), were included. A selection of 396 patients (with the relevant measured biochemical data for this study) was included after pairing groups with mild versus moderate aortic stenosis by age, gender and treatment allocation. After excluding those with missing data a total of 374 patients remained in the current analysis.

Echocardiography and hemodynamic measurements

The standardized echocardiography protocol of the SEAS study was previously published [14,15]. All images were recorded and sent for central, blinded interpretation by qualified technicians at the SEAS echocardiography core laboratory at the Haukeland University Hospital in Bergen, Norway. Captured data was analysed using off-line digital workstations with Image Arena (TomTec Imaging Systems, Unterschleissheim, Germany) software. The American Society of Echocardiography guidelines were used to quantify LV internal dimensions as well as posterior and septal wall thickness along with LV volumes and ejection fraction (determined with the Simpson's method) [16]. LV mass was calculated by using the end-diastolic LV dimensions with an anatomically validated formula [17,18]. LV hypertrophy was determined by calculating the LV mass index for men (≥116 g/m^2) and women (≥104 g/m^2) by dividing LV mass by body surface area [19]. Aortic valve area index (AVAI) was calculated by determining the valve area using the continuity equation with the time velocity/time integral ratio [20] and then indexed for body surface area. Aortic regurgitation was assessed by colour Doppler using 4-point grading systems, previously described by Jones et al. [21]. After echocardiographic examination, clinical blood pressures were measured in supine position.

Biochemical analyses

For this study we determined serum creatinine, serum aspartate aminotransferase and serum high-sensitivity C-reactive protein (CRP) levels with the Konelab autoanalyzer (Thermo Fisher Scientific Oy, Vantaa, Finland). The estimated glomerular filtration rate was determined with the Modification of Diet in Renal Disease (MDRD) Study equation: eGFR $= 175 \times$ (Standardized $S_{cr})^{-1.154} \times$ (age)$^{-0.203} \times$ (0.742 if female). EDTA-coagulated plasma was used to determine fibulin-1 levels by using a sandwich immunoassay [11]. The Elecsys proBNP sandwich immunoassay was used on an Elecsys 2010 (Roche Diagnostics, Mannheim, Germany) to determine the serum NT-proBNP concentration of each participant. Plasma (EDTA) suPAR levels were measured using the suPARnostic ELISA kit (ViroGates, Copenhagen, Denmark).

Statistical analysis

All statistical analyses were performed with the IBM SPSS Statistics, Version 22 (IBM Corporation, Armonk, New York). Non-Gaussian variables (tested by the method of skewness (normal range: −0.8 to 0.8)) were fibulin-1 (0.893), NT-proBNP (2.97), suPAR (1.19), AVAI (borderline, 0.79) and LV mass index (1.07). These variables were logarithmically transformed prior to any statistical analysis. Associations of fibulin-1 with markers of cardiac overload and inflammation were tested for interaction with severity of aortic stenosis, gender and treatment allocation by performing the appropriate interaction terms. X^2 tests were used to compare proportions of dichotomous or categorical variables and independent T-tests to compare the means of continuous variables between groups. An analysis of covariance (ANCOVA) analysis was used to determine fibulin-1's relationship with NT-proBNP and suPAR independent of baseline variables. Pearson correlations between fibulin-1, NT-proBNP, suPAR and echocardiography data were plotted in scatterplot graphs and z-scores were tested. Multiple regression analyses were performed to determine independent relationships between fibulin-1 and main independents of interest (NT-proBNP and suPAR) with the relevant covariates for each model.

Results

The basic clinical characteristics of the study sample are listed in Table 1. The total group was divided according to the predetermined median (0.58 cm^2/m^2) of the AVAI and categorized in a group with mild (≥0.58 cm^2/m^2) versus a group with moderate (<0.58 cm^2/m^2) aortic stenosis. Hemodynamic measures (systolic and diastolic blood pressure) were similar between the groups. The relative wall thickness ($p = 0.002$) and LV mass index ($p = 0.071$) were more pronounced in the moderate aortic stenosis compared to the mild group. Both fibulin-1 ($p = 0.045$) and NT-proBNP ($p = 0.018$) levels were higher in the moderate aortic stenosis group, whereas suPAR levels were similar ($p = 0.44$). After one year, this difference in levels of fibulin-1 (71.5 vs. 67.3 μg/mL), NT-proBNP (179.5 vs. 138.9 ng/L) and suPAR (3.7 vs. 3.6 ng/mL) prevailed (all, $p < 0.05$). Whereas, after four years the differences in fibulin-1 (71.3 vs. 67.7 μg/mL), NT-proBNP (198.8 vs. 159.7 ng/L) and suPAR (3.55 vs. 3.56 ng/mL) were not significantly any more.

In unadjusted analysis, we explored fibulin-1's relationship with echocardiography measures in the total group (Table 2). Fibulin-1 correlated inversely with AVAI at baseline ($p = 0.001$), 1 year follow-up (borderline $p = 0.062$) and 4 year follow-up ($p < 0.001$), but no significant trend was observed with LV mass index, aortic regurgitation, LV ejection fraction and mid-wall shortening (only baseline data available) at any time point. Change in aortic stenosis progression, bicuspid/tricuspid aortic valve myocardial hypertrophy and LV function were not related to baseline fibulin-1 or changes in fibulin-1 (all $p > 0.099$; data not shown). Notably, bicuspid aortic valve ($n = 21$) did not interact with the association of fibulin-1 with NT-proBNP ($\beta = -0.147$; $p = 0.52$) compared to patients with tricuspid valve ($\beta = 0.133$; $p = 0.029$). Similarly, bicuspid aortic valve did not interact with the association of fibulin-1 with suPAR at baseline ($\beta = -0.005$; $p = 0.99$), 1 year ($\beta = 0.323$; $p = 0.396$) and 4 years ($\beta = 0.382$; $p = 0.557$) (interaction data not shown).

Neither gender, AVAI category nor treatment allocation interacted significantly on the association of fibulin-1 with NT-proBNP and suPAR, respectively. In Figure 1, fibulin-1's relationship with NT-proBNP and suPAR were plotted for the total population at baseline, after 1 year and 4 years of treatment. The regression coefficients of fibulin-1 in relation to NT-proBNP and suPAR, strengthened at each follow-up interval (all, $p < 0.001$). Fibulin-1 showed a significant inverse relationship with AVAI at 4 years follow-up only ($r = -0.21$; $p < 0.001$), but a borderline trend was observed between fibulin-1 and AVAI after 1 year follow-up ($p = 0.052$, Figure 2).

Although Simvastatin and Ezetimibe treatment did not influence the correlation of fibulin-1 with NT-proBNP and suPAR, we tested the partially adjusted (age, body mass index and serum creatinine) correlations of fibulin-1 with NT-proBNP, suPAR and echocardiography measures stratified by treatment allocation (Table S1 in File S1). Independently of age, body mass index and creatinine, fibulin-1 significantly correlated with NT-proBNP ($p = 0.001$), suPAR ($p = 0.007$) and AVAI ($p = 0.007$) at baseline. With the exception of no correlation between fibulin-1 and AVAI in the treated group ($p = 0.57$), fibulin-1 significantly correlated with NT-proBNP and suPAR in both placebo vs. treated group (all. $p < 0.01$), and also with AVAI in the placebo group ($p = 0.009$). The same trend was observed after 4 years follow-up, but with stronger correlations and also a borderline

Table 1. Clinical and descriptive characteristics of mild vs. moderate AS patients.

	AVAI ≥0.58 cm^2/m^2 n = 180	AVAI <0.58 cm^2/m^2 n = 194	p-value
Age, yrs.	66.1±9.9	66.3±9.3	0.81
Gender (male/female), n	109/73	130/72	0.37
Body surface area, m^2	1.88±0.21	1.94±0.19	0.002
Treatment vs. Placebo,%	53.3/46.7	48.02/51.98	0.30
Biochemical analyses			
Fibulin-1, μg/mL	67.5±19.7	71.2±16.7	0.045
NT-proBNP, pg/mL	138.9 (30.0–745.8)	179.5 (27.2–1414.6)	0.018
suPAR, ng/mL	3.6±1.11	3.7±1.24	0.44
C-reactive protein, mg/L	0.21 (0.03–1.27)	0.19 (0.03–0.96)	0.37
Serum creatinine, mg/dL	95.2±15.7	97.2±15.5	0.20
Aspartate aminotransferase, U/L	17.7±6.7	16.8±4.02	0.12
γ-glutamyl transferase, U/L	24.9±25.5	23.7±20.9	0.61
Cardiovascular measurements			
Systolic blood pressure, mm Hg	143.2±19.3	144.9±20.0	0.41
Diastolic blood pressure, mm Hg	81.5±9.3	82.2±9.4	0.46
Ejection fraction,%	65.5±8.7	64.7±8.4	0.34
Fractional shortening,%	36.7±6.7	35.9±6.3	0.28
Left ventricular mass index, g/m^2	95.5±26.8	100.6±28.6	0.071
Aortic valve area index, cm^2/m^2	0.75±0.142	0.47±0.074	<0.0001
Relative wall thickness	0.32±0.07	0.34±0.08	0.002

Values are arithmetic mean ± SD, geometric mean (5th and 95th percentiles) or the number of participants indicated as percentage. Left ventricular mass and Aortic valve area were indexed by Body surface area.

Table 2. Pearson correlation coefficients of fibulin-1 with aortic and cardiac measures and relative changes in cardiac measurements.

	Fibulin-1 (log μg/mL)			
	Baseline	**1 Year follow-up**	**4 year follow-up**	**% change in measurement**
Aortic valve area index (log cm^2/m^2)	r = −0.173; p = 0.001	r = −0.103; p = 0.062	r = −0.218; p<0.0001	−4.05
Left ventricular mass index (log g/m^2)	r = −0.078; p = 0.14	r = −0.071; p = 0.19	r = −0.006; p = 0.91	21.99
Left ventricular ejection fraction (%)	r = −0.028; p = 0.61	r = −0.148; p = 0.78	r = −0.091; p = 0.087	1.62
Left ventricular outflow maximum gradient (mm Hg)	r = −0.129; p = 0.001	r = −0.051; p = 0.35	r = −0.143; p = 0.007	0.339
Transaortic time velocity (msec)	r = 0.101; p = 0.045	r = 0.079; p = 0.15	r = 0.082; p = 0.12	28.93
Stress-corrected midwall shortening (%)	r = 0.010; p = 0.85	–	–	–

tendency of fibulin-1 with AVAI in the treated group. Partially adjusted correlations of fibulin-1 with other echocardiography measures are also listed in Table 2s, although no significant relationship existed. ANCOVA was performed to test the relationship of fibulin-1 with NT-proBNP and suPAR at 1 and 4 years follow-up independent of age, treatment allocation and baseline fibulin-1 levels. At 1 year follow-up, fibulin-1 correlated significantly with NT-proBNP (r = 0.218; p<0.001) and suPAR (r = 0.132; p = 0.009) and even stronger correlations were observed at 4 years follow-up (NT-proBNP (r = 0.328; p<0.001) and suPAR (r = 0.166; p = 0.002)).

A multiple regression analysis was performed to show the associations of fibulin-1 with NT-proBNP and suPAR independently of age, gender, serum aspartate aminotransferase, serum creatinine and treatment allocation (Table 3). At baseline fibulin-1 associated inversely with AVAI and aspartate

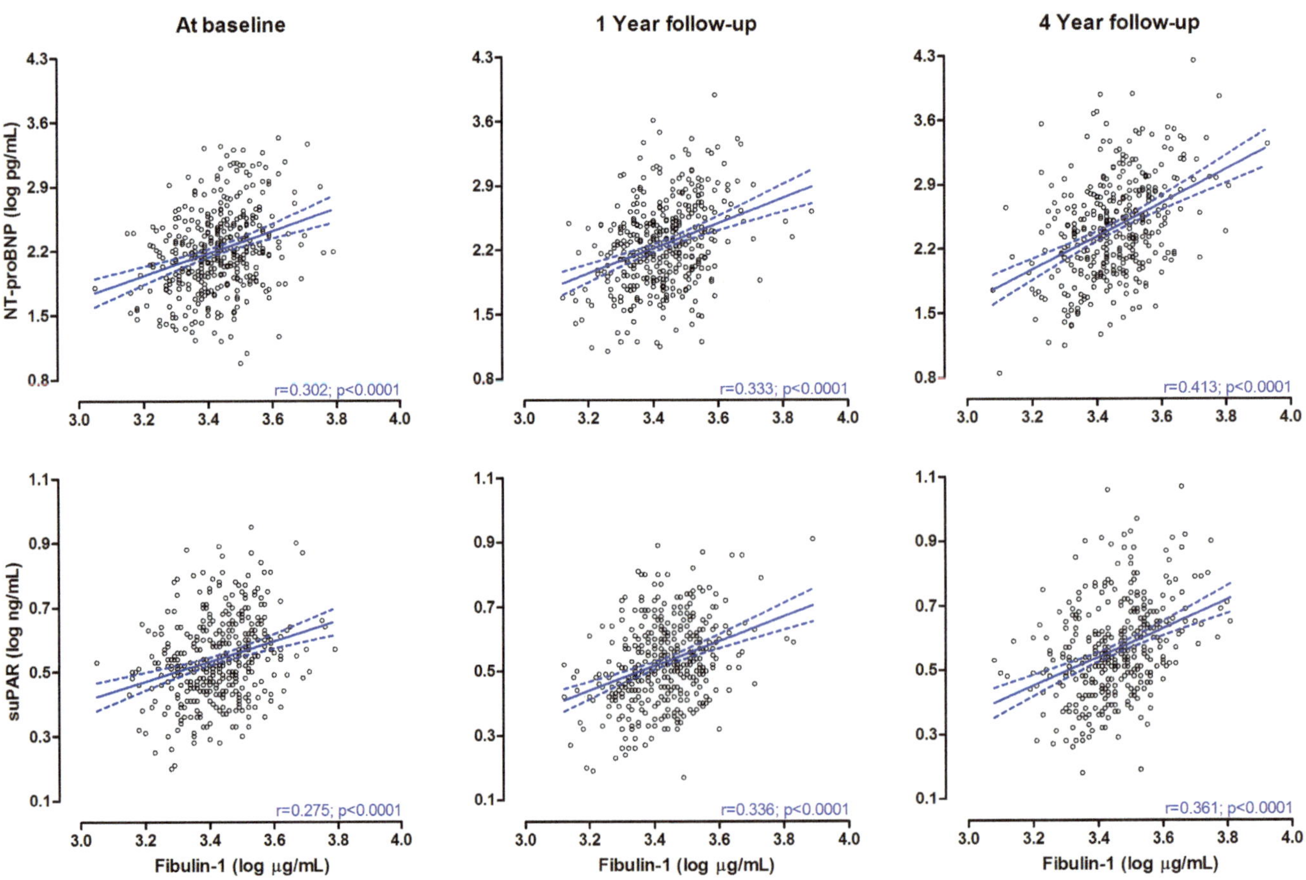

Figure 1. Unadjusted correlations of fibulin-1 with NT-proBNP and suPAR in patients with aortic stenosis during 4 years of follow-up.

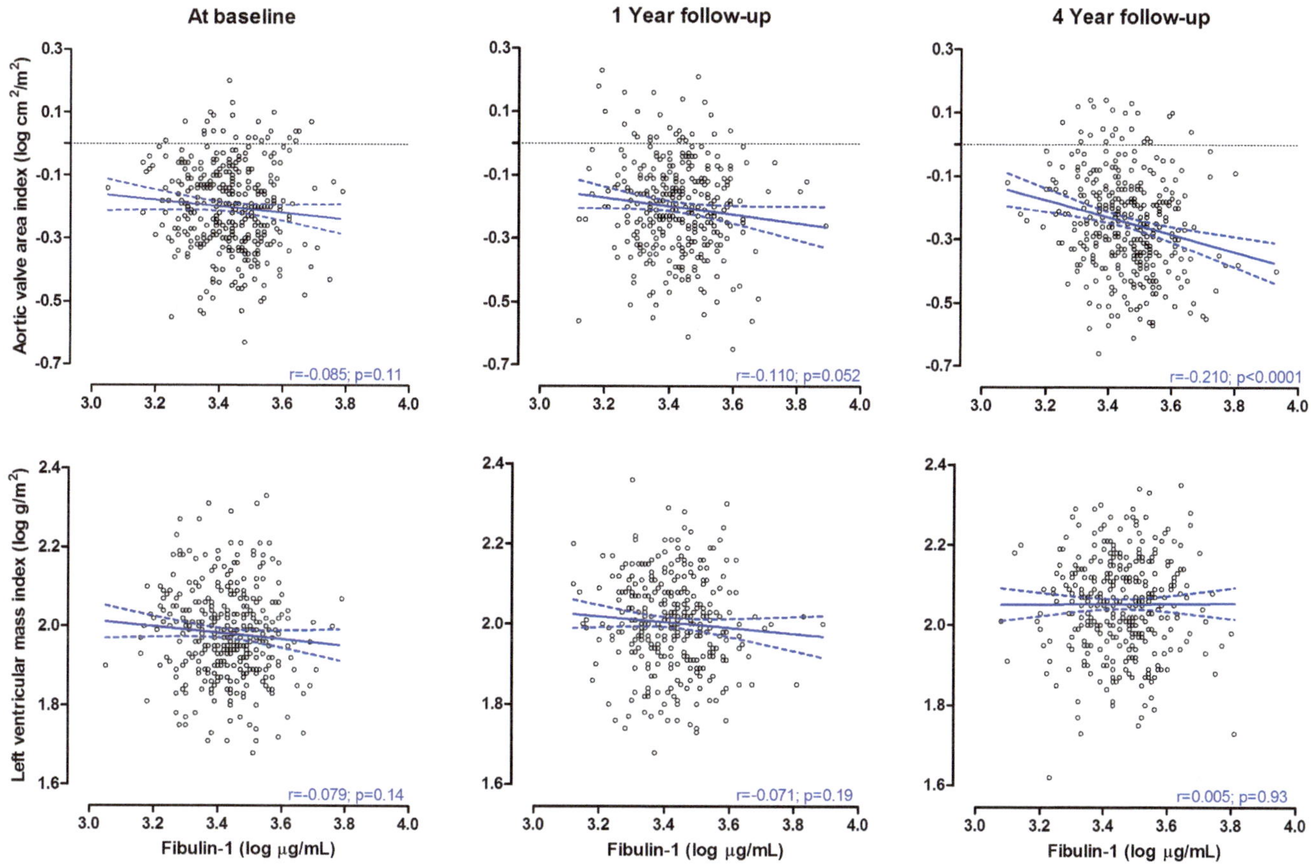

Figure 2. Unadjusted correlations of fibulin-1 with AVAI and LV mass index in patients with aortic stenosis during 4 years of follow-up.

aminotransferase, but not with NT-proBNP and suPAR. After 1 year follow-up period the association of fibulin-1 with NT-proBNP ($\beta = 0.16$; $p = 0.005$) and suPAR ($\beta = 0.16$; $p = 0.006$) became evident and the association with aspartate aminotransferase remained ($\beta = 0.15$; $p = 0.007$), but the significant association with AVAI disappeared ($p = 0.11$). After 4 years the same trend was observed, but with only a borderline association between fibulin-1 and aspartate aminotransferase ($p = 0.067$). In exploratory analysis we performed the same multivariate analysis after dividing the group into higher and lower AVAI category (Tables S2 and S3 in File S1). In the mild AS group (Table S2 in File S1) fibulin-1 associated significantly with NT-proBNP at 4 years follow-up ($p = 0.007$) and with suPAR at both 1 year ($p = 0.040$) and 4 years (0.036) of treatment. In the moderate AS group (Table S3 in File S1) fibulin-1 associated strongly with NT-proBNP at baseline ($p = 0.001$), 1 year ($p = 0.003$) and 4 years ($p = 0.004$) of treatment and with suPAR at both 1 year ($p = 0.003$) and 4 years ($p < 0.001$) follow-up.

Finally, we performed the same regression but using the MDRD Study equation for eGFR instead of serum creatinine only. We observed a significant association between fibulin-1 and NT-proBNP ($\beta = 0.26$; $p < 0.001$) at the first visit after baseline, and with both NT-proBNP ($\beta = 0.25$; $p < 0.001$) and AVAI after 4 years ($\beta = -0.13$; $p = 0.029$).

Discussion

The current study has two new observations: higher fibulin-1 levels were associated with higher suPAR and NT-proBNP levels, especially in patients with lower AVAI; and this association persisted during 4 years of observation independent of age, gender, serum creatinine and treatment intervention. These observations suggest that the association at least partly was due to the increased afterload and inflammation associated with the stenotic aortic valve. The levels of fibulin-1 and NT-proBNP increased independently parallel to increasing severity of the aortic stenosis. The interplay of these biomarkers in aortic stenosis patients indicates the detrimental overload and subsequent adverse changes of the local extracellular matrix scaffold within the myocardium in relation to decreasing aortic valve area.

Although definite mechanisms on fibulin-1's role in extracellular matrix remodelling, especially in clinical situations such as type 2 diabetes, atherosclerosis, cardiac ischemia and heart failure, remain to be elucidated, some evidence exists indicating its role in some of these conditions [8,11]. The undertone of fibulin-1 seems to be driven by potential vascular dysfunction and subsequent extracellular matrix turnover within the cardiovascular tissue. A previous study reported the association between fibulin-1 and NT-proBNP in a healthy cohort of South African men, suggesting that high levels of plasma fibulin-1 along with ventricular secretion of NT-proBNP indicates early morphological changes within blood vessels and cardiac tissue [12]. This is in line with a study

Table 3. Multiple regression analysis of fibulin-1, NT-proBNP and suPAR in patients with AS at baseline and after one and four years of treatment.

Fibulin-1, µg/mL	BASELINE		1 YEAR FOLLOW-UP		4 YEARS FOLLOW-UP	
R^2	0.20		0.24		0.28	
Adjusted R^2	0.19		0.22		0.27	
	Standard β	**p value**	**Standard β**	**p value**	**Standard β**	**p value**
NT-proBNP, pg/mL	0.097	0.079	0.160	0.005	0.224	<0.0001
suPAR, ng/mL	0.053	0.34	0.163	0.006	0.129	0.026
Aortic valve area index, cm^2/m^2	−0.143	0.005	−0.084	0.11	−0.063	0.22
Age, years	0.254	<0.0001	0.166	0.005	0.189	0.001
Gender	0.146	0.011	0.192	0.001	0.187	0.001
Aspartate aminotransferase, U/L	0.161	0.002	0.149	0.007	0.091	0.067
Serum creatinine	0.064	0.26	0.058	0.32	0.098	0.080
Treatment	-	-	−0.026	0.62	−0.010	0.84

Multivariate analysis was performed independently of age, gender, aspartate aminotransferase levels and treatment allocation.

conducted earlier by Cangemi et al. that described the augmented concentrations of fibulin-1 in arterial walls and in plasma of type 2 diabetic patients, and may propose vascular extracellular matrix turnover as shown by their association between fibulin-1 and arteriosclerosis or arterial stiffness [11].

Our study population was clinically diagnosed with asymptomatic aortic stenosis, particularly chosen to evaluate fibulin-1's role in fibrotic and sclerotic processes in relation to cardiac overload and subclinical atherosclerosis-related inflammation. Since this study only evaluated the relationship between biomarkers at baseline and after drug intervention we cannot infer causality. However, this study along with on-going investigations attempts to explain the potential pathway in which these biomarkers are linked. Aortic valve stenosis has similar characteristics with coronary artery disease which include adverse lipid build-up, inflammation and medial calcific lesions [1]. Hemodynamic strain also contributes to valvular thickening, further tightening the orifice of the aortic valve and causing a systolic shunt at the LV outflow [1,22]. It has been shown that LV hypertrophy is related to myocardial sclerosis [23]. However, the link between fibulin-1 and NT-proBNP in our study was unrelated to aortic regurgitation and LV ejection fraction, but linked closely with the AVAI. The lack of association between fibulin-1 and echocardiography data may be due to unrecognised myocardial fibrosis in the asymptomatic and less severe nature of aortic stenosis of this cohort. This hypothesis that fibulin-1 reflects asymptomatic myocardial fibrosis that is not accompanied by LV hypertrophy and/or reduced ejection fraction, give rise to the possibility that fibulin-1 may add prognostic information to the current echocardiographic follow-up in these patients.

Fibulin-1 levels were augmented in our patients with more severe aortic stenosis and this confirms the observation previously described by Scholze et al [24] showing an association to LV systolic load. Since we also found a relationship between fibulin-1 and suPAR along with presented hemodynamic strain in this cohort, our study propose cross-linking between the plasminogen pathway and fibrotic processes within the extracellular matrix. Soluble uPAR has a distinct role in cell adhesion, proliferation and migration between cells in the arterial wall. These cells include endothelial cells, smooth muscle cells and macrophages in atherosclerotic progression [25]. In addition, plasma lipoproteins and molecular pathways involved in thrombosis, fibrinolysis, oxidation and inflammation are regulated by the urokinase-type plasminogen activator (uPA) and its receptor (uPAR) [26,27]. Disproportion in this system leads to disorders in tissue structure and function [25]. Fibulin-1 coincides in the plasminogen system by means of its shared role in cell adhesion, especially from its site of secretion in arterial walls and its interaction with plasma fibrinogen and calcium to promote platelet adhesion [10]. The cross-linking of fibulin-1 with its local extracellular matrix proteins may explain its role within exposed sub-endothelial matrices following vascular disease. In a study earlier this year, NT-proBNP was found to be associated with suPAR, which suggested that hemodynamic strain on the heart is associated with low-grade inflammation [28]. This is due to either systemic inflammation or acute phase responses that contribute to extracellular matrix remodelling within cardiac tissue as a result of increased volume overload [29]. In addition, Eugen-Olsen et al. showed that suPAR associates with an increased risk of cardiovascular disease, cancer, type 2 diabetes and mortality [30]. The interaction between fibulin-1, NT-proBNP and suPAR is therefore warranted to explain the development of sclerotic and fibrotic disease states.

In studies with animals subjected to experimental hypercholesterolemia it was confirmed that elevated lipid accumulation causes both atherosclerosis and contribute to calcification in aortic valves [31–35]. In our study, patients were subjected to lipid lowering treatment or placebo and even with extreme lipid lowering drug interventions, the association of fibulin-1 with both a biomarker of cardiac strain and one of subclinical atherosclerotic inflammation remained after one and four years of treatment, taking into consideration a measure of renal function, gender, age and the liver enzyme aspartate aminotransferase. This result suggests that fibulin-1 may indicate valvular or myocardial fibrosis independent of treatment allocation. Although gender associated significantly in the regression model, it is worthy to mention that suPAR levels are generally higher in women compared to men and that the multiple linearity of this gender difference may reflect an interaction, although our interaction tests revealed no impact of gender. With fibulin-1 connected to both NT-proBNP and suPAR via different physiological pathways and in various disease states, more studies are encouraged to investigate and define the concise mechanism of the relationship between these biomarkers.

Limitations

This study was conducted from a sample selected from the larger SEAS study, since the relevant biomarkers were not available in the entire study population. The study sample was limited to patients with aortic stenosis as defined by aortic valve peak velocities of ≥2.5 and ≤4.0 m/sec by echocardiography. MRI data on aortic stenosis or myocardial fibrosis was not acquired in this study. Other methods for quantifying fibrosis are known, for example late gadolinium enhancement or cardiac magnetic resonance contrast-enhanced T1-mapping. These methods were not available in this study and therefore fibulin-1 may aid as surrogate marker or add to depicting potential fibrosis onset in cardiovascular tissue. Comparing the use of fibulin-1 with known methods is therefore encouraged.

In conclusion, elevated levels of plasma fibulin-1 were associated with aortic stenosis, elevated LV hemodynamic load as indicated by elevated levels of NT-proBNP and soluble uPAR supporting a possible link in cardiovascular extracellular sclerotic processes. This prospective study suggests that fibulin-1 and soluble uPAR are involved in myocardial extracellular matrix turnover as a result of elevated LV overload in patients with aortic stenosis.

Supporting Information

File S1 Supporting tables. Table S1. Partial correlation coefficients of fibulin-1 with NT-proBNP, suPAR and aortic/cardiac measures at baseline and follow-up in patients with aortic stenosis stratified by treatment allocation. **Table S2.** Multiple regression analysis of fibulin-1 and NT-proBNP in patients with mild AS at baseline and after one and four years of treatment. **Table S3.** Multiple regression analysis of fibulin-1 and NT-proBNP in patients with moderate AS at baseline and also after one and four years of treatment.

Author Contributions

Conceived and designed the experiments: MHO KW LMR JE OWN. Performed the experiments: RK MHO. Analyzed the data: RK MHO. Contributed reagents/materials/analysis tools: LMR JE KW WSA OWN. Wrote the paper: RK MHO LMR WSA JE KW AB RW OWN.

References

1. Ramaraj R, Sorrell VL (2008) Degenerative aortic stenosis. British Med J 336: 550–555.
2. Dweck MR, Boon NA, Newby DE (2012) Calcific aortic stenosis: a disease of the valve and the myocardium. J Am Coll Cardiol 60: 1854–1863.
3. Villari B, Vassalli G, Monrad ES, Chiariello M, Turina M, et al. (1995) Normalization of diastolic dysfunction in aortic stenosis late after valve replacement. Circulation 91: 2353–2358.
4. Mandinov L, Eberli FR, Seiler C, Hess OM (2000) Diastolic heart failure. Cardiovasc Res 45(4): 813–825.
5. Rosenhek R, Zilberszac R, Schemper M, Czerny M, Mundigler G, et al. (2010) Natural History of Very Severe Aortic Stenosis. Circulation 121: 151–156.
6. Fay WP, Garg N, Sunkar M (2007) Vascular Functions of the Plasminogen Activation System. Arterioscler Thromb Vasc Biol 27: 1231–1237.
7. Stewart BF, Siscovick D, Lind BK, Gardin JM, Gottdiener JS, et al. (1997) Clinical factors associated with calcific aortic valve disease. JACC 29: 630–634.
8. Hutchinson KR, Stewart JA Jr, Lucchesi PA (2010) Extracellular matrix remodeling during the progression of volume overload-induced heart failure. J Mol Cell Cardiol 48: 564–569.
9. Argraves WS, Tran H, Burgess WH, Dickerson K (1990) Fibulin is an extracellular matrix and plasma glycoprotein with repeated domain structure. J Cell Biol 111(6): 3155–64.
10. Godyna S, Diaz-Ricart M, Argraves WS (1996) Fibulin-1 mediates platelet adhesion via a bridge of fibrinogen. Blood 88(7): 2569–2577.
11. Cangemi C, Skov V, Poulsen MK, Funder J, Twal WO, et al. (2011) Fibulin-1 is a marker for arterial extracellular matrix alterations in type 2 diabetes. Clin Chem 57(11): 1556–65.
12. Kruger R, Schutte R, Huisman HW, Argraves WS, Rasmussen LM, et al. (2012) NT-proBNP is associated with fibulin-1 in Africans: The SAfrEIC study. Atherosclerosis 222: 216–221.
13. Dahl JS, Møller JE, Videbæk L, Poulsen MK, Rudbæk TR, et al. (2012) Plasma fibulin-1 is linked to restrictive filling of the left ventricle and to mortality in patients with aortic valve stenosis. J Am Heart Assoc 1: e003889.
14. Rossebø AB, Pedersen TR, Allen C, Boman K, Chambers JB, et al. (2007) Design and baseline characteristics of the simvastatin and ezetimibe in aortic stenosis (SEAS) study. Am J Cardiol 99: 970–973.
15. Rossebø AB, Pedersen TR, Boman K, Brudi P, Chambers JB, et al. (2008) Intensive lipid lowering with Simvastatin and Ezetimibe in aortic stenosis. N Engl J Med 359: 1343–1356.
16. Lang RM, Bierig M, Devereux RB, Flachskampf FA, Foster E, et al. (2006) Recommendations for chamber quantification. Eur J Echocardiogr 7(2): 79–108.
17. Devereux RB, Alonso DR, Lutas EM, Gottlieb GJ, Campo E, et al. (1986) Echocardiographic assessment of left ventricular hypertrophy: Comparison to necropsy findings. Am J Cardiol 57: 450–458.
18. Perakis AC, Montarello JK, Rosenthal E, Boyd EGCA, Yates AK, et al. (1990) In vitro measurement of stenotic human aortic valve orifice area in a pulsatile flow model. Validation of the continuity equation. Eur Heart J 11: 492–499.
19. Devereux RB, Wachtell K, Gerdts E, Boman K, Nieminen MS, et al. (2004) Prognostic significance of left ventricular mass change during treatment of hypertension. JAMA 292: 2350–2356.
20. Currie PJ, Seward JB, Reeder GS, Vlietstra RE, Bresnahan DR, et al. (1985) Continuous-wave Doppler echocardiographic assessment of severity of calcific aortic stenosis: a simultaneous Doppler-catheter correlative study in 100 adult patients. Circulation 71: 1162–1169.
21. Jones EC, Devereux RB, Roman MJ, Liu JE, Fishman D, et al. (2001) Prevalence and correlates of mitral regurgitation in a population-based sample (the Strong Heart Study). Am J Cardiol 87: 298–304.
22. Cosmi JE, Kort S, Tunick PA, Rosenzweig BP, Freedberg RS, et al. (2002) The risk of the development of aortic stenosis in patients with "benign" aortic valve thickening. Arch Intern Med 162: 2345–2347.
23. Agno FS, Chinali M, Bella JN, Liu JE, Arnett DK, et al. (2005) Aortic valve sclerosis is associated with preclinical cardiovascular disease in hypertensive adults: the Hypertension Genetic Epidemiology Network study. J Hypertens 23: 867–873.
24. Scholze A, Bladbjerg EM, Sidelmann JJ, Diederichsen ACP, Mickley H, et al. (2013) Plasma concentrations of extracellular matrix protein fibulin-1 are related to cardiovascular risk markers in chronic kidney disease and diabetes. Cardiovasc Diabet 12: 6–12.
25. Fuhrman B (2012) The urokinase system in the pathogenesis of atherosclerosis. Atherosclerosis 222(1): 8–14.
26. Nicholl SM, Roztocil E, Davies MG (2006) Plasminogen activator system and vascular disease. Curr Vasc Pharmacol 4(2): 101–16.
27. Noda-Heiny H, Daugherty A, Sobel BE (1995) Augmented urokinase receptor expression in atheroma. Arterioscler Thromb Vasc Biol 15(1): 37–43.
28. Drolet MC, Roussel E, Deshaies Y, Couet J, Arsenault M (2006) A high fat/high carbohydrate diet induces aortic valve disease in C57BL/6J mice. JACC 47: 850–855.
29. Kruger R, Schutte R, Huisman HW, Hindersson P, Olsen MH, et al. (2013) NT-proBNP, C-reactive protein and soluble uPAR in a bi-ethnic male population: the SAfrEIC study. PLoS ONE 8(3): e58506.
30. Eugen-Olsen J, Andersen O, Linneberg A, Ladelund S, Hansen TW, et al. (2010) Circulating soluble urokinase plasminogen activator receptor predicts

cancer, cardiovascular disease, diabetes and mortality in the general population. J Intern Med 268: 296–308.
31. Sackner-Bernstein JD (2000) The myocardial matrix and the development and progression of ventricular remodeling. Curr Cardiol Rep 2: 112–119.
32. Rajamannan NM, Sangiorgi G, Springett M, Arnold K, Mohacsi T, et al. (2001) Experimental hypercholesterolemia induces apoptosis in the aortic valve. J Heart Valve Dis 10: 371–374.
33. Drolet MC, Arsenault M, Couet J (2003) Experimental aortic valve stenosis in rabbits. J Am Coll Cardiol 41: 1211–1217.
34. Weiss RM, Ohashi M, Miller JD, Young SG, Heistad DD (2006) Calcific aortic valve stenosis in old hypercholesterolemic mice. Circulation 114: 2065–2069.
35. Aikawa E, Nahrendorf M, Sosnovik D, Lok VM, Jaffer FA, et al. (2007) Multimodality molecular imaging identifies proteolytic and osteogenic activities in early aortic valve disease. Circulation 115: 377–386.

22

Optimisation of Reference Genes for Gene-Expression Analysis in a Rabbit Model of Left Ventricular Diastolic Dysfunction

Walid Nachar[1], David Busseuil[1], Yanfen Shi[1], Teodora Mihalache-Avram[1], Mélanie Mecteau[1], Eric Rhéaume[1,2], Jean-Claude Tardif[1,2]*

1 Montreal Heart Institute and Université de Montréal, Montreal, Quebec, Canada, 2 Department of Medicine, Université de Montréal, Montreal, Quebec, Canada

Abstract

Left ventricular diastolic dysfunction (LVDD) is characterized by the disturbance of ventricle's performance due to its abnormal relaxation or to its increased stiffness during the diastolic phase. The molecular mechanisms underlying LVDD remain unknown. We aimed to identify normalization genes for accurate gene-expression analysis of LVDD using quantitative real-time PCR (RT-PCR) in a new rabbit model of LVDD. Eighteen rabbits were fed with a normal diet (n = 7) or a 0.5% cholesterol-enriched diet supplemented with vitamin D2 (n = 11) for an average of 14.5 weeks. We validated the presence of LVDD in this model using echocardiography for diastolic function assessment. RT-PCR was performed using cDNA derived from left ventricle samples to measure the stability of 10 genes as candidate reference genes (*Gapdh, Hprt1, Ppia, Sdha, Rpl5, Actb, Eef1e1, Ywhaz, Pgk1, and G6pd)*. Using geNorm analysis, we report that *Sdha*, *Gapdh* and *Hprt1* genes had the highest stability (M <0.2). By contrast, *Hprt1* and *Rpl5* genes were found to represent the best combination for normalization when using the Normfinder algorithm (stability value of 0.042). Comparison of both normalization strategies highlighted an increase of natriuretic peptides (*Bnp* and *Anp*), monocytes chemotactic protein-1 (*Mcp-1*) and NADPH oxidase subunit (*Nox-2*) mRNA expressions in ventricle samples of the hypercholesterolemic rabbits compared to controls ($P<0.05$). This increase correlates with LVDD echocardiographic parameters and most importantly it molecularly validates the presence of the disease in our model. This is the first study emphasizing the selection of stable reference genes for RT-PCR normalization in a rabbit model of LVDD.

Editor: Vincenzo Lionetti, Scuola Superiore Sant'Anna, Italy

Funding: Dr. Jean-Claude Tardif is the principal investigator of this article and he provided the funding from his Canada Research Chair in translational and personalized medicine #950-227725. The funders had no role in study design, data collection and analysis, decision to publish, or preparation of the manuscript.

Competing Interests: The authors have the following interests: The following patents on the theme of HDL and both aortic valve stenosis and diastolic dysfunction were submitted by the Montreal Heart Institute and Drs. Tardif, Rhéaume and Busseuil are mentioned as authors. WO/2010/083611A1 "Method for the prevention and treatment of diastolic dysfunction employing an apolipoproteinA1 (APOA1) mimetic peptide/phospholipid complex". US20130197226 / Pharmaceutical compositions for the treatment of left ventricular diastolic dysfunction comprising an apolipoprotein peptide/phospholipid complex". US20090186808 "Method and compound for the treatment of valvular disease". These patents do not cover the development of a diastolic dysfunction in a rabbit model, nor the use or selection of housekeeping genes. There are no further patents, products in development or marketed products to declare.

* E-mail: jean-claude.tardif@icm-mhi.org

Introduction

Left ventricular diastolic dysfunction (LVDD) accounts for almost half of the cases of heart failure in clinical practice [1]. It is characterized by abnormal left ventricle (LV) relaxation or reduced ventricular compliance, which leads to increased filling pressures [2]. Treatments for LVDD are currently limited to diuretics for symptom relief and to those addressing the underlying cause, including arterial hypertension, myocardial ischemia and aortic valve stenosis (AVS). Many studies have demonstrated the association of hypercholesterolemia with atherosclerosis and plaque formation [3]. However, few studies reported the impairment of cardiac function in humans and animals after exposure to a hypercholesterolemic diet [4–7]. To understand the genetic and molecular mechanisms underlying the cardiac impairments observed in LVDD, numerous studies assessed the expression of genes that might be related to this pathology [8–10]. The level of brain natriuretic peptide (BNP), a neurohormone secreted by the ventricle in response to ventricular volume expansion and increased LV filling pressure, has been shown to be increased in patients with LVDD [11] and animal models with accompanying LV hypertrophy [9,10]. Serum BNP levels have indeed been proposed as a biomarker of LVDD severity [12] and a link between LVDD and LV *Bnp* mRNA expression has been established [9,13]. Oxidative stress and inflammation processes have also been reported to contribute to DD development [14,15]. Indeed, numerous studies showed an increase of the expression of inflammatory genes such as *Mcp-1* or *IL-6* and contributors to oxidative stress such as NADPH oxidase and its subunits in DD cases [9,10]. Although large animal models have been described for LVDD [16], only a limited number of models of experimental LVDD have been described in rabbits. Among these models, the development of LVDD with age or hypercholesterolemia in rabbits has been shown to be similar to the changes seen in humans [4,5,17], making rabbits a valid model to study the mechanisms underlying this pathology.

mRNA quantification by real-time PCR (RT-PCR) remains the most common method used to study gene expression changes associated with different pathologies. RT-PCR is a very sensitive method; however, accurate gene normalization is essential for data interpretation [18,19]. Multiple strategies are available for normalization and can affect the quality of gene-expression studies [19–21]. However, differences between animal models, tissues, cell types, experimental conditions and protocols require the specific evaluation of different reference genes for the selection of the best ones in each experimental setup. Experimental data have clearly demonstrated the value of using multiple reference genes to normalize expression data [21]. The aim of the current study was to identify and validate suitable stable reference genes that can be used for gene-expression studies in a new LVDD rabbit model. These genes may be ultimately used to study gene expression and mechanisms in relation to different possible therapeutic approaches using this model.

Methods

Animals

Animal care and procedures complied with the Canadian Council on Animal Care guidelines and were approved by the Montreal Heart Institute Research Center ethics committee for animal research. To study the effect of the diet on the progression of LVDD, 18 New-Zealand White rabbits (2.91±0.04 kg) were fed with a normal diet (n = 7) or a 0.5% cholesterol-enriched diet supplemented with vitamin D_2 (50 000 IU.day^{-1}) in the drinking water (n = 11) for an average period of 14.5 weeks. Cholesterol-diet rabbits were then fed with a standard diet (without cholesterol and vitamin D_2) to mimic cholesterol-lowering therapy for 2 weeks. Animals were then killed and the LV were removed, flushed with sterile saline, snap frozen in liquid nitrogen and stored at −80°C.

Echocardiography

Examinations were carried out with a phased-array probe 10S (4.5 ~ 11.5 Mega Hertz) using a Vivid 7 Dimension system (GE Healthcare Ultrasound, Horten, Norway). Intra-muscular injections of ketamine (90 mg/kg) and midazolam (0.75 mg/kg) were used for sedation. Complete echocardiography-Doppler examinations were performed at baseline, on the day of the switch to normal diet and on the day of sacrifice to assess several LVDD parameters. Pulsed-wave Doppler was used to record transmitral flow (TMF), left and right pulmonary venous flow in an apical 4-chamber view. Peak velocity during early filling (E), mitral E-wave deceleration time, deceleration rate, peak velocity during active atrial filling (A), and mitral A-wave duration were measured, and E/A ratio was calculated on TMF. Peak velocity of systolic flow (S), diastolic flow (D), reversed atrial flow (Ar), and Ar wave duration were measured, and S/D ratio was calculated on both left and right pulmonary venous flow. Mitral A wave duration minus left (and right) pulmonary venous flow Ar wave duration (A-Ar_{left} and A-Ar_{right} duration) were also calculated from TMF and pulmonary venous flow. Mitral annulus velocities during early filling (Em) and active atrial filling (Am) in both lateral and septal annulus were measured by tissue Doppler imaging. Em/Am and E/Em ratio were calculated. LVDD was classified using previously published criteria [5,22,23]. Special care was taken to obtain similar imaging planes on serial examinations by reviewing previous recordings before the follow-up study. All echocardiographic imaging and measurements were performed throughout the protocol by the same experienced investigator blinded to diet allocation. The average of 3 consecutive cardiac cycles was used for each measurement.

RNA Extraction and cDNA Synthesis

LV tissue (15 to 30 mg) was homogenized in lysis buffer using "PowerGen 125" homogenizer (Fisher Scientific, Ontario, Canada) for 30 seconds. Total RNA was extracted using Qiagen RNeasy Fibrous Tissue Mini Kit (Qiagen, Ontario, Canada), according to manufacturer's instructions. Genomic DNA contamination was removed by RNase-free DNase I digestion during the extraction procedure (according to the RNA extraction kit protocol). The quality and quantity of total RNA was assessed using Agilent RNA 6000 Nano Kit for Bioanalyzer 2100 System (Agilent Technologies, Santa Clara, California, USA). RNA integrity numbers (RIN) were higher than 8.8 for all samples. 700 ng of total RNA were used for first strand synthesis of complementary DNA (cDNA) using High Capacity cDNA Reverse Transcription Kit with RNase inhibitor (Applied Biosystems, California, USA) in a final reaction volume of 20 µl according to manufacturer's instructions.

mRNA Quantification Using Real-time PCR

Quantitative RT-PCR experiments were performed using Stratagene MX 3005P thermal cycler (Agilent Technologies, Santa Clara, California, USA). Final reaction volume was 25 µl and composed of 1X SyberGreen (GoTaq® qPCR Master Mix, Promega Corporation, Madison, WI, USA or Perfecta SyberGreen FastMix®, ROX ™, Quanta BioSciences, Gaithersburg, USA), reference ROX dye, 1 µM of forward and reverse primer, and 2.16 ng of cDNA template. A first incubation was made at 50°C for 2 min followed by an initial denaturation at 95°C for another 2 min. Amplification was then performed during 40 cycles of denaturation at 95 °C for 15 sec and annealing/extension at 60 °C for 1 min. At the end, a dissociation curve was produced to analyze and confirm the specificity of the amplification by observation of a single peak in the curve. Standard curves of five points were produced for each gene to transform sample's Cts to relative expression values. Amplification efficiencies were calculated using MxPro software (version 4.10) to analyze the slopes of the standard curves according to Pfaffl [24] and are presented in Tables 1a and 1b. All samples were run in duplicate and the mean values were used for calculations. PCR products were initially sequenced to confirm the specificity of amplifications. Relative quantities of the unknown samples were normalized against the normalization factor (NF) which was calculated from the geometric means of the expression of the best three and two reference genes selected by geNorm or Normfinder algorithm respectively.

GeNorm analysis determines the pairwise variation of a gene with the other tested genes, through calculation of standard deviation of the log-transformed expression ratios, and defines the internal control gene-stability measure M as the average pairwise variation of a particular gene with all other genes [21]. The gene with the most stable expression gene has the lowest M value. A stepwise exclusion of the least stable gene allows a recalculation of the M values for the rest of genes. To determine the optimal reference gene number for normalization, we considered 0.15 as the cut-off for pairwise variation ($V_n/_{n+1}$), between NF_n and NF_{n+1} as recommended by Vandesompele et al [21].

Normfinder is a mathematical model of gene expression that enables estimation of the overall variation of the candidate normalization genes and of the variation between sample subgroups of the sample set [20]. Indeed, Normfinder selects the

Table 1. Primer sequences and their characteristics for the 10 reference genes whose variation in expression was assessed using RT-PCR.

Gene Symbol	Accession number	Forward primer (5′-3′)	Reverse primer (5′-3′)	PCR efficiency (%)	Amplicon length (bp)	Tm (°C)
Gapdh	NM_001082253	TGGTGAAGGTCGGAGTGAAC	ATGTAGTGGAGGTCAATGAATGG	94.2	121	75.7
Hprt1	NM_001105671	CCTTGGTCAAGCAGTATAATC	GGGCATATCCTACAACAAAC	96.1	135	74.0
Ppia	NM_001082057	ACTTCACACGCCACAATG	TGATCTTCTTGCTGGTCTTG	96.6	273	79.2
Sdha	XM_002723194	GGACCAGGACGCCATCCACTAC	TCCACCGAACGCACGCTGATAG	96.1	124	76.6
Eef1e1	XM_002714163	ACCGCAGAAGAGAAAGCCATAG[23]	AGCGATGTAGCCCATAGTAGAGGA	91.8	190	76.4
G6pd	NM_001171382	GCAGAGTGAGCCCTTCTTC	GCCAGCCACATAGGAGTTG	93.1	85	75.6
Pgk1	XM_002720132	TGTTGGTCGGGCGAAGCAG[23]	CAGTGTCTCCACCGCCGATG	92.2	149	77.9
Rpl5	NM_001195679	GATTGCGTATGCCCGTATAG	CTCCAGTCACCTCCACTTG	98.0	194	76.7
Actb	NM_001101683	CAAGCGTGGCATCCTGAC	CTCGTTGTAGAAGGTGTGGTG	98.0	100	76.5
Ywhaz	XM_002710718	GGTCTGGCCCTTAACTTCTCTGTGTTCTA [25]	GCGTGCTGTCTTTGTATGATTCTTCACTT	103.8	142	73.1

Amplification efficiencies were calculated using MxPro software to analyze the slope of the standard curve according to Pfaffl [24].

best gene for normalization based on its intra- and inter-group variation and combines the two into a stability value. It also determines the best combination of two genes which are chosen with a similar-sized fold change but in the opposite direction.

Reference Gene Selection

Ten candidate genes were tested based on their common use in literature as reference genes [20,21,25]. Gene-specific, intron-spanning whenever possible, primer pairs were designed using Beacon Designer software, version 7.5 (Premier Biosoft International) or adapted from earlier publications [25]. Primer characteristics are described in Tables 1 and 2 for reference genes and genes of interest, respectively. A minimum of two designed primer pairs were tested for optimization. Primers were synthesized by Integrated DNA Technologies Inc (California, USA). Gene expression stability was tested using the geNorm algorithm which is included in the qbase Plus 2 software (version 2.3, Biogazelle, Zwijnaarde, Belgium), and Normfinder which is a free Visual Basic application (VBA) for Excel.

Statistics

Analyses were performed with SAS version 9.3 (SAS Institute Inc., Cary, NC, USA) and Prism graph pad version 5.04. All analyses were conducted at the 0.05 significance level. Data are presented as the mean ± standard error of the mean (SEM). For echocardiographic parameters, analysis of covariance (ANCOVA) adjusted for the baseline value was used to assess the change over the 3 time points in each treatment group and to compare groups at each time points separately. The non-parametric Mann-Whitney test was used to compare mRNA levels of groups. Spearman correlation was used to assess correlations between mRNA and echocardiographic data.

Results

LVDD Characterization Using Echocardiography in a Hypercholesterolemic Rabbit Model

LVDD has previously been observed in hypercholesterolemic rabbits [4]. Given our prior experience with a hypercholesterolemic rabbit model that develops aortic valve stenosis [26], and since LVDD is often associated with aortic valve stenosis, we performed a detailed characterization of diastolic heart function in this animal model using echocardiography. We observed an increase in E wave velocity, E wave deceleration rate, mitral annulus lateral E/Em ratio, septal annulus E/Em ratio and left and right pulmonary vein Ar durations after 14.5 weeks of hypercholesterolemic diet and two weeks after ending this diet compared with the normal diet control group (Table 3). We also report a significant decrease in E wave deceleration time and decreased values of left and right pulmonary vein A-Ar durations in the hypercholesterolemic group at these two time-points compared with the normal group (Figure S1 in File S1). LVDD

Table 2. Primer sequences and their characteristics for the genes of interest whose variation in expression was assessed using RT-PCR.

Gene Symbol	Accession number	Forward primer (5′-3′)	Reverse primer (5′-3′)	PCR efficiency (%)	Amplicon length (bp)	Tm (°C)
Anp	NM_001082262	GTACAACGCCATGTCCAAC	CTTCATCACTCTGCTCACTTAG	95.9	125	74.5
Bnp	XM_002724454	CCTGTGCCCCTGGATGAG	CCGAAGCAGCCTGAGTCC	100.5	80	80.2
Mcp-1	NM_001082294	CAGTGAAGAGGCTAATGAG	GGTTGTGGAATAAGAGGTC	100.2	188	76.2
Nox-2	AF323788	AATGCTTGTGGCTGTGATAAG	TACCAGACTGACTTGAGGATG	98	176	75.9

Amplification efficiencies were calculated using MxPro software to analyze the slope of the standard curve according to Pfaffl [24].

was maintained even after the change for two weeks from a cholesterol-enriched diet to a normal diet, as observed by the negligible changes of diastolic dysfunction-related parameters reported in Table 3.

Real-time PCR and Selection of Reference Genes

To assess mRNA expression from ventricle samples obtained from normal and LVDD rabbits, we used GeNorm and Normfinder algorithms to test the stability of 10 candidate reference genes based on their common use in literature [20,21] (Table 1).

GeNorm analyses are based on pairwise correlation of the expression level for each gene with the rest of the tested genes. An average of expression stability, M value, is given for each gene. The expression of a gene with an M value < 0.5 is considered highly stable. We found that all of the 10 genes tested in the LVs are stably expressed as documented by their average expression stability below 0.5. Among them, the three genes with the lowest M values were *Hprt1* (M = 0.176), *Gapdh* (M = 0.168) and *Sdha* (M = 0.161); see Figure 1 for gene ranking. Pairwise variation (V) analysis, which provides the optimal number of reference genes that should be used in normalization, was also calculated between NF_n and NF_{n+1}. The geometric mean of the three best genes (*Sdha, Gapdh and Hprt1*) is sufficient to calculate the normalization factor, as the geNorm V value obtained for the 2 to 3 best genes ($V_{2-3} = 0.0575$) is lower than 0.15 and inclusion of additional genes would not significantly decrease the variation of the normalization factor (Figure 2).

Normfinder estimates inter- and intra-group variations and assigns a stability value for each gene based on a linear equation of the algorithm (see Methods). The results of Normfinder analysis for stable gene selection were different from those of geNorm. According to Normfinder, *Hprt1* was shown to be the most stable gene (0.049), and *Hprt1* and *Rpl5* represented the best combination of two genes (0.042) (Figure 1).

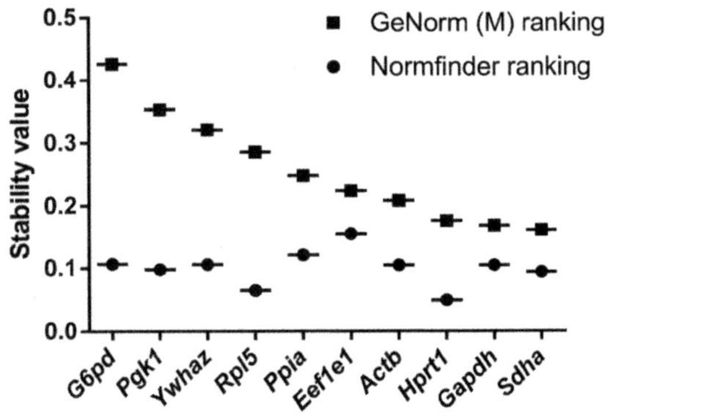

Figure 1. GeNorm and Normfinder ranking of the 10 reference genes tested for the mRNA expression stability in left ventricles of 18 rabbits (normal diet n = 7 and cholesterol diet n = 11). *Sdha, Gapdh* and *Hprt1* are shown as the best 3 genes with the lowest geNorm M value (M = 0.161, M = 0.168 and M = 0.176, respectively). Lower M value corresponds to higher gene stability. However, the use of the Normfinder algorithm results in the selection of *Hprt1* (0.049) as the most stable gene and suggests to use the average of *Hprt1* and *Rpl5* (0.042) as normalization factor.

Quantification of genes of interest: *Bnp, Anp, Mcp-1 and Nox-2* mRNA Expression in LVs

The mRNA expression of the genes of interest was corrected using the reference genes selected from both normalization software (geNorm and Normfinder). Using both combinations suggested by the two software for normalization, we confirm that *Bnp* mRNA expression was induced in LVs from the hypercholesterolemic group compared to the normal group (Figure 3). Indeed, when we normalized against the geometric mean of *Sdha, Gapdh and Hprt1* (selected by geNorm), *Bnp* expression was found to be 5.96 fold increased in the hypercholesterolemic group compared to normals ($P = 0.012$). In agreement with this finding, the use of the geometric mean of *Hprt1* and *Rpl5* (selected by Normfinder) showed a 5.68 fold increase in *Bnp* expression in the hypercholesterolemic group ($P = 0.019$). When using the last gene

Table 3. Statistically significant altered left ventricular diastolic function echocardiographic parameters in hypercholesterolemic compared to normal rabbit groups.

	Baseline		14.5 wks		14.5+2 wks	
	Normal group	Hyperchol group	Normal group	Hyperchol group	Normal group	Hyperchol group
E wave velocity (cm/s)	66.2±4.4	62.6±4.2	67.3±6.3	117.7±6.4***	72.9±2.5	100.9±8.5*
E-wave deceleration time (ms)	35.1 ±1.7	33.9±2.4	32.8±3.3	24.0±2.1*	39.0± 3.4	23.2±2.0***
E-wave deceleration rate (m/s^2)	19.2±1.6	20.4±2.2	20.9±1.3	51.2±3.5***	19.5 + 1.8	46.2±5.2***
Lateral annulus E/Em ratio	6.4±0.6	7.0±0.8	6.8±0.8	12.0 ±1.3*	6.2±0.6	12.7±1.5**
Septal annulus E/Em ratio	6.2±0.5	8.1±0.8	7.4±0.7	10.7±0.8*	8.2±0.5	12.1±0.7*
Left pulmonary vein A- A_r durations (ms)	-4.8±3.3	-2.3±3.6	-7.1±1.5	-26.5±6.5*	-5.1±1.5	-27.6±4.5**
Right pulmonary vein A- A_r durations (ms)	-2.9±3.5	-0.2±3.5	-7.0±2.3	-24.0±3.0**	-3.4±1.5	-23.4±4.9***
Left pulmonary vein A_r duration (ms)	43.2±2.5	39.2±2.7	40.5±1.2	51.4±4.5*	39.7±1.5	53.3±2.7***
Right pulmonary vein A_r duration (ms)	41.2±2.1	35.8±1.6	40.4±2.2	50.1±2.1**	38.1±1.4	51.3±3.3***

Comparison between the normal and hyperchol group at the given time-point. After baseline echocardiographic assessment, the hyperchol group was exposed to a cholesterol-enriched diet + vitamin D for 14.5 weeks before being switched for 2 weeks to a normal diet. E: peak velocity during early filling; Em: mitral annulus velocities during early filling in both lateral and septal annulus; A: peak velocity during active atrial filling; Ar: reversed atrial flow; A-Ar durations: mitral A-wave duration minus left (or right) pulmonary venous flow Ar wave duration. N = 7 for the normal group and n = 7 to 11 for the hyperchol group. *$P<0.05$, **$P<0.01$, ***$P<0.001$ for comparison between the normal and hyperchol group at the given time-point.

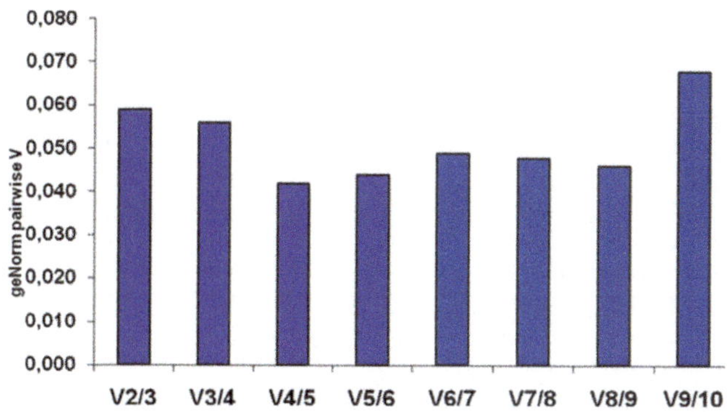

Figure 2. Determination using the geNorm algorithm of the optimal number of reference genes required for effective normalization. Pairwise variation ($V_n/_{n+1}$) calculated between the normalization factors NF_n and NF_{n+1} to assess the optimal number of reference genes to use in normalisation. V<0.15 is considered sufficient to normalise. Here, the use of two to three genes have a $V_2/_3 = 0.0575$, which indicates that the use of two to three genes is sufficient to calculate the normalization factor.

from geNorm classification (*G6pd*), the *Bnp* increase was underestimated (4.2 fold, $P = 0.011$), whereas when normalizing against the last classified gene selected by Normfinder (*Eef1e1*), the *Bnp* increase was overestimated (6.84 fold, $P = 0.011$).

Also *Anp*, *Mcp-1* and *Nox-2* mRNA expressions were found to be increased in the hypercholesterolemic group compared to the normal group (Figure S2 in File S1). Similar results were obtained using both normalization strategies. However, when using *G6pd* for normalization, *Anp* and *Nox-2* expression increases were not significant between groups ($P = 0.109$ and $P = 0.103$, respectively).

Finally, we found that the mRNA expression of *Bnp* correlates with many LVDD-related echocardiographic parameters: transmitral flow E wave velocity, transmitral flow deceleration time, transmitral flow deceleration rate, transmitral flow A duration, left pulmonary vein (A-Ar) duration, right pulmonary vein (A-Ar) duration, mitral annulus lateral E/Em and septal E/Em ratio. Indeed, higher *Bnp* mRNA expression values correspond to higher LVDD severity. Using geNorm or Normfinder reference genes for normalization resulted in very similar correlations of *Bnp* with echocardiographic parameters. In Figure 4, we show some of these

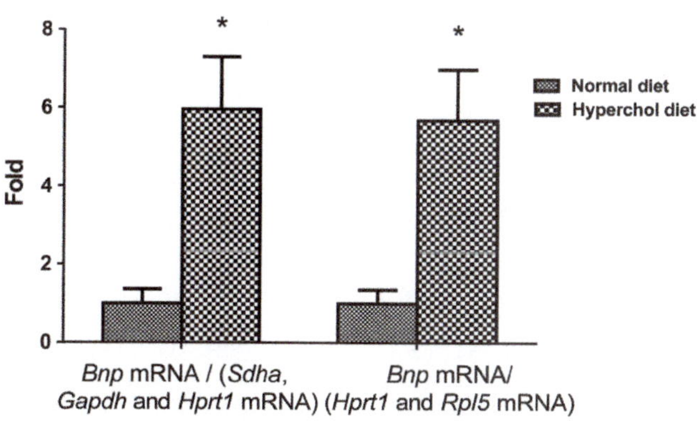

Figure 3. *Bnp* mRNA levels in the normal (n = 7) and high-cholesterol diet (n = 11) groups were normalised against geNorm (on the left) and Normfinder (right)-selected genes. Results shown correspond to mean ± SEM. Non-parametric Mann-Whitney test was used to compare the groups (*$P < 0.02$).

correlations using geometric mean of *Sdha*, *Gapdh* and *Hprt1* as examples.

Discussion

Echocardiographic Validation of a Rabbit Model of LVDD

Multiple echocardiographic parameters (including E-wave velocity, E-wave deceleration time, E-wave deceleration rate, difference in A-Ar durations and E/Em ratios) provide a robust demonstration of diet-induced restrictive LVDD in our rabbit model. Collectively, the changes reflect increased filling pressures, a stiffer LV and severe LVDD [27]. We believe that the proper selection of reference genes in this rabbit model will help further studies to investigate the different mechanisms that may be related to LVDD.

RT-PCR Validation of a Rabbit Model of LVDD

Although hypercholesterolemia has been shown to promote LVDD [28], the mechanisms underlying this progression remain largely unknown. Indeed, some studies reported cellular mechanisms that may be altered in LVDD, including pathways involved in calcium homeostasis as well as extracellular matrix components [29]. Analysis of gene expression is essential to understand the pathways involved in LVDD. RT-PCR is used to validate and determine gene expression because of its high specificity, sensitivity and rapidity. Also, small amounts of samples are needed in such experiments, which facilitate the feasibility of these studies. RT-PCR normalization analysis is crucial for proper interpretation of gene expression data [18–21]. Our study provides the best combination of reference genes (*Sdha*, *Gapdh* and *Hprt1* by geNorm; *Hprt1* and *Rpl5* by Normfinder) that may be used in further mechanistic studies in our animal model. Indeed, these genes are involved in different pathways such as glycolysis, citric acid cycle, purine nucleotide synthesis and ribosomal RNA maturation and have been frequently used as reference genes in earlier studies. Among these studies, we particularly noticed those related to cardiomyocytes and heart failure in general [30–33]. It is important to note that due to the partially completed rabbit genome sequencing, assembly and annotation, finding reference sequences in the rabbit's genome that correspond to reference genes is still difficult compared to humans, mice or rats. For this reason, we validated by sequencing the PCR products for each gene tested here. To our knowledge, this is the first report that gives validated reference genes in a rabbit model of LVDD but our results could also be of use for mRNA assessments from similar hypercholesterolemic rabbit models.

Considering the differences between the two methods used for reference gene selection, it was not surprising to obtain different stability rankings. Indeed, the geNorm algorithm is based on a pairwise variation test, which gives an overall stability of a gene in comparison to the rest of tested genes. However, the Normfinder algorithm estimates inter and intra-group variation and gives a final stability value based on these two parameters. Anderson and colleagues have demonstrated that Normfinder ranking is not similar to geNorm because of the differences between approaches [20]. However, other studies have showed similar classification by using the different approaches [34]. Vandesompele and colleagues concluded that each group has to validate their reference genes regardless of the method used; however, the method used should be reported [19]. When we used the best combinations of reference genes suggested by both methods, we obtained the same results regarding the increase of *Bnp* gene expression. However when using single non-validated potential reference genes (*G6pd* or *Eef1e1*), we showed that the fold increase results obtained were

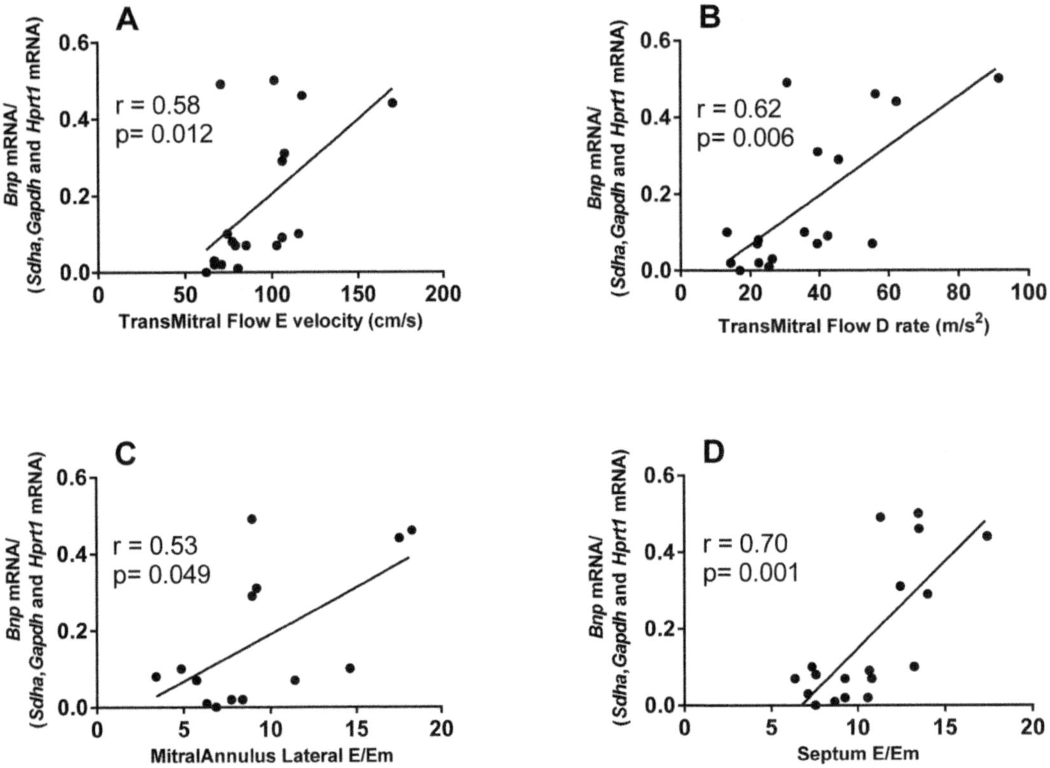

Figure 4. Spearman correlation between normalised *Bnp* mRNA levels (using geNorm selected reference genes) in rabbit left ventricles (normal diet n = 7 and cholesterol diet n = 11) and LVDD parameters determined by echocardiography before sacrifice: transmitral flow E velocity (A), transmitral flow deceleration rate (B), mitral annulus lateral E/Em ratio (C) and mitral annulus septal E/Em ratio (D).

differing by 63%. Similar results and conclusions were obtained with *Anp*, *Mcp-1* and *Nox-2*. The use of a combination of reference genes resulting in stable normalization factors is crucial when changes between groups are not as high as what we observed in the case of *Bnp* mRNA expression. It is frequent in this type of studies to get modest differences between groups for many genes (≈ 2 folds) like *Nox-2* in our present study. In such cases, the validation of the reference genes is even more important.

BNP is a well-documented marker of the evolution of LV dysfunction, with the levels of BNP directly correlating with the severity of LVDD [12,13]. Our findings further confirm this concept with the expression of *Bnp* (and the similar marker of disease *Anp* [10]) mRNA correlating with the echocardiographic results, thereby further validating our model of LVDD in hypercholesterolemic rabbits. Also, the increase of *Mcp-1* and *Nox-2* mRNAs validate the involvement of inflammation and oxidative stress in our model. These additional genes add evidence for the validity of our model as they have been reported to be differentially expressed in LVDD cases [9,10]. Indeed, macrophage recruitment which is mediated in part by *Mcp-1* and adhesion molecules such as intracellular adhesion molecule 1 (ICAM-1) and vascular cell adhesion molecule 1 (VCAM-1), exerts a crucial role in myocardial fibrosis and diastolic dysfunction. Myocardial fibrosis and LVDD were improved by using an *Mcp*-1 neutralizing antibody [35]. Reactive oxygen species (ROS) derived from NADPH subunits such as Nox-2 contribute by several processes to the development of cardiac contractile dysfunction and remodelling [36]. *Gapdh* is often solely used to normalize RT-PCR data in many studies. However, it was clearly shown that *Gapdh* expression is modulated under certain conditions, especially in hypoxia [37,38]. Surprisingly, normalizing only with *Gapdh* in our study yielded the same results in terms of *Bnp* mRNA expression modulation (5.71 fold increase, data not shown) as when using the geometric mean of our best genes combinations. This is probably due to the high stability of this gene in our model (geNorm stability: $M < 0.2$) and because of the large difference in *Bnp* expression seen between the hypercholesterolemic and normal groups. Moreover, it is possible that hypoxia does not play a major role in this LVDD model.

Conclusion

In the present study, we validated a hypercholesterolemic diet rabbit model of LVDD by echocardiography and by RT-PCR. We have identified the best reference genes (for normalization of RT-PCR data) that may be used in further studies to investigate mechanisms underlying LVDD.

Supporting Information

File S1 Figures S1 and S2. Figure S1. Left ventricular diastolic dysfunction parameters assessed by echocardiography in both normal and hypercholesterolemic groups (A) Transmitral flow deceleration time (n = 7 and 11 for normal and hyperchol groups, respectively). (B) E/Em ratio (n = 7 for normal group and n = 10, 8, 7 for hyperchol group at time 0, 14.5 and 16.5 weeks, respectively). The first time-point corresponds to the beginning of the cholesterol-enriched diet for the hyperchol diet rabbit group (baseline); the rabbits from this group were given cholesterol-enriched diet for an average of 14.5 weeks, the time it took to develop significant aortic valve stenosis as defined by higher than 10% decrease in aortic valve area assessed by echocardiography, after which the hyperchol group of rabbits was switched to a normal diet for two weeks before sacrifice. *$P<0.05$; **$P<0.01$; ***$P<0.001$. E: peak velocity during early left ventricular filling, Em: mitral annulus velocity during early left ventricular filling. Figure S2. mRNA levels of *Anp* (A), *Mcp-1* (B) *and Nox-2* (C) in the normal (n = 7) and high-cholesterol diet (n = 11 except for *Anp* where n = 10) groups normalised against geNorm (on the left of each panel) and Normfinder (right)-selected genes. Results shown correspond to mean ± SEM. Non-parametric Mann-Whitney test was used to compare the groups. *$P<0.05$, **$P<0.01$, ***$P<0.001$.

File S2

Acknowledgments

The authors gratefully acknowledge the statistical analysis by Clifford Ekwempe, MSc, at the Montreal Heart Institute Coordinating Center (MHICC). Special thanks to Ekat Kritikou PhD, for scientific review and editing of the current manuscript.

Author Contributions

Conceived and designed the experiments: WN DB ER JCT. Performed the experiments: WN DB YS TMA MM. Analyzed the data: WN DB YS ER JCT. Contributed reagents/materials/analysis tools: JCT. Wrote the paper: WN DB ER JCT.

References

1. Nagueh SF, Appleton CP, Gillebert TC, Marino PN, Oh JK, et al. (2009) Recommendations for the evaluation of left ventricular diastolic function by echocardiography. Eur J Echocardiogr 10: 165–193.
2. Borlaug BA, Kass DA (2006) Mechanisms of diastolic dysfunction in heart failure. Trends Cardiovasc Med 16: 273–279.
3. Ross R, Harker L (1976) Hyperlipidemia and atherosclerosis. Science 193: 1094–1100.
4. Huang Y, Walker KE, Hanley F, Narula J, Houser SR, et al. (2004) Cardiac systolic and diastolic dysfunction after a cholesterol-rich diet. Circulation 109: 97–102.
5. Busseuil D, Shi Y, Mecteau M, Brand G, Gillis MA, et al. (2010) Heart rate reduction by ivabradine reduces diastolic dysfunction and cardiac fibrosis. Cardiology 117: 234–242.
6. Luo TY, Su MJ, Yang YF, Liu YB, Liang HC, et al. (2004) Effect of hypercholesterolemia on myocardial function in New Zealand white rabbits. J Biomed Sci 11: 829–837.
7. Bauersachs J, Hiss K, Fraccarollo D, Laufs U, Ruetten H. (2006) Simvastatin improves left ventricular function after myocardial infarction in hypercholesterolemic rabbits by anti-inflammatory effects. Cardiovasc Res 72: 438–446.
8. Xu Z, Okamoto H, Akino M, Onozuka H, Matsui Y, et al. (2008) Pravastatin attenuates left ventricular remodeling and diastolic dysfunction in angiotensin II-induced hypertensive mice. J Cardiovasc Pharmacol 51: 62–70.
9. Haugen E, Chen J, Wikstrom J, Gronros J, Gan LM, et al. (2007) Parallel gene expressions of IL-6 and BNP during cardiac hypertrophy complicated with diastolic dysfunction in spontaneously hypertensive rats. Int J Cardiol 115: 24–28.
10. Murase T, Hattori T, Ohtake M, Abe M, Amakusa Y, et al. (2012) Cardiac remodeling and diastolic dysfunction in DahlS.Z-Lepr(fa)/Lepr(fa) rats: a new animal model of metabolic syndrome. Hypertens Res 35: 186–193.
11. Irzmanski R, Pawlicki L, Charlusz M, Kowalski J. (2012) Concentration of natriuretic peptides in patients suffering from idiopathic arterial hypertension and left ventricular diastolic dysfunction confirmed by echocardiography. Clin Exp Hypertens 34: 530–540.
12. Lubien E. (2002) Utility of B-Natriuretic Peptide in Detecting Diastolic Dysfunction: Comparison With Doppler Velocity Recordings. Circulation 105: 595–601.
13. Luchner A, Muders F, Dietl O, Friedrich E, Blumberg F, et al. (2001) Differential expression of cardiac ANP and BNP in a rabbit model of progressive left ventricular dysfunction. Cardiovasc Res 51: 601–607.
14. Sciarretta S, Paneni F, Palano F, Chin D, Tocci G, et al. (2009) Role of the renin-angiotensin-aldosterone system and inflammatory processes in the development and progression of diastolic dysfunction. Clin Sci (Lond) 116: 467–477.
15. Sorescu D, Griendling KK. (2002) Reactive oxygen species, mitochondria, and NAD(P)H oxidases in the development and progression of heart failure. Congest Heart Fail 8: 132–140.
16. Dubi S, Arbel Y. (2010) Large animal models for diastolic dysfunction and diastolic heart failure-a review of the literature. Cardiovasc Pathol 19: 147–152.
17. Gan LM, Wikstrom J, Brandt-Eliasson U, Wandt B. (2004) Amplitude and velocity of mitral annulus motion in rabbits. Echocardiography 21: 313–317.
18. Bustin SA, Benes V, Garson JA, Hellemans J, Huggett J, et al. (2009) The MIQE guidelines: minimum information for publication of quantitative real-time PCR experiments. Clin Chem 55: 611–622.
19. Vandesompele J, Kubista M, Pfaffl MW (2009) Reference gene validation software for improved normalization. In: Logan J, Edwards, K, Saunders, N., editor. Real-time PCR: Current technology and applications: Caister Academic Press.
20. Andersen CL, Jensen JL, Orntoft TF. (2004) Normalization of real-time quantitative reverse transcription-PCR data: a model-based variance estimation approach to identify genes suited for normalization, applied to bladder and colon cancer data sets. Cancer Res 64: 5245–5250.
21. Vandesompele J, De Preter K, Pattyn F, Poppe B, Van Roy N, et al. (2002) Accurate normalization of real-time quantitative RT-PCR data by geometric averaging of multiple internal control genes. Genome Biol 3: RESEARCH0034.
22. Khouri SJ, Maly GT, Suh DD, Walsh TE. (2004) A practical approach to the echocardiographic evaluation of diastolic function. J Am Soc Echocardiogr 17: 290–297.
23. Shi Y, Denault AY, Couture P, Butnaru A, Carrier M, et al. (2006) Biventricular diastolic filling patterns after coronary artery bypass graft surgery. J Thorac Cardiovasc Surg 131: 1080–1086.
24. Pfaffl MW. (2001) A new mathematical model for relative quantification in real-time RT-PCR. Nucleic Acids Res 29: e45.
25. Mamo S, Gal AB, Polgar Z, Dinnyes A. (2008) Expression profiles of the pluripotency marker gene POU5F1 and validation of reference genes in rabbit oocytes and preimplantation stage embryos. BMC Mol Biol 9: 67.
26. Busseuil D, Shi Y, Mecteau M, Brand G, Kernaleguen AE, et al. (2008) Regression of aortic valve stenosis by ApoA-I mimetic peptide infusions in rabbits. Br J Pharmacol 154: 765–773.
27. Abraham J, Abraham TP. (2009) The role of echocardiography in hemodynamic assessment in heart failure. Heart Fail Clin 5: 191–208.
28. Talini E, Di Bello V, Bianchi C, Palagi C, Delle Donne MG, et al. (2008) Early impairment of left ventricular function in hypercholesterolemia and its reversibility after short term treatment with rosuvastatin A preliminary echocardiographic study. Atherosclerosis 197: 346–354.
29. Periasamy M, Janssen PM. (2008) Molecular basis of diastolic dysfunction. Heart Fail Clin 4: 13–21.
30. Song W, Lu X, Feng Q. (2000) Tumor necrosis factor-alpha induces apoptosis via inducible nitric oxide synthase in neonatal mouse cardiomyocytes. Cardiovasc Res 45: 595–602.
31. Fatima N, Schooley JF, Jr., Claycomb WC, Flagg TP. (2012) Promoter DNA methylation regulates murine SUR1 (Abcc8) and SUR2 (Abcc9) expression in HL-1 cardiomyocytes. PLoS One 7: e41533.
32. Mohamed BA, Barakat AZ, Zimmermann WH, Bittner RE, Muhlfeld C, et al. (2012) Targeted disruption of Hspa4 gene leads to cardiac hypertrophy and fibrosis. J Mol Cell Cardiol 53: 459–468.
33. Martino A, Cabiati M, Campan M, Prescimone T, Minocci D, et al. (2011) Selection of reference genes for normalization of real-time PCR data in minipig heart failure model and evaluation of TNF-alpha mRNA expression. J Biotechnol 153: 92–99.
34. Willems E, Mateizel I, Kemp C, Cauffman G, Sermon K, et al. (2006) Selection of reference genes in mouse embryos and in differentiating human and mouse ES cells. Int J Dev Biol 50: 627–635.
35. Kai H, Kuwahara F, Tokuda K, Imaizumi T. (2005) Diastolic dysfunction in hypertensive hearts: roles of perivascular inflammation and reactive myocardial fibrosis. Hypertens Res 28: 483–490.
36. Zhao Y, McLaughlin D, Robinson E, Harvey AP, Hookham MB, et al. (2010) Nox2 NADPH oxidase promotes pathologic cardiac remodeling associated with Doxorubicin chemotherapy. Cancer Res 70: 9287–9297.
37. Caradec J, Sirab N, Keumeugni C, Moutereau S, Chimingqi M, et al. (2010) 'Desperate house genes': the dramatic example of hypoxia. Br J Cancer 102: 1037–1043.
38. Caradec J, Sirab N, Revaud D, Keumeugni C, Loric S. (2010) Is GAPDH a relevant housekeeping gene for normalisation in colorectal cancer experiments? Br J Cancer 103: 1475–1476.

Left Ventricular Mass in Dialysis Patients, Determinants and Relation with Outcome. Results from the COnvective TRansport STudy (CONTRAST)

Ira M. Mostovaya[1]*, Michiel L. Bots[2], Marinus A. van den Dorpel[3], Roel Goldschmeding[4], Claire H. den Hoedt[1,3], Otto Kamp[5], Renée Levesque[6], Albert H. A. Mazairac[1], E. Lars Penne[1,7], Dorine W. Swinkels[8], Neelke C. van der Weerd[1,7], Piet M. ter Wee[7,9], Menso J. Nubé[7,9], Peter J. Blankestijn[1], Muriel P. C. Grooteman[7,9]

1 Department of Nephrology, University Medical Center Utrecht, Utrecht, the Netherlands, 2 Julius Center for Health Sciences and Primary Care, University Medical Center Utrecht, Utrecht, the Netherlands, 3 Department of Internal Medicine, Maasstad Hospital, Rotterdam, the Netherlands, 4 Department of Pathology, University Medical Center Utrecht, Utrecht, the Netherlands, 5 Department of Cardiology, Vrije Universiteit Medical Center, Amsterdam, the Netherlands, 6 Department of Nephrology, Centre Hospitalier de l'Université de Montréal St. Luc Hospital, Montréal, Canada, 7 Department of Nephrology, Vrije Universiteit Medical Center, Amsterdam, the Netherlands, 8 Department of Laboratory Medicine, Laboratory of Genetic, Endocrine and Metabolic diseases, Radboud University Medical Centre Nijmegen, the Netherlands, 9 Institute for Cardiovascular Research Vrije Universiteit Medical Center, Vrije Universiteit Medical Center, Amsterdam, the Netherlands

Abstract

Background and Objectives: Left ventricular mass (LVM) is known to be related to overall and cardiovascular mortality in end stage kidney disease (ESKD) patients. The aims of the present study are 1) to determine whether LVM is associated with mortality and various cardiovascular events and 2) to identify determinants of LVM including biomarkers of inflammation and fibrosis.

Design, Setting, Participants, & Measurements: Analysis was performed with data of 327 ESKD patients, a subset from the CONvective TRAnsport STudy (CONTRAST). Echocardiography was performed at baseline. Cox regression analysis was used to assess the relation of LVM tertiles with clinical events. Multivariable linear regression models were used to identify factors associated with LVM.

Results: Median age was 65 (IQR: 54–73) years, 203 (61%) were male and median LVM was 227 (IQR: 183–279) grams. The risk of all-cause mortality (hazard ratio (HR) = 1.73, 95% CI: 1.11–2.99), cardiovascular death (HR = 3.66, 95% CI: 1.35–10.05) and sudden death (HR = 13.06; 95% CI: 6.60–107) was increased in the highest tertile (>260grams) of LVM. In the multivariable analysis positive relations with LVM were found for male gender ($B = 38.8 \pm 10.3$), residual renal function ($B = 17.9 \pm 8.0$), phosphate binder therapy ($B = 16.9 \pm 8.5$), and an inverse relation for a previous kidney transplantation ($B = -41.1 \pm 7.6$) and albumin ($B = -2.9 \pm 1.1$). Interleukin-6 (Il-6), high-sensitivity C-reactive protein (hsCRP), hepcidin-25 and connective tissue growth factor (CTGF) were not related to LVM.

Conclusion: We confirm the relation between a high LVM and outcome and expand the evidence for increased risk of sudden death. No relationship was found between LVM and markers of inflammation and fibrosis.

Trial Registration: Controlled-Trials.com ISRCTN38365125

Editor: Leighton R. James, University of Florida, United States of America

Funding: CONTRAST is partly supported by unrestricted grants from Fresenius Medical Care (The Netherlands) and Gambro Lundia AB (Sweden). Additional support for CONTRAST was also received from Roche, the Netherlands. There are no patents, products in development or marketed products to declare. IM Mostovaya, CH den Hoedt, O Kamp, ML Bots, NC van der Weerd, EL Penne and AHA Mazairac report receiving no lecture fees, no consulting support, or grant support. MPC Grooteman reports research funded by Fresenius, Gambro, and Baxter. PJ Blankestijn reports research funded by Fresenius, Gambro, Roche, Amgen and Novartis, consultant fee and honoraria for lectures from Fresenius, Gambro, Solvay, Medtronic, and Novartis. R Lévesque reports research funded by Amgen Canada. PM ter Wee reports research funded by Abbott, Baxter, Gambro, Fresenius, and Roche; honoraria for lectures received from Amgen, Roche, Genzyme, Fresenius. MJ Nubé reports research funded by Baxter and Fresenius; honoraria for lectures received from Fresenius and Baxter. MA van den Dorpel reports research funded by Amgen.

Competing Interests: The authors have the following interests: CONTRAST is partly supported by unrestricted grants from Fresenius Medical Care (The Netherlands) and Gambro Lundia AB (Sweden). Additional support for CONTRAST was also received from Roche, the Netherlands. There are no patents, products in development or marketed products to declare. IM Mostovaya, CH den Hoedt, O Kamp, ML Bots, NC van der Weerd, EL Penne, and AHA Mazairac report receiving no lecture fees, no consulting support, or grant support. MPC Grooteman reports research funded by Fresenius, Gambro, and Baxter. PJ Blankestijn reports research funded by Fresenius, Gambro, Roche, Amgen, and Novartis; consultant fee and honoraria for lectures from Fresenius, Gambro, Solvay, Medtronic, and Novartis. R Lévesque reports research funded by Amgen Canada. PM ter Wee reports research funded by Abbott, Baxter, Gambro, Fresenius, and Roche; honoraria for lectures received from Amgen, Roche, Genzyme, Fresenius. MJ Nubé reports research funded by Baxter and Fresenius; honoraria for lectures received from Fresenius and Baxter. MA van den Dorpel reports research funded by Amgen.

* E-mail: I.M.Mostovaya@umcutrecht.nl

Introduction

Increased left ventricular mass (LVM) has been well described as a frequent component of end stage kidney disease (ESKD) [1]. In fact, more than seventy percent of patients starting dialysis show left ventricular hypertrophy (LVH) on echocardiography [2]. An increase in left ventricular mass (LVM) is associated with cardiovascular morbidity and mortality [3,4]. Although the relation between LVM and overall mortality and cardiovascular events has been well established in ESKD patients, the association between LVM and certain types of cardiovascular morbidity (such as coronary heart disease: CHD) and mortality (such as sudden death) has not yet been thoroughly investigated.

Several inflammatory biomarkers associated with cardiovascular pathology and morbidity have been described for patients with chronic kidney disease (CKD). High sensitivity C-reactive protein (hsCRP and interleukin-6 (Il-6) are both well accepted markers of inflammation, related to increased risk of death and cardiovascular disease [5]. HsCRP is an acute phase reactant, which has been associated with an increased risk of major cardiovascular disease [6]. HsCRP levels are higher in HD patients than in healthy individuals [7] and have been shown to be independent predictors of LVM indexed for body surface area (LVMi) in CKD patients [8]. Il-6 is a short acting protein secreted by cells of the immune system in response to inflammatory stimuli, and is suspected to be a central regulator in the inflammatory process that leads to atherosclerosis [9]. Several studies have reported the relation between a high Il-6 and increased risk of developing CVD [10–12]. In patient deceased from acute myocardial infarction, Il-6 has been associated with mechanisms of cardiac hypertrophy [13]. Furthermore, Il-6 levels are increased in dialysis patients [7,14].

Connective tissue growth factor (CTGF) is a signalling protein involved in the pathogenesis of renal and cardiac fibrosis [15]. In animal studies CTGF has been described to contribute to development of cardiac hypertrophy [16,17]. CKD patients have a higher plasma CTGF level then healthy individuals, since CTGF is eliminated predominantly by the kidney [18].

Hepcidin-25 is a peptide produced by the liver, which regulates intestinal absorption of iron and its distribution through the body [19]. The gene encoding for hepcidin-25 is regulated in response to anemia, hypoxia and inflammation [20]. Furthermore, hepcidin-25 is related to increased risk of cardiovascular events in chronic hemodialysis patients [21].

Although several studies have described a relationship between hsCRP and left ventricle geometry and function [8,22,23], the relationship between LVM and the four described biomarkers has not been examined in a large population of HD patients.

We hypothesize that a high LVM will be related to a higher risk of mortality and cardiovascular events in our study, as is the case in previously studied dialysis populations. Furthermore we expect to find a positive relation between specific cardiovascular events such as risk of CHD or sudden death and LVM. Regarding hsCRP, Il-6, CTGF and hepcidin-25, since these markers are related to pathophysiological mechanisms that could theoretically promote increase of LVM, we assume to find a positive relation between the magnitude of LVM and hsCRP, Il-6, CTGF and hepcidin-25. Hence, the aims of this study are 1) to determine whether LVM is associated with mortality and various cardiovascular events in our population of ESKD patients and 2) to identify determinants of LVM including biomarkers of inflammation, systemic iron homeostasis and fibrosis in HD patients.

Materials and Methods

Patients

The present study included a subset of patients participating in the CONvective TRAnsport STudy (CONTRAST): 327 hemodialysis patients from 15 dialysis centres (14 Dutch centers and 1 Canadian center). CONTRAST has been designed to investigate the effects of increased convective transport by online HDF as compared with low-flux HD on all-cause mortality and cardiovascular morbidity and mortality (ISRCTN38365125) and included a total of 714 patients [24].

The study was conducted in accordance with the Declaration of Helsinki and approved by the medical ethics review boards of all participating dialysis centres. Written informed consent was obtained from all patients prior to enrolment. The names of the medical ethics committees/review boards that have approved this study are listed in the appendix S1 in File S1.

Data collection

Baseline patient and dialysis characteristics were used for this analysis: information on demography, anthropometrics, medical history, medication and standard laboratory values. A history of cardiovascular disease was defined as a previous acute myocardial infarction, coronary artery bypass graft, percutaneous transluminal coronary angioplasty, angina pectoris, stroke, transient ischemic attack, intermittent claudication, amputation, percutaneous transluminal angioplasty, peripheral bypass surgery and renal percutaneous transluminal angioplasty.

Systolic and diastolic blood pressure was measured before and after three consecutive dialysis sessions at baseline using a standard electronic sphygmomanometer. The average of these measurements was computed and used for analysis.

The primary outcome of CONTRAST was all cause mortality. Cause of death was recorded and subdivided into cardiovascular mortality (fatal myocardial infraction, fatal cerebrovascular accident, fatal decompensatio cordis, a rupture of the abdominal aorta or sudden death) and non-cardiovascular mortality. Sudden death was defined as death within 1 hour of the onset of symptoms as verified by a witness.

The main secondary endpoint was a composite of fatal and non-fatal cardiovascular events. Cardiovascular events were defined as death from cardiovascular causes, non-fatal myocardial infarction, non-fatal stroke, therapeutic coronary procedure (percutaneous transluminal coronary angioplasty and/or stenting), therapeutic carotid procedure (endartrectomy and/or stenting), and vascular intervention not related to vascular access (revascularisation, percutaneous transluminal angioplasty and/or stenting) or amputation. Congestive heart failure was excluded as a cardiovascular event, since the distinction with fluid overload is often difficult to make in patients with end stage renal disease.

Follow up of patients with respect to mortality and non-fatal cardiovascular events was continued even after they stopped with the randomized treatment because of a renal transplant (n = 71), a switch to peritoneal dialysis (n = 5), a move to another non-CONTRAST hospital (n = 11) or a stop of participation for other reasons (n = 58).

An independent Endpoint Adjudication Committee reviewed source documentation for all primary outcome events (deaths), as well as non-fatal cardiovascular events and infections.

Table 1. Demographic, anthropometric, biochemical, hemodynamic and dialysis characteristics of the study population.

	Total Cohort	Echo cor cohort
	n=714	n=327
Demographic data		
Male gender	445 (62%)	200 (61%)
Race, Caucasian	304 (85%)	263 (80%)
Age, years	64.1±13.7	63.0±13.3
Smoking	133 (19%)	66 (20%)
Anthropometrics		
Length (cm)	168±10	168±11
Weight (kg)	72.4±14.4	72.1±14.3
BMI (kg/m^2)	25.4±14.4	25.5±4.9
Body Surface Area (m^2)	1.85 (0.28)*	1.85 (0.30)*
Dialysis Properties		
Dialysis vintage (years)	1.8 (1.0–4.0)*	2.0 (1.0–4.0)*
Duration of dialysis (minutes)	226±23	225±23
Blood flow (mL/minute)	300 (300–348)*	300 (300–350)*
spKt/Vurea	1.40±0.22	1.39±0.20
AV fistula	279 (78%)	260 (80%)
Patients with residual kidney function	186 (52%)	171 (52%)
Comorbidities		
Cardiovascular disease	313 (44%)	146 (45%)
Diabetes	170 (24%)	83 (25%)
Previous kidney transplant	78 (11%)	30 (9%)
Laboratory parameters		
Hemoglobin (g/dL)	11.8±0.40	11.8±1.3
Phosphate (mmol/L)	1.64±0.49	1.67±0.50
Calcium (mmol/L)	2.31±0.18	2.30±0.18
Albumin (g/L)	40.4±3.8	41.2 (37.9–43.5)*
Creatinine (μmol/L), pre-dialysis	861±255	883±252
hsCRP (mg/L)	-	4.0 (1.6–11.9)*
Il-6 (pg/mL)	-	2.0 (1.2 3.8)*
CTGF (nmol/L)	-	3.6 (2.8–4.3)*
Hepcidin -25 (nM)	-	14.2 (6.3–22.4)*
Ferritin (ng/mL)	-	377 (211–597)*
TSAT (%)	-	22 (15–29)*
Medication		
Erythropietin therapy	314 (88%)	295 (91%)
Diuretic therapy	250 (35%)	129 (39%)
Beta-blocker therapy	184 (51%)	174 (53%)
RAS inhibitor therapy	179 (50%)	162 (50%)
Lipid lowering therapy	196 (55%)	152 (47%)
Vitamin D administration	227 (63%)	222 (68%)
Phosphate binding therapy	445 (62%)	194 (59%)
Platelet aggregation therapy or coumarines	111 (34%)	122 (36%)
Iron supplements	476 (67%)	213 (65%)
Hemodynamic measurements		
Systolic blood pressure (mm Hg)	147±21	142±19
Diastolic blood pressure (mm Hg)	75±12	74±10
LVEDD (mm)	-	10 (9–11)*
LVESD (mm)	-	32 (27–38)*
EFLV (%)	-	65 (55–72)*
LVM (g)	-	227 (183–279)*
LVH	-	230 (71%)

*:median and IQR (P25–P75).
AV: arterio-venous;BMI: mody mass index; CTGF: connective tissue growth factor; EFLV: ejection fraction of left ventricle; hsCRP: high sensitivity C-reactive protein; Il-6: interleukin 6; LVEDD: left ventricular end diastolic diameter; LVESD: left ventricular end systolic diameter; LVH: left ventricular hypertrophy; LVM: left ventricular mass; RAS: renin-angiotensin system; TSAT: transferrin saturation.

Laboratory measurements

Standard laboratory samples were analysed in the local laboratories of the participating hospitals by standard laboratory techniques.

Furthermore, in centres where storage of blood samples was logistically feasible, additional blood samples were drawn for the analysis of hsCRP, Il-6, CTGF and hepcidin prior to dialysis. Samples were placed on ice, and centrifuged within 30 min, at 1500 g for 10 minutes, and were stored at −80°C until assayed. A total of 248 patients, out of the 327 who underwent echocardiography, were treated in such centers and therefore had additional measurements of hsCRP, Il-6, CTGF and hepcidin.

High sensitivity CRP, hepcidin-25, CTGF and IL-6 levels were measured centrally. Measurements of the bioactive hepcidin-25 were performed with time of flight mass spectrometry which has been described previously [25]. High sensitivity CRP (mg/L) was measured with a particle-enhanced immunoturbidimetric assay on a Roche-Hitachi analyzer as described elsewhere [21]. IL-6 (pg/mL) was measured with an ELISA (Sanquin, Amsterdam, The Netherlands), details have been described earlier [26]. CTGF levels in plasma were determined by sandwich ELISA, using two specific antibodics (FibroGen Inc., San Francisco, CA, USA) directed against two distinct isotopes in the amino-terminal fragment of CTGF, detecting both full length CTGF and the N-fragment, as shown earlier [18].

Echocardiographic measurements

In 15 centres, patients were requested to undergo 2-dimensional echocardiography next to the standard CONTRAST baseline data collection.

Transthoracic echocardiography studies were performed on a mid-week non-dialysis day by an echocardiographer at the participating local hospital. From the parasternal long axis position the left ventricular end-diastolic diameter (LVEDD), end-systolic diameter (LVESD) as well as the posterior and septal wall thickness were determined. The ultrasound investigations were then assessed by an independent experienced echocardiographer at the core laboratory (VU medical Center, Amsterdam, the Netherlands), who was blinded for other patient data. LVM was calculated using the formula of Devereux and Reickek [27], modified in accordance with the recommendations of the American Society of Echocardiography [28]. LVH was defined as an LVM/height$^{2.7}$ >44g/m$^{2.7}$ for women and >48 g/m$^{2.7}$ for men [3].

Table 2. Hazard ratio of clinical events by LVM in grams divided into tertiles.

	T1: <201	T2: 201<LVM<260	95% CI	T3: >260	95% CI
Crude					
Mortality	1	1.61*	1.01–2.55	2.17*	1.39–3.38
Cardiovascular death	1	2.24	0.90–5.55	3.76*	1.61–8.82
Sudden death	1	8.93*	1.12–71.4	17.8*	2.35–135.0
Cardiovascular events	1	1.47	0.92–2.44	1.66*	1.06–2.67
CHD events	1	1.04	0.51–2.13	1.13	0.56–2.31
Adjusted[a]					
Mortality	1	1.50	0.92–2.10	1.73*	1.11–2.99
Cardiovascular death	1	1.80	0.64–5.07	3.69*	1.35–10.05
Sudden death	1	6.29	0.72–52.70	13.06*	6.60–107.16
Cardiovascular events	1	1.27	0.74–2.18	1.49	0.85–2.60
CHD events	1	1.22	0.71–2.09	1.51	0.87–2.64

*$p<0.05$.
[a]Adjusted with a propensity score containing determinants of LVM (male gender, residual renal function, history of kidney transplantation, albumin, use of RAS-inhibitors, use of phosphate binders, systolic blood pressure) and history of cardiovascular disease, diabetes, height, post-dialysis weight and dialysis modality (intervention).

Data analysis

Data were reported as proportions or as means with standard deviation (SD) or medians with inter-quartile ranges (IQR) when appropriate.

The average percentage of missing values per variable was 7.7%. No data were missing regarding clinical events. Multiple imputation was performed on all variables, where <40% of data were missing. One variable was not imputed due to a higher percentage of missing values, namely blood flow. Imputation was performed to prevent bias in reported estimates and to improve statistical power [29].

To study the independent relation of each variable with LVM, linear regression analysis was used. Patient and dialysis related variables that showed a univariable relation with LVM using a cut-off p-value <0,20 were entered in a multivariate model in consequent groups: demographic data, patient history, dialysis properties, therapeutic parameters and haemodynamic measurements. In addition, height and weight were added into the model upfront.

In a separate analysis, the variables hsCRP, Il-6, hepcidin-25 and CTGF were added to the constructed multivariate model one at a time. The old and new models were compared based on direction of the estimate and the significance of the regression coefficient of the added marker.

The relations between LVM and all-cause mortality, as well as cardiovascular events, cardiovascular death, sudden death and CHD were evaluated by Cox proportional hazards models, involving the time to the first relevant endpoint in any individual patient. For this analysis LVM was both analysed as a linear variable and divided into categories (tertiles). The number of events (in particular sudden death and CHD events) was small, and thus adjusting for all relevant possible confounders would lead to an overfitted model. Propensity scores as opposed to individual variables were used to adjust the models thus omitting the problem of an overfitted model. The propensity score [30] model estimated each individuals probability of having an LVM above the median of the studied population. Propensity score was built using a logistic model including all variables associated with LVM with $p<0.20$. Moreover, height, post-dialysis baseline weight and dialysis modality (intervention) were added into the propensity score model upfront.

Results were considered statistically significant when $p<0.05$ (two-sided). All calculations were made by use of a standard statistical package (SPSS for Windows Version 18.0.1; SPSS Inc. Headquarters, Chicago, Illinois, US).

Results

327 patients participating in CONTRAST underwent echocardiography. Out of this group, in 248 patients blood was collected for a measurement of markers of inflammation and fibrosis. Median age was 65 (IQR: 54–73) years, 203 were male (61%) and the median dialysis vintage was 2.0 (IQR: 1.0–4.0) years. Median LVM was 227 (IQR: 183–279) grams. A total of 230 patients (71%) had LVH. The baseline characteristics of the whole CONTRAST cohort and of the echocardiography population are shown in table 1. The mean follow-up time was 2.0 (minimum 0.1, maximum 6.5) years. Within the group of patients with an LVM measurement 130 (39.8%) patients died from any cause and 116 (35.5%) had a cardiovascular event, out of which 43 (13.1%) were fatal. CHD (angina pectoris or acute myocardial infarction) occurred in 53 (16.2%) patients, of whom 3 (0.9%) died. Sudden death occurred in 24 (7.3%) patients.

Relation to LVM and outcome

Table 2 shows proportional hazard ratios for all-cause mortality, cardiovascular death, sudden death, combined fatal and non-fatal cardiovascular events and CHD events; both crude and adjusted using propensity scores. Risk of all-cause mortality, cardiovascular death and sudden death was increased in the highest tertile (>260grams) of LVM; while no difference in risk was found for overall cardiovascular events and CHD events in the LVM tertiles. Figure 1 shows survival curves for the clinical events described above stratified by LVM tertiles.

As shown in Table S1a and S1b in File S1, when LVM was indexed for BSA or height$^{2.7}$, relations with clinical events were similar.

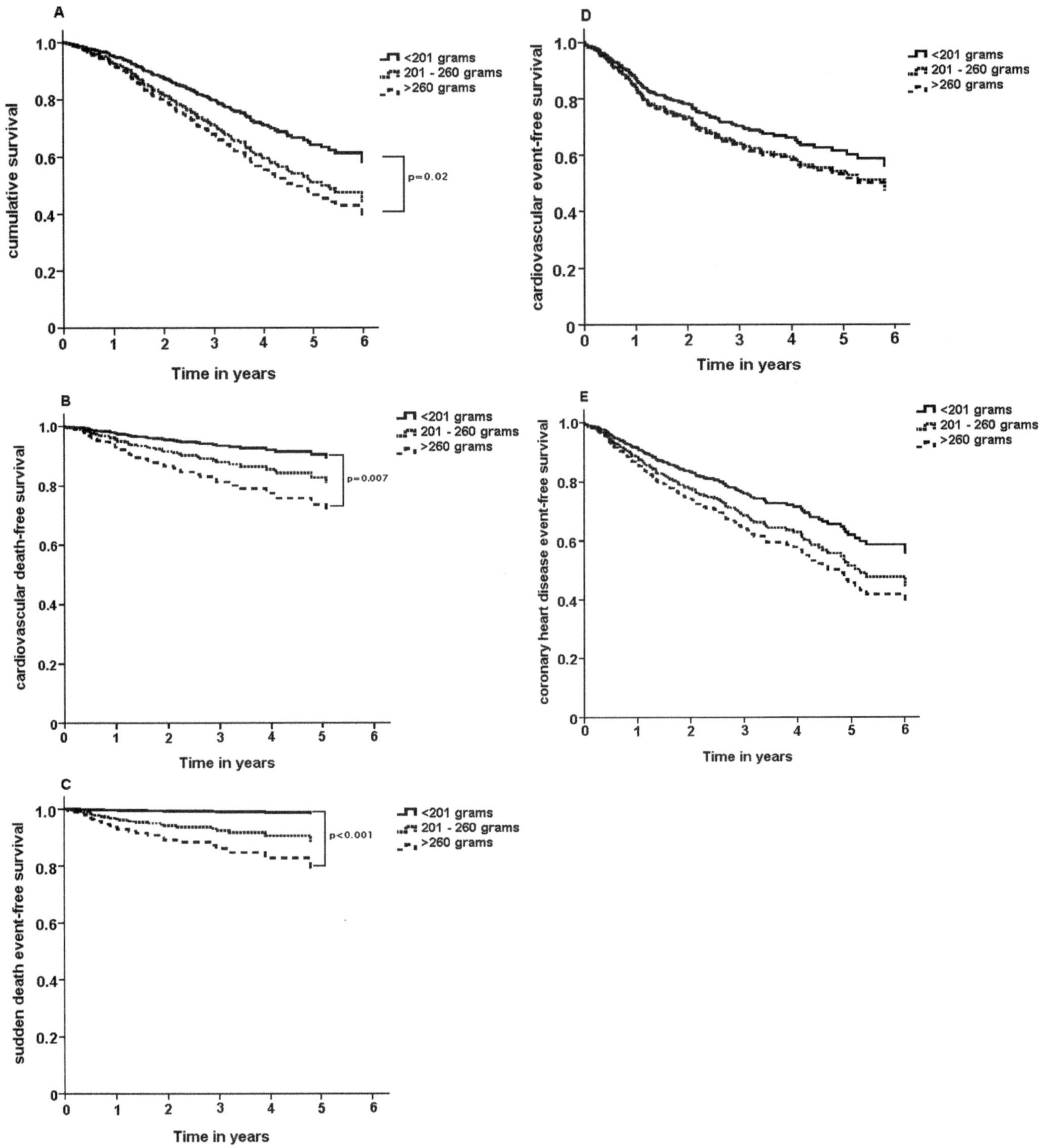

Figure 1. Survival curves for (A) time to death from any cause, (B) cardiovascular death, (C) sudden death, (D) cardiovascular events (both fatal and non-fatal), (E) coronary heart disease events (both fatal and non-fatal, all stratified by LVM tertiles and adjusted using propensity scores.

Determinants of LVM

The univariable and multivariable analysis results of LVM are shown in Table 3. In the multivariate analysis significant positive relations with LVM were found for male gender, presence of residual renal function and phosphate binder therapy. There were inverse relations for a history of kidney transplantation and albumin. The complete-case multivariate regression analysis showed similar results as demonstrated in Table S2 in File S1.

Table 4 shows that hsCRP, Il-6, hepcidin-25 and CTGF were not related to LVM.

Table 3. Determinants of LVM in dialysis patients: univariable and multivariable regression analysis.

	Univariable model		Multivariable model	
Determinant	**B**	**95% CI**	**B**	**95% CI**
Demographic data				
Male gender	56.47	39.03 to 73.90	38.80	18.64 to 58.96
Race, Caucasian	12.92	−9.75 to 35.60		
Age (years)	0.75	0.08 to 1.42		
Smoking	22.20	−0.47 to 44.87		
Dialysis Properties				
Duration of dialysis (hours)	35.14	10.95 to 59.33		
spKt/Vurea	−102.7	−145.7 to −59.75		
AV fistula	17.59	−4.66 to 38.83		
Comorbidities				
Cardiovascular disease	16.54	−1.50 to 34.58		
Diabetes	1.94	−18.45 to 22.37		
Previous kidney transplant	−49.76	−80.38 to −19.01	−41.12	−55.94 to −26.31
Dialysis vintage (years)	−5.45	−8.61 to −2.30		
Residual kidney function	29.28	−11.52 to 47.04	17.88	2.16 to 33.61
Laboratory parameters				
Hemoglobin (g/dL)	−1.00	−12.53 to 10.53		
Phosphate (mmol/L)	0.89	−17.17 to 18.94		
Calcium (mmol/L)	13.37	−32.36 to 63.99		
Calcium*Phosphate	1.28	−6.48 to 9.03		
Albumin (g/L)	−1.99	−4.17 to 0.20	−2.94	−5.08 to −0.81
Creatinin (μmol/L)	−0.02	−0.05 to 0.02		
Therapeutic parameters				
Erythropietin	−9.68	−38.78 to 19.38		
Diuretic	0.97	−18.99 to 20.94		
Beta-blocker	16.26	−1.70 to 34.21		
Alpha-blocker	21.44	−13.64 to 56.51		
RAS inhibitor	21.67	3.82 to 39.51	14.08	−2.46 to 30.62
Lipid lowering therapy	0.95	−17.06 to 18.95		
Vitamin D administration	5.15	−14.16 to 22.45		
Phosphate binder	17.82	−0.420 to 36.05	16.87	0.14 to 33.56
Platelet aggregation inhibitor	10.35	−8.44 to 29.13		
Coumarine derivates	22.50	−14.09 to 59.08		
Iron supplements	22.56	3.81 to 41.32		
Hemodynamic measurements				
Systolic blood pressure (mm Hg)	0.54	0.08 to 1.00	0.37	−0.77 to 0.82

The B reflects the change of total LVM (in grams) related with one unit increment of the determinant.
R^2 of the multivariable model = 0.22.

Discussion

The present study confirmed the relation between a high LVM and outcome [2,4,31,32]. Furthermore we expanded the evidence for a strongly increased risk of sudden death in patients with a high LVM. After confirming that LVM was a strong predictor of cardiovascular and overall mortality we wanted to study what factors determine the magnitude of LVM, and in particular if these determinants were potentially modifiable. In our analysis, factors related to LVM were: male gender, history of kidney transplantation, residual kidney function (RKF), albumin and use of phosphate binders. Thus we did not find determinants of LVM that could easily be altered in daily clinical practice. Lastly, we explored whether novel markers of inflammation, fibrosis and iron homeostasis (hsCRP, Il-6, CTGF and hepcidin-25), which in theory could lead to a higher LVM, were related to LVM in a large population of hemodialysis patients. Apparently, although hsCRP, Il-6, CTGF, hepcidin-25 have previously been found to be associated with cardiovascular damage, no relation exists between these biomarkers and the magnitude of LVM in ESKD patients.

Table 4. Hepcidin, hsCRP, Il-6 and CTGF as determinants of LVM.

	Univariable model		Adding to 'basic' multivariable model		
Determinant	**B**	**95% CI**	**B**	**95% CI**	**ΔR^2**
Hepcidin-25 (nM)	−0.04	−0.46 to 0.38	0.04	−0.38 to 0.45	−0.003
hsCRP (mg/L)	0.22	−0.46 to 0.90	0.07	−0.43 to 0.57	−0.003
Il-6 (pg/mL)	0.03	−0.17 to 0.22	0.06	−0.13 to 0.23	−0.002
CTGF (nmol/L)	0.05	−3.92 to 4.01	0.67	−3.45 to 4.78	−0.001

The B reflects the change of total LVM (in grams) related with one unit increment of the determinant.

LVM and clinical events

A summary of previous papers in which the relation between left ventricular geometry and clinical events was studied in dialysis patients is shown in Table 5. Foley et al studied the relation between LVM and mortality risks in 433 ESKD patients and found a significant linear association between LVM and overall mortality as well as cardiovascular mortality in particular [2]. Zoccali et al studied the prognostic impact of LVM indexed for body surface are or height$^{2.7}$ in 254 dialysis patients and found that both types of LVMi were related to both overall mortality and cardiovascular mortality [31].

We are among the first to describe the relationship between LVM and sudden death specifically in ESKD patients. In fact, ESKD patients in the highest tertile of LVM had an almost 14-fold higher risk of sudden death when compared to the lowest LVM tertile, while their risk of dying from a cardiac cause in general was 'only' increased by a factor 3.5. The underlying mechanism may be through a decrease in myocardial capillary density, diastolic and systolic dysfunction, disturbances in interventricular conduction, chamber dilatation and eventually more compensatory hypertrophy. These processes lead to an increased risk of triggering a fatal arrhythmia [1,33]. Autopsy studies in ESKD patients point to the presence of diffuse inter-myocardiocyte fibrosis specific for this group, which may indicate an electrical instability predisposing to sudden death [34]. The percentage of sudden deaths (56%) from all cardiac deaths in our population was similar to those of earlier studies [33].

For a combination of fatal- and non-fatal cardiovascular events no relation with LVM size was found. To our knowledge, no such relation has been described in earlier literature; although Zoccali et al found a significant relation between LVM indexed for height$^{2.7}$ and fatal- and non-fatal cardiovascular events combined [31]. Since there were only 3 lethal CHD events in our study, this association could not be explored in our population.

Determinants of LVM

Factors related to LVM were: male gender, history of kidney transplantation, residual kidney function (RKF), albumin and use of phosphate binders.

It was a surprising finding that a history of CVD and blood pressure (BP) were not found to be associated with LVM. Regarding the lack of relation between LVM and CVD this could be attributed to the fact that our definition of CVD encompassed several periphery vasculature diseases/interventions, which do not necessarily lead to an enlargement of LVM. Also, many ESKD patients have a high LVM without a history of CVD [2]. While BP is very variable over time in dialysis patients (mostly due to rigorous changes in extracellular volume during and in-between dialysis treatments), our BP results are an average of three pre- and three post-dialysis BP measurements. Hence our BP

Table 5. Summary of previous studies in which the relation between LV geometry and clinical events was examined in dialysis patients.

Author	patient nr	LV measurement	event	Risk measure	Conclusion
Silverberg et al	133	LVMi (g/m^2)	mortality	RR: 2.9 (p = 0.013)	LVH is an important determinant of survival
1989 (33)			CV mortality	RR: 2.7 (0.08)	in incident dialysis patients
Foley et al	433	LVMi (g/m^2)	mortality	RR: 1.003 (p = 0.11)	LVH is highly prevalent in th dialysis
1995 (2)			late (>2 yr) mortality	RR: 1.009 (p<0.001)	population and is a risk factor for mortality
London et al	153	more than 10% decrease	mortality	RR: 0.78 (p = 0.001)	partial regression of LVM has a favorable
2001 (4)		in LVMi (g/height$^{2.7}$)	CV mortality	RR: 0.72 (p = 0.002)	effect on mortlity and CV-mortality
Zoccali et al	254	LVMi (g/m^2)	mortality	HR: 1.01 (p<0.001)/1.03 (p<0.001)	LVM indexed for height$^{2.7}$ provides a more
2001 (32)		LVMi (g/height$^{2.7}$)	CV mortality	HR: 1.01 (p<0.001)/1.03 (p<0.001)	powerful predictor for death and CV events
			CV event	HR: 1.00 (ns)/1.02 (p = 0.004)	compared to LVM indexed for BSA
Zoccali et al	161	in top 75% progression	mortality	HR: 3.07 (p = 0.008)	Changes in LVMi have an independent
2004 (3)		in LVMi (g/height$^{2.7}$)	CV event	HR: 3.02 (p = 0.02)	prognostic value for death and CV events

CV events are defined as a combination of both fatal and non-fatal cardiovascular events.
BSA: body surface area; CV: cardiovascular; HR: hazard ratio; LV: left ventricular; LVH: left ventricular hypertrophy; LVM: left ventricular mass; LVMi: left ventricular mass index; nr: number; RR: relative risk.

measurements could be a poor representative of the total BP burden of a patient (which is truly related to LVM).

The relation between LVM and a history of kidney transplantation [35,36] and albumin [37] is in accordance with earlier literature.

The positive relation between LVM and RKF may be explained by a 'survivor bias': patients that still have RKF have been on dialysis for a shorter period of time. As time passes, the patients with a high LVM are more likely to die, the patient with a lower LVM remain and lose their RKF. In our population, the dialysis vintage differs significantly between patient with RKF (1.92±1.58 years) and without RKF (4.00±3.4 years).

Previous studies on predictors of LVM and LVMi in HD patients identified phosphate and the calcium-phosphate product as patient characteristics associated with LVH [38–40]. In our analysis however, these laboratory values were not significantly related to LVM, while there was a positive association between LVM and use of phosphate binders. The serum calcium and phosphate are well controlled in our dialysis population, and phosphate binders were prescribed to 74% of the patients (mainly sevelamer, a non-calcium containing phosphate binder: 54%). Hyperphosphatemia can lead to vascular calcification and myocardial fibrosis, resulting in increased cardiovascular risk [41]. Thus, it is plausible that in our population the prescription of phosphate binders is a reflection of higher phosphate intake at present and/or hyperphosphatemia in the past, resulting in higher LVM.

Relation between LVM and hsCRP, Il-6, CTGF, hepcidin

We are among the first to investigate the association between LVM and the biomarkers hsCRP, Il-6, CTGF and hepcidin in a population of ESKD patients, which is also large enough to perform appropriate corrections for clinically relevant variables without creating an overfitted model. Although there is a theoretical incentive, as described in the Introduction, to hypothesize that these biomarkers may contribute to LVM, we do not find such a relation in our population. Apparently, although hsCRP, Il-6, CTGF, hepcidin-25 have previously been found to be associated with cardiovascular damage, no relation exists between these biomarkers and the magnitude of LVM in ESKD patients.

In earlier papers concerning LVM and prognosis, LVM was indexed for body surface are, or divided by height$^{2.7}$. It was shown that these indexations, especially LVM/height$^{2.7}$ are better predictors of clinical events than LVM. [3,4]) A downside of ratios is that observed relation may be due to the nominator, the denominator or both. Therefore in the present analyses we chose to use LVM for our analyses only with correction for height and weight in the propensity scores for optimal statistical adjustment. As shown in Tables S1a and S1b in File S1, when LVM was adjusted for height and weight, the relation with clinical events was similar to that of LVM indexed for BSA or height$^{2.7}$.

Strengths and limitations

This study had several limitations. First, 7.7% of data was missing and biomarkers were measured in only 75.5% of the patients. However, since multiple imputation was performed for missing variables included in the multivariable analysis, this prevents the drawing of wrong conclusions due to the fact that data may be missing in specific patients for a reason, and not by chance and by increasing the power of our analyses [29]. Furthermore, our sensitivity analyses of complete cases showed no marked differences with the regression performed on the imputed data. Second, the number of CHD events and sudden deaths was small, thus limiting the precision of our estimates. Third, since cross-sectional data was used to determine variables related to LVM, causality of relations cannot be established. Fourth, measurements of LVM by echocardiography is less precise and reliable than measurement by cardiac magnetic resonance imaging (CMRI) [1]. However, while CMRI is recognized as the "gold standard" for ventricular geometry measurements, it is less often applied in clinical practice since it is more expensive, not widely available and has contra-indications such as claustrophobia and use of cardiac implantable devices [1]. Thus it was not feasible to perform CMRI measurements in our relatively large cohort of dialysis patients. This may have led to misclassification, which generally leads to an underestimation of the magnitude of the relations under study.

The strengths of this study are the large sample size, the concise and prospective data collection, the independent review of source documentation for all primary and secondary outcomes and the double independent analysis of the echocardiography recordings blinded for patient characteristics.

Conclusion

In this study we confirmed the relation between LVM and all-cause mortality. Furthermore we demonstrated a markedly increased risk of sudden death in patients with a high LVM.

No relationship was found for markers of inflammation (except for a negative association with albumin) and fibrosis.

Supporting Information

File S1 Appendix S1, Names of the ethics committees/ institutional review boards. Table S1, (A) Hazard ratio of clinical events by LVMi in grams per m^2 divided into tertiles. (B) Hazard ratio of clinical events by LVMi in grams per height$^{2.7}$ divided into tertiles. **Table S2, Whole-case analysis (n = 289) of determinants of LVM in dialysis patients: univariable and multivariable regression analysis.**

Acknowledgments

The authors are grateful to the patients and nursing staff participating in this project.

Author Contributions

Conceived and designed the experiments: MB MD PW MN PB MG RL. Performed the experiments: MB MD PW MN PB MG CH AM NW LP RL. Analyzed the data: IM MB. Contributed reagents/materials/analysis tools: RG DS OK. Wrote the paper: IM MB PB.

References

1. Glassock RJ, Pecoits-Filho R, Barberato SH (2009) Left ventricular mass in chronic kidney disease and ESRD. Clin J Am Soc Nephrol 4 Suppl 1: S79–S91.
2. Foley RN, Parfrey PS, Harnett JD, Kent GM, Martin CJ, et al (1995) Clinical and echocardiographic disease in patients starting end-stage renal disease therapy. Kidney Int 47: 186–192.
3. Zoccali C, Benedetto FA, Mallamaci F, Tripepi G, Giacone G, et al. (2004) Left ventricular mass monitoring in the follow-up of dialysis patients: prognostic value of left ventricular hypertrophy progression. Kidney Int 65: 1492–1498.
4. London GM, Pannier B, Guerin AP, Blacher J, Marchais SJ, et al. (2001) Alterations of left ventricular hypertrophy in and survival of patients receiving hemodialysis: follow-up of an interventional study. J Am Soc Nephrol 12: 2759–2767.

5. Panichi V, Migliori M, De PS, Taccola D, Bianchi AM, et al. (2000) C-reactive protein as a marker of chronic inflammation in uremic patients. Blood Purif 18: 183–190.
6. Mora S, Musunuru K, Blumenthal RS (2009) The clinical utility of high-sensitivity C-reactive protein in cardiovascular disease and the potential implication of JUPITER on current practice guidelines. Clin Chem 55: 219–228.
7. El-Shehaby AM, El-Khatib MM, Battah AA, Roshdy AR (2010) Apelin: a potential link between inflammation and cardiovascular disease in end stage renal disease patients. Scand J Clin Lab Invest 70: 421–427.
8. Cottone S, Nardi E, Mule G, Vadala A, Lorito MC, et al. (2007) Association between biomarkers of inflammation and left ventricular hypertrophy in moderate chronic kidney disease. Clin Nephrol 67: 209–216.
9. Jones SA, Horiuchi S, Topley N, Yamamoto N, Fuller GM (2001) The soluble interleukin 6 receptor: mechanisms of production and implications in disease. FASEB J 15: 43–58.
10. Ridker PM, Rifai N, Stampfer MJ, Hennekens CH (2000) Plasma concentration of interleukin-6 and the risk of future myocardial infarction among apparently healthy men. Circulation 101: 1767–1772.
11. Biasillo G, Leo M, Della BR, Biasucci LM (2010) Inflammatory biomarkers and coronary heart disease: from bench to bedside and back. Intern Emerg Med 5: 225–233.
12. Vasan RS, Sullivan LM, Roubenoff R, Dinarello CA, Harris T, et al. (2003) Inflammatory markers and risk of heart failure in elderly subjects without prior myocardial infarction: the Framingham Heart Study. Circulation 107: 1486–1491.
13. Kaneko K, Kanda T, Yokoyama T, Nakazato Y, Iwasaki T, et al. (1997) Expression of interleukin-6 in the ventricles and coronary arteries of patients with myocardial infarction. Res Commun Mol Pathol Pharmacol 97: 3–12.
14. Ayerden EF, Ebinc H, Derici U, Aral A, Aybay C, et al. (2009) The relationship between adiponectin levels and proinflammatory cytokines and left ventricular mass in dialysis patients. J Nephrol 22:216–223.
15. Clarkson MR, Gupta S, Murphy M, Martin F, Godson C, et al. (1999) Connective tissue growth factor: a potential stimulus for glomerulosclerosis and tubulointerstitial fibrosis in progressive renal disease. Curr Opin Nephrol Hypertens 8: 543–548.
16. Zhang J, Chang L, Chen C, Zhang M, Luo Y, et al. (2011) Rad GTPase inhibits cardiac fibrosis through connective tissue growth factor. Cardiovasc Res 91: 90–98.
17. Hayata N, Fujio Y, Yamamoto Y, Iwakura T, Obana M, et al. (2008) Connective tissue growth factor induces cardiac hypertrophy through Akt signaling. Biochem Biophys Res Commun 370: 274–278.
18. Gerritsen KG, Peters HP, Nguyen TQ, Koeners MP, Wetzels JF, et al. (2010) Renal proximal tubular dysfunction is a major determinant of urinary connective tissue growth factor excretion. Am J Physiol Renal Physiol 298: F1457–F1464.
19. Fleming RE, Sly WS (2001) Hepcidin: a putative iron-regulatory hormone relevant to hereditary hemochromatosis and the anemia of chronic disease. Proc Natl Acad Sci U S A 98: 8160–8162.
20. Nicolas G, Chauvet C, Viatte L, Danan JL, Bigard X, et al. (2002) The gene encoding the iron regulatory peptide hepcidin is regulated by anemia, hypoxia, and inflammation. J Clin Invest 110: 1037–1044.
21. van der Weerd NC, Grooteman MP, Bots ML, van den Dorpel MA, den Hoedt CH, et al. (2013) Hepcidin-25 is related to cardiovascular events in chronic haemodialysis patients. Nephrol Dial Transplant 28: 3062–3071.
22. Nozari Y, Geraiely B (2011) Correlation between the serum levels of uric acid and HS-CRP with the occurrence of early systolic failure of left ventricle following acute myocardial infarction. Acta Med Iran 49: 531–535.
23. Tatasciore A, Zimarino M, Renda G, Zurro M, Soccio M, et al. (2008) Awake blood pressure variability, inflammatory markers and target organ damage in newly diagnosed hypertension. Hypertens Res 31: 2137–2146.
24. Penne EL, Blankestijn PJ, Bots ML, van den Dorpel MA, Grooteman MP, et al. (2005) Resolving controversies regarding hemodiafiltration versus hemodialysis: the Dutch Convective Transport Study. Semin Dial 18: 47–51.
25. Kroot JJ, Laarakkers CM, Geurts-Moespot AJ, Grebenchtchikov N, Pickkers P, et al. (2010) Immunochemical and mass-spectrometry-based serum hepcidin assays for iron metabolism disorders. Clin Chem 56: 1570–1579.
26. van der Weerd NC, Grooteman MP, Bots ML, van den Dorpel MA, den Hoedt CH, et al. (2012) Hepcidin-25 in chronic hemodialysis patients is related to residual kidney function and not to treatment with erythropoiesis stimulating agents. PLoS One 7: e39783.
27. Devereux RB, Casale PN, Hammond IW, Savage DD, Alderman MH, et al. (1987) Echocardiographic detection of pressure-overload left ventricular hypertrophy: effect of criteria and patient population. J Clin Hypertens 3: 66–78.
28. Schiller NB, Shah PM, Crawford M, DeMaria A, Devereux R, et al. (1989) Recommendations for quantitation of the left ventricle by two-dimensional echocardiography. American Society of Echocardiography Committee on Standards, Subcommittee on Quantitation of Two-Dimensional Echocardiograms. J Am Soc Echocardiogr 2: 358–367.
29. Greenland S, Finkle WD (1995) A critical look at methods for handling missing covariates in epidemiologic regression analyses. Am J Epidemiol 142: 1255–1264.
30. Sjolander A (2009) Propensity scores and M-structures. Stat Med 28: 1416–1420.
31. Zoccali C, Benedetto FA, Mallamaci F, Tripepi G, Giacone G, et al. (2001) Prognostic impact of the indexation of left ventricular mass in patients undergoing dialysis. J Am Soc Nephrol 12: 2768–2774.
32. Silberberg JS, Barre PE, Prichard SS, Sniderman AD (1989) Impact of left ventricular hypertrophy on survival in end-stage renal disease. Kidney Int 36: 286–290.
33. Ritz E, Wanner C (2008) The challenge of sudden death in dialysis patients. Clin J Am Soc Nephrol 3: 920–929.
34. Aoki J, Ikari Y, Nakajima H, Mori M, Sugimoto T, et al. (2005) Clinical and pathologic characteristics of dilated cardiomyopathy in hemodialysis patients. Kidney Int 67: 333–340.
35. Larsson O, Attman PO, Beckman-Suurkula M, Wallentin I, Wikstrand J (1986) Left ventricular function before and after kidney transplantation. A prospective study in patients with juvenile-onset diabetes mellitus. Eur Heart J 7: 779–791.
36. Guizar-Mendoza JM, mador-Licona N, Lozada EE, Rodriguez L, Gutierrez-Navarro M, et al. (2006) Left ventricular mass and heart sympathetic activity after renal transplantation in children and young adults. Pediatr Nephrol 21: 1413–1418.
37. Zoccali C, Mallamaci F, Tripepi G (2003) Traditional and emerging cardiovascular risk factors in end-stage renal disease. Kidney Int Suppl : S105–S110.
38. Achinger SG, Ayus JC (2006) Left ventricular hypertrophy: is hyperphosphatemia among dialysis patients a risk factor? J Am Soc Nephrol 17: S255–S261.
39. Nitta K, Akiba T, Uchida K, Otsubo S, Otsubo Y, et al. (2004) Left ventricular hypertrophy is associated with arterial stiffness and vascular calcification in hemodialysis patients. Hypertens Res 27: 47–52.
40. Chue CD, Edwards NC, Moody WE, Steeds RP, Townend JN, et al. (2012) Serum phosphate is associated with left ventricular mass in patients with chronic kidney disease: a cardiac magnetic resonance study. Heart 98: 219–224.
41. Tonelli M, Pannu N, Manns B (2010) Oral phosphate binders in patients with kidney failure. N Engl J Med 362: 1312–1324.

24

Gender Dimorphism of the Cardiac Dysfunction in Murine Sepsis: Signalling Mechanisms and Age-Dependency

Jianmin Chen[1], Fausto Chiazza[2], Massimo Collino[2], Nimesh S. A. Patel[1], Sina M. Coldewey[3], Christoph Thiemermann[1]*

1 Queen Mary University of London, William Harvey Research Institute, Barts and the London School of Medicine and Dentistry, London, United Kingdom, **2** University of Turin, Department of Drug Science and Technology, Turin, Italy, **3** Jena University Hospital, Department of Anesthesiology and Intensive Care Medicine, Jena, German

Abstract

Development of cardiac dysfunction is associated with increased morbidity and mortality in patients with sepsis. Increasing evidence shows that gender determines the degree of inflammatory response of the host and that females tolerate sepsis better than males. It is unknown whether gender affects the cardiac dysfunction in animals or patients with sepsis. To investigate this, male or female C57BL/6 mice were subjected to either lipopolysaccharide (LPS)/peptidoglycan (PepG) co-administration or cecal ligation and puncture (CLP). At 18 hours after LPS/PepG injection or 24 hours after CLP, cardiac function was evaluated by echocardiography. The septic insult caused a significant cardiac dysfunction in both genders. However, the cardiac dysfunction was significantly less pronounced in females in comparison with males subjected to LPS (3 mg/kg)/PepG (0.1 mg/kg) or CLP. Compared with males injected with LPS (3 mg/kg)/PepG (0.1 mg/kg), western blotting analysis of the myocardium from females injected with LPS/PepG revealed i) profound increases in phosphorylation of Akt and eNOS; ii) significant decreases in phosphorylation of IκBα, nuclear translocation of the NF-κB subunit p65, decreased expression of iNOS and decreased synthesis of TNF-α and IL-6 in the heart. However, the gender dimorphism of the cardiac dysfunction secondary to LPS/PepG was not observed when higher doses of LPS (9 mg/kg)/PepG (1 mg/kg) were used. In conclusion, the cardiac dysfunction caused by sepsis was less pronounced in female than in male mice. The protection of female hearts against the dysfunction associated with sepsis is (at least in part) attributable to cardiac activation of the Akt/eNOS survival pathway, decreased activation of NF-κB, and decreased expression of iNOS, TNF-α and IL-6. It should be noted that the observed gender dimorphism of the cardiac dysfunction in sepsis was not seen when a very severe stimulus (high dose of LPS/PepG co-administration) was used to cause cardiac dysfunction.

Editor: Carmen Infante-Duarte, Charite Universitätsmedizin Berlin, Germany

Funding: JC is supported by a jointly funded PhD-studentship of the China Scholarship Council (grant number 201206240146) and Queen Mary University of London (QMUL). SMC is supported by a Research Fellowship of the German Research Foundation (Deutsche Forschungsgemeinschaft; DFG CO 912/1-1). NSAP is, in part, supported by the Bart's and The London Charity (753/1722). This work is supported, in part, by the William Harvey Research Foundation and by a grant from the University of Turin (Ricerca Locale ex-60% 2013). This work forms part of the research themes contributing to the translational research portfolio of Barts and the London Cardiovascular Biomedical Research Unit, which is supported and funded by the National Institute of Health Research. This work also contributes to the Organ Protection research theme of the Barts Centre for Trauma Sciences, supported by the Barts and The London Charity (Award 753/1722). The funders had no role in study design, data collection and analysis, decision to publish, or preparation of the manuscript.

Competing Interests: The authors have declared that no competing interests exist.

* E-mail: c.thiemermann@qmul.ac.uk

Introduction

Sepsis is one of the most common causes of morbidity and mortality among admissions to the intensive care unit [1,2]. Sepsis is a systemic dysregulated hyperinflammatory and/or anti-inflammatory response to infectious stimuli, such as bacteria, viruses and fungi, which, when excessive, may progress to organ failure and death [3]. Development of myocardial dysfunction is associated with increased morbidity and mortality of sepsis. More than 40% cases of sepsis have cardiovascular impairment [4] and the presence of myocardial dysfunction can increase the mortality rate of affected patients to 70% [5].

There is now good evidence that gender is a key determinant in the degree of the host inflammatory response and even of outcome in patients with sepsis. In a number of clinical and epidemiological studies, a significantly increased survival rate was reported in female patients when compared with male patients with sepsis [6–9]. This may be associated with lower pro-inflammatory and higher anti-inflammatory cytokine levels in female patients [9]. Moreover, healthy female volunteers challenged with either lipopolysaccharide (LPS) or lipoteichoic acid (LTA) showed less pro-inflammatory response than males as demonstrated by lower levels of tumor necrosis factor (TNF)-α, interleukin (IL)-1β, IL-6 and IL-8 in blood [10]. In addition, severely injured male trauma-patients had a higher incidence of sepsis, multiple organ dysfunction syndrome and greater elevations in plasma procalcitonin and IL-6 compared with the equivalent group of females [11]. Further basic research studies also confirmed these clinical data on gender dimorphism following sepsis. These experimental studies suggested that females had immunologic advantage and showed a significantly increased survival rate compared with males following induction of polymicrobial sepsis by cecal ligation and puncture (CLP) [12]. In addition, estrogen treatment attenuated the liver dysfunction and intestine injury caused by sepsis in rats with decreased serum aspartate aminotransferase (AST), alanine aminotransferase (ALT) levels and ameliorated oxidative organ damage [13], while testosterone receptor blockade with flutamide following trauma-hemorrhage restored immune depression and significantly decreased the mortality after a subsequent septic challenge in male animals [14].

However, little is known about the impact of gender dimorphism on cardiac dysfunction caused by sepsis. Moreover, the mechanisms underlying the gender difference in susceptibility of the heart to a septic challenge are not understood. The present study was designed to determine whether the severity of myocardial dysfunction caused by either co-administration of LPS/peptidoglycan (PepG) or polymicrobial sepsis induced by CLP differs in male and female mice. Having found that the cardiac dysfunction associated with sepsis was less pronounced in female than in male mice, we have then investigated the potential signalling pathways that may have contributed to the observed differences.

Materials and Methods

Animals

The animal protocols followed in this study were approved by the Animal Welfare Ethics Review Board (AWERB) of Queen Mary University of London in accordance with the derivatives of both the Home Office guidance on the Operation of Animals (Scientific Procedures Act 1986) published by Her Majesty's Stationery Office and the Guide for the Care and Use of Laboratory Animals of the National Research Council. All surgery was performed under ketamine/xylazine anesthesia and echocardiography was performed under inhalation anesthesia of isoflurane, buprenorphine was administered before surgery as well as 6 hours and 18 hours after surgery to reduce postoperative pain, and all efforts were made to minimize suffering of the animals. This study was carried out on ten week-old male (n = 29) and age-matched female (n = 22) C57BL/6 mice, weighing 20–30 g, and eight month-old male (n = 12) and age-matched female (n = 12) C57BL/6 mice (Charles River Laboratories UK Ltd., Kent, UK), weighing 35–50 g. The animals were allowed to acclimatize to laboratory conditions for a period of at least one week before any experimental procedures were initiated. They were housed in individually ventilated cages lined with an absorbent bedding material with no more than 6 mice per cage. The room temperature and humidity was maintained at 19°C–23°C and 55%, respectively. All animals had free access to a standard diet and water *ad libitum.* The feeding boxes were cleaned and disinfected every 3 days, and the water was changed on a daily basis to prevent infectious diseases. Animals were inspected for signs of illness and/or unusual behaviour by research staff at least once per day. All studies involving animals are reported in accordance with the ARRIVE guidelines for reporting experiments involving animals [15,16].

Model of LPS/PepG-induced Cardiac Dysfunction

Ten week-old male and female C57BL/6 mice received intraperitoneal administration of LPS/PepG (LPS; 3 mg/kg and PepG; 0.1 mg/kg or LPS; 9 mg/kg and PepG; 1 mg/kg in PBS; 5 ml/kg i.p.). Sham-treated mice were not subjected to LPS/PepG, but were otherwise treated the same way. Eighteen hours after LPS/PepG administration, cardiac function was assessed by echocardiography *in vivo.* Mice were then deeply anesthetized i.p. with ketamine/xylazine, and were killed by removing the hearts. Heart samples were stored at −80°C for further analyses. Mice were randomly allocated into eight different groups. The following groups were studied for the low dose LPS/PepG co-administration [LPS (3 mg/kg)/PepG (0.1 mg/kg)] study: (i) Male+vehicle (n = 6); (ii) Female+vehicle (n = 4); (iii) Male+LPS/PepG (n = 7); (iv) Female+LPS/PepG (n = 8). The following groups were studied for the high dose LPS/PepG co-administration [LPS (9 mg/kg)/PepG (1 mg/kg)] study: (i) Male+vehicle (n = 5); (ii) Female+vehicle (n = 4); (iii) Male+LPS/PepG (n = 11); (iv) Female+LPS/PepG (n = 6).

Model of Polymicrobial Sepsis caused by Cecal Ligation and Puncture

Eight month-old male and female C57BL/6 mice were subjected to CLP. Sham-operated mice were not subjected to ligation or perforation of cecum but were otherwise treated the same way. We followed the original CLP protocol introduced by Wichterman and co-workers [17] with slight modifications including analgesia, antibiotic therapy and fluid resuscitation as described previously [18,19]. Based on previous evidence and preliminary data, an 18-G needle was used with the double puncture technique in order to generate reproducible cardiac dysfunction during the early phase of sepsis (24 hours). Briefly, mice were anesthetized i.p. with ketamine (100 mg/kg) and xylazine (10 mg/kg) prepared in the same solution by using 1.5 ml/kg. Buprenorphine (0.05 mg/kg i.p.) was injected additionally to provide adequate analgesia. The rectal temperature of the animals was maintained at 37°C with a homeothermic blanket. The abdomen was opened via a 1.5 cm midline incision, and the cecum exposed. The cecum was ligated just below the ileocecal valve and punctured at both opposite ends. After a small amount of fecal matter was extruded from both ends, the cecum was placed back in its anatomical position and the abdomen was sutured. Ringer's solution was given s.c. for resuscitation directly after surgery (1 ml/mouse) and 6 hours and 18 hours after surgery (0.5 ml/mouse). Antibiotic (Imipenem/Cilastin; 20 mg/kg s.c.) and analgesia (buprenorphine; 0.05 mg/kg i.p.) was administered 6 hours and 18 hours after surgery. At 24 hours after CLP, cardiac function was assessed by echocardiography *in vivo.* Mice were then deeply anesthetized i.p. with ketamine/xylazine, and were killed by removing the hearts. Heart samples were stored at −80°C for further analyses. Mice were randomly allocated into four different groups: (i) Male+sham-operation (n = 4); (ii) Female+sham-operation (n = 4); (iii) Male+CLP (n = 8); (iv) Female+CLP (n = 8).

Assessment of Cardiac Function *in vivo*

Cardiac function was assessed in mice by echocardiography *in vivo* as reported previously [18,19]. At 18 hours after LPS/PepG co-administration or 24 hours after CLP, anesthesia was induced with 3% isoflurane and maintained at 0.5 to 0.7% for the duration of the procedure. Before assessment of cardiac function, mice were allowed to stabilize for at least 10 minutes. During echocardiography the heart rate was obtained from ECG tracing and the temperature was monitored with a rectal thermometer. Two-dimensional and M-mode echocardiography images were recorded using a Vevo-770 imaging system (VisualSonics, Toronto, Ontario, Canada). Percentage fractional area change (FAC) was assessed from a two-dimensional trace and percentage EF and fractional shortening (FS) were calculated from the M-mode measurements in the parasternal short axis view at the level of the papillary muscles.

Western Blot Analysis

Semi-quantitative western blot analyses were carried out in mouse heart tissues as described previously [20]. We assessed the degree of phosphorylation of Akt on Ser^{473}, endothelial nitric oxide synthase (eNOS) on Ser^{1177}, inhibitor of κB (IκB) α on $Ser^{32/36}$, as well as the nuclear translocation of the p65 subunit of nuclear factor (NF)-κB (nucleus/cytosol ratio) and inducible nitric oxide synthase (iNOS) expression. Briefly, mouse heart samples were homogenized in 10% homogenization buffer and centrifuged at 4000 RPM for 5 minutes at 4°C. Supernatants were removed and centrifuged at 14 000 RPM at 4°C for 40 minutes to obtain the cytosolic fraction. The pelleted nuclei were re-suspended in extraction buffer and centrifuged at 14 000 RPM for 20 minutes at 4°C. The resulting supernatants containing nuclear proteins were carefully removed, and protein content was determined on both nuclear and cytosolic extracts using a bicinchoninic acid (BCA) protein assay following the manufacturer's directions (Therma Fisher Scientific, Rockford, IL). Proteins were separated by 8% sodium dodecyl sulphatepolyacrylamide gel electrophoresis (SDS-PAGE) and transferred to a polyvinyldenedifluoride (PVDF) membrane, which was then incubated with a primary antibody (rabbit anti-total Akt, dilution 1:1000; mouse anti-pAkt Ser^{473}, dilution 1:1000; rabbit anti-total eNOS, dilution 1:200; goat anti-peNOS Ser^{1177}, dilution 1:200; mouse anti-total IκBα, dilution 1:1000; mouse anti-IκBα $pSer^{32/36}$, dilution 1:1000; rabbit anti-NF-κ*B* p65, dilution 1:1000; rabbit anti-total iNOS, dilution 1:200). Blots were then incubated with a secondary antibody conjugated with horseradish peroxidase (dilution 1:10000) for 30 minutes at room temperature and developed with the ECL detection system. The immunoreactive bands were visualized by autoradiography. Densitometric analysis of the bands was performed using the Gel Pro Analyzer 4.5, 2000 software (Media Cybernetics, Silver Spring, MD, USA). Each group was then adjusted against corresponding sham data to establish relative protein expression when compared with sham animals.

Quantitative Determination of Tissue TNF-α and IL-6 by ELISA

The expressions of TNF-α and IL-6 in mouse heart samples were determined using mouse TNF-α and IL-6 immunoassay kits (R&D Systems, Minneapolis, MN), respectively, and have been normalized to the protein content.

Statistics

All values described in the text and figures are presented as mean ± standard error of the mean (SEM) of n observations, where n represents the number of animals studied. Statistical analysis was performed using GraphPad Prism 6.0 (GraphPad Software, San Diego, California, USA). Two-way ANOVA followed by Sidak's multiple comparisons test was used to compare intergroup differences. Comparing results were considered statistically significant when $P<0.05$.

Materials

Unless otherwise stated, all compounds in this study were purchased from Sigma-Aldrich Company Ltd (Poole, Dorset, UK). All solutions were prepared using non-pyrogenic saline [0.9% (w/v) NaCl; Baxter Healthcare Ltd, Thetford, Norfolk, UK]. Antibodies for immunoblot analysis were purchased from Santa Cruz Biotechnology, Inc. (Heidelberg, Germany).

Results

Gender Dimorphism of Cardiac Dysfunction in Response to LPS (3 mg/kg)/PepG (0.1 mg/kg) Co-administration

To determine the gender difference of cardiac dysfunction caused by LPS/PepG, left ventricular function was assessed using echocardiography at 18 hours after intraperitoneal injection of LPS (3 mg/kg)/PepG (0.1 mg/kg) or PBS (5 mg/kg). Mice injected with LPS/PepG had a lower body temperature and a lower heart rate in comparison to sham-treated mice (male sham/female sham versus male+LPS/PepG/female+LPS/PepG; $P<0.05$; Table 1). In sham-treated mice, there was no difference of EF, FS or FAC between male and female mice ($P>0.05$; Figure 1A–D). When compared to sham-treated mice, LPS/PepG caused a significant reduction in EF ($P<0.05$; Figure 1A–B), FS ($P<0.05$; Figure 1A, 1C) and FAC ($P<0.05$; Figure 1A, 1D) in both male and female mice, indicating the development of cardiac dysfunction *in vivo*. However, female mice subjected to LPS/PepG exhibited significantly higher EF, FS and FAC in comparison with male mice ($P<0.05$; Figure 1A–D), indicating the cardiac dysfunction caused by LPS/PepG was less pronounced in female than in male animals.

Gender Dimorphism of Cardiac Dysfunction in Response to CLP-induced Polymicrobial Sepsis

The murine model of CLP with fluid resuscitation and antibiotic treatment offers a clinically relevant model of abdominal polymicrobial human sepsis. Cardiac dysfunction induced by polymicrobial sepsis caused by CLP was only observed in 8 month-old male mice [19]. We sought to confirm the above observed gender difference of cardiac dysfunction in the CLP animal model in 8 month-old male and female mice. Left ventricular function was assessed using echocardiography at 24 hours after CLP or sham surgery. Mice that underwent CLP had a lower body temperature and a lower heart rate in comparison to sham-operated mice (male sham/female sham versus male+CLP/female+CLP; $P<0.05$; Table 1). In sham-operated mice, there was no difference of EF, FS or FAC between male and female mice ($P>0.05$; Figure 1E–H). When compared to sham-treated mice, polymicrobial sepsis induced by CLP caused a significant reduction in EF ($P<0.05$; Figure 1E–F), FS ($P<0.05$; Figure 1E, 1G) and FAC ($P<0.05$; Figure 1E, 1H) in both male and female mice, indicating the development of cardiac dysfunction *in vivo*. However, female mice that underwent CLP exhibited significantly higher EF, FS and FAC in comparison with male mice ($P<0.05$; Figure 1E–H), indicating the cardiac dysfunction induced by CLP was less pronounced in female than in male animals.

Gender Dimorphism of the Phosphorylation of Akt in the Hearts of Mice Subjected to LPS (3 mg/kg)/PepG (0.1 mg/kg) Co-administration

The potential underlying mechanisms behind the observed gender dimorphism of cardiac dysfunction were investigated by semi-quantitative western blot analysis of the mouse heart subjected to LPS/PepG at 18 hours. When compared to male sham-treated mice, female sham-treated mice showed a higher degree of phosphorylation of Akt on Ser^{473} in heart tissue, but these data were not significant ($P>0.05$; Figure 2A). Exposure of male mice to LPS/PepG for 18 hours caused a small and non-significant increase in the phosphorylation of Akt on Ser^{473} ($P>0.05$; Figure 2A). However, exposure of female mice to LPS/PepG for 18 hours induced a significant increase in the phosphorylation

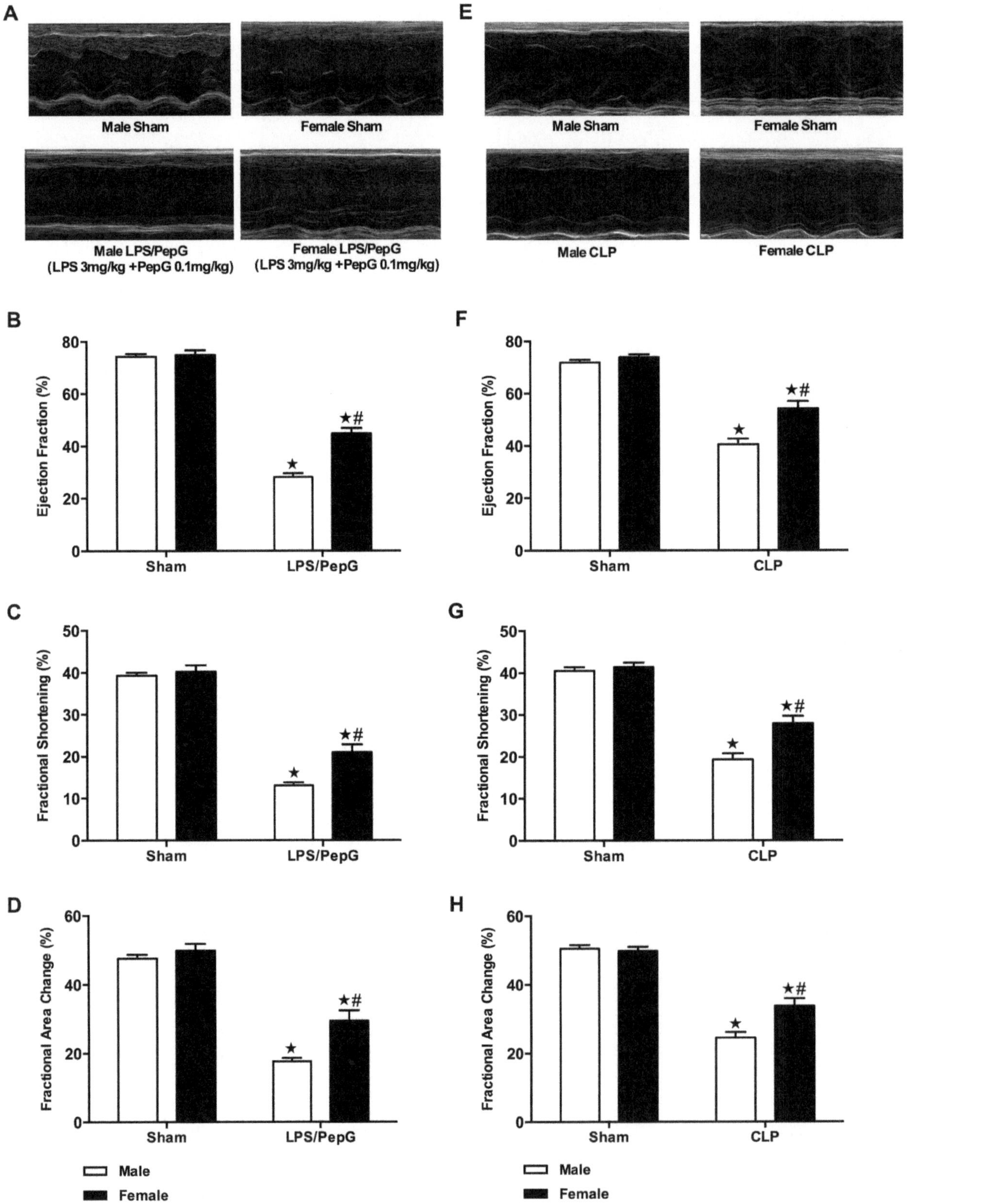

Figure 1. Gender dimorphism of cardiac dysfunction in mice subjected to LPS (3 mg/kg)/PepG (0.1 mg/kg) co-administration and in mice that underwent CLP. Panel **A–D**: Male or female mice received either LPS (3 mg/kg)/PepG (0.1 mg/kg) or PBS intraperitoneally. Cardiac function was assessed at 18 hours. (**A**) Representative M-mode echocardiograms; percentage (%) (**B**) ejection fraction (EF); (**C**) fractional shortening (FS); and (**D**) fractional area of change (FAC). The following groups were studied: Male+vehicle (n = 6); Female+vehicle (n = 4); Male+LPS/PepG (n = 7); Female+LPS/PepG (n = 8). Panel **E–H:** Male or female mice were subjected to CLP or sham-operation. Cardiac function was assessed at 24 hours. (**E**) Representative M-mode echocardiograms; % (**F**) EF; (**G**) FS; and (**H**) FAC. The following groups were studied: Male+sham-operation (n = 4); Female+

sham-operation (n = 4); Male+CLP (n = 8); Female+CLP (n = 8). Panel **A–H**: Data are expressed as means ± SEM for n number of observations. ★$P<0.05$ versus the respective sham group, #$P<0.05$ versus male LPS/PepG or CLP group.

of Akt on Ser^{473} compared with either female sham-treated mice or male LPS/PepG-treated mice ($P<0.05$; Figure 2A).

Gender Dimorphism of the Phosphorylation of eNOS in the Hearts of Mice Subjected to LPS (3 mg/kg)/PepG (0.1 mg/kg) Co-administration

When compared to male sham-treated mice, female sham-treated mice showed a higher degree of phosphorylation of eNOS on Ser^{1177} in heart tissue, but these data were not significant ($P>0.05$; Figure 2B). Exposure of male mice to LPS/PepG for 18 hours caused a small and not significant increase in the phosphorylation of eNOS on Ser^{1177} ($P>0.05$; Figure 2B). However, exposure of female mice to LPS/PepG for 18 hours induced a significant increase in the phosphorylation of eNOS on Ser^{1177} compared with either female sham-treated mice or male LPS/PepG-treated mice ($P<0.05$; Figure 2B).

Gender Dimorphism of the Phosphorylation of IκBα in the Hearts of Mice Subjected to LPS (3 mg/kg)/PepG (0.1 mg/kg) Co-administration

In sham-treated mice, there was no difference in the phosphorylation of IκBα on $Ser^{32/36}$ between male and female hearts ($P>0.05$; Figure 3A). When compared to sham-treated mice, both male and female mice subjected to LPS/PepG demonstrated significant increases in the phosphorylation of IκBα on $Ser^{32/36}$ in heart tissue ($P<0.05$; Figure 3A). However, the increase in IκBα phosphorylation on $Ser^{32/36}$ caused by LPS/PepG was significantly less pronounced in hearts obtained from female than male mice ($P<0.05$; Figure 3A).

Gender Dimorphism of Nuclear Translocation of the p65 NF-κB Subunit in the Hearts of Mice Subjected to LPS (3 mg/kg)/PepG (0.1 mg/kg) Co-administration

In sham-treated mice, there was no difference of nuclear translocation of the p65 NF-κB subunit between male and female hearts ($P>0.05$; Figure 3B). When compared to sham-treated mice, both male and female mice subjected to LPS/PepG demonstrated significant increases in the nuclear translocation of the p65 NF-κB subunit in heart tissue ($P<0.05$; Figure 3B). However, female mice subjected to LPS/PepG exhibited a significantly attenuated response in the nuclear translocation of the p65 NF-κB subunit in comparison with male mice ($P<0.05$; Figure 3B), indicating an important role of gender in LPS/PepG induced activation of NF-κB.

Gender Dimorphism of the Expression of iNOS in the Hearts of Mice Subjected to LPS (3 mg/kg)/PepG (0.1 mg/kg) Co-administration

In sham-treated mice, we detected a faint expression of iNOS protein, but there was no difference of iNOS expression between male and female hearts ($P>0.05$; Figure 3C). When compared to sham-treated mice, LPS/PepG caused significant increases in the expression of iNOS protein in the heart ($P<0.05$; Figure 3C). However, in hearts from female mice subjected to LPS/PepG, the levels of iNOS protein were significantly lower than in hearts from male mice subjected to LPS/PepG ($P<0.05$; Figure 3C).

Table 1. Gender dimorphism of heart rate and temperature of mice responses to septic insults.

Parameter	Male		Female	
	Sham	**LPS (3 mg/kg)/ PepG (0.1 mg/kg)**	**Sham**	**LPS (3 mg/kg)/ PepG (0.1 mg/kg)**
Number	6	7	4	8
Heart Rate (bpm)	543.33±23.23	486.14±15.07*	569.25±16.44	505.75±12.16*
Temperature (°C)	35.38±0.31	30.38±0.87*	35.62±0.46	32.24±0.94*
	Sham	**CLP**	**Sham**	**CLP**
Number	4	8	4	8
Heart Rate (bpm)	537.25±25.76	481.13±11.98*	546.75±10.06	494.25±18.69*
Temperature (°C)	35.02±0.52	31.19±0.67*	35.45±0.32	32.08±0.81*
	Sham	**LPS (9 mg/kg)/ PepG (1 mg/kg)**	**Sham**	**LPS (9 mg/kg)/ PepG (1 mg/kg)**
Number	5	11	4	6
Heart Rate (bpm)	550.50±26.34	456.72±12.08*	570.75±20.14	448.17±28.53*
Temperature (°C)	35.52±0.44	29.16±0.63*	35.90±0.48	29.70±1.03*

Heart rate and temperature were recorded at 18 hours in mice subjected to LPS/PepG co-administration and at 24 hours in mice that underwent CLP. Bpm, beats per minute. Data are expressed as means ± SEM for n number of observations.
*$P<0.05$ versus the respective sham group,
#$P<0.05$ versus male LPS/PepG or CLP group.

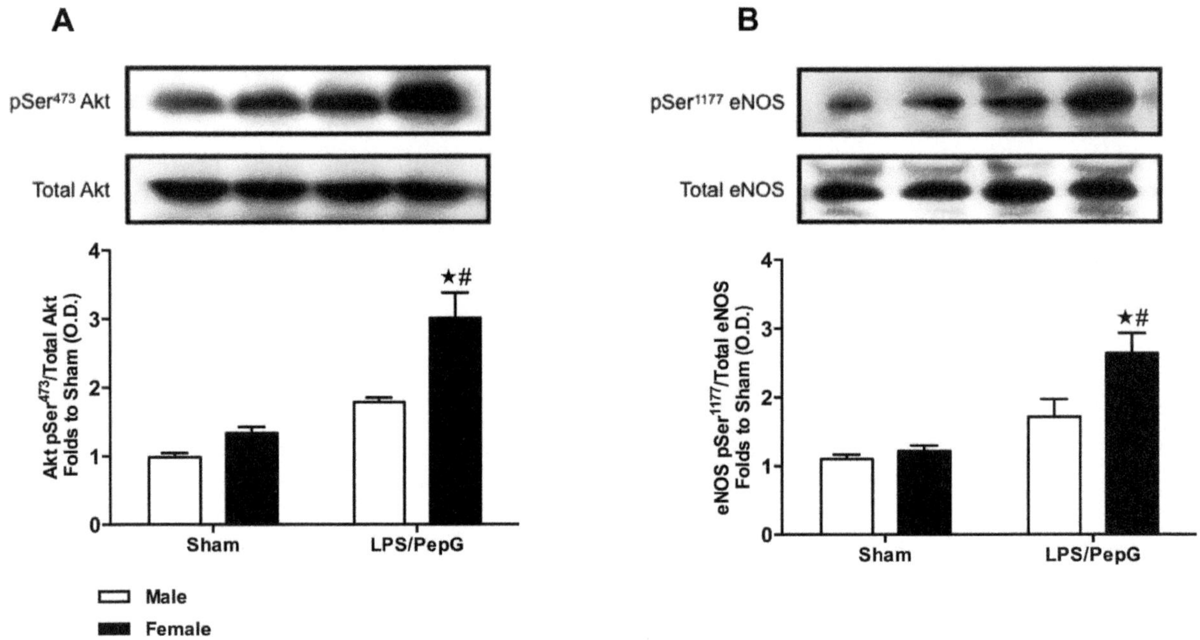

Figure 2. Gender dimorphism of the phosphorylation of Akt and eNOS in the hearts of mice subjected to LPS (3 mg/kg)/PepG (0.1 mg/kg) co-administration. Male or female mice received either LPS (3 mg/kg)/PepG (0.1 mg/kg) or PBS. Signalling events in heart tissue were assessed at 18 hours. Densitometric analysis of the bands is expressed as relative optical density (O.D.) of (**A**) phosphorylated Akt (pSer^{473}) corrected for the corresponding total Akt content and normalized using the related sham band; (**B**) phosphorylated eNOS (pSer^{1177}), corrected for the corresponding total eNOS content and normalized using the related sham band. Each analysis (**A–B**) is from a single experiment and is representative of three to four separate experiments. Data are expressed as means ± SEM for n number of observations. ★$P<0.05$ versus the respective sham group, #$P<0.05$ versus male LPS/PepG group.

Gender Dimorphism of the Expression of TNF-α and IL-6 in the Hearts of Mice Subjected to LPS (3 mg/kg)/PepG (0.1 mg/kg) Co-administration

When compared to male sham-treated mice, female sham-treated mice showed a lower TNF-α and IL-6 expressions in heart tissue, but these data were not significant ($P>0.05$; Figure 3D–E). When compared to sham-treated mice, both male and female mice subjected to LPS/PepG demonstrated significant increases in the expression of TNF-α and IL-6 in heart tissue ($P<0.05$; Figure 3D–E). However, female mice subjected to LPS/PepG exhibited a significantly attenuated response in the expression of TNF-α and IL-6 in comparison with male mice after LPS/PepG challenge ($P<0.05$; Figure 3D–E).

Gender Dimorphism of Cardiac Dysfunction was Blunted in Response to High Dose of LPS (9 mg/kg)/PepG (1 mg/kg) Co-administration

To further investigate whether the gender dimorphism still exists under increased inflammatory stimulus, left ventricular function was assessed using echocardiography at 18 hours after intraperitoneal injection of LPS (9 mg/kg)/PepG (1 mg/kg) or vehicle. Mice injected with LPS/PepG had a lower body temperature and a lower heart rate in comparison to sham-treated mice (male sham/female sham versus male+LPS/PepG/female+LPS/PepG; $P<0.05$; Table 1). In sham-treated mice, there was no difference in EF, FS or FAC between male and female mice ($P>0.05$; Figure 4A–D). When compared to sham-treated mice, LPS/PepG caused a significant reduction in EF ($P<0.05$; Figure 4A–B), FS ($P<0.05$; Figure 4A, 4C) and FAC ($P<0.05$; Figure 4A, 4D) in both male and female mice, indicating the development of cardiac dysfunction *in vivo*. When compared to male LPS/PepG-treated mice, female mice subjected to LPS/PepG showed a significant increase in FAC ($P<0.05$; Figure 4A, 4D), but this was not significant for EF ($P>0.05$; Figure 4A–B) and FS ($P>0.05$; Figure 4A, 4C), indicating that gender dimorphism of the cardiac dysfunction after septic insult was abrogated by the severe injury induced by high dose of LPS (9 mg/kg)/PepG (1 mg/kg) co-administration.

Discussion

We describe here for the first time that the myocardial dysfunction caused by LPS/PepG is less pronounced in female than in male mice *in vivo*. This finding is in agreement with the previous reports showing that the cardiac dysfunction caused by myocardial ischemia/reperfusion injury [21], trauma-hemorrhage [22] and burns [23] is also less pronounced in females than in males. Estrogen modulates a number of acute injury-related myocardial responses; specifically estrogen protects the heart against the injury and dysfunction caused by trauma-hemorrhage [24] and ischemia/reperfusion injury (in isolated hearts subjected to global ischemia and in hearts undergoing LAD occlusion *in vivo*) [25,26]. Although we provide clear evidence that female hearts show less dysfunction than male murine hearts when challenged with LPS/PepG, we wished to confirm this finding by using a more clinically relevant model of polymicrobial sepsis with antibiotic therapy and fluid-resuscitation caused by CLP in middle-aged mice (8 month-old) [18,19]. The age of mice was selected based on the knowledge that 8 month-old female C57BL/6 mice are pre-ovarian failure and still have an active estrus cycle [27]. Most notably, we demonstrate here that the cardiac function in female mice subjected to polymicrobial sepsis induced by CLP was significantly less pronounced than the cardiac dysfunction

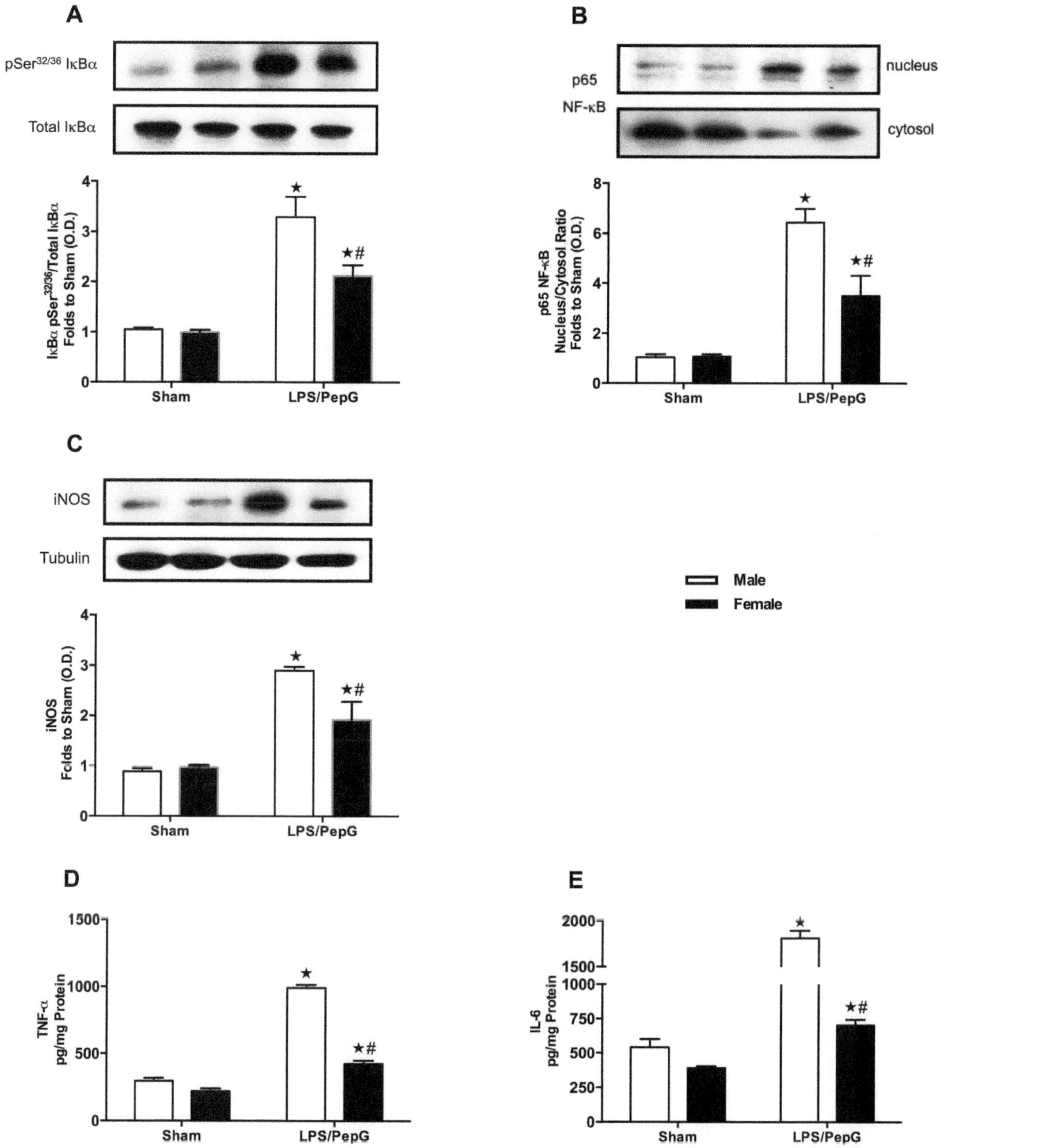

Figure 3. Gender dimorphism of the phosphorylation of IκBα, nuclear translocation of the p65 NF-κB subunit, expression of iNOS, TNF-α and IL-6 in the hearts of mice subjected to LPS (3 mg/kg)/PepG (0.1 mg/kg) co-administration. Male or female mice received either LPS (3 mg/kg)/PepG (0.1 mg/kg) or PBS. Signalling events in heart tissue were assessed at 18 hours. Densitometric analysis of the bands is expressed as relative optical density (O.D.) of (**A**) phosphorylated IκBα (pSer$^{32/36}$) corrected for the corresponding total IκBα content and normalized using the related sham band; (**B**) NF-κB p65 subunit levels in both, cytosolic and nuclear fractions expressed as a nucleus/cytosol ratio normalized using the related sham bands; (**C**) iNOS expression corrected for the corresponding tubulin band, and (**D**) TNF-α expression in heart tissue of mice subjected to LPS/PepG; (**E**) IL-6 expression in heart tissue of mice subjected to LPS/PepG. Each analysis (**A–E**) is from a single experiment and is representative of three to four separate experiments. Data are expressed as means ± SEM for n number of observations. ★$P<0.05$ versus the respective sham group, #$P<0.05$ versus male LPS/PepG group.

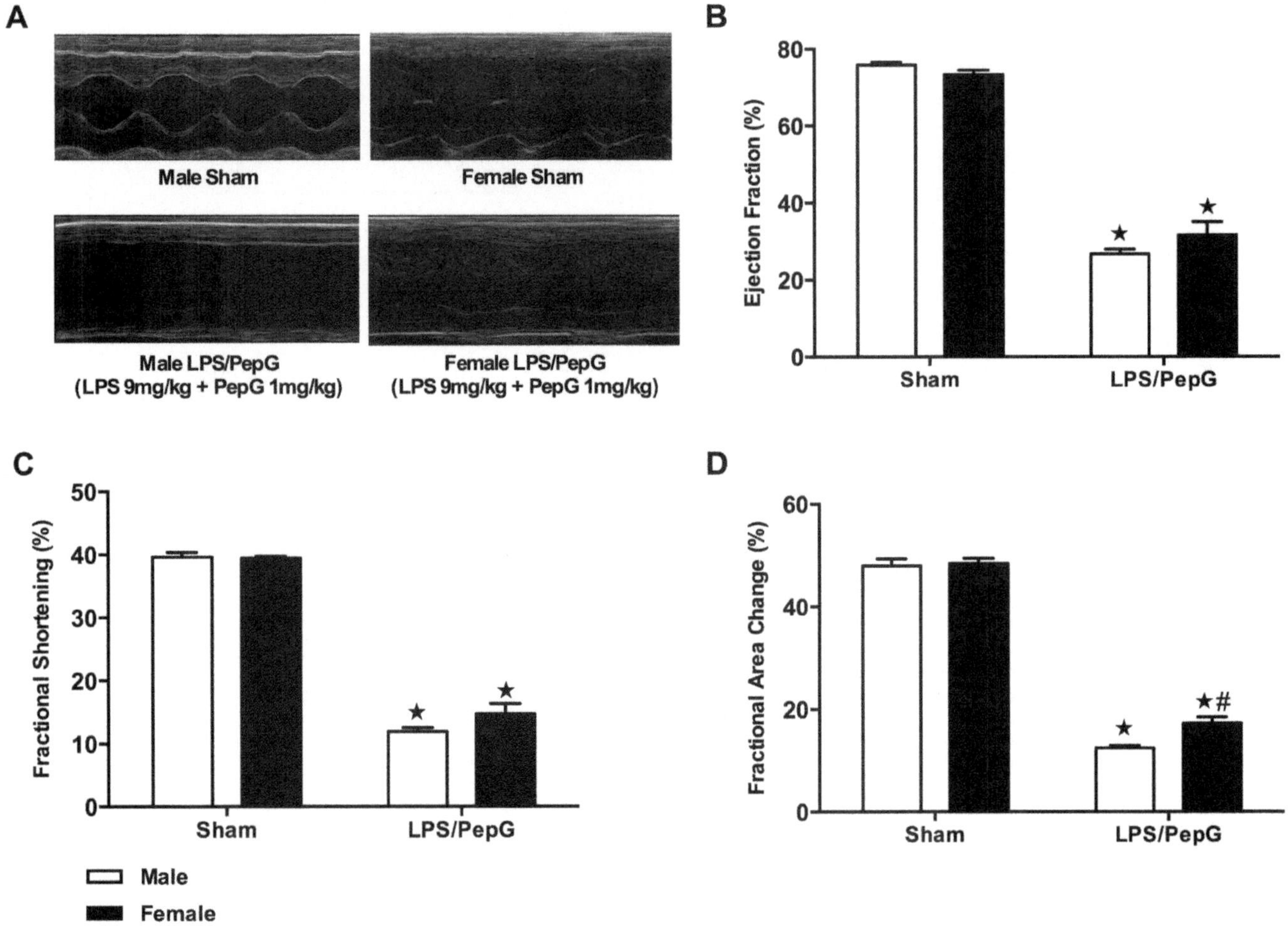

Figure 4. Gender dimorphism of cardiac dysfunction was blunted in response to high dose of LPS (9 mg/kg)/PepG (1 mg/kg) co-administration. Panel **A–D**: Male or female mice received either LPS (9 mg/kg)/PepG (1 mg/kg) or PBS intraperitoneally. Cardiac function was assessed at 18 hours. (**A**) Representative M-mode echocardiograms; percentage (%) (**B**) ejection fraction (EF); (**C**) fractional shortening (FS); and (**D**) fractional area of change (FAC). The following groups were studied: Male+vehicle (n = 5); Female+vehicle (n = 4); Male+LPS/PepG (n = 11); Female+LPS/PepG (n = 6). Data are expressed as means ± SEM for n number of observations. ★$P<0.05$ versus the respective sham group, #$P<0.05$ versus male LPS/PepG group.

observed in male mice. Taken together, these findings indicate that the hearts of young or older female mice exhibit less cardiac dysfunction in response to polymicrobial sepsis or co-administration of LPS/PepG.

To obtain a better insight into the mechanisms underlying the observed gender dimorphism of the cardiac response to sepsis, we investigated the phosphorylation of Akt, eNOS and IκBα, nuclear translocation of NF-κB subunit p65, iNOS expression, as well as TNF-α and IL-6 expression in murine hearts; When compared to the hearts of male mice subjected to LPS/PepG, hearts of female mice subjected to LPS/PepG showed i) profound increases in phosphorylation of Akt and eNOS; ii) reductions in phosphorylation of IκBα and nuclear translocation of the NF-κB subunit p65, iii) reduced expression of the pro-inflammatory cytokines TNF-α and IL-6, and iv) reduced expression of iNOS.

Akt is a member of the phosphoinositide 3-kinases (PI3K) signal transduction enzyme family, activation of which protects the heart against injury [28,29]. Here we demonstrate that co-administration of LPS/PepG to female rather than male mice leads to a greater increase in Akt-phosphorylation and, hence, activity in the heart of female animals. Indeed, a greater increase in cardiac Akt phosphorylation in female when compared to male hearts also accounts for the reduced cardiac injury caused by ischemia-reperfusion in female mice. Most notably, when the Akt-pathway is blocked, the degree of cardiac injury in male and female mice was identical. Thus, activation of cardiac Akt (presumably by estradiol) protects female hearts against cardiac injury and dysfunction [30]. Estradiol activates cardiac Akt, which in turn also leads to a reduction in the cardiac dysfunction caused by trauma-hemorrhage [24,29]. Blockade of the Akt pathway also abrogated the salutary effects of estradiol on cardiac function following trauma-hemorrhage [24]. Moreover, activation of Akt mediates the inhibition by estradiol of the TNF-α expression and NF-κB activation caused by LPS in cardiomyocytes [31]. In the present study, we found a small increase in cardiac Akt activity in female than in male sham hearts. In line with this finding, one previous study showed that young women possess higher levels of Akt in the myocardium compared to comparably aged men or postmenopausal women, and that sexually mature female mice have elevated Akt kinase activity in nuclear extracts of hearts than male mice [32]. The hypothesis that cardiac Akt activity is modulated by estrogen is also supported by the finding that the

Akt activation in cardiomyocytes was reduced in ovariectomized rats [33]. In addition, activation of the PI3K/Akt signalling cascade by estrogen was observed in rat cardiomyocytes [29]. A few studies have been conducted to explain the exact mechanism by which estrogen induces Akt activation. Estrogen receptor α has been shown to bind with the p85 α regulatory subunit of PI3K in a ligand-dependent manner in human endothelial cells; increased estrogen receptor associated PI3K activity induced by estrogen leads to the activation of Akt and eNOS in human endothelial cells [34]. Another study has shown that the direct interaction between estrogen receptor and the PI3K regulatory subunit p85 in a time-dependent manner was consistent with the temporal profile for Akt phosphorylation in neurons [35]. Additionally, in cardiomyocytes, estrogen stimulated Akt activation and prevented DNA fragmentation [29]. Thus, we propose that the higher cardiac activation of Akt in female mice importantly contributes to the improvement in cardiac dysfunction in sepsis.

Activation of Akt is known to modulate eNOS activity through phosphorylation of eNOS at Ser^{1177} [36,37]. Indeed, the present study reported an increase in eNOS phosphorylation in female than in male hearts, which was correlated with the expression pattern of Akt. Augmentation of eNOS activity was shown to decrease sepsis-related increases in neutrophil-endothelial cell interaction and potentially maintain microvascular patency in sepsis [38]. There is good evidence that estrogen modulates activation of eNOS. Estrogen receptor α has been implicated in increased PI3K/Akt and eNOS activation induced by estrogen in human endothelial cells [34]. Another study demonstrated that estrogen stimulation of the eNOS promoter was mediated via increased activity of the transcription factor Sp1 (which is essential for the activity of the human eNOS promoter) [39]. Moreover, estradiol treatment in guinea pigs increased eNOS mRNA in skeletal muscle, suggesting an increase in eNOS activity [40]. In line with these findings, data from the present study indicate that less vulnerability of female hearts to sepsis may be mediated in part by an increased activity of eNOS, secondary to the activation of PI3K/Akt pathway.

NF-κB controls the transcription of a large number of genes, particularly those involved in inflammatory and acute stress responses, such as cytokines, chemokines, cell adhesion molecules, apoptotic factors, and other mediators [41]. IκBα inactivates NF-κB by masking the nuclear localization signals of the NF-κB proteins and by sequestering NF-κB as an inactive complex in the cytoplasm [41,42]. Phosphorylation of IκBα by IκB kinase (IKK) leads to the dissociation of IκBα from NF-κB, which liberates NF-κB to enter the nucleus and activates the expression of NF-κB target genes [41]. Up-regulation of NF-κB has been linked to the development of myocardial dysfunction following the onset of sepsis [19,43]. Inhibition of NF-κB activation results in improved myocardial function after septic challenge [18]. Additionally, the dimer of estrogen and its receptor can bind to NF-κB in osteoblasts following IL-1β exposure, further, NF-κB is proved to be one of the targets for estrogen receptor, resulting in reduced IL-6 promoter activity [44]. In murine splenic macrophages, estradiol inhibited TNF-α and IL-6 production was associated with a decreased LPS-induced NF-κB-binding activity [44]. Thus, our present results indicate that less myocardial dysfunction in females subjected to LPS/PepG could be importantly due to the decreased activation of NF-κB (secondary to the reduced activation of IκBα and, hence, nuclear translocation) in murine hearts. Activation of NF-κB may also mediate myocardial dysfunction through induction of expression of its target gene iNOS, which plays an important role in sepsis-related hypotension and impaired left ventricular function [45,46]. Indeed, in the present study, iNOS expression was increased in male hearts, which correlates with their exacerbated cardiac dysfunction under septic insult.

In addition to causing the expression of iNOS, NF-κB activation also leads to a pronounced increase in production of inflammatory mediators such as TNF-α and IL-6 [47]. In turn, TNF also activates NF-κB through TNF-receptor-associated factors, this increases cytokine production, thus forming a feed-forward mechanism and amplifying the inflammatory reaction [48]. There is good evidence that those inflammatory cytokines play a significant role in the pathogenesis of sepsis-induced cardiac dysfunction [49,50]. Moreover, clinical studies showed that stimulation of healthy females with LPS or LTA led to lower TNF-α and IL-6 levels in blood than males [10]. Female patients with sepsis had a higher survival rate, which was correlated with lower TNF-α and higher IL-10 levels [9], while male trauma-patients showed higher IL-6 level than females [11]. In experimental studies, cardiomyocyte TNF-α and IL-6 release was markedly lower in female than male rats following burn injury [23]. In addition, female hearts expressed less myocardial TNF-α in isolated hearts subjected to ischemia/reperfusion injury [21] or LPS treatment [51]. Others have suggested that elevated plasma TNF-α and IL-6 induced by trauma-hemorrhage was prevented by estradiol treatment in rats [24,52]. Consistent with these findings, in our study, female mice, which had better cardiac function following septic insult, expressed less myocardial TNF-α and IL-6 than male mice subjected to LPS/PepG co-administration.

Our study demonstrated that the gender dimorphism of cardiac dysfunction in response to septic insults was abolished by the severe injury induced by high dose of LPS (9 mg/kg)/PepG (1 mg/kg) co-administration. This is in line with a report that the inflammatory cytokine response differed more strongly between blood from men and women after low-concentration of LPS stimulation compared with a higher stimulus concentration [10]. Population-based studies on sex dimorphism in mortality after sepsis showed inconsistent results. Some studies reported increased mortality in males [7,8], while other studies demonstrated mortality from severe sepsis/sepsis was not affected by gender [53,54]. The inconsistency may have resulted from multiple factors such as pre-existing co-morbidities. More importantly, our observations of gender dimorphism in cardiac dysfunction responses to different severities of injury may partially explain the conflicting clinical data.

It could be argued that the present study did not provide information about proestrus/estrus or diestrus state of estrus cycle in female mice subjected to septic insults. In this regard, a recent study showed that female mice with CLP survived better than male mice that underwent CLP, but the higher survival in females did not correspond to any specific estrus phase [55]. Furthermore, it has been demonstrated vaginal cytology does not reflect changes of circulating estrogens in females and that the estrus cycle cannot be predicted by vaginal smears [56]. Moreover, we did not notice a lot of variations in data obtained from female mice in our study. Therefore, estrus cycle phases were not monitored in this study.

Conclusion

Our findings provide for the first time a very clear indication of a gender dimorphism in the sepsis-induced cardiac dysfunction *in vivo* and we have shown that female mice have less cardiac dysfunction than male mice subjected to either co-administration of LPS/PepG in young mice or CLP in older mice. We report here that female hearts subjected to sepsis have a greater activation of Akt/eNOS, and less activation of NF-κB, which in turn results in reduced expression of the proinflammaroy cytokines TNF-α and IL-6 as well as iNOS. We propose that the above pro-survival and anti-inflammatory signalling events contribute to the reduced cardiac dysfunction in female mice with sepsis.

Author Contributions

Conceived and designed the experiments: CT NSAP JC. Performed the experiments: JC FC MC SMC. Analyzed the data: JC CT NSAP FC MC SMC. Contributed to the writing of the manuscript: JC CT NSAP SMC MC.

References

1. Angus DC, Linde-Zwirble WT, Lidicker J, Clermont G, Carcillo J, et al. (2001) Epidemiology of severe sepsis in the United States: analysis of incidence, outcome, and associated costs of care. Crit Care Med 29:1303–1310.
2. Padkin A, Goldfrad C, Brady AR, Young D, Black N, et al. (2003) Epidemiology of severe sepsis occurring in the first 24 hrs in intensive care units in England, Wales, and Northern Ireland. Crit Care Med 31:2332–2338.
3. Hotchkiss RS, Monneret G, Payen D (2013) Immunosuppression in sepsis: a novel understanding of the disorder and a new therapeutic approach. Lancet Infect Dis 13:260–268.
4. Fernandes CJ Jr, Akamine N, Knobel E (1999) Cardiac troponin: a new serum marker of myocardial injury in sepsis. Intensive Care Med 25:1165–1168.
5. Blanco J, Muriel-Bombin A, Sagredo V, Taboada F, Gandia F, et al. (2008) Incidence, organ dysfunction and mortality in severe sepsis: a Spanish multicentre study. Crit Care 12: R158.
6. Bone RC (1992) Toward an epidemiology and natural history of SIRS (systemic inflammatory response syndrome). JAMA 268:3452–3455.
7. Ghuman AK, Newth CJ, Khemani RG (2013) Impact of gender on sepsis mortality and severity of illness for prepubertal and postpubertal children. J Pediatr 163:835–840 e831.
8. Melamed A, Sorvillo FJ (2009) The burden of sepsis-associated mortality in the United States from 1999 to 2005: an analysis of multiple-cause-of-death data. Crit Care 13: R28.
9. Schroder J, Kahlke V, Staubach KH, Zabel P, Stuber F (1998) Gender differences in human sepsis. Arch Surg 133:1200–1205.
10. Aulock SV, Deininger S, Draing C, Gueinzius K, Dehus O, et al. (2006) Gender difference in cytokine secretion on immune stimulation with LPS and LTA. J Interferon Cytokine Res 26:887–892.
11. Oberholzer A, Keel M, Zellweger R, Steckholzer U, Trentz O, et al. (2000) Incidence of septic complications and multiple organ failure in severely injured patients is sex specific. J Trauma 48:932–937.
12. Zellweger R, Wichmann MW, Ayala A, Stein S, DeMaso CM, et al. (1997) Females in proestrus state maintain splenic immune functions and tolerate sepsis better than males. Crit Care Med 25:106–110.
13. Sener G, Arbak S, Kurtaran P, Gedik N, Yegen BC (2005) Estrogen protects the liver and intestines against sepsis-induced injury in rats. J Surg Res 128:70–78.
14. Angele MK, Wichmann MW, Ayala A, Cioffi WG, Chaudry IH (1997) Testosterone receptor blockade after hemorrhage in males. Restoration of the depressed immune functions and improved survival following subsequent sepsis. Arch Surg 132:1207–1214.
15. Kilkenny C, Browne WJ, Cuthill IC, Emerson M, Altman DG (2010) Improving bioscience research reporting: the ARRIVE guidelines for reporting animal research. PLoS Biol 8: e1000412.
16. McGrath JC, Drummond GB, McLachlan EM, Kilkenny C, Wainwright CL (2010) Guidelines for reporting experiments involving animals: the ARRIVE guidelines. Br J Pharmacol 160:1573–1576.
17. Wichterman KA, Baue AE, Chaudry IH (1980) Sepsis and septic shock a review of laboratory models and a proposal. J Surg Res 29:189–201.
18. Coldewey SM, Rogazzo M, Collino M, Patel NS, Thiemermann C (2013) Inhibition of IkappaB kinase reduces the multiple organ dysfunction caused by sepsis in the mouse. Dis Model Mech 6:1031–1042.
19. Khan AI, Coldewey SM, Patel NS, Rogazzo M, Collino M, et al. (2013) Erythropoietin attenuates cardiac dysfunction in experimental sepsis in mice via activation of the beta-common receptor. Dis Model Mech 6:1021–1030.
20. Collino M, Pini A, Mugelli N, Mastroianni R, Bani D, et al. (2013) Beneficial effect of prolonged heme oxygenase 1 activation in a rat model of chronic heart failure. Dis Model Mech 6:1012–1020.
21. Wang M, Baker L, Tsai BM, Meldrum KK, Meldrum DR (2005) Sex differences in the myocardial inflammatory response to ischemia-reperfusion injury. Am J Physiol Endocrinol Metab 288: E321–326.
22. Szalay L, Shimizu T, Suzuki T, Yu HP, Choudhry MA, et al. (2006) Estradiol improves cardiac and hepatic function after trauma-hemorrhage: role of enhanced heat shock protein expression. American journal of physiology Regulatory, integrative and comparative physiology 290: R812–818.
23. Horton JW, White DJ, Maass DL (2004) Gender-related differences in myocardial inflammatory and contractile responses to major burn trauma. Am J Physiol Heart Circ Physiol 286: H202–213.
24. Hsu JT, Kan WH, Hsieh CH, Choudhry MA, Bland KI, et al. (2009) Mechanism of salutary effects of estrogen on cardiac function following trauma-hemorrhage: Akt-dependent HO-1 up-regulation. Crit Care Med 37:2338–2344.
25. Kim YD, Chen B, Beauregard J, Kouretas P, Thomas G, et al. (1996) 17 beta-Estradiol prevents dysfunction of canine coronary endothelium and myocardium and reperfusion arrhythmias after brief ischemia/reperfusion. Circulation 94:2901–2908.
26. Kolodgie FD, Farb A, Litovsky SH, Narula J, Jeffers LA, et al. (1997) Myocardial protection of contractile function after global ischemia by physiologic estrogen replacement in the ovariectomized rat. J Mol Cell Cardiol 29:2403–2414.
27. Nelson JF, Felicio LS, Randall PK, Sims C, Finch CE (1982) A longitudinal study of estrous cyclicity in aging C57BL/6J mice: I. Cycle frequency, length and vaginal cytology. Biol Reprod 27:327–339.
28. Rajesh KG, Suzuki R, Maeda H, Yamamoto M, Yutong X, et al. (2005) Hydrophilic bile salt ursodeoxycholic acid protects myocardium against reperfusion injury in a PI3K/Akt dependent pathway. J Mol Cell Cardiol 39:766–776.
29. Yu HP, Hsieh YC, Suzuki T, Choudhry MA, Schwacha MG, et al. (2007) The PI3K/Akt pathway mediates the nongenomic cardioprotective effects of estrogen following trauma-hemorrhage. Ann Surg 245:971–977.
30. Bae S, Zhang L (2005) Gender differences in cardioprotection against ischemia/reperfusion injury in adult rat hearts: focus on Akt and protein kinase C signaling. J Pharmacol Exp Ther 315:1125–1135.
31. Liu CJ, Lo JF, Kuo CH, Chu CH, Chen LM, et al. (2009) Akt mediates 17beta-estradiol and/or estrogen receptor-alpha inhibition of LPS-induced tumor necresis factor-alpha expression and myocardial cell apoptosis by suppressing the JNK1/2-NFkappaB pathway. J Cell Mol Med 13:3655–3667.
32. Camper-Kirby D, Welch S, Walker A, Shiraishi I, Setchell KD, et al. (2001) Myocardial Akt activation and gender: increased nuclear activity in females versus males. Circ Res 88:1020–1027.
33. Ren J, Hintz KK, Roughead ZK, Duan J, Colligan PB, et al. (2003) Impact of estrogen replacement on ventricular myocyte contractile function and protein kinase B/Akt activation. Am J Physiol Heart Circ Physiol 284: H1800–1807.
34. Simoncini T, Hafezi-Moghadam A, Brazil DP, Ley K, Chin WW, et al. (2000) Interaction of oestrogen receptor with the regulatory subunit of phosphatidylinositol-3-OH kinase. Nature 407:538–541.
35. Mannella P, Brinton RD (2006) Estrogen receptor protein interaction with phosphatidylinositol 3-kinase leads to activation of phosphorylated Akt and extracellular signal-regulated kinase 1/2 in the same population of cortical neurons: a unified mechanism of estrogen action. J Neurosci 26:9439–9447.
36. Dimmeler S, Fleming I, Fisslthaler B, Hermann C, Busse R, et al. (1999) Activation of nitric oxide synthase in endothelial cells by Akt-dependent phosphorylation. Nature 399:601–605.
37. Fulton D, Gratton JP, McCabe TJ, Fontana J, Fujio Y, et al. (1999) Regulation of endothelium-derived nitric oxide production by the protein kinase Akt. Nature 399:597–601.
38. Khan R, Kirschenbaum LA, LaRow C, Berna G, Griffin K, et al. (2010) Augmentation of platelet and endothelial cell eNOS activity decreases sepsis-related neutrophil-endothelial cell interactions. Shock 33:242–246.
39. Kleinert H, Wallerath T, Euchenhofer C, Ihrig-Biedert I, Li H, et al. (1998) Estrogens increase transcription of the human endothelial NO synthase gene: analysis of the transcription factors involved. Hypertension 31:582–588.
40. Weiner CP, Lizasoain I, Baylis SA, Knowles RG, Charles IG, et al. (1994) Induction of calcium-dependent nitric oxide synthases by sex hormones. Proc Natl Acad Sci U S A 91:5212–5216.
41. Senftleben U, Karin M (2002) The IKK/NF-kappa B pathway. Crit Care Med 30: S18–26.
42. Jacobs MD, Harrison SC (1998) Structure of an IkappaBalpha/NF-kappaB complex. Cell 95:749–758.
43. Kapoor A, Shintani Y, Collino M, Osuchowski MF, Busch D, et al. (2010) Protective role of peroxisome proliferator-activated receptor-beta/delta in septic shock. Am J Respir Crit Care Med 182:1506–1515.
44. Stein B, Yang MX (1995) Repression of the interleukin-6 promoter by estrogen receptor is mediated by NF-kappa B and C/EBP beta. Mol Cell Biol 15:4971–4979.
45. Barth E, Radermacher P, Thiemermann C, Weber S, Georgieff M, et al. (2006) Role of inducible nitric oxide synthase in the reduced responsiveness of the myocardium to catecholamines in a hyperdynamic, murine model of septic shock. Crit Care Med 34:307–313.
46. Thiemermann C, Vane J (1990) Inhibition of nitric oxide synthesis reduces the hypotension induced by bacterial lipopolysaccharides in the rat in vivo. Eur J Pharmacol 182:591–595.
47. Brown MA, Jones WK (2004) NF-kappaB action in sepsis: the innate immune system and the heart. Front Biosci 9:1201–1217.
48. Miyamoto S, Verma IM (1995) Rel/NF-kappa B/I kappa B story. Adv Cancer Res 66:255–292.
49. Natanson C, Eichenholz PW, Danner RL, Eichacker PQ, Hoffman WD, et al. (1989) Endotoxin and tumor necrosis factor challenges in dogs simulate the cardiovascular profile of human septic shock. J Exp Med 169:823–832.

50. Parrillo JE, Burch C, Shelhamer JH, Parker MM, Natanson C, et al. (1985) A circulating myocardial depressant substance in humans with septic shock. Septic shock patients with a reduced ejection fraction have a circulating factor that depresses in vitro myocardial cell performance. J Clin Invest 76:1539–1553.
51. Zhu H, Shan L, Peng T (2009) Rac1 mediates sex difference in cardiac tumor necrosis factor-alpha expression via NADPH oxidase-ERK1/2/p38 MAPK pathway in endotoxemia. J Mol Cell Cardiol 47:264–274.
52. Hsieh YC, Frink M, Hsieh CH, Choudhry MA, Schwacha MG, et al. (2007) Downregulation of migration inhibitory factor is critical for estrogen-mediated attenuation of lung tissue damage following trauma-hemorrhage. Am J Physiol Lung Cell Mol Physiol 292: L1227–1232.
53. Mahmood K, Eldeirawi K, Wahidi MM (2012) Association of gender with outcomes in critically ill patients. Crit Care 16: R92.
54. Wichmann MW, Inthorn D, Andress HJ, Schildberg FW (2000) Incidence and mortality of severe sepsis in surgical intensive care patients: the influence of patient gender on disease process and outcome. Intensive Care Med 26:167–172.
55. Drechsler S, Weixelbaumer K, Raeven P, Jafarmadar M, Khadem A, et al. (2012) Relationship between age/gender-induced survival changes and the magnitude of inflammatory activation and organ dysfunction in post-traumatic sepsis. PLoS One 7: e51457.
56. Weixelbaumer KM, Drechsler S, Wehrenpfennig P, Khadem A, Bahrami S, et al. (2014) Estrus cycle status defined by vaginal cytology does not correspond to fluctuations of circulating estrogens in female mice. Shock 41:145–153.

25

Clinical Significance of Markers of Collagen Metabolism in Rheumatic Mitral Valve Disease

Tanima Banerjee[1], Somaditya Mukherjee[1], Sudip Ghosh[1], Monodeep Biswas[2], Santanu Dutta[3], Sanjib Pattari[4], Shelly Chatterjee[1], Arun Bandyopadhyay[1]*

1 Department of Cell Biology and Physiology, CSIR-Indian Institute of Chemical Biology, Kolkata, WB, India, **2** Department of Cardiology, Geisinger Community Medical Center and Wright Center for Graduate Medical Education, Scranton, Pennsylvania, United States of America, **3** Department of Cardio-thoracic and Vascular Surgery, Institute of Post Graduate Medical Education and Research, SSKM Hospital, Kolkata, WB, India, **4** Department of Pathology, Rabindra Nath Tagore International Institute of Cardiac Sciences, Kolkata, WB, India

Abstract

Background: Rheumatic Heart Disease (RHD), a chronic acquired heart disorder results from Acute Rheumatic Fever. It is a major public health concern in developing countries. In RHD, mostly the valves get affected. The present study investigated whether extracellular matrix remodelling in rheumatic valve leads to altered levels of collagen metabolism markers and if such markers can be clinically used to diagnose or monitor disease progression.

Methodology: This is a case control study comprising 118 subjects. It included 77 cases and 41 healthy controls. Cases were classified into two groups- Mitral Stenosis (MS) and Mitral Regurgitation (MR). Carboxy-terminal propeptide of type I procollagen (PICP), amino-terminal propeptide of type III procollagen (PIIINP), total Matrix Metalloproteinase-1(MMP-1) and Tissue Inhibitor of Metalloproteinase-1 (TIMP-1) were assessed. Histopathology studies were performed on excised mitral valve leaflets. A p value <0.05 was considered statistically significant.

Results: Plasma PICP and PIIINP concentrations increased significantly ($p<0.01$) in MS and MR subjects compared to controls but decreased gradually over a one year period post mitral valve replacement ($p<0.05$). In MS, PICP level and MMP-1/TIMP-1 ratio strongly correlated with mitral valve area ($r=-0.40$; $r=0.49$ respectively) and pulmonary artery systolic pressure ($r=0.49$; $r=-0.49$ respectively); while in MR they correlated with left ventricular internal diastolic ($r=0.68$; $r=-0.48$ respectively) and systolic diameters ($r=0.65$; $r=-0.55$ respectively). Receiver operating characteristic curve analysis established PICP as a better marker ($AUC=0.95$; 95% $CI=0.91-0.99$; $p<0.0001$). A cut-off >459 ng/mL for PICP provided 91% sensitivity, 90% specificity and a likelihood ratio of 9 in diagnosing RHD. Histopathology analysis revealed inflammation, scarring, neovascularisation and extensive leaflet fibrosis in diseased mitral valve.

Conclusions: Levels of collagen metabolism markers correlated with echocardiographic parameters for RHD diagnosis.

Editor: Utpal Sen, University of Louisville, United States of America

Funding: This work is supported by grants from Council of Scientific and Industrial Research (CSIR), New Delhi, India (NWP 0004, MLP 115) to AB. TB and SM are recipients of fellowships from CSIR, New Delhi. The funders had no role in study design, data collection and analysis, decision to publish, or preparation of the manuscript.

Competing Interests: The authors have declared that no competing interests exist.

* E-mail: arunb@iicb.res.in

Introduction

Rheumatic Heart Disease (RHD) is a chronic acquired disorder of heart. It is a major public health concern in Low and Middle Income Countries (LMICs) having a global prevalence of at least 15.6 million cases, with 282,000 new cases and demanding 233,000 deaths each year [1]. It results as a sequelae of Acute Rheumatic Fever (ARF), caused by autoimmune reactions following untreated *Streptococcus pyogenes* throat infection in genetically susceptible individuals [2]. Acute rheumatic fever is a common health problem in developing countries [3]. It is estimated that around 12 million people, mainly children, suffer from the disease worldwide [4]. It is predicted that RHD would continue to cause high mortality and morbidity in LMICs and hence requires improved diagnostic and treatment strategies for disease management [5]. Based on WHO Global Burden of Disease, RHD has been categorized as a Neglected Tropical Disease (NTD) [6]. In India, Rheumatic heart disease is responsible for 30–40% cardiovascular disease related hospital admissions [7].

Although ARF causes pancarditis, it primarily affects endocardium and repeated episodes of autoimmune reactions cause chronic inflammation and scarring in valvular apparatus. Mitral valve is most commonly affected followed by aortic valve. The tricuspid and pulmonary valves are usually less severely affected. RHD in mitral valve manifests most commonly as mitral stenosis followed by mitral regurgitation or combination of both producing hemodynamic burden on heart causing clinical features like dyspnoea, palpitation and heart failure [8]. Management involves medical and surgical interventions for symptom alleviation and periodic clinical monitoring usually with transthoracic echocardiogram. In fact for prevention of heart failure and improvement of symptoms surgery is the treatment of choice. However till date, no biochemical indicators are available for prediction, diagnosis and management of the disease.

Fibrillar collagens (types I and III) arethe major components of the myocardial extracellular matrix. These are synthesized and secreted by fibroblasts as procollagen precursors. During the maturation process, the amino (N) terminal and carboxy (C) terminal propeptides are cleaved to yield triple helical monomers. The carboxy-terminal propeptide of type I procollagen (PICP) is released into the bloodstream during the synthesis of type I collagen. Therefore, PICP is considered to be a marker of type I collagen synthesis. Similarly amino terminal propeptide of type III collagen (PIIINP) is released into circulation during type III collagen synthesis. Fibrillar collagens are substrates for matrix metalloproteinases (MMPs), an endogenous family of zinc dependent enzymes which are responsible for extracellular matrix remodelling with tissue destruction under various pathophysiological conditions. Among them, MMP-1 has the highest affinity for fibrillar collagens. It is mainly secreted by fibroblasts and is able to initiate type I collagenolysis. Active form of MMP-1 can be regulated by its interaction with tissue inhibitor of matrix metalloproteinase-1 (TIMP-1), also expressed in the fibroblasts [9]. Marginal increase in serum PICP has been reported in various heart diseases like hypertensive heart disease [10,11] cardiomyopathy and heart failure [12,13]. But clinical significance of collagen metabolism markers, produced by structural remodelling of ECM in rheumatic valve has not yet been explored.

Methods

Study Population

The study population consisted of 118 subjects aged between 15 and 65 years. Rheumatic heart disease subjects who visited Cardio thoracic and vascular surgery (CTVS) department of the Institute of Post Graduate Medical Education and Research- Seth Sukhlal Karnani Memorial Hospital (IPGME&R-SSKM), Kolkata, India from January 2010 to July 2012 were recruited into the study as cases.

Blood was collected from 72 RHD subjects in their chronic stage before surgical intervention (Pre-op) and out of them, 8 subjects were included again after valve replacement surgery (Post-op). In addition, for random validation, 5 post-op subjects were also included whose post-operative echocardiographic analysis could not be performed (Figure S1; Tables S1, S2 in File S1). Subjects with diabetes, hypertension, renal failure, metabolic bone disease, liver failure, severe systemic illness, rheumatoid arthritis or any organic heart disease except rheumatic heart disease were excluded from the studyafter careful clinical examination and relevant investigations. Patients with features of overt heart failure (LVEF<50%) were also not included.

Forty one healthy individuals with no evidence or family history of cardiac illness or past history of rheumatic fever or any medication use were selected as controls and underwent the same clinical examination and investigation protocols. All control subjects included in the study were normotensive, had normal cardiac function and lipid profile and also had normal fasting blood glucose levels. Most of the subjects who were recruited earlier have again been included in this study for comparing the different markers of collagen metabolism in mitral stenosis and regurgitation respectively which was not shown previously [14].

Echocardiography

Two-dimensional transthoracic echocardiography with targeted M-mode and Doppler were performed using commercially available systems by trained cardiologists.Echocardiographic diagnosis of RHD conformed to the recommendation of the 2012 World Heart Federation criteria [15]. All measurements were made by blinded observers and mean of the three readings were recorded. Left atrial dimension and left ventricular dimension both at systole and diastole were recorded. Mitral valve area (MVA) was measured by planimetry and pressure half time (PHT) methods. The mean of these two readings were taken in subjects with mitral valve disease. Pulmonary artery systolic pressure (PASP) was also measured in these subjects. Ejection fraction was calculated by Simpson's method.None of the subjects had left ventricular systolic dysfunction as defined by an ejection fraction ≤50%. Doppler measurements of pressure gradients across valves was analyzed to assess the haemodynamic severity of lesions [15]. To assess LV hypertrophy, LV mass was calculated following the recommendations of the American Society of Echocardiography and European Association of Echocardiography using the Devereux formula: 0.89 (1.04 [LV internal diameter + posterior wall thickness + interventricular septal thickness]^3 - [LV internal diameter]^3) + 0.6 g. Relativewall thickness was estimated using the formula 2×posterior wall thickness/LV internal diameter in diastole [16]. RHD subjects were classified as Predominantly Mitral Stenosis (MS) with or without mild or moderate stenotic or regurgitant lesions (e.g; Aortic Stenosis, Aortic Regurgitation etc.) and Predominantly Mitral Regurgitation (MR) with mild or moderate other lesions [17].

Clinical Examination

Clinical examination was performed by trained physicians and the data recorded in a structured pro forma. The patients' symptoms were recorded as per the New York Heart Association (NYHA) functional class. Systolic blood pressure (SBP) and diastolic blood pressure (DBP) were measured using standard cuff equipment at the clinic. Pulse rate including any irregularity was noted. Most recent electrocardiograms (ECGs) were reviewed. Cardio-thoracic ratio was measured from the chest skiagram performed in the subjects.

Biochemical Determinations

Peripheral venous blood samples were drawn from healthy and chronic RHD subjects during clinical assessment and immediately subjected to plasma isolation. Each sample was centrifuged for 10 minutes at 4°C. The plasma was then separated into aliquots and stored at −80°C before analysis. Plasma concentrations of PICP (Takara Bio Inc. Shiga, Japan), PIIINP (Uscn Life Science Inc. Wuhan, P.R. China), total MMP-1 (AnaSpec, San Jose, CA, USA) and total TIMP-1 (R&D Systems, Minneapolis, MN, USA) were determined by enzyme immunoassay (EIA) using commercial assay systemsas per the manufacturer's instructions. Duplicate measurements were taken and the results averaged.The intra-assay and inter-assay variations for determining PICP concentrations were 6% and 5% respectively. The inter-assay and intra-assay coefficients of variation were <12% and <10% for MMP-1 and 4.9% and 3.9% for TIMP-1,respectively.Due to technical limitations, total MMP-1 and TIMP-1 were assessed in 17 controls and 42 subjects, PIIINP was measured in 34 controls and 63subjects and PICP was measured in 41 controls and 66 subjects.

Histopathology

Anterior leaflets of mitral valvetissue samples, from subjects undergoing valve replacement and from post-mortem control subjects without any known history of cardiovascular disease were collected and fixed in 10% formalin. Samples were then embedded in paraffin and 5 μm thick sections were prepared according to standard procedure. Tissue sections were either stained with hematoxylin - eosin (HE stain, Sigma Chemical Co., St Louis, MO, USA) as described earlier [18] or with Masson Trichrome to examine fibrosis. Sections were examined under an Olympus BX51 (Olympus Corporation, Tokyo, Japan) microscope and images were captured with a digital camera attached to it. Picrosirius red -0.1% Sirius red F3B solution in picric acid (Direct Red 80; Sigma Chemical Co., St. Louis, MO, USA) staining was also performed in valve leaflets to examine the collagen content and alignment and infer type of collagen. Stained sections therefore were observed using a binocular polarized light microscope (Nikon Eclipse binocular polarising microscope, LV 100 POL, Japan) with the same exposure time for each section. Under polarized light, birefringence is specific for collagen where red colour shows fibrillar type I collagen and yellow green colour indicates reticular type III collagen [19].

Immunohistochemistry

Immunohistochemical staining of formalin fixed paraffin embedded tissue sections were performed following the protocol described in [20,21]. First sections were deparaffinized in xylene twice for 2 min each, followed by serial hydration steps in alcohol: 100% for 3 min, 95% for 1 min, 70% for 1 min. Sections were then sequentially rinsed in running tap water and phosphate buffer saline (PBS) for 2 min each, followed by antigen retrieval in citrate buffer. Tissue areas were marked and the sections were washed with PBS in 0.2% Triton X-100, thrice for 5 min, followed by blocking in 5% BSA at room temperature for 2 hours. Staining was performed by incubating the sections with anti-collagen type I primary antibody (C-2456), (Sigma Chemical Co., St. Louis, MO, USA) overnight at 4°C followed by washing three times with PBS. Secondary antibody conjugated with Alexa Fluor, (Molecular Probes, Life Technologies, Grand Island, NY, USA) was incubated at room temperature for 1 hour followed by washing thrice with PBS. Finally coverslips were mounted with Prolong Gold anti-fade reagent (Molecular Probes, Life Technologies, Grand Island, NY, USA) and visualized under a laser scanning confocal system (Leica Microsystem, GmbH, Wetzlar, Germany).

Statistical Analysis

Data are expressed as mean ± standard error of mean (SEM) for continuous variables, while frequencies define categorical variables. Using Microcal Origin 8.0 software (Origin Lab, Northampton,USA) normal distribution of all continuous variables was tested using the 1-sample Kolmogorov-Smirnov test. Categorical variables were analysed by Chi square (χ^2) or Fisher's exact test. Differences between the two groups of RHD subjects were tested by Student's *t*- test for unpaired and paired data. One way Analysis of Variance (ANOVA) followed by Post-hoc tests was used to compare biomarker levels among controls and the two groups of subjects. Non-parametric tests were used when required.The correlation between quantitative normal variables

Table 1. Baseline Characteristics.

Variables	Control (n = 41)	Case (n = 72)	p value
Age (years)	32.34±1.34	34.26±1.50	0.64
Male/Female	26/25	27/45	0.15
Clinical Presentation data			
Pulse (bpm)	75.32±1.87	81.25±1.56	0.03
SBP (mm Hg)	117.22±1.90	112.86±2.01	0.15
DBP (mmHg)	79.88±1.40	72.86±1.45	0.002
NYHA class			
I	41(100%)	28(38.89%)	<0.0001
II	0	29(40.28%)	NA
III	0	11(15.28%)	NA
IV	0	4(5.56%)	NA
Echocardiographic parameters (Normal range)			
LA (20–40 mm)	30.41±0.53	54.25±1.48(n = 65)	<0.0001
LVIDd (35–56 mm)	42.80±0.76	51.77±1.19	<0.0001
LVIDs (24–42 mm)	27.39±0.54	34.70±0.82	<0.0001
LVPW (6–11 mm)	8.61±0.13	8.81±0.19(n = 70)	0.59
IVSD (6–11 mm)	8.71±0.14	9.07±0.21(n = 70)	0.29
EF (%)	66.95±0.59	58.60±0.82	<0.0001
Fractional shortening (%)	35.79±0.94	32.64±0.83	0.006
Relative Wall Thickness	0.41±0.01	0.36±0.01(n = 70)	0.0002
Left Ventricle Mass (Kg)	0.12±0.004	0.18±0.008(n = 70)	<0.0001

BPM beats per minute; DBP diastolic blood pressure; EF ejection fraction; IVSD inter-ventricular septal diameter; LA left atrium; LVIDd left ventricular internal diameter diastolic; LVIDs left ventricular internal diameter systolic; LVPW left ventricular posterior wall; n number of subjects; NA not applicable; NYHA New York Heart Association; SBP systolic blood pressure. Values indicate mean ± standard error of mean. p<0.05 considered significantly different between two groups.

was analysed by linear regression using Microsoft Excel 2010. Receiver operating characteristics (ROC) curves, prepared using GraphPad Prism software 5.30 (GraphPad, San Diego,California,USA) assessed the overall performance of plasma biomarkers. A two-tailed p value ≤0.05 was considered statistically significant.

Ethics Statement

The study protocol which conformed to the principles of the Declaration of Helsinki for biomedical research, was approved by the Institutional Review Boards of the Indian Institute of Chemical Biology, Kolkata and IPGME&R-SSKM, Kolkata, India. Written informed consent was obtained from all subjects before participation in the study.

Table 2. Baseline Patient Characteristics.

Variables	Predominantly MS (n = 42)	Predominantly MR (n = 30)	p value
Age(years)	37.55±1.81	29.67±2.35	0.009
Male/Female	20/22	7/23	0.04
Clinical Presentation data			
H/o Rheumatic Fever	29(69%)	20(66.67%)	1.00
Pulse (bpm)	79.38±2.09	83.87±2.30	0.16
SBP(mm Hg)	112.29±2.70	113.67±3.05	0.74
DBP(mmHg)	73.95±2.05	71.33±1.96	0.38
CT ratio(n-58)	0.56±0.02(n = 25)	0.63±0.04(n = 12)	0.14
Atrial fibrillation	15(35.71%)	7(23.33%)	0.31
Premature atrial complex	1	0	NA
NYHA class			
I	19(45.24%)	9(30%)	0.23
II	16(38.09%)	13(43.33%)	0.81
III	6(14.29%)	5(16.67%)	1.00
IV	1(2.38%)	3(10%)	0.30
Medicine use			
Diuretics	29(69.05%)	24(80%)	0.42
Spironolactone	9(21.43%)	9(30%)	0.42
ACE inhibitors	1(2.38%)	13(43.33%)	<0.0001
ARBs	0	0	NA
β blockers	8(19.05%)	3(10%)	0.34
Digoxin	27(64.29%)	20(66.67%)	1.00
Warfarin	21(50%)	10(33.33%)	0.23
Variables	**Predominantly MS (n = 42)**	**Predominantly MR (n = 30)**	**p value**
Echocardiographic parameters (Normal range)			
LA (20–40 mm)	51.56±1.36(n = 37)	57.81±2.81(n = 28)	0.04
LVIDd (35–56 mm)	45.89±1.04	59.79±1.58	<0.0001
LVIDs (24–42 mm)	31.83±0.82	38.92±1.27	<0.0001
LVPW (6–11 mm)	8.73±0.28(n = 40)	8.91±0.25	0.63
IVSD (6–11 mm)	9.08±0.31(n = 40)	9.07±0.26	0.97
EF (%)	56.98±1.08	60.88±1.18	0.02
PASP (mm Hg)	57.85±3.83(n = 24)	55±5.15(n = 12)	0.66
MVA (sq.mm)	84±3(n = 40)	226±23(n = 11)	<0.0001
Fractional shortening(%)	31.13±0.94	34.76±1.44	0.03
Relative Wall Thickness	0.39±0.02(n = 40)	0.31±0.01	0.002
Left Ventricle Mass(Kg)	0.14±0.007(n = 40)	0.23±0.014	<0.0001

ACE angiotensin converting enzymes; ARB angiotensin receptor blocker; bpm beats per minute; CT cardio-thoracic; DBP diastolic blood pressure; EF ejection fraction; H/o history of; IVSD inter-ventricular septal diameter; LA left atrium; LVIDd left ventricular internal diameter diastolic; LVIDs left ventricular internal diameter systolic; LVPW left ventricular posterior wall; MVA mitral valve area; n number of subjects; NA not applicable; NYHA New York Heart Association; PASP pulmonary artery systolic pressure; SBP systolic blood pressure. Values indicate mean ± standard error of mean.
$p<0.05$ considered significantly different between two groups.

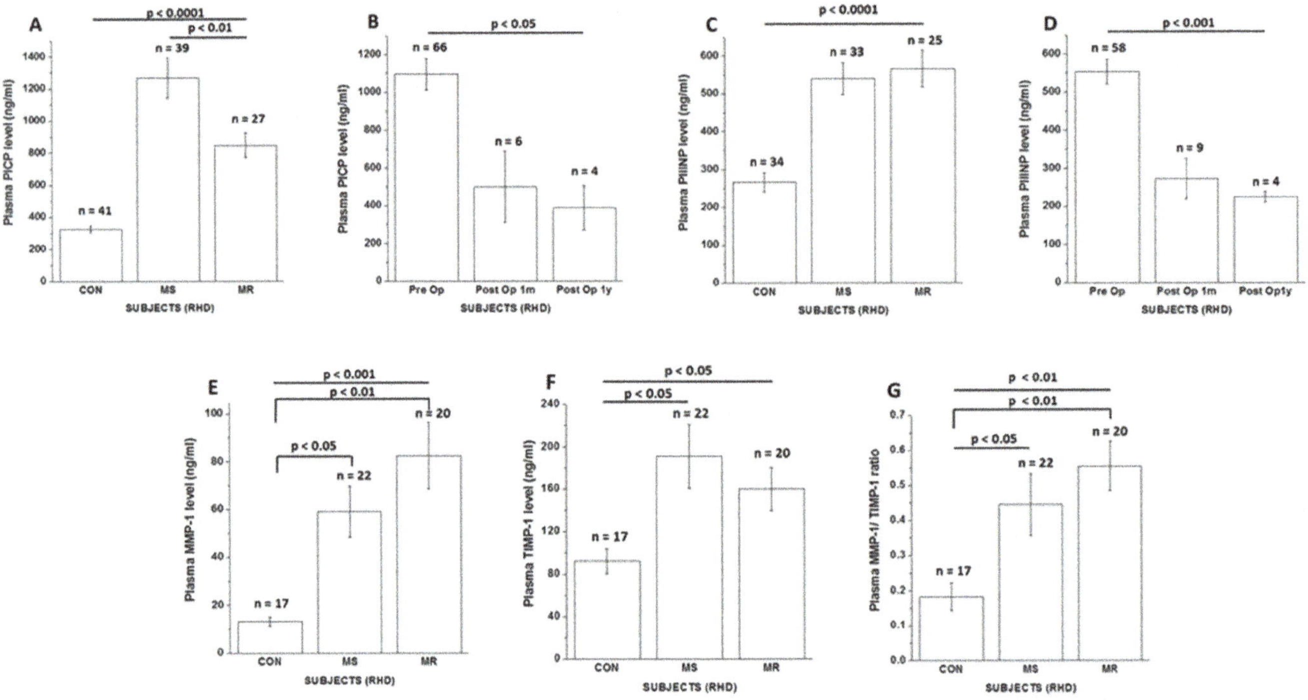

Figure 1. Plasma concentrations of circulating biomarkers of collagen turnover in normal, MS and MR subjects. (A) Mean plasma PICP in control, MS and MR subjects before (Pre Op) valve replacement surgery. (B) Progressive reduction in plasma PICP concentration one month and one year or above following mitral valve replacement. (C) Mean plasma PIIINP in control, MS and MR subjects before (Pre Op) valve replacement surgery. (D) Progressive decrease in plasma PIIINP concentration one month and one year or more after mitral valve replacement. (E) Mean plasma concentration of total MMP-1 in control, MS and MR subjects. (F) Mean TIMP-1 concentration in control, MS and MR subjects. (G) Plasma MMP-1/TIMP-1 ratio in control, MS and MR subjects.

Results

Baseline Characteristics Analysis

Baseline characteristics of subjects recruited into the study are presented in Tables 1 and 2 respectively. Table 1 shows that almost an equal percentage of males and females comprised the control group. Heart rate, Diastolic Blood Pressure (DBP) and all the echocardiographic parameters except Left Ventricular Posterior Wall (LVPW) and Interventricularseptal Diameter (IVSD) were significantly different ($p<0.05$) between the control and patient groups. As shown in Table 2, about 63% of RHD subjects (45 of 72 subjects) were female. Around 52% of MS subjects were females while in the MR group about 77% of the subjects were females.The clinical and demographic variables were comparable between the RHD subgroups except for age. About 69% patients had a previous history of Acute Rheumatic Fever.39% RHD subjects were in NYHA class I,40% belonged to NYHA class II,15% belonged to class III and the remaining 6% in class IV. All control subjects belonged to NYHA class I (Table 1). None of the controls under study had any history of medication intake during the course of study. On the other hand, 74%, 25% and 65% of the RHD subjects were taking diuretics (furosemide, torsemide), spironolactone and digoxin respectively. 15% were on beta blockers, 19% had history of intake of ACE inhibitors and 43% of subjects were on anticoagulant therapy (Table 2). All RHD subjects included in the study were under rigorous penicillin prophylaxis to prevent recurrent episodes of acute rheumatic fever.

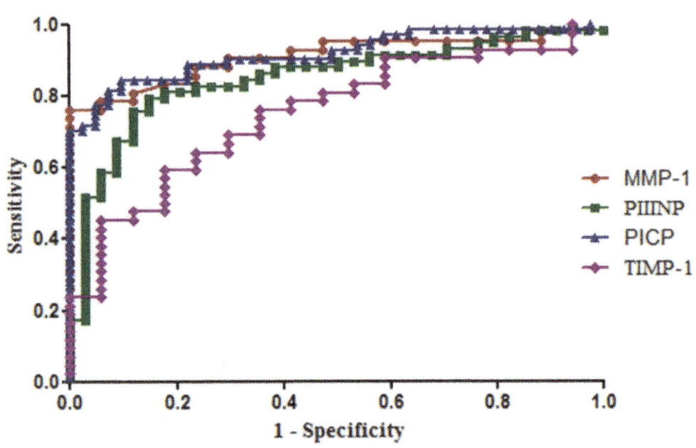

Figure 2. Receiver operating characteristics curve for biomarkers in rheumatic heart disease subjects.

Among the echocardiographic parameters, Left atrial (LA) diameter, Mitral Valve Area (MVA), Left ventricular ejection fraction (EF), Left ventricular internal diameter in diastole (LVIDd), left ventricular internal diameter in systole (LVIDs), Left Ventricle (LV) Mass and Fractional Shortening (FS) were significantly higher in MR subjects ($p<0.05$) compared to MS subjects. Relative Wall Thickness (RWT) also differed between the two groups of RHD subjects (Table 2).

Circulating markers of collagen metabolism are elevated in Rheumatic Mitral Valve Disease

Plasma PICP levels were significantly different among the three groups of subjects as assessed by one-way ANOVA ($p<0.0001$; Figure 1A). Post-hoc tests reveal that PICP levels were significantly

Table 3. Overall Performance of Different Parameters According to ROC Curves for Prediction of RHD.

Biomarkers	Cut Off	Sensitivity (%)	Specificity (%)	AUC	p value	LR	95% CI	PPV	NPV
PICP (ng/ml)	>459	90.9	90.2	0.95	<0.0001	9.32	0.91 to 0.99	0.94	0.86
PIIINP (ng/ml)	>351	81	82.3	0.85	<0.0001	4.59	0.77 to 0.93	0.89	0.72
MMP-1 (ng/ml)	>21.8	83.3	82.3	0.91	<0.0001	4.72	0.84 to 0.98	0.95	0.68
TIMP-1 (ng/ml)	>105	69	70.6	0.75	0.003	2.35	0.62 to 0.88	0.89	0.72

p <0.05 considered significantly different.
AUC, area under curve; CI, confidence interval; LR, likelihood ratio; MMP-1, matrix metalloproteinase -1; NPV, negative predictive value; PICP, carboxy terminal propeptide of type I collagen; PIIINP, amino terminal propeptide of type III collagen; PPV, positive predictive value; TIMP-1, tissue inhibitor of matrix metalloproteinase-1.

($p<0.01$) higher in MS (1265±125 ng/ml, n = 39) and MR (848±74 ng/ml, n = 27) subjects than controls (324±18 ng/ml, n = 41).Level of PICP also differed significantly between MS and MR subjects ($p<0.01$). Significant decrease in circulating PICP levels was observed one month (2.2 fold) and one year (3 fold) post mitral valve replacement surgery (p = 0.02; Figure 1B).

Figure 1C showed the distribution of plasma PIIINP levels in MS and MR patients along with control subjects. Patients with RHD showed higher PIIINP levels ($p<0.0001$). Plasma PIIINP concentration was significantly different ($p<0.01$) between MS (539±42 ng/ml, n = 33) and controls and between MR (565±48 ng/ml, n = 25) subjects and controls (266±24 ng/ml, n = 34) but not between MS and MR subjects. The extent of reduction in circulating PIIINP levels post mitral valve replacement surgery was also significant over a one month (2.1 fold) and a one year (2.6 fold) period ($p<0.001$; Figure 1D). Again, when paired comparisons were performed, PIIINP level (547±99 ng/ml) decreased significantly one month post -surgery (212±14 ng/ml, Δ pre -post = 257%, n = 6, $p<0.01$; Figure S2).

Total plasma MMP-1 values showed a significantly different distribution across the groups (p = 0.0002). Compared to controls, total MMP- 1 level (13±1.9 ng/ml, n = 17) increased significantly in subjects with MS (59±10 ng/ml, n = 22, $p<0.05$) and MR (82±14 ng/ml, n = 20, $p<0.01$; Figure 1E). Total TIMP-1 levels varied significantly among the three groups (p = 0.02; Figure 1F). Compared to controls (92±12 ng/ml, n = 17), levels were significantly higher in MS (191±30 ng/ml, n = 22; $p<0.05$) but not in MR patients (160±21 ng/ml, n = 20). Also MMP-1/TIMP-1 ratio, an index of MMP-1 activity was significantly different among the three groups (p = 0.003; Figure 1G). The ratio increased in both MS and MR groups by about 2.5 fold and 3.1 fold respectively, compared to controls. There was no significant difference in the levels of collagen metabolism markers between male and female subjects in both MS and MR categories (Table S3 in File S1). It was also observed that TIMP-1 and PICP levels were significantly higher in MS and MR subjects respectively with atrial fibrillation ($p<0.05$; Table S4 in File S1).

Assessment of diagnostic accuracy of indices of collagen metabolism

As shown in Figure 2, ROC curve analysis demonstrates plasma PICP, total MMP-1 and PIIINP as significant predictors of rheumatic heart disease (Table 3).PICP performed better than MMP-1, PIIINP or TIMP-1 with AUC of 0.95 (Table 3). Overall, the cut off value of PICP showed the best sensitivity and specificity for predicting valve fibrosis (Table 3). Thus the likelihood of presenting severe mitral valve disease of rheumatic originwas 9.32 times higher for subjects with PICP values >459 ng/ml, 4.59 times higher for subjects with PIIINP values >351 ng/ml, 4.72 times higher for subjects with MMP-1 values >21.8 ng/ml and 2.35 times higher for subjects with TIMP-1 values >105 ng/ml (Table 3). The sensitivity of PICP was 92% in Mitral Stenosis (AUC = 0.97) and 89% in Mitral Regurgitation (AUC = 0.91). The sensitivity of PIIINP was 82% in Mitral Stenosis(AUC = 0.84) and 80% in Mitral Regurgitation (AUC = 0.86). However the sensitivity of MMP-1 was found to be 90% in MR (AUC = 0.97) while it was about 77% in Mitral Stenosis (AUC = 0.85). The sensitivities of TIMP-1 were comparable between Mitral Stenosis and Mitral Regurgitation patients (AUC = 0.75 in both) (Tables 4 and 5 respectively.)

Relationship of Collagen Metabolism Markers with severity determinants in Predominantly Mitral Stenosis

In MS patients, plasma PICP showed a strong inverse correlation with MVA while MMP-1/TIMP-1 ratio showed a strong positive association with it (Figure 3A, 3B). Plasma PICP levels also correlated positively with PASP while MMP-1/TIMP-1

Table 4. Overall Performance of Different Parameters According to ROC Curves for Prediction of Mitral Stenosis.

Biomarkers	Cut Off	Sensitivity (%)	Specificity (%)	AUC	p value	LR	95% CI	PPV	NPV
PICP (ng/ml)	>489.3	92.3	92.7	0.97	<0.0001	12.6	0.95 to 1.00	0.92	0.93
PIIINP (ng/ml)	>351.4	81.8	82.4	0.84	<0.0001	4.64	0.73 to 0.94	0.82	0.82
MMP-1 (ng/ml)	>19.94	77.3	76.5	0.85	0.0002	3.28	0.73 to 0.98	0.81	0.72
TIMP-1 (ng/ml)	>108	68.2	70.6	0.75	0.007	2.32	0.60 to 0.91	0.75	0.63

p<0.05 considered significantly different.
AUC, area under curve; CI, confidence interval; LR, likelihood ratio; MMP-1, matrix metalloproteinase -1; NPV, negative predictive value; PICP, carboxy terminal propeptide of type I collagen; PIIINP, amino terminal propeptide of type III collagen; PPV, positive predictive value; TIMP-1, tissue inhibitor of matrix metalloproteinase-1.

Table 5. Overall Performance of Different Parameters According to ROC Curves for Prediction of Mitral Regurgitation.

Biomarkers	Cut Off	Sensitivity (%)	Specificity (%)	AUC	p value	LR	95% CI	PPV	NPV
PICP (ng/ml)	>457	88.9	87.8	0.91	<0.0001	7.29	0.82 to 0.99	0.83	0.91
PIIINP (ng/ml)	>341.7	80	79.4	0.86	<0.0001	3.89	0.76 to 0.96	0.74	0.84
MMP-1 (ng/ml)	>23.49	90	88.24	0.97	<0.0001	7.65	0.93 to 1.02	0.9	0.88
TIMP-1 (ng/ml)	>105.1	70	70.6	0.75	0.009	2.38	0.59 to 0.91	0.82	0.67

$p < 0.05$ considered significantly different.
AUC, area under curve; CI, confidence interval; LR, likelihood ratio; MMP-1, matrix metalloproteinase -1; NPV, negative predictive value; PICP, carboxy terminal propeptide of type I collagen; PIIINP, amino terminal propeptide of type III collagen; PPV, positive predictive value; TIMP-1, tissue inhibitor of matrix metalloproteinase-1.

ratio correlated inversely (Figures 3C, 3D). Plasma PICP showed inverse associations with LVPW and IVSD respectively while MMP-1/TIMP-1 ratio inversely correlated with EF and FS and positively with LVIDs (Table S5 in File S1) in this group. Total MMP-1 levels correlated positively with LVIDs and inversely with EF and FS. PIIINP levels were found to positively associate with EF (Table S5 in File S1) and weakly correlated with MVA or PASP (Figures 3A, 3C).

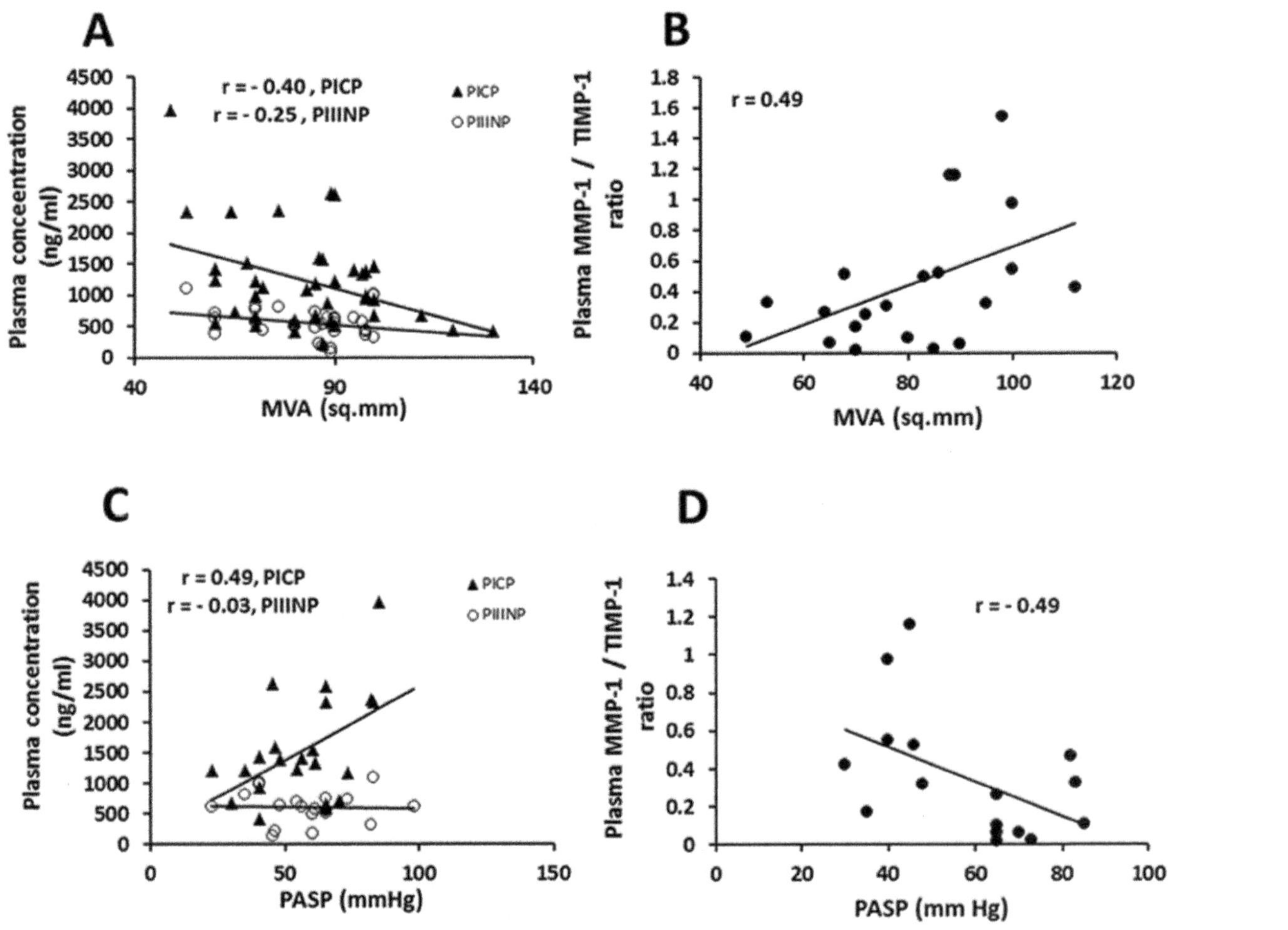

Figure 3. Relationship between plasma markers of collagen metabolism and severity of rheumatic mitral stenosis. (A) Inverse correlations of plasma PICP ($y = -17.241x+2654.1$; $p = 0.01$) and PIIINP ($y = -4.6576x+938.36$; $p = 0.15$) concentration with mitral valve area(MVA). (B) Direct correlation ($y = 0.0127x-0.582$; $p = 0.03$) between plasma MMP-1/TIMP-1 ratio and MVA. (C) Direct correlation of plasma PICP ($y = 24.155x+186.83$; $p = 0.02$) and almost no correlation of plasma PIIINP ($y = -0.4083+634.78$; $p = 0.91$) with pulmonary artery systolic pressure (PASP). (D) Inverse correlation ($y = -0.0091x+0.8791$; $p = 0.05$) between plasma MMP-1/TIMP-1 ratio and PASP.

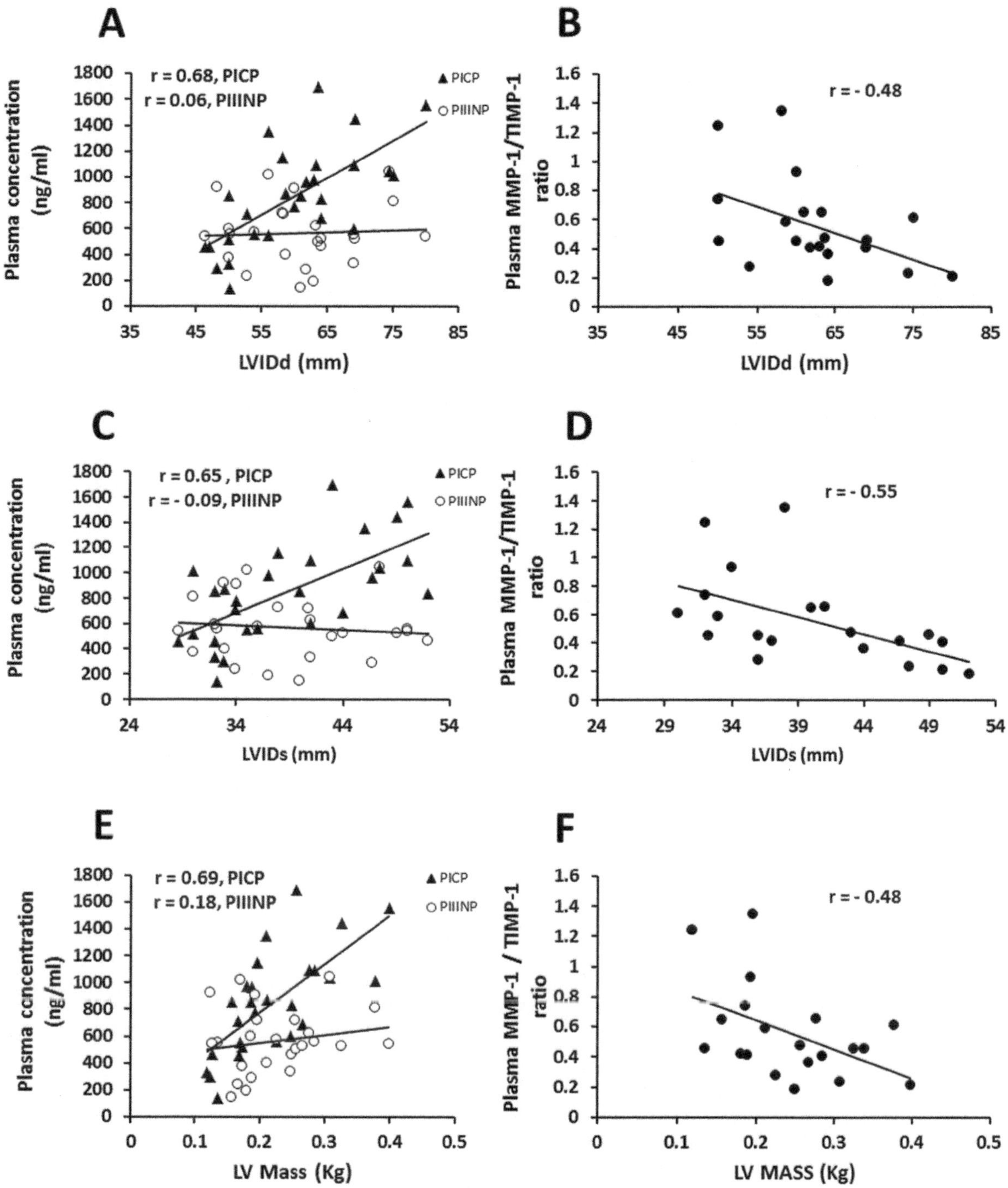

Figure 4. Relationship between plasma PICP levels and hemodynamic parameters in rheumatic mitral regurgitation. (A) Direct correlation of plasma PICP ($y = 28.83x - 875.54$; $p = 0.0001$) and no correlation of plasma PIIINP ($y = 1.5469x + 471.72$; $p = 0.79$) with left ventricular diameter at diastole (LVIDd). (B) Inverse correlation ($y = -0.0181x + 1.6878$; $p = 0.04$) between plasma MMP-1/TIMP-1 ratio and ventricular diameter at diastole (LVIDd). (C) Direct correlation of plasma PICP ($y = 34.933x - 506.05$; $p = 0.0002$) and no correlation of plasma PIIINP ($y = -3.3609x + 697.11$; $p = 0.64$) with left ventricular internal diameter at systole (LVIDs). (D) Inverse correlation($y = -0.0241x + 1.523$; $p = 0.01$) between plasma MMP-1/TIMP-1 ratioand LVIDs. (E) Direct correlation of plasma PICP ($y = 3620.7x + 53.656$; $p < 0.0001$) and weak correlation of plasma PIIINP ($y = 593.3x + 430.94$; $p = 0.39$) with left ventricular mass (LVM). (F) Inverse correlation ($y = -1.9248x + 1.0243$; $p = 0.03$) between plasma MMP-1/TIMP-1 ratio and LVM.

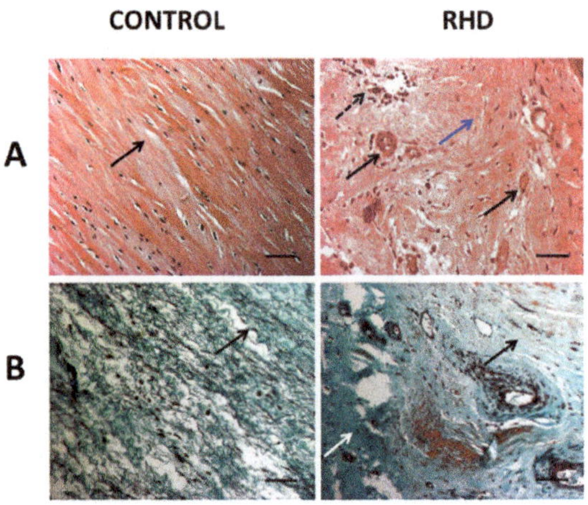

Figure 5. Histopathology of heart valve. (A) Representative images (100× magnification) of hematoxylin-eosin stained sections of 1 normal heart valve (control) and 3 rheumatic valve samples (RHD). Rheumatic mitral valve tissue section shows abundance of inflammatory cells (arrow head), fibrosis (blue arrow) and neovascularisation (black arrow). Normal mitral valve section shows wavy arrangement of collagen fibres (black arrow). Scale bar represents 50 μm. (B) Representative images (100×) of Masson's trichrome stained cross sections showing dense collagen deposition (arrow) in mitral valve tissue of RHD patient compared to loose parallel pattern of collagen (arrow) in normal heart valve. Scale bar represents 50 μM.

Relationship of Collagen Metabolism Markers with severity determinants in Predominantly Mitral Regurgitation

In MR patients circulating PICP strongly associated with LVIDd, LVIDs and LV mass while MMP-1/TIMP-1 ratio showed strong inverse relationship with the above parameters (Figures 4A to 4F). Plasma PICP correlated positively with LA diameter and negatively with relative wall thickness while circulating PIIINP levels showed a strong positive association with PASP in this group (Table S6 in File S1) and weak correlation with LVIDs. Plasma TIMP-1 levels however, did not correlate significantly with any of the echocardiographic parameters in MS and MR.

Histopathology Analysis

Gross examination of HE stained mitral valve sections from the RHD subjects showed thickening of valve leaflets with irregular margins. Microscopic examination showed enhanced degree of fibrosis and neovascularisation (arrows marked in Figure 5A). Focal perivascular mild infiltration of lymphocytes and plasma cells were prominent, thus confirming inflammatory aetiology in those subjects. In contrast, normal valve was composed of loose collagen tissue with absence of blood vessels and inflammatory cells (Figure 5A).

Masson trichrome staining shows collagen deposition in valve leaflets of RHD subjects and controls. Normal mitral valve shows loose parallel arrangement of collagen fibres whereas diseased valve shows dense and extensive collagen fibres, predominantly arranged in random pattern (Figure 5B). A representative picture illustrating the relative abundance of collagens type I (red colour) and type III (green colour) in the mitral valve leaflets of the subjects under polarized light is shown in Figure 6A. The abnormal accumulation of fibrous tissue was seen as a scattered deposition of collagen type I (red deposition) in diseased valve leaflets leading to a marked disarray of the ECM architecture. The extent of total collagen ($p<0.05$), collagen type I deposition as well as collagen type I/type III ratio was higher ($p<0.0001$) in the rheumatic mitral valve than normal valve (Figures 6B–6E). This is further supported by immunofluorescence analysis of mitral valve leaflets using anti-collagen I antibody which clearly showed increased and scattered collagen I deposition in RHD subjects (Figure 6F).

Discussion

In present perspective, 2D Doppler echocardiography has proved to be an essential diagnostic tool not only in clinically determined RHD but also in subclinical RHD [22,23]. In this form of RHD, features of valve damage like annular dilatation, prolapsed leaflet, trivial-mild regurgitation could be detected on echocardiography without clinical symptoms or signs of RHD. However, role of echocardiography to confirm diagnosis of subclinical RHD still remains controversial, especially in a developing country like India. There is also a considerable degree of overlap between normal and pathological findings on echocardiography in detecting subclinical RHD. In India where burden of rheumatic fever cases is large and highly skilled echo-Doppler facilities are available only in limited number of centres, accurate diagnosis of RHD would be difficult [15,24,25]. However, the acute management of such patients and the duration of secondary prophylaxis would not change significantly, even if a diagnosis of subclinical carditis were made. In the present study we have mainly focused on early cases of established RHD where timely determination of severity and prognostication may alter therapeutic strategies, and prevent further progression to advanced stages with low cardiac performance.

Mitral valve leaflets are composed of 74% type I, 24% of type III and 2% of type V collagen. Fibrous tissues intermixed with elastic fibres form the extracellular matrix (ECM) of valvular apparatus covered by a layer of endothelial cells [26]. Fibrosis is the hallmark of structural remodelling, resulting from chronic inflammatory rheumatic process in valvular apparatus. Fibrosis results from extensive deposition of collagen induced by mechanical overload combined with the action of other pro fibrotic factors or tissue damage.

A significantly raised plasma concentration of PICP observed in both MS (377%) and MR (245%) could be explained by anincreased production and deposition of collagen over heart valves by myofibroblasts [27,28]. During inflammatory process like chronic RHD, cytokines are released which lead to differentiation of valvular interstitial cells (VICs) to activated myofibroblasts [27]. VICs are the most abundant cells in valve leaflets which produce various kinds of extracellular matrix (ECM) proteins including collagen. They also produce ECM degrading enzymes like MMPs. The above finding is also supported by collagen birefringence under polarized light whichindicates a 186% increase in Type I collagen in diseased valve tissue than control. Earlier report have shown increased deposition of collagen on excised RHD valves [29]. Elevated plasma level of PIIINP in MS (200%) and MR (212%) in the present study gets supported by previous studies which have shown that activated myofibroblasts result in fibrosis through increased production of both type I and type III collagen [30]. Active role of VICs in producing MMPs like collagenases (MMP-1, MMP-13) and gelatinases (MMP-2, MMP-9) have also been reported [31]. High level of total MMP-1 in MS (446%) and MR (624%) in our study indicated that in addition to increased level of markers of synthesis, collagen degrading enzymes are also raised in RHD.

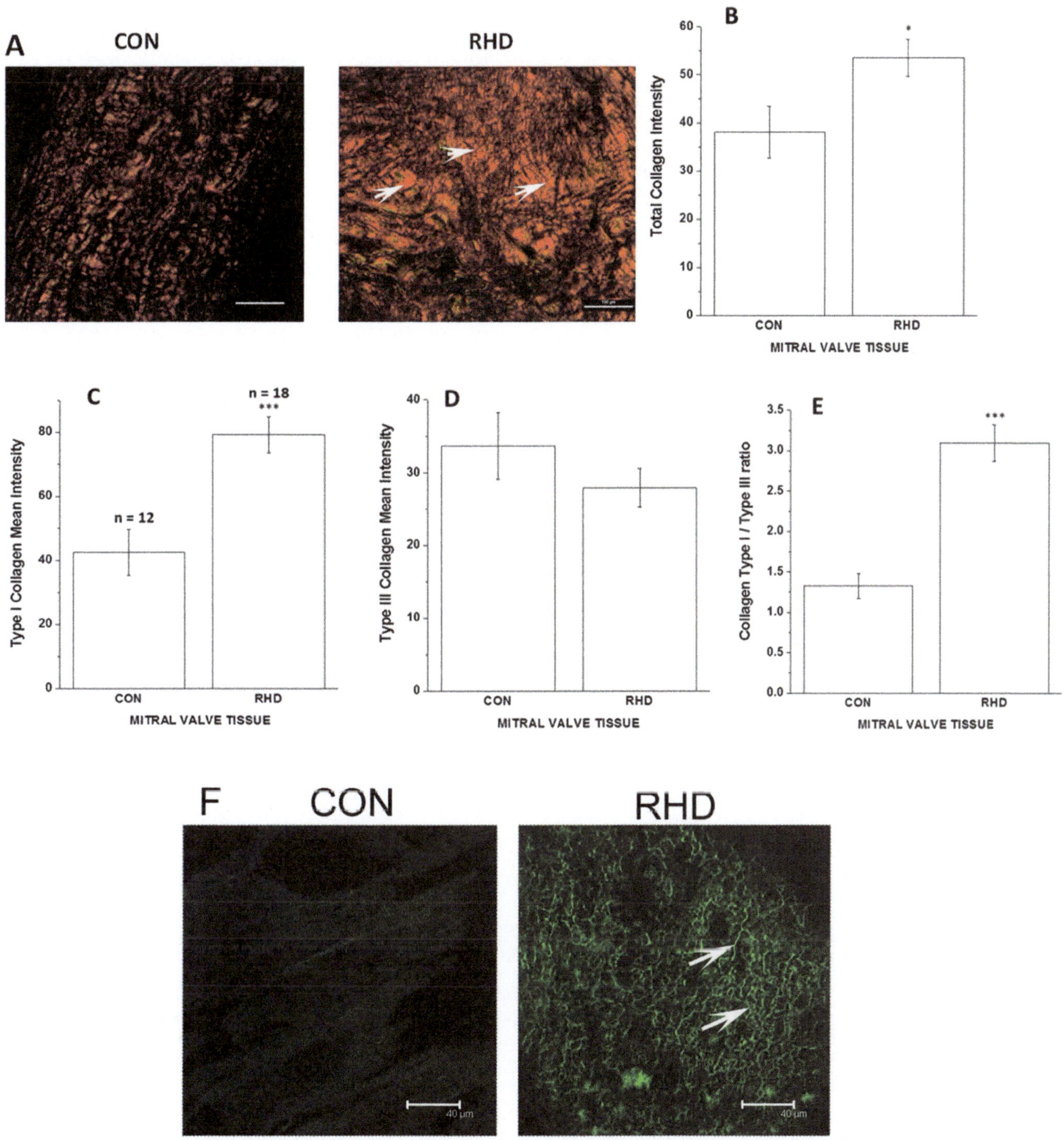

Figure 6. Assessment of collagen deposition by picrosirius red staining and immunostaining methods. (A) Representative images (20× magnification) of picrosirius red stained sections of 1 normal heart valve (control) and 3 rheumatic mitral valve samples (RHD). Stained sections were observed using a binocular polarized light microscope. Under polarized light, birefringence is specific for collagen where red colour shows fibrillar type I collagen and yellow green colour indicates reticular type III collagen. Arrow indicates scattered deposition of collagen type I in diseased valve Scale bar represents 100 µm. (B) Total collagen intensity in control vs. RHD mitral valve tissue sections. (C) Type I collagen mean intensity in control vs. RHD mitral valve cross sections. (D) Type III collagen mean intensity in control vs. RHD mitral valve cross sections. (E) Ratio of Type I to Type III collagen in control vs. RHD mitral valve sections.(F) Representative images of immuno stained sections of 1 normal heart valve (control) and 3 rheumatic mitral valve samples (RHD) showing (arrow marked) collagen type 1 deposition. Scale bar represents 45 µm. *$p<0.05$ vs. control,***$p<0.0001$ vs. control. Here "n" denotes total number of tissue sections.

Rheumatic mitral stenosis occurs due to thickening of the mitral valve leaflets and fusion of commissures and chordae tendineae. Earlier it was reported that PICP may determine clinical severity in mitral stenosis since it inversely correlated with MVA and positively correlated with PASP in mitral stenosis with mild or no mitral regurgitation [14]. But the association of other markers of ECM remodelling like PIIINP and MMP-1/TIMP-1 ratio with the above parameters were not dealt with previously. Besides, the relationship between biochemical markers of collagen metabolism and haemodynamic parameters in mitral regurgitation remained to be established in greater detail. Therefore in this study, previous data of PICP of some of the individuals have been included to compare its performance with PIIINP and collagenolytic markers. However unlike PICP, PIIINP showed weak correlation with MVA and PASP in MS. Since PIIINP is not cleaved completely during the conversion of procollagen type III into collagen type III and part of it is released during fiber degradation, PIIINP can be considered to be a marker of both collagen synthesis and degradation. Hence, it is weakly associated with echocardiographic parameters in both MS and MR. In MS, correlation of MMP-1/TIMP-1 ratio with MVA and PASP followed an opposite trend to that shown by PICP, indicating that collagen synthesis on mitral valve is more favoured compared to degradation with disease progression in MS. Besides valvular apparatus, atrial fibrosis may also have some contribution to altered levels of collagen metabolism markers in MS subjects. Such atrial fibrosis is supposed to be responsible for atrial fibrillation found in rheumatic mitral stenosis [32].

In rheumatic mitral regurgitation primary morphological change occur in mitral valvular apparatus which leads to secondary remodelling in LV. This includes post inflammatory thickening and fusion of the mitral valve leaflets at the commissures along with scar retraction producing an eccentrically located funnel shaped orifice. It results in reduced valve motion in both systole and diastole. Such restrictive mechanism of regurgitation is unique to rheumatic heart disease and differs from degenerative valvular regurgitation [26]. Left ventricular (LV) dilatation and eccentric hypertrophy in mitral regurgitation are secondary remodelling due to haemo-dynamic volume overload on LV produced by primary morphological change in the mitral valve in RHD. In compensated phase of mitral regurgitation, with increase in end diastolic volume, there is a compensatory dilatation of ventricle. This eccentric hypertrophy initially helps to maintain high stroke volume in compensated phase. But in decompensated phase, progressive ventricular dilatation causes increase in wall stress with tissue damage and contractile dysfunction [33,34].

Ultrastructurally in volume overload states, sarcomere replication in series causes myocyte lengthening (Frank-Starling mechanism) resulting in ventricular dilatation. Besides, dilatation or eccentric hypertrophy in mitral regurgitation is also contributed by alteration in collagen cross linking and break down of collagen weave by MMP activation. This is entirely different from pressure overload states where an extensive production and deposition of collagen occurs in the ventricle itself [35]. Therefore it is likely that in spite of progressive ventricular dilatation due to collagen weave degradation (secondary remodelling), there is an elevation in plasma level of PICP in MR and it also directly associates with LVIDd, LVIDs and LV mass. It may be due to extensive fibrosis on valvular apparatus (primary event) that occurs concomitantly and progressively with ventricular dilatation. However elevation in plasma PICP concentration is somewhat compromised in MR particularlysince degradation activity is increased in MR. This is evident from a significant increase in MMP-1 level in MR compared to MS subjects as mentioned earlier.This also explains an inverse correlation of MMP-1/TIMP-1 ratio with the above LV parameters in MR.

Significant decrease in plasma PICP and PIIINP levels following mitral valve replacement after one month and one year strongly suggest contribution of mitral valve apparatus in altered levels of collagen metabolism markers in RHD. Thus fibrotic state of the mitral valve precedes the occurrence of myocardial dysfunction and overt heart disease. This information might be helpful for the development of diagnostic and therapeutic strategies by targeting structural remodelling of the heart valves in RHD.

Though in our present study we have shown a 141% higher deposition of total interstitial collagen on rheumatic mitral valve, due to technical limitations, histological alterations and collagen distribution in other parts of cardiac tissue could not be shown. It would be interesting if some controls with same hemodynamic status (heart valve disease) but not related to RHD were considered in order to better appreciate the specificity of our findings. Also the presence of a larger multi-centric population would have helped to validate the current findings.

Adequate information and improved data on chronic diseases of developing nations such as rheumatic heart disease are lacking presumably because limited research activities are carried out worldwide on such diseases. This may be attributed to the rare incidence of RHD in many of the developed nations around the world today. Hence a disease like RHD that still remains a public health burden in LMICs lacks sufficient attention globally. Antibiotic prophylaxis is recommended as the most effective approach for control of recurrent attacks of ARF; yet most of the cases progress to chronic RHD. Echocardiography has an established role not only in diagnosis but also determines severity of RHD. However it is costly and only available in limited tertiary health care facilities. As a result due to lack of monitoring most of them progress to advanced RHD with low ejection fraction. Sometimes other than conservative medical treatment, even surgery may not be considered a possible option in them. So there is a need for a biomarker that would correlate with the echocardiographic progression of valve damage and would decide therapeutic interventions much earlier. Result of our present study based on biomarkers of collagen metabolism is a step forward towards that goal. As our study has shown that increased fibrosis correlates with echo parameters of advanced disease, attempts could be made for development of cardiac specific antifibrotic medication that may prevent permanent morphological damage of heart valves. However it may be mentioned that the target population for carrying out active surveillance programme in endemic regions with the help of collagen metabolism markers needs to be defined clearly in further studies as collagen is a ubiquitous protein and degradation products may be detectable in a variety of other conditions. Moreover procuring and preserving blood samples and rapid detection in field may be cumbersome with available technologies. Finally, undertaking cross country research collaboration initiatives involving multiple centres would help to provide new insights for better understading and management of the disease.

Supporting Information

Figure S1 Flow Chart of Study Design.

Figure S2 Comparison of plasma PIIINP level of the same RHD subjects (n = 6) before surgery and one month after mitral valve replacement.

File S1 Table S1. Characteristics of randomly collected post-operative RHD subjects. Table S2. Preoperative Echocardiographic Characteristics of randomly collected post-operative RHD subjects. Table S3 Level of collagen metabolism markers in male and female subjects with Mitral Stenosis and Mitral Regurgitation lesions. Table S4 Level of collagen metabolism markers in subjects with and without Atrial Fibrillation in Mitral Stenosis and Mitral Regurgitation groups. Table S5 Association of collagen metabolism markers with continuously distributed variables in subjects with Mitral Stenosis. Table S6. Association of collagen metabolism markers with continuously distributed variables in subjects with Mitral Regurgitation.

Acknowledgments

The authors are grateful to Professor P. K. Mitra, MD, IPGMER, SSKM Hospital, Kolkata, India for the initiatives and clinical support during the entire study. The authors are thankful to Dr. D.C. Pal (Department of Geological Sciences, Jadavpur University) for providing Nikon Eclipse polarising microscope facility.

Author Contributions

Conceived and designed the experiments: AB SM TB MB SG. Performed the experiments: TB SM SC SG. Analyzed the data: TB SM MB SG SP SD AB. Contributed reagents/materials/analysis tools: AB. Wrote the paper: AB SM TB SG MB SP.

References

1. Marijon E, Mirabel M, Celermajer DS, Jouven X (2012) Rheumatic Heart Disease. Lancet 379:953–964.
2. GuilhermeL, Köhler KF, Postol E, Kalil J (2011) Genes, autoimmunity and pathogenesis of rheumatic heart disease. Ann Pediatr Cardiol 4:13–21.
3. Eisenberg MJ (1993) Rheumatic heart disease in the developing world: prevalence, prevention, and control. Euro Heart J 14:122–128.
4. World health organization(2004) 2001 Report of a WHO Expert Consultation. Geneva,13–19.
5. Steer AC, Carapetis JR.(2009) Prevention and treatment of rheumatic heart disease in the developing world. Nat Rev Cardiol 6:689–698.
6. World Health Organization (2011) Projections of mortality and burden of disease, 2004–2030; standard DALYs (3% discounting, age weights) -baseline scenario; 2008; WHO regions.
7. Kadir IS, Barker TA, Clarke B, Denley H, Grötte GJ (2004) Recurrent acute rheumatic fever: a forgotten diagnosis? Ann ThoracSurg 78:699–701.
8. Carabello BA (2005) Modern management of mitral stenosis. Circulation 112:432–7.
9. López B, González A, Díez J (2010) Circulating biomarkers of collagen metabolism in cardiac diseases. Circulation 121:1645–1654.
10. QuerejetaR, López B, González A, Sánchez E, Larman M, et al. (2004) Increased collagen type I synthesis in subjects with heart failure of hypertensive origin: relation to myocardial fibrosis. Circulation 110:1263–1268.
11. Querejeta R,Varo N, López B, Larman M, Artiñano E, et al. (2000) Serum carboxy-terminal propeptide of procollagen type I is a marker of myocardial fibrosis in hypertensive heart disease. Circulation 101:1729–1735.
12. López B, Querejeta R, González A, Sánchez E, LarmanM, et al. (2004) Effects of loop diuretics on myocardial fibrosis and collagen type I turnover in chronic heart failure. J Am Coll Cardio l43:2028–2035.
13. MartosR, Baugh J, LedwidgeM, O'Loughlin C, Conlon C, et al. (2007) Diastolic heart failure: evidence of increased myocardial collagen turnover linked to diastolic dysfunction. Circulation 115:888–895.
14. Banerjee T, Mukherjee S, Biswas M, Dutta S, Chatterjee S, et al. (2012) Circulating carboxy-terminal propeptide of type I procollagen is increased in rheumatic heart disease Int J Cardiol 156:117–119.
15. Reményi B,Wilson N, Steer A, Ferreira B, Kado J, et al. (2012) World Heart Federation criteria for echocardiographic diagnosis of rheumatic heart disease—an evidence-based guideline.Nat Rev Cardio 19:297–309.
16. Ganau A, Devereux RB, Roman MJ, de Simone G, Pickering TG, et al. (1992) Patterns of left ventricular hypertrophy and geometric remodelling in essential hypertension. J Am Coll Cardiol 19:1550–1558.
17. Lancellotti P, Moura L, Pierard LA, Agricola E, Popescu BA, et al.(2010) European Association of Echocardiography Recommendations for the assessment of valvular regurgitation.Part2:mitral and tricuspid regurgitation(native valve disease). Eur J Echocardiogr 11:307–32
18. Ghose Roy S, Mishra S, Ghosh G, Bandyopadhyay A (2007) Thyroid hormone induces myocardial matrix degradation by activating matrix metalloproteinase-1. Matrix Biol 26:269–279.
19. Zhang H,Sun L, Wang W, Ma X (2006) Quantitative analysis of fibrosis formation on the microcapsule surface with the use of picro-sirius red staining, polarized light microscopy, and digital image analysis. J Biomed Mater Res A76:120–125.
20. Hara M, Noiseux N, Bindokas V P (2005) High resolution optical imaging of infarction in intact organs. Biotechniques 39:373–376.
21. Yeghiazarians Y, Zhang Y, Prasad M, Shih H, Saini S, et al. (2009) Injection of bone marrow cell extract into infarcted hearts results in functional improvement comparable to intact cell therapy. Mol Ther 17:1250–1256.
22. Marijon E, Ou P, Celermajer DS, Ferreira B, Mocumbi AO, Jani D, Paquet C, Jacob S, Sidi D, Jouven X. (2007) Prevalence of rheumatic heart disease detected by echocardiographic screening. N Engl J Med 357:470–476.
23. Marijon E, Ou P, Celermajer DS, Ferreira B, Mocumbi AO, et al. (2008) Echocardiographic screening for rheumatic heart disease. Bull World Health Organ 86:84.
24. Narula J, Kaplan EL (2001) Echocardiographic diagnosis of rheumatic fever. Lancet 358:2000.
25. Brand A, Dollberg S, Keren A (1992) The prevalence of valvular regurgitation in children with structurally normal hearts: a colour Doppler echocardiographic study. American Heart Journal 123:177–180.
26. McCarthy KP, Ring L, RanaBS (2010) Anatomy of the mitral valve: understanding the mitral valve complex in mitral regurgitation. Eur J Echocardiogr 11:i3–i9.
27. Walker GA, Masters KS, Shah DN, Anseth KS, Leinwand LA (2004) Valvularmyofibroblast activation by transforming growth factor-beta: implications for pathological extracellular matrix remodelling in heart valve disease. Circ Res 95:253–260.
28. Khan R, Sheppard R (2006) Fibrosis in heart disease: understanding the role of transforming growth factor-beta in cardiomyopathy, valvular disease and arrhythmia. Immunology 118:10–24.
29. Leong SW, Soor GS, Butany J, Henry J, Thangaroopan M, et al. (2006) Morphological findings in 192 surgically excised native mitral valves. Can J Cardiol 22:1055–1061.
30. González A, López B, QuerejetaR, Díez J. (2002) Regulation of myocardial fibrillar collagen by angiotensin II.A role in hypertensive heart disease? J Mol Cell Cardiol 34:1585–1593.
31. Rabkin E, Aikawa M, Stone JR,Fukumoto Y, Libby P, et al. (2001) Activated interstitial myofibroblasts express catabolic enzymes and mediate matrix remodeling in myxomatous heart valves. Circulation 104:2525–2532.
32. Boldt A,Wetzel U, Lauschke J, Weigl J, Gummert J, et al. (2004) Fibrosis in left atrial tissue of patients with atrial fibrillation with and without underlying mitral valve disease. Heart 90:400–405.
33. Gaasch WH, Meyer TE. (2008) Left ventricular response to mitral regurgitation: implications for management. Circulation 118:2298–2303.
34. Marciniak A, Claus P, Sutherland GR, Marciniak M, Karu T, et al. (2007) Changes in systolic left ventricular function in isolated mitral regurgitation.A strain rate imaging study. Eur Heart J 28:2627–2636.
35. Lorell BH, Carabello BA. (2000) Left ventricular hypertrophy: pathogenesis, detection, and prognosis. Circulation 102:470–479.

Permissions

All chapters in this book were first published in PLOS ONE, by The Public Library of Science; hereby published with permission under the Creative Commons Attribution License or equivalent. Every chapter published in this book has been scrutinized by our experts. Their significance has been extensively debated. The topics covered herein carry significant findings which will fuel the growth of the discipline. They may even be implemented as practical applications or may be referred to as a beginning point for another development.

The contributors of this book come from diverse backgrounds, making this book a truly international effort. This book will bring forth new frontiers with its revolutionizing research information and detailed analysis of the nascent developments around the world.

We would like to thank all the contributing authors for lending their expertise to make the book truly unique. They have played a crucial role in the development of this book. Without their invaluable contributions this book wouldn't have been possible. They have made vital efforts to compile up to date information on the varied aspects of this subject to make this book a valuable addition to the collection of many professionals and students.

This book was conceptualized with the vision of imparting up-to-date information and advanced data in this field. To ensure the same, a matchless editorial board was set up. Every individual on the board went through rigorous rounds of assessment to prove their worth. After which they invested a large part of their time researching and compiling the most relevant data for our readers.

The editorial board has been involved in producing this book since its inception. They have spent rigorous hours researching and exploring the diverse topics which have resulted in the successful publishing of this book. They have passed on their knowledge of decades through this book. To expedite this challenging task, the publisher supported the team at every step. A small team of assistant editors was also appointed to further simplify the editing procedure and attain best results for the readers.

Apart from the editorial board, the designing team has also invested a significant amount of their time in understanding the subject and creating the most relevant covers. They scrutinized every image to scout for the most suitable representation of the subject and create an appropriate cover for the book.

The publishing team has been an ardent support to the editorial, designing and production team. Their endless efforts to recruit the best for this project, has resulted in the accomplishment of this book. They are a veteran in the field of academics and their pool of knowledge is as vast as their experience in printing. Their expertise and guidance has proved useful at every step. Their uncompromising quality standards have made this book an exceptional effort. Their encouragement from time to time has been an inspiration for everyone.

The publisher and the editorial board hope that this book will prove to be a valuable piece of knowledge for researchers, students, practitioners and scholars across the globe.

List of Contributors

Chun-Ho Yun
Division of Radiology, Department of Internal Medicine, Mackay Memorial Hospital, Taipei, Taiwan

Tze-Fan Chao, Kang-Ling Wang, Yenn-Jiang Lin, Shih-Lin Chang, Li-Wei Lo, Yu-Feng Hu and ShihAnn Chen
Division of Cardiology, Department of Medicine, Taipei Veterans General Hospital, Taipei, Taiwan
Institute of Clinical Medicine, and Cardiovascular Research Center, National Yang-Ming University, Taipei, Taiwan

Yau-Huei Lai, Chih_Hsuan Yen, Chung-Lieh Hung, Jen-Yuan Kuo and Hung-I Yeh
Division of Cardiology, Department of Internal Medicine, Mackay Memorial Hospital, Taipei, Taiwan
Department of Medicine, Mackay Medical College, and Mackay Medicine Nursing and Management College, Taipei, Taiwan

Sergey Gurevich, Samuel C. Volo, Anika Afroz, Maya Petashnick, Agnes Kim, Richard B. Devereux and Peter M. Okin
Greenberg Cardiology Division/Department of Medicine, Weill Cornell Medical College, New York, New York, United States of America

Jonathan D. Kochav
Greenberg Cardiology Division/Department of Medicine, Weill Cornell Medical College, New York, New York, United States of America
Duke University School of Medicine, Durham, North Carolina, United States of America

Jiwon Kim
Greenberg Cardiology Division/Department of Medicine, Weill Cornell Medical College, New York, New York, United States of America
Memorial Sloan Kettering Cancer Center Department of Medicine, New York, New York, United States of America

Jonathan W. Weinsaft
Greenberg Cardiology Division/Department of Medicine, Weill Cornell Medical College, New York, New York, United States of America
Department of Radiology, Weill Cornell Medical College, New York, New York, United States of America
Memorial Sloan Kettering Cancer Center Department of Medicine, New York, New York, United States of America

Charles Mady and Vera M. C. Salemi
Cardiomyopathy Unit of the Heart Institute (InCor) do Hospital das Clínicas da Faculdade de Medicina da Universidade de São Paulo, São Paulo, Brazil

Maria C. Irigoyen, Leandro E. Souza, Cristiano Mostarda, Raquel N. La Fuente, Georgia O. Candido and Pamella R. M. Souza
Hypertension Unit of the Heart Institute (InCor) do Hospital das Clínicas da Faculdade de Medicina da Universidade de São Paulo, São Paulo, Brazil

Leandro E. Souza
Federal University of São Paulo, Biosciences Department, Santos, São Paulo, Brazil

Raquel A. Sirvente
Cardiomyopathy Unit of the Heart Institute (InCor) do Hospital das Clínicas da Faculdade de Medicina da Universidade de São Paulo, São Paulo, Brazil
Hypertension Unit of the Heart Institute (InCor) do Hospital das Clínicas da Faculdade de Medicina da Universidade de São Paulo, São Paulo, Brazil

Florian Schwarz and Dominik Zinsser
Institute for Clinical Radiology, Hospital of the Ludwig Maximilian University of Munich, Munich, Germany

Philipp Lange and Martin Greif
Medical Clinic I - Cardiology, Hospital of the Ludwig Maximilian University of Munich, Munich, Germany

Peter Boekstegers
HELIOS Klinikum Siegburg, HELIOS Kliniken GmbH, Siegburg, Germany

Christoph Schmitz
Department of Cardiac Surgery, Hospital of the Ludwig Maximilian University of Munich, Munich, Germany

Maximilian F. Reiser and Hans C. Becker
Institute for Clinical Radiology, Hospital of the Ludwig Maximilian University of Munich, Munich, Germany
DZHK (German Centre for Cardiovascular Research), Partner Site Munich Heart Alliance, Munich, Germany

Christian Kupatt
Medical Clinic I - Cardiology, Hospital of the Ludwig Maximilian University of Munich, Munich, Germany
DZHK (German Centre for Cardiovascular Research), Partner Site Munich Heart Alliance, Munich, Germany

Ahmadou M. Jingi
Department of Internal Medicine and Specialties, Faculty of Medicine and Biomedical Sciences, University of Yaoundé I, Yaoundé, Cameroon

Jean Jacques N. Noubiap
Internal Medicine Unit, Edéa Regional Hospital, Edéa, Cameroon

Philippe Kamdem
Centre Médical de la Trinité, Bafoussam, Cameroon

Samuel Kingue
Department of Internal Medicine and Specialties, Faculty of Medicine and Biomedical Sciences, University of Yaoundé I, Yaoundé, Cameroon
Department of Internal Medicine, Yaoundé General Hospital, Yaoundé, Cameroon

Fatiha Imestouren, Aurelie Armougon and André Leke
Neonatal Intensive Care Unit, Amiens University Hospital, Amiens, France

Lucie Razafimanantsoa
Pediatric Cardiology, Amiens University Hospital, Amiens, France

Mahdi Mahmoudzadeh and Fabrice Wallois
NSERM U1105, GRAMFC, Jules Verne University of Picardie, Amiens, France

Sabrina Goudjil and Guy Kongolo
Neonatal Intensive Care Unit, Amiens University Hospital, Amiens, France
NSERM U1105, GRAMFC, Jules Verne University of Picardie, Amiens, France

Michal Mor, Wesam Mulla, Sigal Elyagon and Shani Dror
Cardiac Arrhythmia Research Laboratory, Department of Physiology and Cell Biology, Faculty of Health Sciences, Ben-Gurion University of the Negev, Beer-Sheva, Israel

Noah Liel-Cohen
Cardiology Department, Soroka University Medical Center, Beer-Sheva, Israel

Hovav Gabay
Cardiac Arrhythmia Research Laboratory, Department of Physiology and Cell Biology, Faculty of Health Sciences, Ben-Gurion University of the Negev, Beer-Sheva, Israel
Department of Emergency Medicine, Recanati School for Community Health Professions, Faculty of Health Sciences and PREPARED Center for Emergency Response Research, Ben-Gurion University of the Negev, Beer-Sheva, Israel

Yoram Etzion
Cardiac Arrhythmia Research Laboratory, Department of Physiology and Cell Biology, Faculty of Health Sciences, Ben-Gurion University of the Negev, Beer-Sheva, Israel
Division of Internal Medicine, Soroka University Medical Center, Beer-Sheva, Israel

Zhang-Wei Chen, Ju-Ying Qian, Jian-Ying Ma and Jun-Bo Ge
Department of Cardiology, Zhongshan Hospital affiliated to Fudan University, Shanghai, China

Ying-Hua Chen
Department of Endocrinology Medicine, East Hospital affiliated to Tongji University, Shanghai, China

Ran Chen, Bei Wang, Ming-Ming Ma, Yuan Yang, Bo-Wen Zhao
Department of Diagnostic Ultrasound and Echocardiography, Sir Run Run Shaw Hospital, Zhejiang University College of Medicine and Sir Run Run Shaw Institute of Clinical Medicine of Zhejiang University, Hangzhou, China

Xia Wu
Department of Radiology, Sir Run Run Shaw Hospital, Zhejiang University College of Medicine and Sir Run Run Shaw Institute of Clinical Medicine of Zhejiang University, Hangzhou, China

Li-Jun Shen
Department of Ultrasound, The First People's Hospital, Hangzhou Xiao Shan District, Hangzhou, China

Jingmin Zhou, Xiaotong Cui, Xuejuan Jin, Jun Zhou, Jie Cui, Hongmin Zhu, Aijun Sun, Kai Hu and Junbo Ge
Shanghai Institute of Cardiovascular Diseases, Zhongshan Hospital, Fudan University, Shanghai, China

Hanying Zhang, Bixiao Tang
Fengjing Community Health Center, Jinshan District, Shanghai, China

Michael Fu
Section of Cardiology, Department of Medicine, Sahlgrenska University Hospital/ Östra Hospital, University of Gothenburg, Gothenburg, Sweden

Hans Herlitz
Section of Nephrology, Department of Medicine, Sahlgrenska University Hospital/Östra Hospital, University of Gothenburg, Gothenburg, Sweden

Brice Stéphane Reynolds
Unité de Recherche Clinique, Université de Toulouse, INP, Ecole Nationale Vétérinaire de Toulouse, Toulouse, France

Emilie Trehiou-Sechi and Carolina Carlos Sampedrano
Unité de Cardiologie d'Alfort, Centre Hospitalier Universitaire Vétérinaire d'Alfort, Université Paris-Est, Ecole Nationale Vétérinaire d'Alfort, Maisons-Alfort, France

Patrick Nguyen
Nutrition and Endocrinology Unit, LUNAM Université, Oniris, National College of Veterinary Medicine, Food Science and Engineering, Nantes, France

Didier Concordet
UMR 1331 Toxalim, INRA, Université de Toulouse, INP, Ecole Nationale Vétérinaire de Toulouse, Toulouse, France

Isabelle Testault
Atlantia Veterinary Hospital, Nantes, France

Jonathan Elliott
Department of Comparative Biomedical Sciences, Royal Veterinary College, Royal College Street, Camden, London, United Kingdom

Jérôme Abadie
Department of Pathology LUNAM Université, Oniris, National College of Veterinary Medicine, Food Science and Engineering, Nantes, France

Vincent Biourge
Centre de Recherches, Royal Canin SAS, Aimargues, France

Valérie Chetboul
Unité de Cardiologie d'Alfort, Centre Hospitalier Universitaire Ve´te´ rinaire d'Alfort, Université Paris-Est, Ecole Nationale Vétérinaire d'Alfort, Maisons-Alfort, France
INSERM, U955, Equipe 03, Créteil, France

Yong-Won Shin
Department of Neurology, Laboratory for Neurotherapeutics, Biomedical Research Institute, Seoul National University Hospital, Seoul, South Korea

Jeong-Min Kim
Department of Neurology, Chung-Ang University Medical Center, College of Medicine, Chung-Ang University, Seoul, South Korea

Young Dae Cho and Moon Hee Han
Department of Radiology, Seoul National University Hospital, Seoul, South Korea

Keun-Hwa Jung, Soon-Tae Lee, Kon Chu, Manho Kim and Sang Kun Lee
Department of Neurology, Laboratory for Neurotherapeutics, Biomedical Research Institute, Seoul National University Hospital, Seoul, South Korea
Program in Neuroscience, Neuroscience Research Institute of SNUMRC, College of Medicine, Seoul National University, Seoul, South Korea

Jae-Kyu Roh
Department of Neurology, Laboratory for Neurotherapeutics, Biomedical Research Institute, Seoul National University Hospital, Seoul, South Korea
Department of Neurology, Armed Forces Capital Hospital, Seongnam, Gyeunggido, South Korea

Lin Ling and Xiangjun Yang
Department of Cardiology, the First Affiliated Hospital of Soochow University, Suzhou, China

Yan Cheng
Department of Cardiology, The Affiliated Wuxi People's Hospital of Nanjing Medical University, Wuxi, China

Liucheng Ding
The Second Affiliated Hospital of Nanjing Medical University, Nanjing, China

Jiansong Yuan and Shubin Qiao
Department of Cardiology, State Key Laboratory of Cardiovascular Disease, Fuwai Hospital, National Center for Cardiovascular Disease, Peking Union Medical College and Chinese Academy of Medical Sciences, Beijing, China

Shi Chen
Department of Cardiology, West China Hospital, Sichuan University, Chengdu, Sichuan, China

Fujian Duan, Jiafen Zhang and Hao Wang
Department of Echocardiography, State Key Laboratory of Cardiovascular Disease, Fuwai Hospital, National Center for Cardiovascular Disease, Peking Union Medical College and Chinese Academy of Medical Sciences, Beijing, China

Samarjit Das, Nathaniel Campbell and Charles Steenbergen
Department of Pathology, Johns Hopkins University, Baltimore, Maryland, United States of America

Venugopal Chenna
Departments of Pathology and Translational Molecular Pathology, Houston, Texas, United States of America

Djahida Bedja
Department of Cardiology, Johns Hopkins University, Baltimore, Maryland, United States of America
Australian School of Advanced Medicine, Macquarie University, Sydney, Australia

Brittany Dunkerly
Department of Pathology, Johns Hopkins University, Baltimore, Maryland, United States of America
Notre Dame of Maryland University, Baltimore, Maryland, United States of America

Anirban Maitra
Department of Pathology, Johns Hopkins University, Baltimore, Maryland, United States of America
Departments of Pathology and Translational Molecular Pathology, Houston, Texas, United States of America
Department of Oncology, Johns Hopkins University, Baltimore, Maryland, United States of America

Erwan Donal and Gaëlle Kervio
Service de Cardiologie et CIC-IT 804, CHU de Rennes & Laboratoire Traitement du Signal et de l'Image, INSERM U1099, Rennes, France

Loïc Biére, Gwenola Terrien, Alain Furber, Serge Willoteaux and Fabrice Prunier
L'UNAM Université, Angers, France
Université Angers, UPRES EA3860, Laboratoire Cardioprotection, Remodelage et Thrombose, CHU Angers, Service de Cardiologie, Angers, France

Doron Aronson, Morad Nakhleh, Tawfiq Zeidan-Shwiri and Michael Mutlak
Department of Cardiology, Rambam Medical Center, Haifa, Israel

Peretz Lavie and Lena Lavie
Lloyd Rigler Sleep Apnea Research Laboratory, The Ruth and Bruce Rappaport Faculty of Medicine, Technion, Israel Institute of Technology, Haifa, Israel

Maria C. Serrano
Division of Pediatric Cardiology, Department of Pediatrics, University of Miami, Jackson Memorial Hospital, Miami, Florida, United States of America

Davis Johansen and Kirsti Ytrehus
Cardiovascular Research Group, Department of Medical Biology, Faculty of Health Science, UiT - The Arctic University of Norway, Tromsø, Norway

Nils Thomas Songstad
Women's Health and Perinatology Research Group, Institute of Clinical Medicine, Faculty of Health Sciences, UiT - The Arctic University of Norway, Tromsø, Norway,
Department of Pediatrics, University Hospital of Northern Norway, Tromsø, Norway,

Vasilis Sitras and Ganesh Acharya
Women's Health and Perinatology Research Group, Institute of Clinical Medicine, Faculty of Health Sciences, UiT - The Arctic University of Norway, Tromsø, Norway

Department of Obstetrics and Gynecology, University Hospital of Northern Norway, Tromsø, Norway

Wenche Stueflotten, Johanna Andreassen and Svend Aakhus
Department of Cardiology, Oslo University Hospital Rikshospitalet, Oslo, Norway

Arne Yndestad
Research Institute of Internal Medicine, Oslo University Hospital Rikshospitalet, Oslo, Norway

Kristin Godang
Department of Endocrinology, Oslo University Hospital Rikshospitalet, Oslo, Norway

Rolf Svendsmark
Department of Radiology, Oslo University Hospital Rikshospitalet, Oslo, Norway

Erik Gjertsen
Department of Internal Medicine, Drammen Hospital, Vestre Viken Hospital Trust; Drammen, Norway

Kaspar Broch
Department of Cardiology, Oslo University Hospital Rikshospitalet, Oslo, Norway
Faculty of Medicine, University of Oslo, Oslo, Norway

Erik T. Askevold
Department of Cardiology, Oslo University Hospital Rikshospitalet, Oslo, Norway
Research Institute of Internal Medicine, Oslo University Hospital Rikshospitalet, Oslo, Norway

Hans-Jørgen Smith
Department of Radiology, Oslo University Hospital Rikshospitalet, Oslo, Norway
Faculty of Medicine, University of Oslo, Oslo, Norway

Thor Ueland
Research Institute of Internal Medicine, Oslo University Hospital Rikshospitalet, Oslo, Norway
Faculty of Medicine, University of Oslo, Oslo, Norway

Pål Aukrust
Research Institute of Internal Medicine, Oslo University Hospital Rikshospitalet, Oslo, Norway
Section of Clinical Immunology and Infectious Diseases, Oslo University Hospital Rikshospitalet, Oslo, Norway
Faculty of Medicine, University of Oslo, Oslo, Norway

Lars Gullestad
Department of Cardiology, Oslo University Hospital Rikshospitalet, Oslo, Norway
Faculty of Medicine, University of Oslo, Oslo, Norway
K. G. Jebsen Cardiac Research Centre and Center for Heart Failure Research, Faculty of Medicine, University of Oslo, Oslo, Norway

Bianca C. Bernardo, Xiao-Ming Gao, Yow Keat Tham, Helen Kiriazis, Catherine E. Winbanks, Jenny Y. Y. Ooi, Esther J. H. Boey, Paul Gregorevic and Xiao-Jun Du
Baker IDI Heart and Diabetes Institute, Melbourne, Victoria, Australia

Susanna Obad
Santaris Pharma, Horsholm, Denmark

Sakari Kauppinen
Department of Haematology, Aalborg University Hospital, Copenhagen, Denmark

Ruby C. Y. Lin
Ramaciotti Centre for Genomics, School of Biotechnology & Biomolecular Sciences, University of New South Wales, Sydney, New South Wales, Australia

Julie R. McMullen
Baker IDI Heart and Diabetes Institute, Melbourne, Victoria, Australia
Departments of Medicine Monash University, Clayton, Victoria, Australia
Departments of Physiology, Monash University, Clayton, Victoria, Australia

Lars M. Rasmussen
Department of Clinical Biochemistry and Pharmacology, Centre for Individualized Medicine in Arterial Diseases (CIMA), Odense University Hospital, Odense, Denmark

William S. Argraves
Medical University of South Carolina, Department of Cell Biology, Charleston, South Carolina, United States of America

Jesper Eugen-Olsen
Clinical Research Centre 136, Hvidovre Hospital, Copenhagen, Denmark

Olav W. Nielsen
Department of Cardiology, Bispebjerg Hospital, Copenhagen, Denmark

Adam Blyme
Department of Cardiology, Glostrup Hospital, Copenhagen, Denmark

Ronnie Willenheimer
Lund University and Heart Health Group, Malmö, Sweden,

Kristian Wachtell
Department of Medicine, Glostrup Hospital, Copenhagen, Denmark

Ruan Kruger and Michael H. Olsen
Hypertension in Africa Research Team (HART), North-West University, Potchefstroom, South Africa
The Cardiovascular and Metabolic Preventive Clinic, Department of
Endocrinology, Centre for Individualized Medicine in Arterial Diseases (CIMA), Odense University Hospital, Odense, Denmark,

Walid Nachar, David Busseuil, Yanfen Shi, Teodora Mihalache-Avram and Mélanie Mecteau
Montreal Heart Institute and Université de Montré al, Montreal, Quebec, Canada

Eric Rhéaume and Jean-Claude Tardif
Montreal Heart Institute and Université de Montréal, Montreal, Quebec, Canada
Department of Medicine, Université de Montréal, Montreal, Quebec, Canada

Ira M. Mostovaya, Albert H. A. Mazairac and Peter J. Blankestjin
Department of Nephrology, University Medical Center Utrecht, Utrecht, the Netherlands

Michiel L. Bots
Julius Center for Health Sciences and Primary Care, University Medical Center Utrecht, Utrecht, the Netherlands

Marinus A. van den Dorpel
Department of Internal Medicine, Maasstad Hospital, Rotterdam, the Netherlands

Roel Goldschmeding
Department of Pathology, University Medical Center Utrecht, Utrecht, the Netherlands

Otto Kamp
Department of Cardiology, Vrije Universiteit Medical Center, Amsterdam, the Netherlands
Renée Levesque
Department of Nephrology, Centre Hospitalier de l'Université de Montréal St. Luc Hospital, Montréal, Canada

Dorine W. Swinkels
Department of Laboratory Medicine, Laboratory of Genetic, Endocrine and Metabolic diseases, Radboud University Medical Centre Nijmegen, the Netherlands

Claire H. den Hoedt
Department of Nephrology, University Medical Center Utrecht, Utrecht, the Netherlands
Department of Internal Medicine, Maasstad Hospital, Rotterdam, the Netherlands

E. Lars Penne and Neelke C. van der Weerd
Department of Nephrology, University Medical Center Utrecht, Utrecht, the Netherlands
Department of Nephrology, Vrije Universiteit Medical Center, Amsterdam, the Netherlands

Piet M. ter Wee, Menso J. Nube and Muriel P. C. Grooteman
Department of Nephrology, Vrije Universiteit Medical Center, Amsterdam, the Netherlands
Institute for Cardiovascular Research Vrije Universiteit Medical Center, Vrije Universiteit Medical Center, Amsterdam, the Netherlands

Jianmin Chen, Nimesh S. A. Patel and Christoph Thiemermann
Queen Mary University of London, William Harvey Research Institute, Barts and the London School of Medicine and Dentistry, London, United Kingdom

Fausto Chiazza and Massimo Collino
University of Turin, Department of Drug Science and Technology, Turin, Italy

Sina M. Coldewey
Jena University Hospital, Department of Anesthesiology and Intensive Care Medicine, Jena, German

Tanima Banerjee, Somaditya Mukherjee, Sudip Ghosh, Shelly Chatterjee and Arun Bandyopadhyay
Department of Cell Biology and Physiology, CSIR-Indian Institute of Chemical Biology, Kolkata, WB, India

Monodeep Biswas
Department of Cardiology, Geisinger Community Medical Center and Wright Center for Graduate Medical Education, Scranton, Pennsylvania, United States of America

Santanu Dutta
Department of Cardio-thoracic and Vascular Surgery, Institute of Post Graduate Medical Education and Research, SSKM Hospital, Kolkata, WB, India

Sanjib Pattari
Department of Pathology, Rabindra Nath Tagore International Institute of
Cardiac Sciences, Kolkata, WB, India

Index